ATLAS OF TUMOR PATHOLOGY

Third Series
Fascicle 17

TUMORS OF THE SALIVARY GLANDS

by

GARY L. ELLIS, D.D.S.
Armed Forces Institute of Pathology and
Department of Veteran Affairs Special Reference
Laboratory for Pathology, Washington, D.C.

PAUL L. AUCLAIR, D.M.D., M.S.
Captain, United States Navy, Dental Corps
Armed Forces Institute of Pathology
Washington, D.C.

Published by the
ARMED FORCES INSTITUTE OF PATHOLOGY
Washington, D.C.

Under the Auspices of
UNIVERSITIES ASSOCIATED FOR RESEARCH AND EDUCATION IN PATHOLOGY, INC.
Bethesda, Maryland
1996

Accepted for Publication
1995

Available from the American Registry of Pathology
Armed Forces Institute of Pathology
Washington, D.C. 20306-6000
ISSN 0160-6344
ISBN 1-881041-26-3

ATLAS OF TUMOR PATHOLOGY

EDITOR
JUAN ROSAI, M.D.
Department of Pathology
Memorial Sloan-Kettering Cancer Center
New York, New York 10021-6007

ASSOCIATE EDITOR
LESLIE H. SOBIN, M.D.
Armed Forces Institute of Pathology
Washington, D.C. 20306-6000

EDITORIAL ADVISORY BOARD

EDITORS' NOTE

The Atlas of Tumor Pathology has a long and distinguished history. It was first conceived at a Cancer Research Meeting held in St. Louis in September 1947 as an attempt to standardize the nomenclature of neoplastic diseases. The first series was sponsored by the National Academy of Sciences-National Research Council. The organization of this Sisyphean effort was entrusted to the Subcommittee on Oncology of the Committee on Pathology, and Dr. Arthur Purdy Stout was the first editor-in-chief. Many of the illustrations were provided by the Medical Illustration Service of the Armed Forces Institute of Pathology, the type was set by the Government Printing Office, and the final printing was done at the Armed Forces Institute of Pathology (hence the colloquial appellation "AFIP Fascicles"). The American Registry of Pathology purchased the Fascicles from the Government Printing Office and sold them virtually at cost. Over a period of 20 years, approximately 15,000 copies each of nearly 40 Fascicles were produced. The worldwide impact that these publications have had over the years has largely surpassed the original goal. They quickly became among the most influential publications on tumor pathology ever written, primarily because of their overall high quality but also because their low cost made them easily accessible to pathologists and other students of oncology the world over.

Upon completion of the first series, the National Academy of Sciences-National Research Council handed further pursuit of the project over to the newly created Universities Associated for Research and Education in Pathology (UAREP). A second series was started, generously supported by grants from the AFIP, the National Cancer Institute, and the American Cancer Society. Dr. Harlan I. Firminger became the editor-in-chief and was succeeded by Dr. William H. Hartmann. The second series Fascicles were produced as bound volumes instead of loose leaflets. They featured a more comprehensive coverage of the subjects, to the extent that the Fascicles could no longer be regarded as "atlases" but rather as monographs describing and illustrating in detail the tumors and tumor-like conditions of the various organs and systems.

Once the second series was completed, with a success that matched that of the first, UAREP and AFIP decided to embark on a third series. A new editor-in-chief and an associate editor were selected, and a distinguished editorial board was appointed. The mandate for the third series remains the same as for the previous ones, i.e., to oversee the production of an eminently practical publication with surgical pathologists as its primary audience, but also aimed at other workers in oncology. The main purposes of this series are to promote a consistent, unified, and biologically sound nomenclature; to guide the surgical pathologist in the diagnosis of the various tumors and tumor-like lesions; and to provide relevant histogenetic, pathogenetic, and clinicopathologic information on these entities. Just as the second series included data obtained from ultrastructural (and, in the more recent Fascicles, immunohistochemical) examination, the third series will, in addition, incorporate pertinent information obtained with the newer molecular biology techniques. As in the past, a continuous attempt will be made to correlate, whenever possible, the nomenclature used in the Fascicles with that proposed by the World Health Organization's International Histological Classification of Tumors. The format of the third series has been changed in order to incorporate additional items and to ensure a consistency of style throughout. Close cooperation between the various authors and their respective liaisons from the editorial board will be emphasized to minimize unnecessary repetition and discrepancies in the text and illustrations.

To its everlasting credit, the participation and commitment of the AFIP to this venture is even more substantial and encompassing than in previous series. It now extends to virtually all scientific, technical, and financial aspects of the production.

The task confronting the organizations and individuals involved in the third series is even more daunting than in the preceding efforts because of the ever-increasing complexity of the matter at hand. It is hoped that this combined effort—of which, needless to say, that represented by the authors is first and foremost—will result in a series worthy of its two illustrious predecessors and will be a suitable introduction to the tumor pathology of the twenty-first century.

Juan Rosai, M.D.
Leslie H. Sobin, M.D.

PREFACE AND ACKNOWLEDGMENTS

In Fascicle 10, Tumors of the Major Salivary Glands, of the second series of the Atlas of Tumor Pathology, A. C. Thackray and R. B. Lucas noted that it had been 20 years since the publication of the first Fascicle on the subject written by Foote and Frazell. They further commented that Foote and Frazell had established a solid foundation upon which to build and further refine classification and nomenclature for salivary gland disease. That second series Fascicle appeared shortly after the first Histological Typing of Salivary Gland Tumours was published by the World Health Organization (WHO) in 1972, and Thackray and Lucas used that classification as the basis for their discussion and elaboration on salivary gland tumors and diseases. It now has been over 20 years since publication of the second series Fascicle written by Thackray and Lucas, and in 1991 the WHO published an updated second edition of the Histological Typing of Salivary Gland Tumours. Like the second series Fascicle, this third series Fascicle builds upon the work of its predecessor and conforms to the classification presented in the recent edition of the WHO monograph on salivary gland tumors with only a few minor exceptions. Additions and modifications of the classification of salivary gland tumors, especially malignant neoplasms, have been greater during the last 20 years than during the preceding 20 years between the first and second series Fascicles. In addition, while the second series Fascicle limited the discussion to only tumors of the major salivary glands, this third series Fascicle includes tumors of both major and minor salivary glands. While most types of neoplasms and diseases that affect the major salivary glands also affect the minor salivary glands and vice versa, there are some important differences.

The recent edition of the WHO monograph provides a short definition and brief description of each entity. In this Fascicle we provide an in depth discussion and description of the clinicopathologic parameters of each tumor and disease. One of the principal objectives and attributes of the Atlas of Tumor Pathology has been to liberally illustrate the spectrum of each tumor or disease. Recent developments in color printing technology now allow extensive use of color photographs in this Fascicle. It is anticipated that color illustrations will better correlate with the microscopic images used for tissue diagnosis.

Morphometry, flow cytometry, immunohistochemistry, gene rearrangement studies, and other molecular biologic methodologies are exciting new areas that are being developed into diagnostic procedures in the pathology laboratory. Where these methodologies are applicable to salivary gland disease they are included. However, histomorphologic evaluation remains the principal and most useful method for diagnosis of salivary gland tumors and is the emphasis of this Fascicle. Differential diagnosis is emphasized in the discussion of most tumors.

In addition to information published in the literature, the experience of the authors and data from cases in the files at the Armed Forces Institute of Pathology (AFIP) are presented in this Fascicle. From time to time comments have been made to the authors that the AFIP's experience has a bias for male patients and unusual tumors because it is a military institution and a consultative center for second opinions. This is true. In this Fascicle the male bias of patients at military and VA medical centers has been eliminated in discussions on incidence rates in the sexes by including data only on cases that were received from civilian laboratories, which represent about 80 percent of our referrals. The AFIP does receive many challenging, unusual, and rare tumors; however, it also receives a large number of more typical and common salivary gland tumors. The AFIP's experience with common salivary gland neoplasms as a proportion of all neoplasms is similar to that of other recently published investigations. In many laboratories, salivary gland tumors constitute only a very small portion of the surgical specimens, and many pathologists desire confirmation of their diagnoses from other pathologists, such as those at the AFIP. Almost all investigative centers have some biases, recognized or unrecognized. The AFIP receives many consultation requests from small to medium sized community hospitals and laboratories, which we believe may be a more representative population base than that of some large medical centers. The AFIP experience is perhaps the largest base of experience in the world and worthy of description and analysis.

We recognize that as classification systems evolve and expand, historical information and archived material is less valuable if based upon old classification systems and not retrospectively updated. Therefore, in reviewing the AFIP experience in this Fascicle, only data on cases reviewed since 1985 have been included since the current classification scheme has been in use since then and the authors have personally reviewed most of these cases.

We are indebted to the many pathologists who have generously contributed the thousands of cases that form the basis for this atlas and have been invaluable in understanding the broad morphologic spectrum of these tumors. Many contributors have also provided follow-up information and additional material that contribute to our knowledge of the biologic behavior of these tumors. While our contributors are too numerous to name individually, we wish to express our sincere thanks to each of them.

Special appreciation is extended to Dr. Irving Dardick, Department of Pathology, University of Toronto, for his enthusiastic willingness to share from his superb collection of electron micrographs. We are likewise indebted to the generosity of Dr. Carol F. Adair, Department of Otolarynology, Armed Forces Institute of Pathology (AFIP), Dr. Michael R. Henry, Department of Laboratory Medicine, Division of Anatomic Pathology, National Naval Medical Center, Bethesda, Maryland; Sally-Beth Buckner, Department of Cellular Pathology, AFIP, and Dr. Yener S. Erozan, Department of Pathology, Johns Hopkins Hospital, Baltimore, Maryland for allowing us to review and photograph their outstanding collections of salivary gland FNA smears.

We thank Mr. Luther Duckett from the Photography Division, Center for Medical Illustrations, AFIP for allowing us to share many enjoyable hours with him at the photomicroscope. His talented eyes focused nearly every photomicrograph used in this atlas, and we appreciate his patience and diligence. We are also very appreciative for the anatomic illustrations provided by Venetia Valiga, Center for Medical Illustrations, AFIP.

We thank Dr. Leslie Sobin, Department of Gastrointestinal Pathology, AFIP for his support and vote of confidence in this and other projects.

We express deep appreciation to each of our colleagues in the Department of Oral Pathology, AFIP, for sharing their insights on the diseases discussed in this publication and for helping us remain focused on our ultimate goal in this project of helping improve patient care. Accurate diagnosis is the beginning of appropriate treatment. Similarly, we thank our colleagues in the American Academy of Oral and Maxillofacial Pathology for providing a forum for reporting, debating, and scrutinizing the concepts about salivary gland tumors put forth by the pathlogy community.

The gratitude we have for the support and caring provided by our families can not be adequately expressed.

Gary L. Ellis, D.D.S.

Paul L. Auclair, D.M.D.

TUMORS OF THE SALIVARY GLANDS

Contents

TUMORS OF THE SALIVARY GLANDS

1
THE NORMAL SALIVARY GLANDS

The salivary gland system is comprised of three paired, large aggregations of exocrine glandular tissue known collectively as the major salivary glands and numerous small aggregations of glands scattered nonuniformly in the mucosa of the oral cavity, the minor salivary glands. The salivary glands produce the fluids that constitute oral saliva. Since the seromucous glands of the nasal cavity, larynx, and bronchi do not contribute to the saliva, by definition they are not salivary glands; however, they are morphologically

and functionally similar to oral minor salivary glands. The major salivary glands are the parotid, submandibular (submaxillary), and sublingual glands, and each is described below.

Salivary gland tissue consists of branching tubules or ducts that have the principal secretory cells, the acinar cells, at the branch end and an opening into the oral cavity at the other end of a single collecting duct (fig. 1-1). However, all salivary glands are not identical, morphologically or functionally. There are two types of acinar

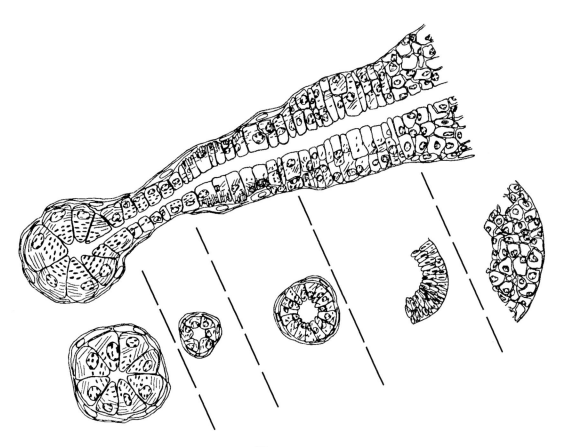

Figure 1-1
SCHEMATIC OF A BASIC SALIVARY GLAND UNIT
Cytomorphologic features of various portions of the salivary system from the secretory end piece to the oral cavity are illustrated. From left to right are the acinus, intercalated duct, striated duct, excretory duct, and oral cavity.

Table 1-1

ACINAR CELL TYPES IN VARIOUS SALIVARY GLANDS

Salivary Gland	Type of Acini*
Parotid	Serous
Submandibular	Serous and mucous
Sublingual	Mucous and serous
Palate	Mucous
Tongue	Mucous and serous
Lip	Mucous
Buccal mucosa	Mucous

*Predominant type first.

cells, serous and mucous, whose secretions differ; the chemical composition of the saliva is dependent on the relative proportion of these two cell types, which varies among the salivary glands (Table 1-1).

DEVELOPMENT

Salivary gland development begins in the fifth to sixth week of embryonic life when the parotid gland primordia appear. Chronologically, this is followed by the appearance of the submandibular primordia at the end of the sixth week and the sublingual primordia at about the seventh to eighth week (16,20,21). The numerous intraoral minor salivary glands develop during the third month of gestation (16). The salivary gland primordia begin as buds of proliferative epithelium from the primitive stomodeum (oral cavity). The stomodeal epithelium is part ectoderm and part endoderm. The parotid gland primordia develop from the oral ectoderm while the submandibular and sublingual gland primordia probably arise from endoderm (16,21). This appears to have little significance regarding neoplasia, however. The parotid gland epithelial buds form between the maxillary and mandibular processes of the mandibular arch in the area of the future right and left cheeks. The primordia of the submandibular glands grow from the floor of the oral cavity between the lower jaw and tongue, the linguogingival groove, on each side of the midplane. The sublingual gland primordia arise as several epithelial buds adjacent to the developing submandibular glands (fig. 1-2). The epithelial buds continue to proliferate as strands into the underlying oral ectomesenchyme, which increases in cellularity around the developing glands and has a role in the lobular organization of the glands and encapsulation of the parotid and submandibular glands (16,21).

At the end of each solid epithelial cord of the developing salivary glands the terminal bulb, a cluster of epithelia, forms. Clefts develop in the terminal bulbs, and these newly formed bulbs proliferate into the ectomesenchyme as branches from the original cord. This process of cord-like proliferation, bulb formation, bulb clefting, and further proliferation continues in a repetitive manner (16). Each new cord of epithelium remains contiguous with the preceding cord such that continuity with the oral epithelium is maintained. Initially, the epithelial cords and bulbs are without lumens. Lumen formation occurs first in the epithelial cords and progresses to the terminal bulbs. Concurrent cellular differentiation results in the characteristic cellular features of excretory ducts, striated ducts, intercalated ducts, and acini (see below) (16). The proximal branched cords become excretory and main ducts, the distal branched cords become striated ducts, and the luminized terminal bulbs become intercalated ducts and acini. After luminization but before cellular differentiation the terminal bulbs are referred to as terminal tubules and saccules (fig. 1-3). The epithelium of the terminal tubules and saccules has two layers: an inner luminal layer of cells which differentiates into acinar and intercalated duct cells and an outer layer which differentiates into myoepithelial cells (16). Complete maturation of the salivary glands does not occur until after birth (21).

At about the third month of gestation the parotid gland is colonized by lymphocytes that eventually develop into several intraparotid and periparotid lymph nodes and lymphoid nodules. These appear to lack the complete organization of a lymph node (21).

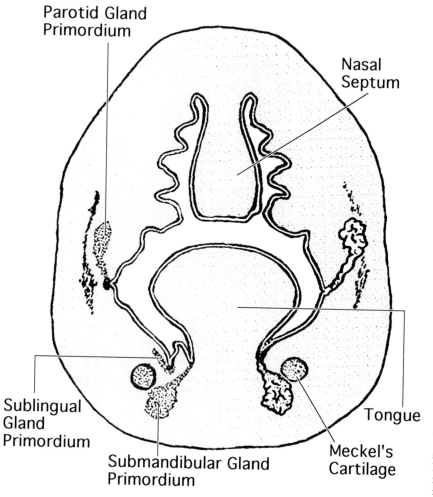

Parotid Gland
Primordium

Nasal
Septum

Sublingual
Gland
Primordium

Submandibular Gland
Primordium

Meckel's
Cartilage

Tongue

Figure 1-2
EMBRYONIC DEVELOPMENT
OF SALIVARY GLANDS

Top: The origin of the parotid gland, submandibular gland, and sublingual gland from the epithelial lining of the primitive stomodeum is illustrated in the schematic drawing of the oral cavity of a 9-week-old embryo.

Bottom: Photomicrograph in section through fetal tongue, linguogingival groove, and buccal mucosa shows the proliferative epithelial cord of the developing parotid gland (arrow).

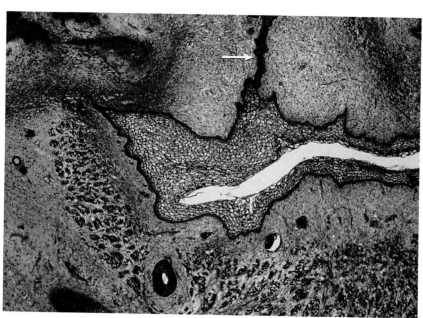

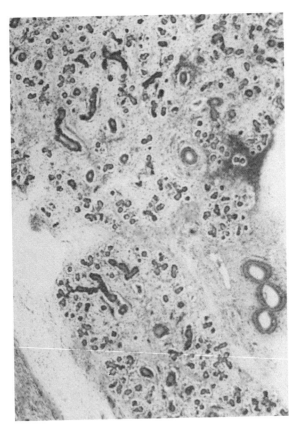 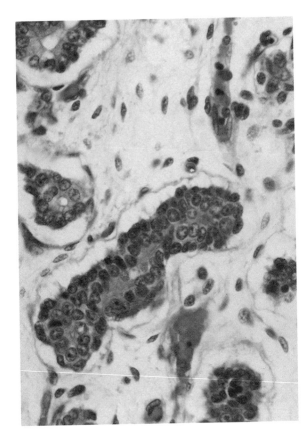

Figure 1-3
FETAL PAROTID GLAND

Left: The primitive epithelial ducts and tubules are mostly undifferentiated and within a very loose, but moderately cellular, fibrous stroma in a 25-week-old fetus.

Right: At high magnification the terminal tubules are a double layer of epithelial cells. The outer layer will differentiate into myoepithelial and basal cells, and the inner cells will become ductal and serous acinar cells.

GROSS ANATOMY

Parotid Gland. The parotid gland is the largest of the salivary glands and in adults weighs 15 to 30 g (16,21). It is roughly triangular shaped, with the apex just inferior to the angle of the mandible and the more superior base along the zygomatic arch. The anterior portion of the gland lies along the posterior edge of the ramus of the mandible and slightly overlays the posterior edge of the masseter muscle. Posteriorly, the gland is bounded by the ear, the mastoid process, and the anterior edge of the sternocleidomastoid muscle (fig. 1-4). The deep, medial portion of the gland extends into the parapharyngeal area and is confined by the styloid process and stylomandibular ligament; styloglossus, stylohyoid, stylopharyngeal, and digastric muscles; and carotid sheath. Anteriorly, this deep portion of the gland lies against the medial pterygoid muscle (fig. 1-5). Laterally, the gland is only covered by skin and subcutaneous adipose tissue. Fibrous and adipose tissue from the deep cervical fascia encapsulate the gland. The gland is in close contact or embraces several important structures including the internal jugular vein and branches, external carotid arteries and branches, lymph nodes, auriculotemporal branch of the trigeminal nerve, and the facial nerve (12,16,20,21).

The secretions of the gland flow through a duct system that converges to a single duct, the Stensen duct, which is 4 to 7 cm long. This duct exits the gland along its anterior edge, traverses across the lateral surface of the masseter muscle, penetrates the buccal fat pad and buccinator muscle just anterior to the anterior edge of the masseter muscle,

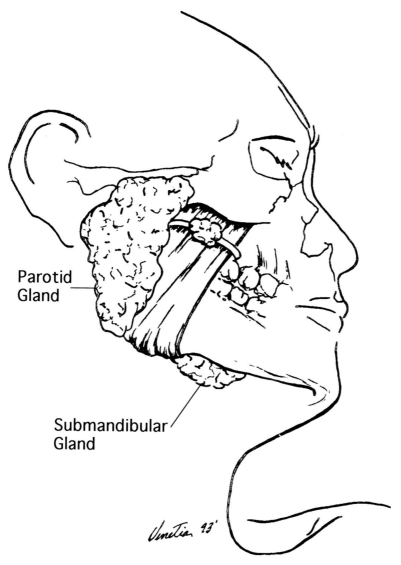

Figure 1-4
ANATOMIC RELATIONSHIP
OF PAROTID AND
SUBMANDIBULAR GLANDS
This lateral view of the head shows the anatomic position and relationship of the parotid and submandibular glands to the ear, zygomatic arch, mandible, and masseter muscle. The parotid gland duct (Stensen's duct) crosses the masseter muscle and penetrates the buccal tissues. Lobules of accessory parotid tissue are located along the course of the duct.

Parotid Gland

Submandibular Gland

and opens into the oral cavity on the buccal mucosa opposite the maxillary second molar. Accessory parotid gland tissue is found along the anterior portion of the gland and the Stensen duct in about 20 percent of people (fig. 1-4) (21).

Although anatomically the parotid gland is a single contiguous structure, surgically it is convenient to conceptualize a superficial (or lateral) and a deep (or medial) lobe that are separated by the course of the facial nerve through the gland (12,20). Most neoplasms occur in the superficial portion of the gland. The facial (cranial VII) nerve emerges from the stylomastoid foramen and immediately enters the posteromedial sur-

face of the parotid gland. As it enters the gland, the nerve divides into two main trunks that further branch and then course in superior, anterior, and inferior directions in a generally similar mediolateral plane. The posterior edge of the ramus of the mandible also impinges upon the gland, and the gland narrows from the superficial to the deep portions. For tumors that arise in the deep portion of the gland the path of least resistance for expansion is into the parapharyngeal space; these tumors manifest as pharyngeal swellings rather than the facial swellings that develop with the more common tumors of the superficial lobe (fig. 1-5) (20).

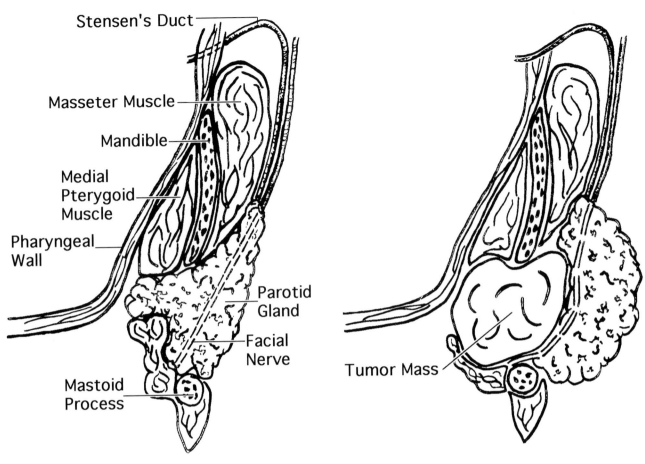

Figure 1-5
ANATOMIC RELATIONSHIP OF PAROTID GLAND

Left: This illustration represents a horizontal section through the lateral portion of the pharynx and mandible at the level of the mastoid process. The parotid gland is traversed by the facial nerve, and the deep portion of the gland narrows and is bounded by the posterior of the ramus of the mandible, muscles of the styloid process, and medial pterygoid muscle.

Right: Tumors that arise within the deep portion of the gland may expand into the lateral pharyngeal space and produce swelling of the lateral pharyngeal wall.

Secretomotor innervation of the parotid gland is by parasympathetic nerve fibers via the ninth cranial nerve, although after a complicated course the nerve fibers enter the gland by way of the otic ganglion and auriculotemporal nerve (2,12). Sympathetic fibers accompany the blood vessels. Interruption of the parasympathetic nerve pathways results in atrophy of the gland (2,12). Blood supply and drainage are via branches of the external carotid artery and retromandibular vein (20,21).

The intimate relationship between parenchymal and lymphoid tissue in the parotid gland is unique among salivary gland tissues. During embryonic development the parotid is seeded with lymphoid cells that develop into several lymph nodes within and around the parenchymal tissue (fig. 1-6) (21). In a study of parotid glands from 10 adult cadavers, McKean et al. (24) found that the number of parotid lymph nodes varied from 3 to 24 per gland. Over 90 percent were lateral to the facial nerve in the superficial portion of the gland. These lymph nodes drain the anterolateral portion of the auricle and external auditory meatus, skin of the temporal and frontotemporal region, root of the nose, eyelids and conjunctiva, tympanic cavity, and the parotid gland itself (35). They drain into the deep cervical lymph nodes along the anterior aspect of the sternocleidomastoid muscle.

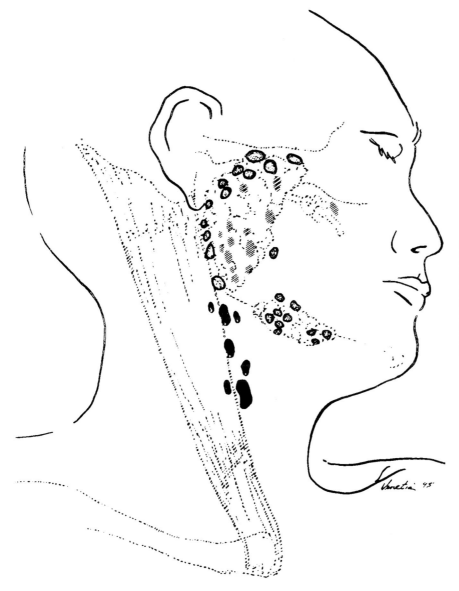

Figure 1-6
GLANDULAR
LYMPH NODES
The parotid gland has several periparotid (dark outline) and intraparotid (shaded) lymph nodes that drain portions of the ear, temporal region, lateral face, eyelids, and conjunctiva. They in turn drain into the internal jugular lymph nodes. The submandibular lymph nodes are all extraglandular.

Submandibular Gland. The submandibular gland is the second largest salivary gland and weighs approximately 7 to 15 g (16,20,21). It occupies a large portion of the submandibular triangle, which is formed by the inferior border of the mandible and the anterior and posterior bellies of the digastric muscle (fig. 1-4). Superiorly, the submandibular space is bounded by the mylohyoid muscle. The posterior extension of the submandibular gland rises upward and around the posterior edge of this muscle and into the sublingual space of the floor of the oral cavity (fig. 1-7) (16,20). Like the parotid gland, the duct system converges into a single main excretory duct, the Wharton duct, that extends about 5 cm from the superior portion of the gland in an anterior direction in the lingual sulcus to an opening, the sublingual caruncula, adjacent to the lingual frenum in the anterior floor of the mouth. The openings of the paired submandibular glands are only a few millimeters apart (fig. 1-8) (20,21). The submandibular gland is enveloped in a fine fibrous capsule. There are no lymph nodes within this capsule, but three to six lymph nodes lie adjacent to the gland in the submandibular triangle (fig. 1-6) (25). These lymph

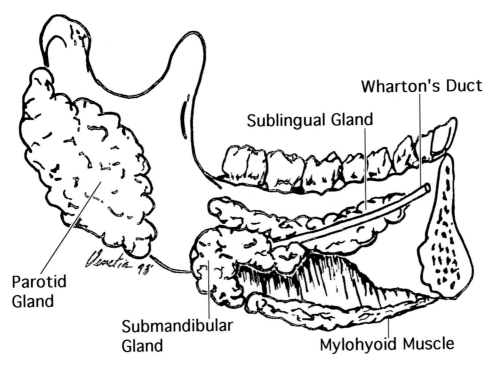

Figure 1-7
ANATOMIC RELATIONSHIP OF THE MAJOR SALIVARY GLANDS
This illustration of the medial surface of the mandible and mylohyoid muscle shows the relationship of the submandibular, sublingual, and parotid glands. The submandibular duct (Wharton's duct) runs anteriorly to the anterior floor of the mouth.

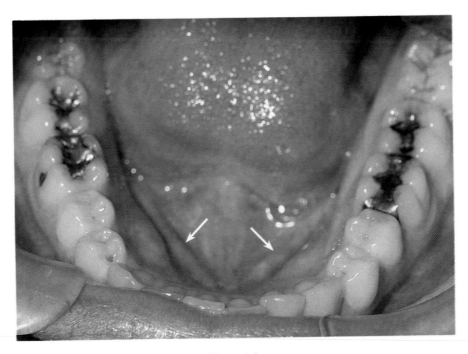

Figure 1-8
WHARTON'S DUCT
The right and left submandibular ducts (arrows) course anteriomedially in the floor of the mouth to openings at the lingual carunculae, which are only a few millimeters apart.

nodes receive afferent vessels from the nose, lips, gums, lateral part of the floor of the mouth, anterior and lateral portions of the tongue, and the submandibular gland and send efferent vessels into the deep cervical lymph nodes along the internal jugular vein and sternocleidomastoid muscle (25,35). The blood supply and drainage of the gland is by the lingual and facial arteries and the anterior facial vein (20). The gland is innervated by parasympathetic secretomotor fibers of the facial nerve and sympathetic nerves (21). Unlike the parotid gland, no large nerves course through the parenchyma of the submandibular gland.

Sublingual Gland. The sublingual gland is the smallest of the major salivary glands and weighs about 2 to 4 g (16,20,21). It lies above the mylohyoid muscle in the lingual sulcus of the floor of the mouth between the tongue and the sublingual fossa of the mandible (fig. 1-7). Its superior aspect is covered only by oral mucosa. Unlike the parotid and submandibular glands, the sublingual gland has several ducts that connect to the oral cavity. The largest of these ducts, the Bartholin duct, opens into the submandibular duct just posterior to sublingual caruncula (16). The several smaller ducts that open directly into the oral cavity are known as the Rivinus ducts (16,21). The blood supply is from the sublingual and submental arteries, and venous drainage is via tributaries of the external jugular vein (21). Innervation is from parasympathetic fibers of the facial nerve (21).

Minor Salivary Glands. It is estimated that there are 500 to 1000 lobules of minor salivary gland tissue dispersed within the mucosa of the oral cavity (16,20). These intraoral glands usually are not clinically evident although salivary lobules often can be palpated in the lips. For the most part, the gland lobules are 1 to 5 mm in size and separated from one another by connective tissue, but glands in the posterior hard palate are more numerous and more confluent. Most lobules have individual excretory ducts that open into the oral cavity, but the duct orifices are not usually perceptible on the normal oral mucosa.

HISTOLOGY

Parotid Gland. Within the parotid gland the main excretory duct branches into smaller interlobular ducts, which in turn branch into many, even smaller, intralobular striated ducts. The striated ducts likewise divide into numerous intercalated ducts, which are connected to the terminal secretory structures, the acini. The acini of the parotid gland are nearly 100 percent serous, although occasionally a few mucous type acini can be found (fig. 1-9). The serous acinar cells are arranged in small, roughly spherical clusters of three to six cells in a two-dimensional plane of section. Each acinus surrounds a tiny lumen, although it is frequently not discernible in the plane of section, and the acinus itself is surrounded by a basement membrane. The serous cells are roughly triangular or trapezoidal shaped with the narrowest part of the cells at the luminal surface. The abundant cytoplasm contains numerous basophilic zymogen granules, the secretory granules (fig. 1-9), but the number of cytoplasmic granules varies with the secretory phase of the cell. The granules stain with periodic acid–Schiff (PAS) and are resistant to diastase digestion (fig. 1-9), but they are unreactive with mucicarmine stain. The nuclei are uniform, round, and located in the basal half of the cells.

The intercalated ducts are longer and more conspicuous in the parotid gland than in any of the other salivary glands, but their small size in comparison to the acini and striated ducts makes them more difficult to discern. The intercalated ducts are lined by low cuboidal cells with scant cytoplasm and uniform round nuclei (fig. 1-10). Since their nuclei are about the same size as the nuclei of acinar cells, the nuclear/cytoplasmic ratio is much greater in intercalated duct cells than acinar cells. The cytoplasm is amphophilic to eosinophilic.

Located between the basal surface of acinar and intercalated duct cells and the basement membrane are myoepithelial cells. Some investigators also have reported myoepithelial cells in association with striated and interlobular excretory ducts (5,8). These are flattened, stellate, and spindle-shaped cells with cellular processes that extend in basket-like fashion around the acini and intercalated ducts. The myoepithelial cells have histologic and ultrastructural features of both epithelium and smooth muscle and are believed to have contractile properties that aid in the secretion of saliva. These cells are very difficult to visualize in routine hematoxylin and eosin–stained tissue sections.

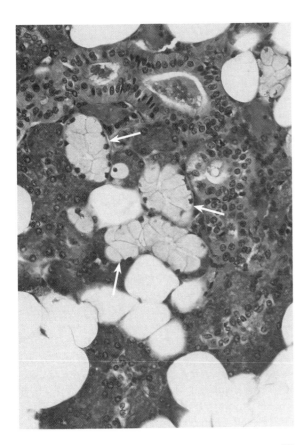
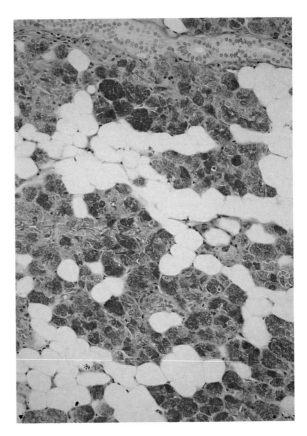

Figure 1-9
PAROTID GLAND ACINI

Left: Clusters of large, pale-staining mucous cells (arrows) occasionally are present in the parotid gland, but the acini are overwhelmingly of serous type. Each serous acinus is composed of several pyramidal-shaped cells with basal nuclei and basophilic cytoplasmic granules.

Right: The serous cell granules are PAS positive and resistant to diastase digestion. (PAS stain)

Figure 1-10
INTERCALATED DUCT

The cells of the intercalated duct (arrow) are small in comparison to the acinar cells and are cuboidal with pale-stained cytoplasm and central nuclei. A small lumen is evident.

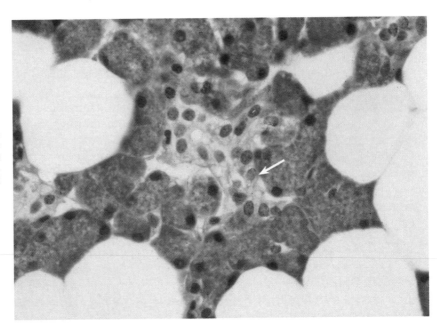

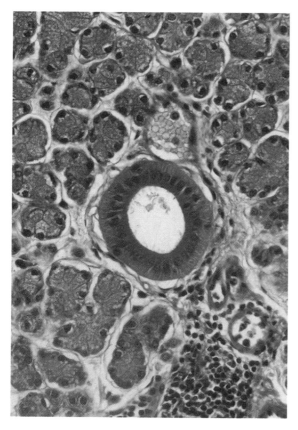

Figure 1-11
STRIATED DUCT
The striated duct is larger than an acinus and much larger than the intercalated duct. The ductal cells are eosinophilic columnar cells with central nuclei and vertical cytoplasmic striations due to folds in the basal plasma membranes.

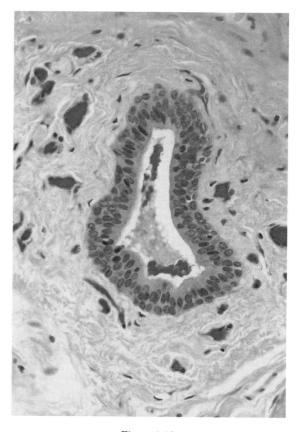

Figure 1-12
INTERLOBULAR EXCRETORY DUCT
This small, interlobular excretory duct is lined by pseudostratified columnar epithelium and embedded in dense fibrous connective tissue.

The striated ducts are much larger than the intercalated ducts: the diameter is about three to six times the size of an acinus. Striated ductal cells are columnar and intensely eosinophilic. The nuclei are uniform and round and located in the center or luminal half of the cells. The fine vertical striations, for which the cells are named, can be seen with high-magnification light microscopy in the basal half to two thirds of the cells (fig. 1-11). These striations are due to prominent basal folds in the plasma membranes. The striated duct cells react more intensely with phosphotungstic acid–hematoxylin stain than other cellular constituents because they contain a large number of mitochondria. Occasional myoepithelial cells and scattered basal cells are located between the striated cells and basement membrane.

For the most part, interlobular and extraglandular excretory ducts are lined by pseudostratified columnar epithelium (fig. 1-12). Small basal cells are distributed along the basement membrane, and occasional goblet-type mucous cells are intermingled among the pseudostratified columnar cells. As the excretory duct approaches and merges with the oral mucosal epithelium, the ductal epithelium becomes stratified squamous type.

The glandular parenchyma is segregated into varying sized lobules by septa of fibrous tissue, which also forms a capsule around the entire gland. A variable amount of fat is found in both intralobular and extralobular locations. The clusters of acinar cells are closely apposed and very dense in young persons, but with advancing

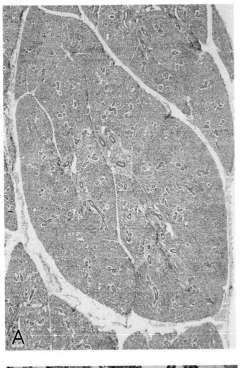

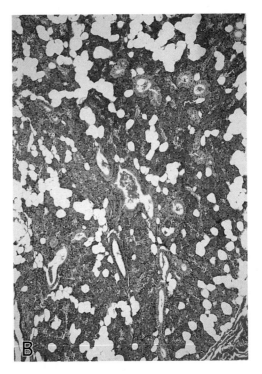

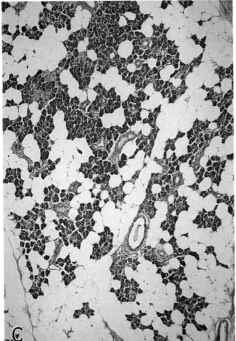

Figure 1-13
INTRAGLANDULAR ADIPOSE
TISSUE IN PAROTID GLAND

A: The parotid gland from a neonate contains no discernible adipose tissue.

B: There is a moderate amount of intralobular adipose tissue in parotid tissue from a middle-aged adult.

C: The intraparotid adipose tissue is quite prominent in the gland from an elderly person.

age the amount of interstitial adipose tissue increases while the parenchymal tissue decreases (fig. 1-13). Since the secretory capacity of the parotid gland exceeds normal requirements, the decreasing parenchyma/fat ratio rarely results in xerostomia unless some intercurrent disease alters the function of the gland.

Lymphoid tissue in the form of small, unstructured nodules and lymph nodes is found scattered within and around the parotid gland

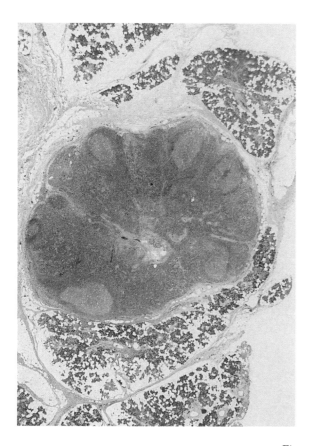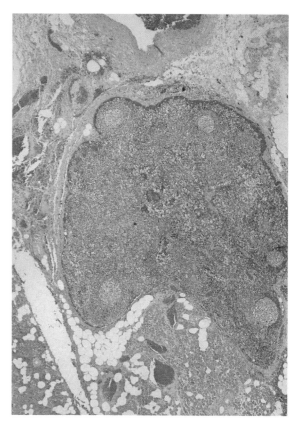

Figure 1-14
PAROTID LYMPH NODES
These intraparotid (left) and periparotid (right) lymph nodes are encapsulated and have subcapsular sinuses and germinal centers. Even the periparotid lymph node (right) is within the capsule and in contact with parenchymal tissue of the parotid gland.

(fig. 1-14). Some of the small lymphoid nodules lack capsules and subcapsular and medullary sinuses of true lymph nodes. Periglandular lymph nodes lie within the capsule of the gland. McKean et al. (24) found that only about one fourth of the parotid lymph nodes, which were distinguished from unstructured lymphoid nodules, had germinal centers. Glandular tissue is frequently entrapped in the medullary region of these lymph nodes.

Foci of sebaceous glands or small collections of sebaceous cells are infrequently seen in parotid gland tissue in routinely examined surgical pathology specimens (fig. 1-15). If thorough serial sections of whole parotid glands were examined, foci of sebaceous cells would probably be found in the majority. Therefore, sebaceous cells can be considered a normal, albeit minor, constituent of parotid glands, but their significance is unknown.

Large peripheral nerves in contact with or in close proximity to parotid parenchymal tissue represent the facial nerve and its branches (fig. 1-16).

Submandibular Gland. The lobular architecture and parenchyma of the acini, intercalated ducts, striated ducts, interlobular ducts, and main excretory duct of the submandibular gland are similar to the parotid gland. Unlike the acini of the parotid gland, which are mostly serous, mucous cells constitute a more significant portion of submandibular gland acini (about 10 percent) (fig. 1-17). Acini with mucous cells are generally a mixture of mucous and serous cells. The serous cells are typically arranged as crescent-shaped caps (demilunes) at the periphery of the mucous acinar cells. The mucous cells have abundant, clear to faintly basophilic, finely granular to furrowed cytoplasm with basally oriented, round nuclei. The intercalated ducts

Figure 1-15
SEBACEOUS CELLS
IN PAROTID GLAND
The cells in two foci of sebaceous differentiation (arrows) are large with central nuclei and clear reticulated cytoplasm that is unreactive with mucicarmine stain. Small foci of sebaceous cells occur frequently in the parotid gland. (Mucicarmine stain)

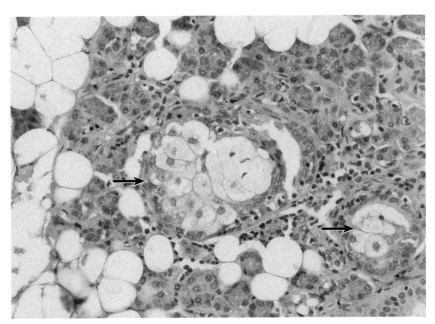

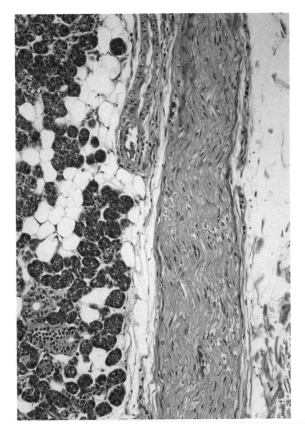
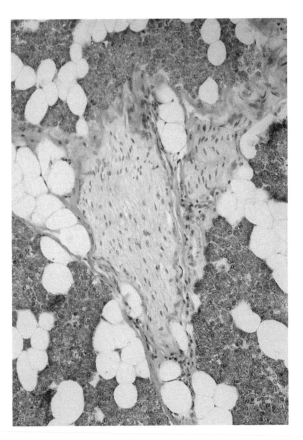

Figure 1-16
FACIAL NERVE BRANCHES IN PAROTID GLAND
A relatively large nerve lies adjacent to a lobule of parotid glandular tissue (left) while a smaller nerve branch is within a lobule and in contact with serous acini (right).

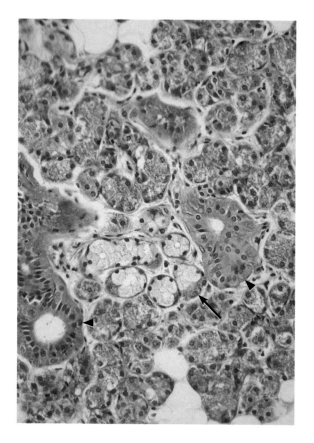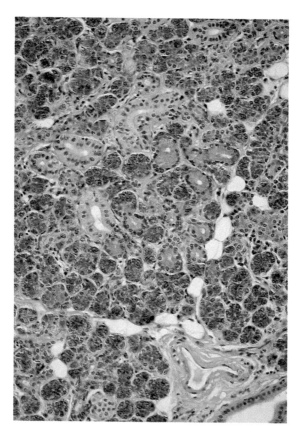

Figure 1-17
SUBMANDIBULAR GLAND ACINI
Left: In the submandibular gland mucous acini comprise about 10 percent of the acinar tissue. Serous cells are frequently located at the periphery of mucous acini as crescent-shaped cells (arrow). The striated ducts (arrowheads) are more prominent and the intercalated ducts are shorter than those in the parotid gland.
Right: The mucous cells are highlighted among the serous acini as rose pink cells. (Mucicarmine stain)

are shorter and less discernible while the striated ducts are more conspicuous than their counterparts in the parotid gland. Again, the myoepithelial cells are obscure in routine-stained tissue sections. For any specific age group, the amount of intraglandular adipose tissue is less than in the parotid gland. Lymph nodes, lymphoid nodules, and large peripheral nerves are not present within the gland.

Sublingual Gland. Unlike the parotid and submandibular glands, most of the acini of the sublingual gland are mixed type, composed of mucous cells with serous cell demilunes (fig. 1-18). These secretory end pieces are frequently elongated rather than spherical like acini in the parotid and submandibular glands. The lobular architecture is less organized and both the intercalated ducts and striated ducts are shorter than

in either of the other major salivary glands. Similar to the submandibular gland, lymphoid tissue and large peripheral nerves are not usually evident within the substance of the gland. Several collecting ducts connect to the oral mucosa and submandibular gland duct.

Minor Salivary Glands. The minor intraoral salivary glands are scattered within the oral mucosal and submucosal tissues of the buccal mucosa, lips, floor of mouth, hard and soft palates, tonsillar pillars, and tongue as small lobules of mostly mucous type exocrine glands (fig. 1-19). The anterior hard palate and gingiva are generally devoid of salivary glands, but the retromolar mandibular ridge does contain salivary glands. In the tongue, salivary gland tissue located on the anterior ventral portion is of mucous type, and is called the Blandin and Nunn glands; in

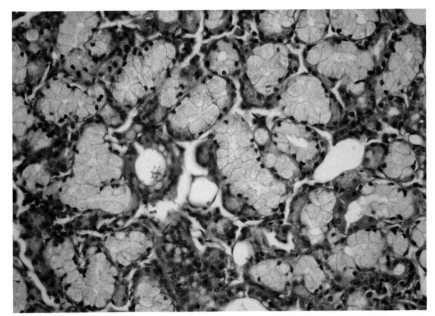

Figure 1-18
SUBLINGUAL GLAND ACINI
The sublingual gland acini are typically elongated tubules of mucous cells with serous cell demilunes.

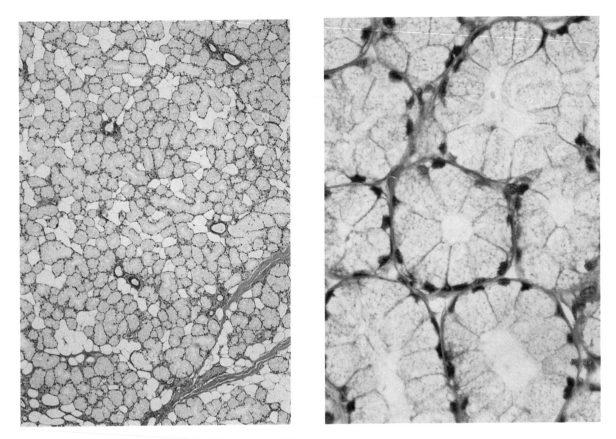

Figure 1-19
MINOR SALIVARY GLANDS OF THE PALATE
Left: The palate contains the largest foci of intraoral salivary gland tissue, which is composed of mucous acini but no striated ducts.
Right: At high magnification the mucous acini are round with central lumens. The mucous cells are pyramidal with very pale granular cytoplasm and nuclei located next to the basal plasma membranes.

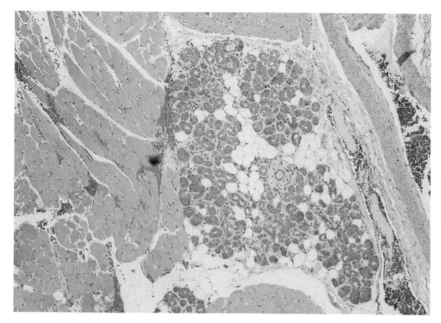

Figure 1-20
MINOR SALIVARY GLANDS
IN TONGUE
The minor salivary glands are small aggregates of unencapsulated mucous or serous glands. In the tongue they are in intimate contact with the striated muscle tissue.

the region of the circumvallate papillae on the posterior dorsal and lateral portion, it is serous and called the von Ebner glands. The minor glands are mostly unencapsulated and lie in close contact with the structures around them, especially the muscles of the tongue and lips (fig. 1-20). This intramuscular, unencapsulated morphology is a factor to be considered in histologic evaluation of invasive growth and malignancy in minor salivary gland neoplasms.

ULTRASTRUCTURE

Acinar Cells. At the ultrastructural level, the most notable feature of serous acinar cells is the presence of numerous cytoplasmic secretory granules that are located predominantly in the apical portion of the cell (fig. 1-21). These are round, membrane-bound structures of varying electron density and diameter. The number of granules depends upon the secretory phase of the cell. Basal and lateral to the nucleus is the extensive array of the rough endoplasmic reticulum and Golgi region; mitochondria are modestly numerous. Basal lamina is located along the basal surface. When the cell is not distended with secretory product, the basal plasma membrane has numerous folds. In addition to the luminal surface, microvilli extend into the intercellular space, which is continuous with the

lumen. In the intercellular space are complex interdigitations of plasma membranes of adjacent cells. There are junctional complexes at the apical end of the cells and desmosomal attachments at sites along the lateral borders (7,16,22).

Mucous acinar cells are similar to serous cells but the secretory droplets are often larger, more irregularly shaped, and more electron lucent. The number and size of secretory droplets and the prominence of the Golgi apparatus and endoplasmic reticulum vary with the functional stage of the cell. The secretory droplets often fuse to form very large droplets. A rough endoplasmic reticulum, Golgi apparatus, and mitochondria are usually located in the basal portion of the cell. The lateral intercellular interdigitations are less complex than those of serous cells. The basal plasma membrane folds are more complex in mucous cells of the submandibular and sublingual glands than in mucous cells of the minor salivary glands, but minor salivary gland mucous cells have more complex lateral interdigitations (7,16,22).

Myoepithelial Cells. Myoepithelial cells are situated between the basal plasma membrane of the acinar and intercalated duct cells, and perhaps even striated and excretory ducts, and the basal lamina. They have a flattened, elongated shape with extension of several cytoplasmic processes over the acinar and duct cells. Myoepithelial cells adjacent to duct cells have fewer

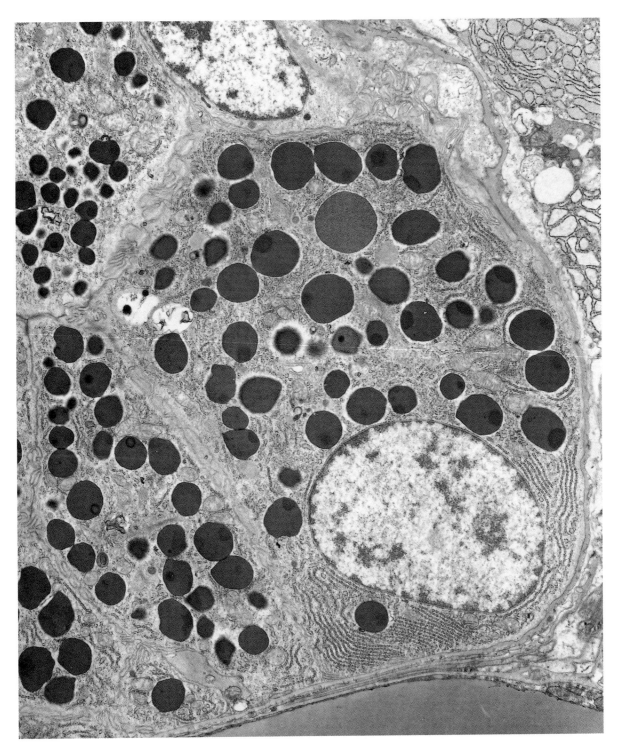

Figure 1-21
ULTRASTRUCTURE OF THE SEROUS ACINAR CELL

Variable-sized secretory granules occupy most of the apical portion of the cytoplasmic compartment. Parallel arrays of rough endoplasmic reticula lie adjacent to the basally located, round nucleus. The intercellular space contains interdigitations of adjacent cells and represents a canaliculus that is connected to the acinar lumen and is actually the beginning of the duct system (X11,300).

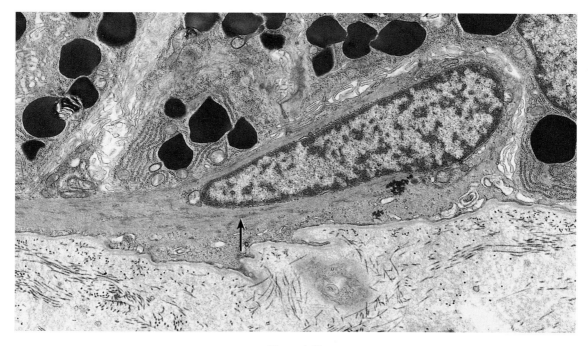

Figure 1-22
ULTRASTRUCTURE OF THE MYOEPITHELIAL CELL
The myoepithelial cell lies between the basal lamina and the basal plasma membranes of the acinar cells. The cell body is flattened and the nucleus is elongated. In the cytoplasm are numerous microfilaments with focal dense bodies (arrow) (X13,300).

cytoplasmic processes and the nuclei are elongated or irregularly shaped. The cytoplasmic processes and the basal portion of the cell bodies contain numerous microfilaments with focal densities, which are similar to those of smooth muscle cells (fig. 1-22). Pinocytotic vesicles are present along the basal plasma membranes. Mitochondria, an endoplasmic reticulum, Golgi vesicles, and lysosomes are concentrated about the nuclei. Desmosomes attach the myoepithelial cells to the acinar and ductal cells, and tonofilaments are present in some cells (8).

Intercalated Duct Cells. Intercalated duct cells have none of the special or characteristic ultrastructural features that are seen in acinar, myoepithelial, and striated duct cells. Some cells in proximity to acinar cells contain a few secretory granules; otherwise, within the scant cytoplasm is a basally located rough endoplasmic reticulum, an apically located Golgi region, and mitochondria. The lateral cell membranes interdigitate with adjacent cells, and there are few microvilli on the luminal surface. The cells are connected by junctional complexes and a few desmosomes (fig. 1-23) (16,22).

Striated Duct Cells. The cytoplasmic striations evident with light microscopy are due to extensive vertical folds in the basal plasma membrane of these tall columnar cells. Numerous mitochondria are in the cytoplasmic compartment between the folds (fig. 1-24). Laterally, the basal folds form a complex interdigitation with plasma membrane folds of adjacent cells. Around the centrally located nuclei are small amounts of endoplasmic reticulum and a Golgi complex. The cells have junctional complexes and desmosomes on their lateral surfaces and short microvilli on their luminal surface (7,16,22).

IMMUNOHISTOCHEMISTRY

Fixation and preparation of tissue specimens influences the results of immunohistochemical studies and may explain some of the variability of features reported by different investigators. Fresh frozen tissue specimens are often more sensitive to immunostaining than formalin-fixed and paraffin-embedded tissue, and some antigens are preserved better in one fixative than another. Still, in most laboratories formalin fixation is standard

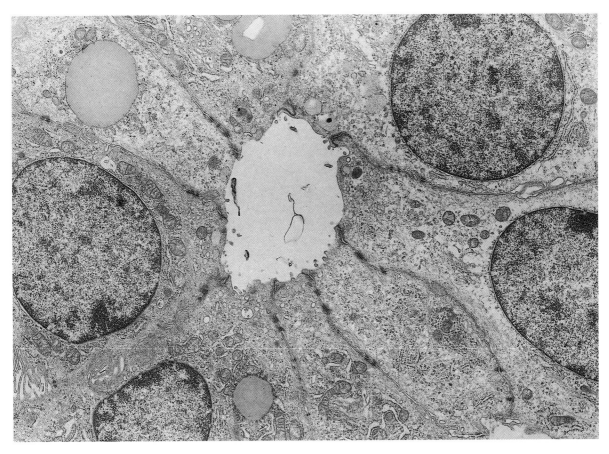

Figure 1-23
ULTRASTRUCTURE OF AN INTERCALATED DUCT CELL
The relatively small cytoplasmic compartment contains a round nucleus, mitochondria, lipid vacuoles, and an endoplasmic reticulum. There are a few short microvilli on the luminal surface, and intercellular connections are apical junctional complexes with several desmosomes (X6,000).

for most tissues. In routinely formalin-fixed and paraffin-embedded tissue preparations of normal salivary glands at the Armed Forces Institute of Pathology (AFIP), immunohistochemical staining with a cocktail of monoclonal antibodies (AE1/AE3 and CK1) for high and low molecular weight keratin intermediate filaments has resulted in intense reactivity in intercalated, striated, and excretory duct luminal cells but only weak or no reactivity in acinar and myoepithelial cells (fig. 1-25). Others have reported similar experiences with cytokeratin expression (17,23,27,28,33). Some studies have shown that among the several subtypes of cytokeratins, keratin 14 is specific to myoepithelial and ductal basal cells (3,8,9,11,39). Controversy over immunoreactivity for S-100 protein in normal salivary

gland tissue exists: some investigators have reported that such immunoreactivity is a marker for myoepithelial cells (6,15,19); others, including those at the AFIP, have found little or no reactivity for S-100 protein in normal salivary glands (9,36); still others have reported reactivity for S-100 protein in acinar and ductal cells as well as myoepithelial cells (18,30,38). At the AFIP, immunoreactivity for S-100 protein has been observed in myoepithelial and intercalated duct cells in salivary gland tissue under stress, i.e., non-neoplastic salivary gland tissue adjacent to expanding neoplasms (fig. 1-26). Dardick et al. (9) found that the rich network of unmyelinated nerves in the interstitial tissues around the glandular parenchyma, rather than the myoepithelium, immunostains for S-100 protein. Normal

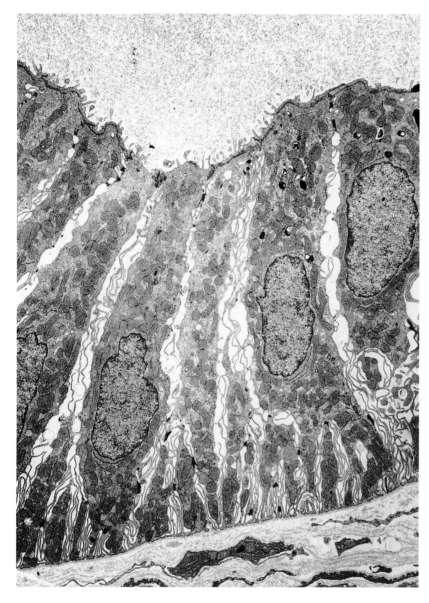

Figure 1-24
ULTRASTRUCTURE OF A
STRIATED DUCT CELL
The basal plasma membranes have prominent vertical folds, and there are numerous mitochondria. The lateral surfaces have processes that interdigitate with adjacent cells. Apical junctional complexes and desmosomes connect adjoining cells (X6,000).

myoepithelial cells do react with anti-smooth muscle actin antibodies (fig. 1-27) (9,11,17,18,28, 45). Some investigators have reported that normal myoepithelial cells react with anti-vimentin, anti-myosin, and anti-glial fibrillary acidic protein antibodies (6,13,17,23,28,33,38,45); others have reported negative results (3,10,28,30).

Normal serous cells have demonstrated immunoreactivity for alpha-amylase, transferrin, and lactoferrin (fig. 1-28) (26,29,40,42–44). In addition to cytokeratin, intercalated duct cells are reactive with antibodies to lysozyme, transferrin, and lactoferrin (26,34,42,44). Crocker and

Egan (6) reported that normal salivary gland is reactive for alpha-1-antitrypsin but not alpha-1-antichymotrypsin; others, however, have reported the opposite (43,44).

Fibronectin, type IV collagen, laminin, and tenascin have been found in the basement membrane region of acinar and ductal salivary tissues with immunohistochemical studies (4,37,41). A report of immunoreactivity to estradiol and progesterone in excretory duct cells suggests that salivary gland tissue may be a target tissue for estrogen (32). Prolactin binding sites also have been described in striated duct cells (1,31).

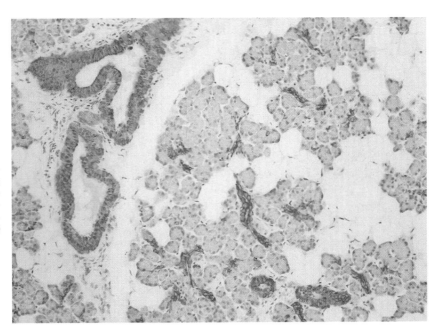

Figure 1-25
IMMUNOHISTOCHEMICAL
STAINING OF
SALIVARY GLANDS
Intercalated, striated, and interlobular ducts react intensely with an
anticytokeratin monoclonal antibody cocktail, but acinar and myoepithelial cells are mostly unreactive. (Avidin-biotin peroxidase stain)

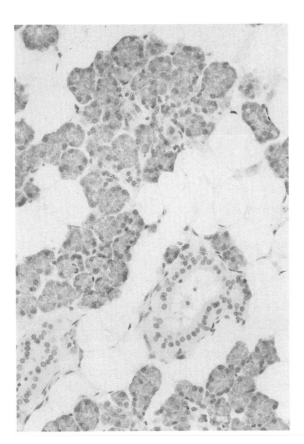

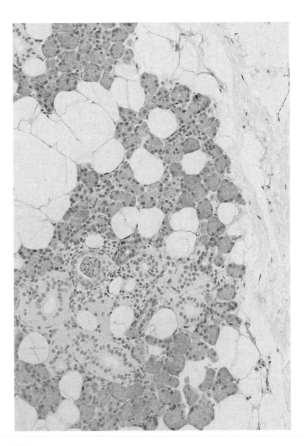

Figure 1-26
IMMUNOHISTOCHEMICAL STAINING OF SALIVARY GLANDS
Left: This normal, formalin-fixed parotid tissue is unreactive for S-100 protein.
Right: In this parotid tissue adjacent to a mixed tumor, some of the myoepithelial and intercalated duct cells are immunoreactive for S-100 protein. (Avidin-biotin peroxidase stain)

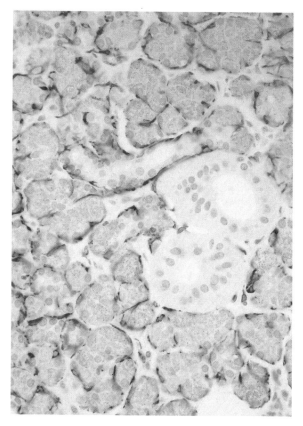

Figure 1-27
IMMUNOHISTOCHEMICAL STAINING
OF SALIVARY GLANDS
The normally hardly noticeable, elongated and flattened myoepithelial cells at the periphery of the acini, intercalated ducts, and striated ducts have become conspicuous due to their immunostaining for alpha-smooth muscle actin. (Avidin-biotin peroxidase stain)

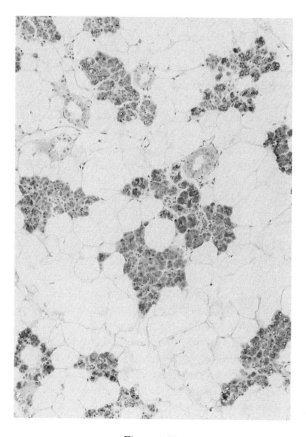

Figure 1-28
IMMUNOHISTOCHEMICAL STAINING
OF SALIVARY GLANDS
The serous acinar cells immunostain for alpha-amylase. (Avidin-biotin peroxidase stain)

PHYSIOLOGY

The primary function of the salivary glands is to produce saliva. Both parasympathetic and sympathetic stimulation increase the production of saliva, but parasympathetic stimulation is the more dominant (2,14). The principal function of saliva is to lubricate the oral mucosa and aid in the swallowing of food, but the constituents of saliva also function in enzymatic digestion of food, antimicrobial defense, buffering of acids released by bacteria into the oral environment, remineralization of enamel, and mediation of taste (2,7,14).

Saliva is about 99.5 percent water and has a specific gravity of 1.002 to 1.012. The remaining constituents are electrolytes, organic analytes (mostly protein components of blood), and macromolecules (2). About 600 to 1500 ml of saliva are produced each day, but the level of production is cyclical. Less than 5 percent of saliva is produced during sleep, and about 80 to 90 percent is produced in response to gustatory and masticatory stimuli (2,7). The parotid gland produces most of the saliva and is followed in production capacity by the submandibular gland. The sublingual and minor salivary glands contribute about 10 to 15 percent of the saliva (7).

The fluid component of saliva is produced by osmotic perfusion of blood plasma through the interstitium and acinar cells by means of active electrolyte movement into the lumen by the acinar cells, while macromolecules are released from the secretory granules of the acinar cells (2,7). The secretory granules discharge their contents into the lumen of the acinus by exocytosis, i.e., the membranes of the granules fuse with portions of the luminal plasma membranes of the acinar cells. Within the acinar lumens the saliva has a sodium and chloride ion concentration similar to blood and interstitial fluid, but sodium and chloride ions are actively reabsorbed and potassium and carbonate ions are secreted by the ductal cells, principally the striated ductal cells, which results in a hypotonic saliva (7). During periods of increased saliva production, the flow of saliva is so rapid that the ductal cells are unable to alter the ion concentrations as effectively. Therefore, the sodium and chloride concentrations are higher and the potassium and carbonate concentrations are lower in active rather than in quiescent periods of salivary secretion (14).

Serous cells produce a thin, watery fluid that contains alpha-amylase, an enzyme that begins the digestion of food as it is masticated in the oral cavity and digests starches. The mucous acini generate a more viscous, mucinous saliva that is higher in glycoproteins and provides a protective lubricating film on the oral mucosa (7).

Saliva provides a flushing mechanism to remove bacteria from the oral environs. In addition, saliva contains several antimicrobial agents such as IgA immunoglobulin, lactoferrin, lysozyme, and peroxidases. IgA agglutinates microorganisms and facilitates the cleansing action of saliva; lactoferrin deprives bacteria of essential iron; and lysozyme hydrolyzes bacterial cell walls (7). IgA is produced by plasma cells in the interstitial tissue of the salivary glands and is actively transported into the salivary secretions by the acinar and ductal epithelial cells, which produce and attach a secretory part to it (2).

The pH of saliva is about 6.0 to 7.4 (14). This pH is nonconducive to the growth of pathogenic oral bacteria; the carbonate ions buffer acids produced by oral bacteria that can demineralize enamel of teeth. Saliva also contains high concentrations of calcium and phosphate ions that assist in the remineralization of enamel (7). The concentration of calcium in saliva from the submandibular gland is nearly twice as high as in saliva from the parotid gland (2). Proline-rich salivary proteins prevent spontaneous precipitation of calcium phosphate (7).

Several hormone-like polypeptides have been identified in salivary gland cells and saliva, but their specific functions or significance have not been clarified. Some of these include kallikrein, renin, epidermal growth factor, and nerve growth factor (2). Kallikrein may have a role in the vascular hemodynamics of the salivary glands: kallikrein secreted by salivary cells is converted to bradykinin, which is a strong vasodilator (14). The blood flow to actively secreting salivary gland tissue may be 10 times as much as to contracting skeletal muscle (2).

REFERENCES

1. Abbey LM, Witorsch RJ. Prolactin binding in normal human minor salivary gland tissue: an immunohistochemical study. Oral Surg Oral Med Oral Pathol 1984;58:682–7.
2. Batsakis JG. Physiology. In: Cummings CW, Frederickson JM, Harker LA, Krause CJ, Schuller DE, eds. Otolaryngology—head and neck surgery. 2nd ed. St. Louis: CV Mosby, 1993:986–96.
3. Burns BF, Dardick I, Parks WR. Intermediate filament expression in normal parotid glands and pleomorphic adenomas. Virchows Arch [A] 1988;413:103–12.
4. Caselitz J, Schmitt P, Seifert G, Wustrow J, Schuppan D. Basal membrane associated substances in human salivary glands and salivary gland tumours. Pathol Res Pract 1988;183:386–94.
5. Chaudhry AP, Cutler LS, Yamane GM, Labay GR, Sunderraj M, Manak JR Jr. Ultrastructure of normal human parotid gland with special emphasis on myoepithelial distribution. J Anat 1987;152:1–11.
6. Crocker J, Egan MJ. Immunohistochemistry of salivary gland tumors. Ear Nose Throat J 1989;68:130–6.
7. Dale AC. Salivary glands. In: Ten Cate AR, ed. Oral histology: development, structure, and function. 2nd ed. St. Louis: CV Mosby, 1985:303–31.
8. Dardick I, Rippstein P, Skimming L, Boivin M, Parks WR, Dairkee SH. Immunohistochemistry and ultrastructure of myoepithelium and modified myoepithelium of the ducts of human major salivary glands: histogenetic implications for salivary gland tumors. Oral Surg Oral Med Oral Pathol 1987;64:703–15.

9. Dardick I, Stratis M, Parks WR, DeNardi FG, Kahn HJ. S-100 protein antibodies do not label normal salivary gland myoepithelium. Histogenetic implications for salivary gland tumors. Am J Pathol 1991;138:619–28.

10. de Araújo VC, de Araújo NS. Vimentin as a marker of myoepithelial cells in salivary gland tumors. Eur Arch Otorhinolaryngol 1990;247:252–5.

11. Draeger A, Nathrath WB, Lane EB, Sundström BE, Stigbrand TI. Cytokeratins, smooth muscle actin and vimentin in human normal salivary gland and pleomorphic adenomas. Immunohistochemical studies with particular reference to myoepithelial and basal cells. APMIS 1991;99:405–15.

12. Graney DO, Jacobs JR, Kern R. Anatomy. In: Cummings CW, Fredrickson JM, Harker LA, Krause CJ, Schuller DE, eds. Otolaryngology—head and neck surgery. 2nd ed. St. Louis: CV Mosby, 1993:977–85.

13. Gustafsson H, Virtanen I, Thornell LE. Glial fibrillary acidic protein and desmin in salivary neoplasms. Expression of four different types of intermediate filament proteins within the same cell type. Virchows Arch [Cell Pathol] 1989;57:303–13.

14. Guyton AC. Textbook of medical physiology. 8th ed. Philadelphia: WB Saunders, 1991:711–3.

15. Hara K, Ito M, Takeuchi J, Iijima S, Endo T, Hidaka H. Distribution of S-100b protein in normal salivary glands and salivary gland tumors. Virchows Arch [A] 1983;401:237–49.

16. Hiatt JL, Sauk JJ. Embryology and anatomy of the salivary glands. In: Ellis GL, Auclair PL, Gnepp DR, eds. Surgical pathology of the salivary glands. Philadelphia: WB Saunders, 1991:2–9.

17. Hirano T, Gluckman JL, deVries EJ. The expression of alpha vascular smooth-muscle actin in salivary gland tumors. Arch Otolaryngol Head Neck Surg 1990;116:692–6.

18. Jones H, Moshtael F, Simpson RH. Immunoreactivity of alpha smooth muscle actin in salivary gland tumours: a comparison with S100 protein. J Clin Pathol 1992;45:938–40.

19. Kahn HJ, Baumal R, Marks A, Dardick I, van Nostrand AW. Myoepithelial cells in salivary gland tumors. An immunohistochemical study. Arch Pathol Lab Med 1985;109:190–5.

20. Kaplan MJ, Johns ME. Malignant neoplasms. In: Cummings CW, Fredrickson JM, Harker LA, Krause CJ, Schuller DE, eds. Otolaryngology—head and neck surgery. 2nd ed. St. Louis: CV Mosby, 1993:1043–78.

21. Martinez-Madrigal F, Micheau C. Histology of the major salivary glands. Am J Surg Pathol 1989;13:879–99.

22. Martinez-Madrigal F, Micheau C. Major salivary glands. In: Sternberg SS, ed. Histology for Pathologists. New York: Raven Press, 1992:457–78.

23. Matsushima R, Nakayama I, Shimizu M. Immunohistochemical localization of keratin, vimentin and myosin in salivary gland tumors. Acta Pathol Jpn 1988;38:445–54.

24. McKean ME, Lee K, McGregor IA. The distribution of lymph nodes in and around the parotid gland: an anatomical study. Br J Plast Surg 1985;38:1–5.

25. McVay CB. Anson & McVay surgical anatomy. 6th ed. Philadelphia: WB Saunders, 1984:255.

26. Mitani H, Murase N, Mori M. Immunohistochemical demonstration of lysozyme and lactoferrin in salivary pleomorphic adenomas. Virchows Arch [Cell Pathol] 1989;57:257–65.

27. Mori M, Ninomiya T, Okada Y, Tsukitani K. Myoepitheliomas and myoepithelial adenomas of salivary gland origin. Immunohistochemical evaluation of filament proteins, S-100 alpha and beta, glial fibrillary acidic proteins, neuron-specific enolase, and lactoferrin. Pathol Res Pract 1989;184:168–78.

28. Morinaga S, Nakajima T, Shimosato Y. Normal and neoplastic myoepithelial cells in salivary glands: an immunohistochemical study. Hum Pathol 1987;18:1218–26.

29. Morley DJ, Hodes JE, Calland J, Hodes ME. Immunohistochemical demonstration of ribonuclease and amylase in normal and neoplastic parotid glands. Hum Pathol 1983;14:969–73.

30. Nakazato Y, Ishida Y, Takahashi K, Suzuki K. Immunohistochemical distribution of S-100 protein and glial fibrillary acidic protein in normal and neoplastic salivary glands. Virchows Arch [A] 1985;405:299–310.

31. Ninomiya T, Orito T, Tsukitani K, Mori M, Imanishi Y. Immunoreactive prolactin in lesions and tumours of salivary glands. Acta Histochem 1988;84:41–50.

32. Ozono S, Onozuka M, Sato K, Ito Y. Immunohistochemical localization of estradiol, progesterone, and progesterone receptor in human salivary glands and salivary adenoid cystic carcinomas. Cell Struct Funct 1992;17:169–75.

33. Saku T, Okabe H, Yagi Y, Sato E, Tsuda N. A comparative study on the immunolocalization of keratin and myosin in salivary gland tumors. Acta Pathol Jpn 1984;34:1031–40.

34. Sehested M, Barfoed C, Krogdahl A, Bretlau P. Immunohistochemical investigation of lysozyme, lactoferrin, alpha 1-antitrypsin, alpha 1-antichymotrypsin and ferritin in parotid gland tumors. J Oral Pathol 1985;14:459–65.

35. Sessions RB, Hudkins CP. Malignant cervical adenopathy. In: Cummings CW, Fredrickson JM, Harker LA, Krause CJ, Schuller DE, eds. Otolaryngology—head and neck surgery. 2nd ed. St. Louis: CV Mosby, 1993:1605–15.

36. Siar CH, Ng KH. Immunohistochemical study of the distribution of S-100 protein in pleomorphic adenomas of minor salivary glands. J Nihon Univ Sch Dent 1992;34:96–105.

37. Skalova A, Leivo I. Basement membrane proteins in salivary gland tumours. Distribution of type IV collagen and laminin. Virchows Arch [A] 1992;420:425–31.

38. Stead RH, Qizilbash AH, Kontozoglou T, Daya AD, Riddell RH. An immunohistochemical study of pleomorphic adenomas of the salivary gland: glial fibrillary acidic protein-like immunoreactivity identifies a major myoepithelial component. Hum Pathol 1988;19:32–40.

39. Su L, Morgan PR, Harrison DL, Waseem A, Lane EB. Expression of keratin mRNAs and proteins in normal salivary epithelia and pleomorphic adenomas. J Pathol 1993;171:173–81.

40. Sumitomo S, Kumasa S, Tatemoto Y, Ookusa Y, Mori M. Immunohistochemical localization of amylase in sialoadenitis and salivary gland tumors. J Oral Pathol 1986;15:381–5.

41. Sunardhi-Widyaputra S, van Damme B. Immunohistochemical expression of tenascin in normal human salivary glands and in pleomorphic adenomas. Pathol Res Pract 1993;189:138–43.

42. Takahashi H, Fujita S, Tsuda N, Tezuka F, Okabe H. Iron-binding proteins in adenoid cystic carcinoma of salivary glands: an immunohistochemical study. Tohoku J Exp Med 1991;163:1–16.

43. Takahashi H, Tsuda N, Fujita S, Tezuka F, Okabe H. Immunohistochemical investigation of vimentin, neuron-specific enolase, alpha 1-antichymotrypsin and alpha 1-antitrypsin in adenoid cystic carcinoma of the salivary gland. Acta Pathol Jpn 1990;40:655–64.

44. Takahashi H, Tsuda N, Tezuka F, Okabe H. Difference of immunohistochemical reactions in epithelial cells of adenolymphoma. J Oral Pathol 1988;17:287–92.

45. Zarbo RJ, Bacchi CE, Gown AM. Muscle-specific protein expression in normal salivary glands and pleomorphic adenomas: an immunocytochemical study with biochemical confirmation. Mod Pathol 1991;4:621–6.

2
CLASSIFICATION

This third series of the Atlas of Tumor Pathology is testament to the fact that concepts and classification of tumors continuously undergo modification as research provides new insights that have prognostic and therapeutic relevance. A review of the classification of salivary gland neoplasms that was formulated by Foote and Frazell (1) in the first series Fascicle on salivary gland tumors in 1954 (Table 2-1) reveals that some categories have withstood the test of time and remain current while other categories have been modified or no longer exist. For example, the category malignant mixed tumor has been redefined into three distinct neoplasms: carcinoma ex mixed tumor, carcinosarcoma, and metastasizing mixed tumor. The categories pseudoadamantine adenocarcinoma, anaplastic adenocarcinoma, solid adenocarcinoma, and mucous cell adenocarcinoma are no longer recognized. Benign lymphoepithelial lesion is now regarded as a type of autoimmune sialadenitis rather than a neoplasm. On the other hand, Foote and Frazell's category of acinic cell adenocarcinoma later became modified to acinic cell tumor in the second series Fascicle in 1974 (3) and the World Health Organization's (WHO's) first classification in 1972 (4), because it was thought that not all acinar cell neoplasms had malignant potential. However, in the revised WHO classification in 1991 (2) and in this Fascicle, the original concept of Foote and Frazell has been acknowledged as more appropriate, and the term acinic cell adenocarcinoma is used once again.

The second series Fascicle on salivary gland tumors by Thackray and Lucas (3) was published 20 years after the first one, and it has now been over 20 years since the publication of the second series Fascicle. Classification terms are here modified, added to, or deleted (Table 2-2). Adenolymphoma is a term that appeared in the second series Fascicle instead of papillary cystadenoma lymphomatosum in the first series Fascicle. Adenolymphoma is considered an inappropriate term for a benign salivary neoplasm by most American pathologists, and European pathologists apparently disfavor the term papillary cystadenoma lymphomatosum. Therefore, the long-used synonym, Warthin's tumor, has been adopted by the WHO and this Fascicle. Tubular adenoma and trabecular adenoma have been deleted as specific terms while canalicular adenoma has been distinguished from basal cell adenoma and added to the classification. Clear cell adenoma in the second series Fascicle is now recognized as a malignant neoplasm and more appropriately classified as epithelial-myoepithelial carcinoma. Two new categories of benign epithelial neoplasms are cystadenomas and ductal papillomas, which include sialadenoma papilliferum, inverted ductal papilloma, and intraductal papilloma. Most modifications to the second series Fascicle have occurred among the malignant epithelial neoplasm. Acinar cell and mucoepidermoid neoplasms are now clearly recognized as carcinomas and the ambiguous terms acinic

Table 2-1

CLASSIFICATION OF FOOTE AND FRAZELL*

Benign
　　Mixed tumor
　　Papillary cystadenomata lymphomatosa
　　Oxyphil adenoma
　　Sebaceous cell adenoma
　　Benign lymphoepithelial lesion
　　Unclassified

Malignant
　　Malignant mixed tumor
　　Mucoepidermoid tumor
　　Squamous cell carcinoma
　　Adenocarcinoma
　　　　Adenoid cystic
　　　　Trabecular or solid
　　　　Anaplastic
　　　　Mucous cell
　　　　Pseudoadamantine
　　　　Acinic cell
　　Unclassified

*From reference 1.

27

Table 2-2

CLASSIFICATION OF THACKRAY AND LUCAS*

Adenomas
   Pleomorphic adenoma
   Monomorphic adenoma
      Adenolymphoma
      Oxyphilic adenoma
      Tubular adenoma
      Clear cell adenoma
      Basal cell adenoma
      Trabecular adenoma
      Sebaceous adenoma
      Sebaceous lymphadenoma

Mucoepidermoid tumor

Acinic cell tumor

Carcinomas
   Adenoid cystic carcinoma
   Adenocarcinoma
   Epidermoid carcinoma
   Undifferentiated carcinoma
   Carcinoma in pleomorphic adenoma
   Malignant lymphoepithelial lesion

Connective tissue and other tumors
   Benign
      Hemangioma
      Lymphangioma
      Lipoma
      Neurinoma
   Sarcoma
   Lymphoma

Metastatic tumors

*From reference 3.

cell tumor and mucoepidermoid tumor have been replaced. Recognition of the category of neoplasm called polymorphous low-grade adenocarcinoma may be the most important addition to the classification of salivary gland neoplasms. Other additions to malignant epithelial neoplasms are basal cell adenocarcinoma, cystadenocarcinoma, salivary duct carcinoma, sebaceous carcinomas, oncocytic carcinoma, and mucinous adenocarcinoma. Sialoblastoma is a recently defined term for congenital and infantile salivary gland neoplasms that appear to cover a histologic spectrum from benign to malignant; this entity has not previously been listed in a classification of salivary gland neoplasms. With the relatively recent delineation of the concept of mucosal-associated lymphoid tissue (MALT) and the fact that salivary glands, especially the parotid gland, contain a component of this extranodal lymphoid tissue, the incidence and classification of lymphomas of the salivary glands has acquired new parameters. There are several common and uncommon non-neoplastic, pathologic conditions that are often clinically difficult to distinguish from neoplastic disease and are discussed in this Fascicle. Among these is the cystic and lymphoid sialadenopathy associated with human immunodeficiency virus (HIV) infection and acquired immunodeficiency syndrome (AIDS) that did not exist at the time of publication of the last Fascicle.

The previous Fascicle on tumors of the major salivary glands essentially amplified the classification presented in the WHO's Histological Typing of Salivary Gland Tumours that had been published 2 years earlier (4). Similarly, this Fascicle closely conforms with the recent second edition of the WHO's Histological Typing of Salivary Gland Tumours (2). By intent, the descriptions and illustrations of the entities presented in the WHO monographs are brief and limited. This Fascicle provides more detailed and informative discussions and more fully illustrates the clinicopathologic spectrum of each entity. In addition to sialoblastoma, which is only mentioned in the WHO classification as embryonal carcinoma in the category of "other carcinomas," there are a few other differences. Clear cell adenocarcinoma is not a category in the WHO classification, and, presumably, homogeneous clear cell malignant neoplasms in that classification are incorporated in the category epithelial-myoepithelial carcinoma. This Fascicle identifies a group of clear cell carcinomas with clinicopathologic features that appear to be distinct from epithelial-myoepithelial carcinomas. The WHO monograph mentions carcinosarcoma and metastasizing pleomorphic adenoma as types of carcinoma in pleomorphic adenoma; however, that definition is inadequate, so these two tumors are classified separately in this Fascicle. In addition to sebaceous lymphadenoma, there is a small group of similar neoplasms that lack sebaceous differentiation.

These are classified as lymphadenomas and include tumors both with and without sebaceous differentiation.

The following is the classification system of salivary gland tumors used in this third series Fascicle.

BENIGN EPITHELIAL NEOPLASMS
Mixed tumor (pleomorphic adenoma)
Myoepithelioma
Warthin's tumor
Basal cell adenoma
Canalicular adenoma
Oncocytoma
Cystadenoma
Ductal papillomas
    Sialadenoma papilliferum
    Inverted ductal papilloma
    Intraductal papilloma
Lymphadenomas and sebaceous adenomas
Sialoblastoma

MALIGNANT EPITHELIAL NEOPLASMS
Mucoepidermoid carcinoma
Adenocarcinoma
Acinic cell adenocarcinoma
Adenoid cystic carcinoma
Polymorphous low-grade adenocarcinoma
Malignant mixed tumors
    Carcinoma ex mixed tumor
    Carcinosarcoma
    Metastasizing mixed tumor
Squamous cell carcinoma
Basal cell adenocarcinoma
Epithelial-myoepithelial carcinoma
Clear cell adenocarcinoma
Cystadenocarcinoma
Undifferentiated carcinomas
    Small cell undifferentiated carcinoma
    Large cell undifferentiated carcinoma
    Lymphoepithelial carcinoma
Oncocytic carcinoma
Salivary duct carcinoma
Sebaceous adenocarcinoma and
    lymphadenocarcinoma
Myoepithelial carcinoma
Adenosquamous carcinoma
Mucinous adenocarcinoma

MESENCHYMAL NEOPLASMS
Benign
Sarcomas

MALIGNANT LYMPHOMAS

METASTATIC TUMORS

NON-NEOPLASTIC TUMOR-LIKE CONDITIONS

REFERENCES

1. Foote FW Jr, Frazell EL. Tumors of the major salivary glands, 1st Series, Fascicle 11. Atlas of Tumor Pathology. Washington, D.C.: Armed Forces Institute of Pathology, 1954.
2. Seifert G, Sobin LH. Histological typing of salivary gland tumours. World Health Organization international histological classification of tumours. 2nd ed. New York: Springer-Verlag 1991.
3. Thackray AC, Lucas RB. Tumors of the major salivary glands. Atlas of Tumor Pathology, 2nd Series, Fascicle 10. Washington, D.C.: Armed Forces Institute of Pathology, 1974.
4. Thackray AC, Sobin LH. Histological typing of salivary gland tumours. International histological classification of tumours No. 7. Geneva: World Health Organization, 1972.

3

SALIVARY GLAND TUMORS: GENERAL CONSIDERATIONS

INCIDENCE

A review of the literature shows that the annual incidence of salivary gland tumors throughout the world varies from about 0.4 to 6.5 cases per 100,000 people (3). An increased regional incidence among certain patients has been noted (31): the incidence among the Inuit living in the Canadian Arctic was 13.5 cases per 100,000 people between 1950 and 1966; while it has since declined, it is still significantly higher than the overall average (2,28,69). Salivary gland tumors account for between 2 to 6.5 percent of all neoplasms of the head and neck (1,47,82,87).

ETIOLOGY

Information on the etiology of salivary gland tumors is limited, but several risk factors have been identified. These include radiation exposure, genetic predisposition (30), tobacco use, exposure to certain industrial chemicals, and viruses.

Evidence that exposure of the salivary glands to ionizing radiation increases the risk of developing salivary tumors is substantial. Studies of Japanese who were exposed to radiation following the explosion of the atomic bombs on Hiroshima and Nagasaki have shown a 3.5- to 11-fold increase in relative risks (6,7,60,94,95). Therapeutic radiation has been linked to an annual incidence of salivary gland tumors per 100,000 people as high as 77 cases compared to 0.6 cases in the nonexposed control group (33,71–73,79). Because the salivary glands concentrate iodine, patients treated with ^{131}I may be at increased risk (29,62,90). Excessive use of medical or dental diagnostic radiographs may also have a role in tumor initiation (34,50,65–67). No correlation of increased risks with radon levels has been found (53) but one has been suggested with increased exposure to ultraviolet radiation (90).

A possible etiologic association of lymphoepithelial carcinoma with Epstein-Barr virus has been observed (35,41,68). Other viruses with a possible etiologic role include polyoma virus; cytomegalovirus; type B and C particles similar to those associated with murine breast tumors

and murine leukemia, respectively; and human papilloma virus types 16 and 18 (17,20,46,74).

Although in some older studies no association of increased risk of developing tumors of the salivary glands was found with either heavy smoking or alcohol consumption (36,101), several recent studies show an association of smoking with Warthin's tumor (39,45,55,77). Occupations associated with increased risk of salivary carcinoma include asbestos mining, manufacturing of rubber and related products, plumbing, and some types of woodworking (25,51,52,91). In a study assessing the possible etiologic role of environmental dusts, nutrition, and lifestyles, Dietz and colleagues (18) found the highest relative risks of developing a parotid tumor were in those patients who had increased exposure to nickel, chromium, asbestos, and cement dusts.

DEMOGRAPHIC AND CLINICAL FEATURES

An overview of several large series of salivary gland neoplasms shows that between 64 and 80 percent of all primary epithelial tumors occur in the parotid glands, 7 to 11 percent occur in the submandibular glands, less than 1 percent occur in the sublingual glands, and 9 to 23 percent occur in the minor glands (3,19,21,75,82). Between 54 and 79 percent of all tumors are benign and 21 to 46 percent are malignant. This variability appears to be related to the type of cases referred to the treatment center, particularly for tumors that occur in minor rather than major glands. Malignant tumors account for 15 to 32 percent of parotid tumors, 41 to 45 percent of submandibular tumors, 70 to 90 percent of sublingual tumors, and about 50 percent of minor gland tumors (3,19,21,75,82).

The peak incidence of salivary gland tumors occurs in the sixth and seventh decades of life (3,21). The average ages of patients with benign and malignant tumors is about 46 and 47 years, respectively. The incidence of mixed tumors, mucoepidermoid carcinomas, and acinic cell adenocarcinomas peaks in the third and fourth decades (3). In children (defined as under 17 years of age) mucoepidermoid carcinoma is the most common malignant salivary gland tumor (3,4,12,13,16,37,42,44,76,78). Compared to adult patients, a greater proportion of all salivary gland tumors in children are mesenchymal tumors, and a greater proportion of the epithelial tumors are malignant (4,12,37,44,59,78). In all age groups, females are more frequently affected than males, but there is some gender variation according to the tumor type (3,21,82).

In most large series, mixed tumors account for about 50 percent of all benign and malignant salivary gland tumors (3,21,75,82), but in one study, they represented 74 percent (19). The second most common benign tumor is Warthin's tumor, representing 4 to 14 percent of all tumors. Mucoepidermoid carcinoma is the most common malignancy in some studies (3,19,82); in others, adenoid cystic carcinoma (21) and carcinoma ex mixed tumor (75) are most frequent. Adenocarcinoma, not otherwise specified and acinic cell adenocarcinoma also comprise a significant proportion of the carcinomas in these studies. Because of its relatively recent description, the frequency of polymorphous low-grade adenocarcinoma has not been established: in the Armed Forces Institute of Pathology (AFIP) Salivary Gland Registry it represents 4 percent of all tumors accessioned since 1985 and since that time is the fourth most common epithelial malignancy behind mucoepidermoid carcinoma; adenocarcinoma, not otherwise specified; and acinic cell adenocarcinoma. It is noteworthy that in this Registry, malignant lymphoma and metastatic disease together represent over 9 percent of all tumors presenting in the major glands; others have also found these categories to represent a substantial proportion of all major gland tumors (3,57).

Variations in the incidence of specific types of tumors have been noted in certain geographic regions. For instance, in studies of patients from a region in Denmark and from central Pennsylvania, Warthin's tumor accounted for about 30 percent of all parotid tumors (55,64), a figure about seven times higher than reported in most series. Studies of British patients have shown the frequency of mucoepidermoid carcinoma to be considerably lower (2.1 percent) than the predominant worldwide range of 5 to 15 percent (21,22,56,96). Similarly, in some regions of the world there is variation in site distribution and

a greater proportion of tumors arise in the submandibular gland and minor glands of the palate than in the parotid gland (61).

SITE-SPECIFIC TUMOR DIFFERENCES

Large studies of salivary gland tumors have shown that a greater proportion of malignant tumors occur in the minor glands than in the major glands (3,19,21,75,82). This proportion varies, however, among individual minor gland sites. In the AFIP material reviewed since 1985, 66 percent of salivary gland tumors in the lower lip were malignant compared to 31 percent of those in the upper lip. About 50 percent of palatal tumors were malignant, but in the tongue, retromolar area, and floor of the mouth 80, 93, and 93 percent, respectively, were malignant.

There is also a difference in the incidence of specific forms of salivary gland tumors in the major and minor glands. Canalicular adenomas and polymorphous low-grade adenocarcinomas occur almost exclusively in minor gland sites. Warthin's tumors, on the other hand, are nearly always found in the parotid glands. Only rarely do oncocytoma, carcinoma ex mixed tumor, and basal cell adenocarcinoma involve the minor glands. Likewise, acinic cell adenocarcinoma and epithelial-myoepithelial carcinoma are less often encountered in minor than major gland sites.

Mixed tumors in the major glands are usually surrounded by well-developed capsular connective tissue, but mixed tumors of the minor glands frequently lack this feature. Instead, in minor gland sites mixed tumors are often juxtaposed against salivary acini and ducts without a capsule. This can cause concern for malignancy. Similarly, because minor salivary gland tissue in the tongue is normally located between fascicles of skeletal muscle, benign tumors arising from such tissue may erroneously appear invasive.

The architectural and cytomorphologic features of salivary gland tumors arising from minor and major sites are nearly identical. Exceptions are mixed tumors and myoepitheliomas of the minor glands, which are more often predominantly composed of neoplastic plasmacytoid epithelial cells than their counterparts in the major glands. Awareness of this difference helps preclude misinterpretation of such tumors as plasmacytomas.

MICROSCOPIC GRADING

The microscopic grade of salivary gland carcinomas has been shown to be an independent predictor of behavior and often plays an important role in optimizing treatment (23,32,58,85,88,92). There is often a positive correlation between grade and clinical stage. While the grading of specific tumors is discussed in detail in their respective sections, an introductory overview is presented here.

At the risk of oversimplification, there are essentially four methods of grading salivary gland tumors. For most carcinomas there is only a single grade; for these, classification alone determines the grade. For example, the diagnosis of acinic cell adenocarcinoma, basal cell adenocarcinoma, or polymorphous low-grade adenocarcinoma indicates low-grade biologic behavior. Similarly, the diagnosis of salivary duct carcinoma, primary squamous cell carcinoma, or undifferentiated carcinoma denotes high-grade tumors. The next three methods are uniquely applied to individual tumors: grading of adenocarcinoma, not otherwise specified, is based on evaluation of cytomorphologic features; separation of adenoid cystic carcinoma into intermediate-grade and high-grade types is based, respectively, on the recognition of the predominant growth either as cribriform-tubular or solid; and specific grading criteria are applied to mucoepidermoid carcinoma that combine the presence or absence of growth characteristics and cytomorphologic features. The carcinomatous element of carcinoma ex mixed tumor is graded according to whichever of these methods is most applicable.

CLINICAL STAGING

The current system for the clinical staging of major salivary gland carcinomas is largely based on studies by Spiro and colleagues and Levitt et al. (49,83,86). These investigators have shown that prognosis largely depends on the size of the primary tumor and the presence or absence of local neoplastic extension. Local extension is defined as clinical or macroscopic evidence of invasion of skin, soft tissues, bone, or nerve. Microscopic evidence alone is not enough for staging purposes. Other, less important variables are palpability of suspected metastasis to the re-

gional lymph nodes and the presence or absence of distant metastasis. Regional nodes include those within or immediately adjacent to the salivary gland and the deep cervical lymph nodes.

These proposed criteria were accepted by the American Joint Committee on Cancer and the International Union Against Cancer with only minor modifications and are shown in Table 3-1 (5,27). The clinical parameters include tumor size, local extension of tumor, metastasis to regional nodes, and distant metastases. Because it was shown that local extension is far less ominous in smaller tumors, a suffix is appended to each T category. T1 and T2 lesions with local extension and T3 tumors without local extension are all considered stage II tumors.

Although there are no comparable staging guidelines for tumors of the intraoral minor glands, Spiro et al. (84) applied the criteria used for epidermoid carcinoma of the oral cavity, pharynx, larynx, and sinus to mucoepidermoid carcinoma with some success. These investigators have since applied these same criteria to various types of salivary carcinomas in 353 patients and found survival correlated closely with the stage of tumor: the 10-year survival was 83, 53, 35, and 24 percent for patients with stage I through stage IV disease, respectively (88).

Although not included as a staging criterion, facial nerve involvement has been shown by some investigators to have prognostic value (23,63,81).

DIAGNOSTIC IMAGING

Imaging of the salivary glands provides a noninvasive method of evaluating salivary gland disease that may preoperatively establish intraglandular or extraglandular origin, the relationship of the lesion to the facial nerve, and, in some cases, establish benignancy or malignancy. While plain radiography demonstrates sialoliths and sialography often provides diagnostic information about ductal inflammatory diseases of the salivary glands, computed tomography (CT), ultrasonography, CT sialography, and magnetic resonance imaging (MRI) are generally more useful for the evaluation of neoplastic disease (8,10,15,26,40,43,54,70,97–100). In patients not suspected of having inflammatory or infectious disease, however, MRI provides several advantages in salivary gland imaging over other methods. It

Table 3-1
STAGING SYSTEM FOR MAJOR SALIVARY GLANDS*

PRIMARY TUMOR (T)
- TX   Primary tumor cannot be assessed
- T0   No evidence of primary tumor
- T1** Tumor 2 cm or less in greatest diameter
- T2** Tumor more than 2 cm but not more than 4 cm in greatest dimension
- T3** Tumor more than 4 cm but not more than 6 cm in greatest dimension
- T4** Tumor more than 6 cm in greatest dimension

REGIONAL LYMPH NODES (N)
- NX   Regional lymph nodes cannot be assessed
- N0   No regional lymph node metastasis
- N1   Metastasis in a single ipsilateral lymph node, 3 cm or less in greatest dimension
- N2   Metastasis in a single ipsilateral lymph node, more than 3 cm but not more than 6 cm in greatest dimension; or in multiple ipsilateral lymph nodes, none more than 6 cm in greatest dimension; or in bilateral or contralateral lymph nodes, none more than 6 cm in greatest dimension
  - N2a   Metastasis in a single ipsilateral lymph node more than 3 cm but not more than 6 cm in greatest dimension
  - N2b   Metastases in multiple ipsilateral lymph nodes, none more than 6 cm in greatest dimension
  - N2c   Metastases in bilateral or contralateral lymph nodes, none more than 6 cm in greatest dimension
- N3   Metastasis in a lymph node more than 6 cm in greatest dimension

DISTANT METASTASIS (M)
- MX   Presence of distant metastasis cannot be assessed
- M0   No distant metastasis
- M1   Distant metastasis

STAGE GROUPING

Stage	T	N	M
Stage I	T1a	N0	M0
	T2a	N0	M0
Stage II	T1b	N0	M0
	T2b	N0	M0
	T3a	N0	M0
Stage III	T3b	N0	M0
	T4a	N0	M0
	Any T (except T4b)	N1	M0
Stage IV	T4b	Any N	M0
	Any T	N2,N3	M0
	Any T	Any N	M1

*Table modified from Beahrs OH, Henson DE, Utter RV, Myers MT, eds. Manual for staging of cancer, 3rd ed. Philadelphia: JB Lippincott, 1988:52.
** All T categories are subdivided into either (a) no local extension or (b) local extension. Local extension is clinical or macroscopic evidence of invasion of skin, soft tissues, bone, or nerve.

does not have the associated risks of CT related to the radiation exposure and contrast media. Furthermore, because it provides excellent contrast with soft tissues, it allows better evaluation of the tumor interface with normal tissues (9,11,93).

With MRI, the signal of the T1-weighted image of normal parotid gland is intermediate between fat, which is white, and muscle, which is darker; the submandibular gland, however, usually less fatty than the parotid, is closer to

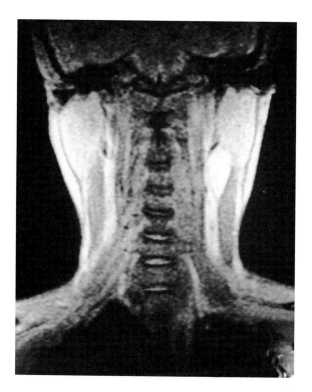 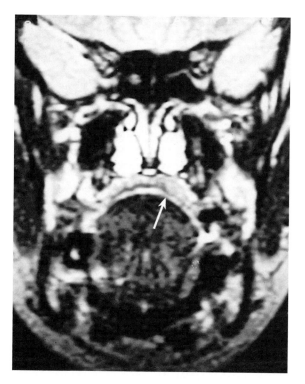

Figure 3-1
MRI OF METASTATIC AND OCCULT PRIMARY ADENOID CYSTIC CARCINOMA

Left: This patient presented with a neck mass that was shown to be a cervical lymph node containing metastatic adenoid cystic carcinoma. The tumor was distinct and separate from the parotid gland which, in this T1-weighted image, shows a bright signal.

Right: Although intraoral clinical examination of the patient failed to reveal mucosal evidence of disease, the T2-weighted image reveals the primary tumor in the soft palate (arrow). (Courtesy of Drs. Mahmood F. Mafee, Washington, DC, and Jiraporn Laothamatas, Bangkok, Thailand.)

muscle in signal intensity. The signal of the parotid approaches that of fat as the parenchyma undergoes fatty infiltration with age. In most patients the interface of tumor with fat is best seen with T1 images. However, because tumors may be close in intensity to muscle with T1 images and because most salivary gland tumors are brighter on T2 than T1 images (fig. 3-1), the T2-weighted image highlights the interface of the tumor with muscle more clearly (93). Some investigators have found the use of the short tau inversion recovery sequences (STIR) provides advantages that include a higher degree of contrast between normal and neoplastic tissue, reduced motion artifact, suppressed signal from fat, and detection of very small recurrences (14).

The lack of tumor confinement by fascial boundaries suggests malignancy unless previous surgery has been performed that may have disrupted the integrity of the fascia. Hypercellular tumors usually show less difference in intensities between the T1- and T2-weighted images than less cellular tumors (80). Because the T2 signal intensity increases with higher water content, fluid-containing cystic spaces and vascular lesions demonstrate high signal intensity on T2 images (24,48,93). Therefore, non-neoplastic cystic lesions, including human immunodeficiency virus (HIV)-related parotid cysts and lymphadenopathy; cystic tumors such as Warthin tumors, cystadenomas, and cystadenocarcinomas; and prominently cystic mucoepidermoid carcinomas often show bright areas on T2 images (38).

REFERENCES

1. Abiose BO, Oyejide O, Ogunniyi J. Salivary gland tumours in Ibadan, Nigeria: a study of 295 cases. Afr J Med Sci 1990;19:195–9.

2. Albeck H, Nielsen NH, Hansen HE, et al. Epidemiology of nasopharyngeal and salivary gland carcinoma in Greenland. Arctic Med Res 1992;51:189–95.

3. Auclair PL, Ellis GL, Gnepp DR, Wenig BM, Janney CG. Salivary gland neoplasms: general considerations. In: Ellis GL, Auclair PL, Gnepp DR, eds. Surgical pathology of the salivary glands. Philadelphia: WB Saunders, 1991:135–64.

4. Baker SR, Malone B. Salivary gland malignancies in children. Cancer 1985;55:1730–6.

5. Beahrs OH, Henson DE, Hutter RV, Myers MH. Manual for staging of cancer. 3rd ed. Philadelphia: JB Lippincott, 1988:51–6.

6. Belsky JL, Tachikawa K, Cihak RW, Yamamoto T. Salivary gland tumors in atomic bomb survivors, Hiroshima-Nagasaki, 1957 to 1970. JAMA 1972;219:864–8.

7. Belsky JL, Takeichi N, Yamamoto T, et al. Salivary gland neoplasms following atomic radiation: additional cases and reanalysis of combined data in a fixed population, 1957-1970. Cancer 1975;35:555–9.

8. Bogaert J, Hermans R, Baert AL. Pleomorphic adenoma of the parotid gland. J Belge Radiol 1993;76:307–10.

9. Byrne MN, Spector JG, Garvin CF, Gado MH. Preoperative assessment of parotid masses: a comparative evaluation of radiologic techniques to histopathologic diagnosis. Laryngoscope 1989;99:284–92.

10. Califano L, Zupi A, Giardino C. Accuracy in the diagnosis of parotid tumours. J Craniomaxillofac Surg 1992;20:354–9.

11. Casselman JW, Mancuso AA. Major salivary gland masses: comparison of MR imaging and CT. Radiology 1987;165:183–9.

12. Castro EB, Huvos AG, Strong EW, Foote FW Jr. Tumors of the major salivary glands in children. Cancer 1972;29:312–7.

13. Catania VC, Bozzetti F, Santangelo A, Salvadori B. Parotid gland tumors in infants and children. Tumori 1977;63:195–8.

14. Chaudhuri R, Bingham JB, Crossman JE, Gleeson MJ. Magnetic resonance imaging of the parotid gland using the STIR sequence. Clin Otolaryngol 1992;17:211–7.

15. Corr P, Cheng P, Metreweli C. The role of ultrasound and computed tomography in the evaluation of parotid masses. Australas Radiol 1993;37:195–7.

16. Dahlqvist A, Ostberg Y. Malignant salivary gland tumours in children. Acta Otolaryngol (Stockh) 1982;94:175–9.

17. Dawe CJ. Tumours of the salivary and lachrymal glands, nasal fossa and maxillary sinuses. IARC Sci Publ 1979;23:91–133.

18. Dietz A, Barm B, Gewelke U, Sennewald E, Heller WD, Maier H. Zur epidemiologie der parotistumoren. Eine fallkontrollstudie. HNO 1993;41:83–90.

19. Eneroth CM. Salivary gland tumors in the parotid gland, submandibular gland, and the palate region. Cancer 1971;27:1415–8.

20. Epstein J, Scully C. Cytomegalovirus: a virus of increasing relevance to oral medicine and pathology. J Oral Pathol Med 1993;22:348–53.

21. Eveson JW, Cawson RA. Salivary gland tumours. A review of 2410 cases with particular reference to histological types, site, age and sex distribution. J Pathol 1985;146:51–8.

22. Eveson JW, Cawson RA. Tumours of the minor (oropharyngeal) salivary glands: a demographic study of 336 cases. J Oral Pathol 1985;14:500–9.

23. Frankenthaler RA, Byers RM, Luna MA, Callender DL, Wolf P, Goepfert H. Predicting occult lymph node metastasis in parotid cancer. Arch Otolaryngol Head Neck Surg 1993;119:517–20.

24. George CD, Ng YY, Hall-Craggs MA, Jones BM. Parotid haemangioma in infants: MR imaging at 1.5T. Pediatr Radiol 1991;21:483–5.

25. Graham S, Blanchet M, Rohrer T. Cancer in asbestos-mining and other areas of Quebec. JNCI 1977;59:1139–45.

26. Hebert G, Ouimet-Oliva D, Nicolet V, Bourdon F. Imaging of the salivary glands. Can Assoc Radiol J 1993;44:342–9.

27. Hermanek P, Sobin LH. TNM classification of malignant tumours. 4th ed. New York: Springer-Verlag, 1987:30–2.

28. Hildes JA, Schaefer O. The changing picture of neoplastic disease in the western and central Canadian Arctic (1950-1980). Can Med Assoc J 1984;130:25–32.

29. Hoffman DA, McConahey WM, Fraumeni JF Jr, Kurland LT. Cancer incidence following treatment of hyperthyroidism. Int J Epidemiol 1982;11:218–24.

30. Holloway SM, Sofaer JA. Coefficients of relationship by isonymy among oral cancer registrations in Scottish males. Community Dent Oral Epidemiol 1992;20:284–7.

31. Horn-Ross PL, West DW, Brown SR. Recent trends in the incidence of salivary gland cancer. Int J Epidemiol 1991;20:628–33.

32. Kane WJ, McCaffrey TV, Olsen KD, Lewis JE. Primary parotid malignancies. A clinical and pathologic review. Arch Otolaryngol Head Neck Surg 1991;117:307–15.

33. Kaste SC, Hedlund G, Pratt CB. Malignant parotid tumors in patients previously treated for childhood cancer: clinical and imaging findings in eight cases. Am J Roentgenol 1994;162:655–9.

34. Katz AD, Preston-Martin S. Salivary gland tumors and previous radiotherapy to the head or neck. Report of a clinical series. Am J Surg 1984;147:345–8.

35. Kärja J, Syrjnen S, Usenius T, Vornanen M, Collan Y. Oral cancer in children under 15 years of age. A clinicopathologic and virologic study. Acta Otolaryngol (Stockh) 1988;449:145–9.

36. Keller AZ. Residence, age, race and related factors in the survival and associations with salivary tumors. Am J Epidemiol 1969;90:269–77.

37. Kessler A, Handler SD. Salivary gland neoplasms in children: a 10-year survey at the Children's Hospital of Philadelphia. Int J Pediatr Otorhinolaryngol 1994;29:195–202.

38. Kirshenbaum KJ, Nadimpalli SR, Friedman M, Kirshenbaum GL, Cavallino RP. Benign lymphoepithelial parotid tumors in AIDS patients: CT and MR findings in nine cases. Am J Neuroradiol 1991;12:271–4.

39. Kotwall CA. Smoking as an etiologic factor in the development of Warthin's tumor of the parotid gland. Am J Surg 1992;164:646–7.

40. Kress E, Schulz HG, Neumann T. Die diagnostik der erkrankungen der grossen kopfspeicheldrusen durch sonographie, sialographie und CT-sialographie. Ein methodenvergleich. HNO 1993;41:345–51.

41. Krishnamurthy S, Lanier AP, Dohan P, Lanier JF, Henle W. Salivary gland cancer in Alaskan natives, 1966-1980. Hum Pathol 1987;18:986–96. (Published erratum appears in Hum Pathol 1988;19(3):328.)

42. Krolls SO, Trodahl JN, Boyers RC. Salivary gland lesions in children. A survey of 430 cases. Cancer 1972;30:459–69.

43. Kurabayashi T, Ida M, Ohbayashi N, Ishii J, Sasaki T. Criteria for differentiating superficial from deep lobe tumours of the parotid gland by computed tomography. Dentomaxillofac Radiol 1993;22:81–5.

44. Lack EE, Upton MP. Histopathologic review of salivary gland tumors in childhood. Arch Otolaryngol Head Neck Surg 1988;114:898–906.

45. Lamelas J, Terry JH Jr, Alfonso AE. Warthin's tumor: multicentricity and increasing incidence in women. Am J Surg 1987;154:347–51.

46. Lamey PJ, Waterhouse JP, Ferguson MM. Animal model of human disease. Pleomorphic salivary adenoma. Virally induced pleomorphic salivary adenoma in the CFLP mouse. Am J Pathol 1982;109:129–32.

47. Leegaard T, Lindeman H. Salivary-gland tumours. Clinical picture and treatment. Acta Otolaryngol Suppl (Stockh) 1969;263:155–9.

48. Levine E, Wetzel LH, Neff JR. MR imaging and CT of extrahepatic cavernous hemangiomas. AJR Am J Roentgenol 1986;147:1299–304.

49. Levitt SH, McHugh RB, Gmez-Marin O, et al. Clinical staging system for cancer of the salivary gland: a retrospective study. Cancer 1981;47:2712–24.

50. Maillie HD, Gilda JE. Radiation-induced cancer risk in radiographic cephalometry. Oral Surg Oral Med Oral Pathol 1993;75:631–7.

51. Mancuso TF, Brennan MJ. Epidemiological considerations of cancer of the gallbladder, bile ducts and salivary glands in the rubber industry. J Occup Med 1970;12:333–41.

52. Milham S Jr. Cancer mortality pattern associated with exposure to metals. Ann N Y Acad Sci 1976;271:243–9.

53. Miller AS, Harwick RD, Alfaro-Miranda M, Sundararajan M. Search for correlation of radon levels and incidence of salivary gland tumors. Oral Surg Oral Med Oral Pathol 1993;75:58–63.

54. Minami M, Tanioka H, Oyama K, et al. Warthin tumor of the parotid gland: MR-pathologic correlation. AJNR Am J Neuroradiol 1993;14:209–14.

55. Monk JS Jr, Church JS. Warthin's tumor. A high incidence and no sex predominance in central Pennsylvania. Arch Otolaryngol Head Neck Surg 1992;118:477–8.

56. Morgan MN, Mackenzie DH. Tumours of salivary glands. A review of 204 cases with 5-year follow-up. Br J Surg 1968;55:284–8.

57. O'Brien CJ, Malka VB, Mijailovic M. Evaluation of 242 consecutive parotidectomies performed for benign and malignant disease. Aust N Z J Surg 1993;63:870–7.

58. O'Brien CJ, Soong SJ, Herrera GA, Urist MM, Maddox WA. Malignant salivary tumors—analysis of prognostic factors and survival. Head Neck Surg 1986;9:82–92.

59. Ogata H, Ebihara S, Mukai K. Salivary gland neoplasms in children. Jpn J Clin Oncol 1994;24:88–93.

60. Ohkita T, Takahashi H, Takeichi N, Hirose F. Prevalence of leukaemia and salivary gland tumours among Hiroshima atomic bomb survivors. In: Late biological effects of ionizing radiation. Vol I. Vienna, International Atomic Energy Agency, 1978:71–81.

61. Onyango JF, Awange DO, Muthamia JM, Muga BI. Salivary gland tumours in Kenya. East Afr Med J 1992;69:525–30.

62. Palmer JA, Mustard RA, Simpson WJ. Irradiation as an etiologic factor in tumours of the thyroid, parathyroid and salivary glands. Can J Surg 1980;23:39–42.

63. Pedersen DE, Overgaard J, Sogaard H, Elbrond O, Overgaard M. Maligne parotistumorer. Behandlingsresultater og prognose hos 110 konsekutive patienter. Ugeskr Laeger 1993;155:2255–9.

64. Poulsen P, Jorgensen K, Grontved A. Benign and malignant neoplasms of the parotid gland: incidence and histology in the Danish County of Funen. Laryngoscope 1987;97:102–4.

65. Preston-Martin S. Prior x-ray therapy for acne related to tumors of the parotid gland. Arch Dermatol 1989;125:921–4.

66. Preston-Martin S, Thomas DC, White SC, Cohen D. Prior exposure to medical and dental x-rays related to tumors of the parotid gland. JNCI 1988;80:943–9.

67. Preston-Martin S, White SC. Brain and salivary gland tumors related to prior dental radiography: implications for current practice. J Am Dent Assoc 1990;120:151–8.

68. Saw D, Lau WH, Ho JH, Chan JK, Ng CS. Malignant lymphoepithelial lesion of the salivary gland. Hum Pathol 1986;17:914–23.

69. Schaefer O, Hildes JA, Medd LM, Cameron DG. The changing pattern of neoplastic disease in Canadian Eskimos. In: Shephard RJ, Itoh S, eds. Circumpolar health. Toronto: Univ of Toronto Press 1976:277–83.

70. Schlakman BN, Yousem DM. MR of intraparotid masses. AJNR Am J Neuroradiol 1993;14:1173–80.

71. Schneider AB, Favus MJ, Stachura ME, Arnold MJ, Frohman LA. Salivary gland neoplasms as a late consequence of head and neck irradiation. Ann Intern Med 1977;87:160–4.

72. Schneider AB, Shore-Freedman E, Ryo UY, Bekerman C, Favus M, Pinsky S. Radiation-induced tumors of the head and neck following childhood irradiation. Prospective studies. Medicine (Baltimore) 1985;64:1–15.

73. Schneider AB, Shore-Freedman E, Weinstein RA. Radiation-induced thyroid and other head and neck tumors: occurrence of multiple tumors and analysis of risk factors. J Clin Endocrinol Metab 1986;63:107–12.

74. Scully C. Viruses and salivary gland disease: are there associations? Oral Surg Oral Med Oral Pathol 1988;66:179–83.

75. Seifert G, Miehlke A, Haubrich J, Chilla R. Diseases of the salivary glands: diagnosis, pathology, treament, facial nerve surgery. Stuttgart: Georg Thieme Verlag, 1986:171–9.

76. Seifert G, Okabe H, Caselitz J. Epithelial salivary gland tumors in children and adolescents. Analysis of 80 cases (Salivary Gland Register 1965-1984). ORL J Otorhinolaryngol Relat Spec 1986;48:137–49.

77. Shah D, Williams E, Brooks SE. Warthin's tumour in Jamaica. Incidence, electron microscopy and immunoenzyme studies. West Indian Med J 1990;39:225–32.

78. Shikhani AH, Johns ME. Tumors of the major salivary glands in children. Head Neck Surg 1988;10:257–63.

79. Shore-Freedman E, Abrahams C, Recant W, Schneider AB. Neurilemomas and salivary gland tumors of the head and neck following childhood irradiation. Cancer 1983;51:2159–63.

80. Som PM, Biller HF. High-grade malignancies of the parotid gland: identification with MR imaging. Radiology 1989;173:823–6.

81. Spiro IJ, Wang CC, Montgomery WW. Carcinoma of the parotid gland. Analysis of treatment results and patterns of failure after combined surgery and radiation therapy. Cancer 1993;71:2699–705.

82. Spiro RH. Salivary neoplasms: overview of a 35-year experience with 2,807 patients. Head Neck Surg 1986;8:177–84.

83. Spiro RH, Hajdu SI, Strong EW. Tumors of the submaxillary gland. Am J Surg 1976;132:463–8.

84. Spiro RH, Huvos AG, Berk R, Strong EW. Mucoepidermoid carcinoma of salivary gland origin. A clinicopathologic study of 367 cases. Am J Surg 1978;136:461–8.

85. Spiro RH, Huvos AG, Strong EW. Adenocarcinoma of salivary origin. Clinicopathologic study of 204 patients. Am J Surg 1982;144:423–31.

86. Spiro RH, Huvos AG, Strong EW. Cancer of the parotid gland. A clinicopathologic study of 288 primary cases. Am J Surg 1975;130:452–9.

87. Spiro RH, Koss LG, Hajdu SI, Strong EW. Tumors of minor salivary origin. A clinicopathologic study of 492 cases. Cancer 1973;31:117–29.

88. Spiro RH, Thaler HT, Hicks WF, Kher UA, Huvos AH, Strong EW. The importance of clinical staging of minor salivary gland carcinoma. Am J Surg 1991;162:330–6.

89. Spitz MR, Batsakis JG. Major salivary gland carcinoma. Descriptive epidemiology and survival of 498 patients. Arch Otolaryngol 1984;110:45–9.

90. Spitz MR, Sider JG, Newell GR, Batsakis JG. Incidence of salivary gland cancer in the United States relative to ultraviolet radiation exposure. Head Neck Surg 1988;10:305–8.

91. Swanson GM, Belle SH. Cancer morbidity among woodworkers in the US automotive industry. J Occup Med 1982;24:315–9.

92. Szanto PA, Luna MA, Tortoledo ME, White RA. Histologic grading of adenoid cystic carcinoma of the salivary glands. Cancer 1984;54:1062–9.

93. Tabor EK, Curtin HD. MR of the salivary glands. Radiol Clin North Am 1989;27:379–92.

94. Takeichi N, Hirose F, Yamamoto H. Salivary gland tumors in atomic bomb survivors, Hiroshima, Japan. I. Epidemiologic observations. Cancer 1976;38:2462–8.

95. Takeichi N, Hirose F, Yamamoto H, Ezaki H, Fujikura T. Salivary gland tumors in atomic bomb survivors, Hiroshima, Japan. II. Pathologic study and supplementary epidemiologic observations. Cancer 1983;52:377–85.

96. Thackray AC, Lucas RB. Tumors of the major salivary glands. Atlas of Tumor Pathology, 2nd Series, Fascicle 10. Washington, D.C.: Armed Forces Institute of Pathology, 1974:125–6.

97. Traxler M, Hajek P, Solar P, Ulm C. Magnetic resonance in lesions of the parotid gland. Int J Oral Maxillofac Surg 1991;20:170–4.

98. Traxler M, Schurawitzki H, Ulm C, et al. Sonography of nonneoplastic disorders of the salivary glands. Int J Oral Maxillofac Surg 1992;21:360–3.

99. Van Mieghem F, Corthouts B, Degryse H, De Schepper A. Computed tomography of major salivary gland tumors. A retrospective study of 31 cases. J Belge Radiol 1991;74:193–9.

100. Weber AL. Imaging of the salivary glands. Curr Opin Radiol 1992;4:117–22.

101. Williams RR, Horm JW. Association of cancer sites with tobacco and alcohol consumption and socioeconomic status of patients: interview study from the Third National Cancer Survey. JNCI 1977;58:519–24.

❖❖❖

4

BENIGN EPITHELIAL NEOPLASMS

MIXED TUMOR
(PLEOMORPHIC ADENOMA)

Definition. Mixed tumor is a benign, epithelial-derived tumor composed of cells that demonstrate both epithelial and mesenchymal differentiation. The epithelial differentiation manifests as well-formed ductal structures with closely associated nonductal cells that frequently include spindle, round, stellate, plasmacytoid, polygonal, and clear forms. The nonductal element demonstrates varying degrees of myxoid, hyaline, cartilaginous, or osseous differentiation. In the major salivary glands the tumors are usually encapsulated but in the minor glands they usually are not. The terms mixed tumor and pleomorphic adenoma are used synonymously; the former emphasizes the "mixture" of epithelial and mesenchymal elements while the latter denotes the considerable morphologic diversity that these adenomas exhibit.

General Features. Mixed tumor is the most common neoplasm of salivary gland origin. In four large published series, mixed tumors represented 45 to 74 percent of all salivary gland tumors (25,27,75,76). At the Armed Forces Institute of Pathology (AFIP) mixed tumors comprise 28 percent of all benign and malignant salivary gland tumors and 30 percent of all parotid neoplasms seen since 1985. They constitute 60 percent of the benign tumors from all salivary gland sites: 61 percent of major gland tumors and 54 percent of minor gland tumors. Other large series of cases from several different countries have shown a greater incidence (27,28,30,41,76,87, 92). The most common intraoral site is the palate, with a nearly equal incidence in the hard and soft palates, but other common locations are the upper lip and the buccal mucosa. Rarely, mixed tumors are presumed to have arisen from ectopic salivary gland tissue present in lymph nodes, mandible, or maxilla (3,55).

Mixed tumors are usually solitary, but, infrequently, a second metachronous or synchronous mixed tumor develops in a different gland. The most common associated salivary gland neoplasm is Warthin's tumor, but association with mucoepidermoid carcinoma, acinic cell adeno-

carcinoma, and adenoid cystic carcinoma has been described (33).

The average age of patients with mixed tumors is about 43 years (27). Nearly 40 percent of cases at the AFIP developed in individuals less than 40 years of age. Most patients in this latter group were 20 to 39 years old, but mixed tumor is the most common salivary gland tumor in children and adolescents (43). Women are more likely to be affected than men (27,86).

The presence of both epithelial and stromal-rich elements has led to considerable discussion about the histogenesis of mixed tumors. Immunohistochemical and ultrastructural evidence suggest that this tumor is entirely of epithelial origin and that the mesenchymal areas are composed predominantly of cells that represent neoplastic modified myoepithelial cells (12,14,17). The characteristic morphologic diversity occurs because the epithelial element expresses ductal and myoepithelial differentiation, produces variable quantities of mucopolysaccharide matrix, and undergoes chondroid and osseous metaplasia (15,16).

Clinical Features. Mixed tumors are typically slow-growing, asymptomatic, discrete masses that may become large if untreated. Large tumors often form a single but irregularly nodular mass that stretches the overlying skin or mucosa (fig. 4-1). Recurrent lesions frequently occur as multiple nodules that are less mobile than initial lesions (fig. 4-2). Except for predominantly myxoid lesions, mixed tumors are firm and only slightly compressible.

In the parotid gland mixed tumors are usually mobile and most often present in the lower pole of the superficial (lateral) lobe of the gland. Occasionally they arise in the deep lobe of the gland, expand into the parapharyngeal space (fig. 4-3), and produce swelling in the region of the tonsillar fossa, soft palate, or lateral pharynx (1,34). Rarely, facial paralysis occurs, apparently as a result of extrinsic compression of the facial nerve (2,64).

Mixed tumors of the palate are typically located lateral to the midline and only rarely appear as midline masses (fig. 4-4). Because tumors of the hard palate are confined by mucosa

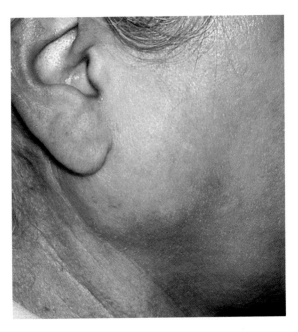

Figure 4-1
MIXED TUMOR OF PAROTID
The preauricular mass had enlarged to this size over a period of 5 years. (Courtesy of Dr. Charles E. Tomich, Indianapolis, IN.)

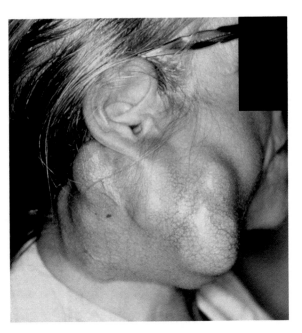

Figure 4-2
RECURRENT MIXED TUMOR
The characteristic multinodular growth of recurrent mixed tumor is obvious in this parotid mass. (Courtesy of Dr. Lewis R. Eversole, Los Angeles, CA.)

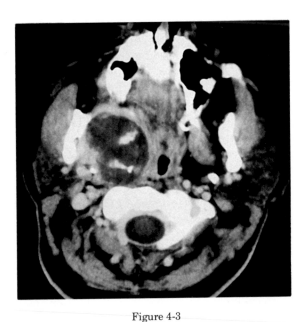

Figure 4-3
MIXED TUMOR OF DEEP LOBE OF PAROTID
Computed tomography revealed a large mixed tumor located medial to the mandibular ramus. The tumor had prominent osseous and cartilaginous elements that initially led to diagnosis as an osteochondroma.

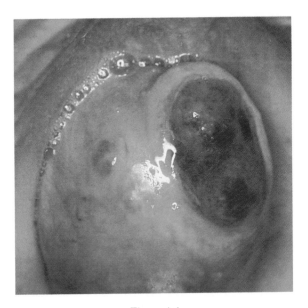

Figure 4-4
MIXED TUMOR OF PALATE
Most mixed tumors involve only one side of the palate because there are few minor glands in the midline. In this case the tumor appears symmetrical on either side of the midline. Large intraoral tumors are susceptible to trauma-related ulceration, as illustrated here. (Courtesy of F. J. Kratochvil, Bethesda, MD.)

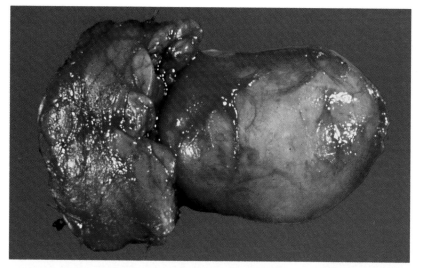

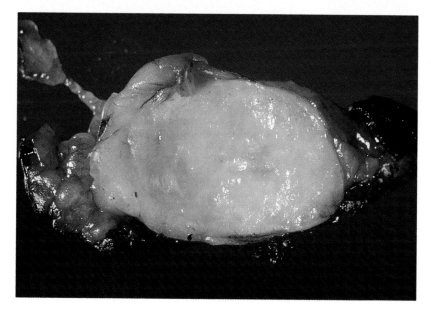

Figure 4-5
MIXED TUMOR
Top: This tumor of the sub-mandibular gland has a smooth, glistening capsular surface.
Bottom: The cut surface of this circumscribed parotid tumor has a homogeneous tan or tan-white surface and is partially encompassed by a thin fibrous capsule. (Courtesy of Department of Anatomic Pathology, Walter Reed Army Medical Center, Washington, DC.)

that is tightly bound to palatal bone, mobility is very limited in this site. Mixed tumors in other minor gland sites, such as the upper lip or buccal mucosa, are mobile and covered by normal mucosa unless traumatized.

Gross Findings. Typically, mixed tumor is an irregular, round to ovoid mass with well-defined borders (fig. 4-5). In the major glands an incomplete fibrous capsule is usually evident that varies in thickness and separates the tumor from the gland, but some mixed tumors are unencapsulated. Mixed tumors that originate from the glands in the oral mucosa frequently have only a poorly developed or no capsule, al-

though these tumors usually readily separate from surrounding tissue during surgery.

The cut surface of the neoplastic tissue is mostly homogeneously tan to white but often has shiny, partly translucent zones that represent myxochondroid or cartilaginous areas (fig. 4-6). Tumors larger than 1 cm often have numerous protuberances which give them a lobulated appearance. Hemorrhage and infarction are occasionally seen and are usually secondary to prior surgical manipulation, such as biopsy or fine-needle aspiration. Recurrent parotid tumors have multiple, often discrete, nodules distributed throughout connective tissue, fat, and salivary gland (fig. 4-7).

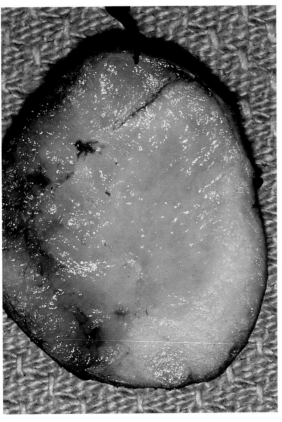

Figure 4-6
MIXED TUMOR
The translucent central zone represents myxochondroid tissue. There is a small rim of normal gland along the margin on the left, but elsewhere the tumor is close to the margins.

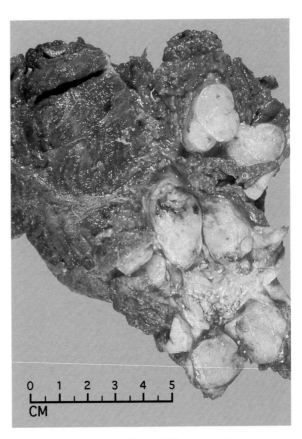

Figure 4-7
RECURRENT MIXED TUMOR
Grossly, the presence of multiple individual nodules are typical of recurrent mixed tumors.

Microscopic Findings. Mixed tumors are renowned for their cytomorphologic and architectural diversity. Despite their protean histopathology, each tumor shares with others the essential diagnostic feature of being composed of both epithelial and mesenchymal-like tissues (fig. 4-8). The proportion of each of these elements varies widely and one or the other is often predominant. Because of its diverse appearance, some investigators subclassify mixed tumors on the basis of the proportion of the mesenchymal-like and epithelial elements (73). The *cellular type* of mixed tumor is one in which the epithelial element predominates whereas the *myxoid type* is composed largely of a myxomatous or myxochrondromatous mesenchymal-like element. This distinction has no therapeutic significance but helps emphasize the broad morphologic spectrum possible within this neoplasm. Most mixed tumors have a myxoid component that comprises 30 percent or more of the neoplasm; only 12 to 15 percent have an epithelial element that constitutes more than 80 percent of the entire tumor (74).

The thickness of the fibrous capsule of parotid and submandibular mixed tumors is variable and is sometimes thin or even absent (fig. 4-9). This capsular tissue occasionally contains small finger-like extensions or small islands of neoplastic epithelial cells (fig. 4-10). Prominently myxoid tumors often have incomplete capsules, and tumor tissue is juxtaposed against normal gland. This is characteristic of mixed tumors in the minor glands where a capsule is rarely well developed.

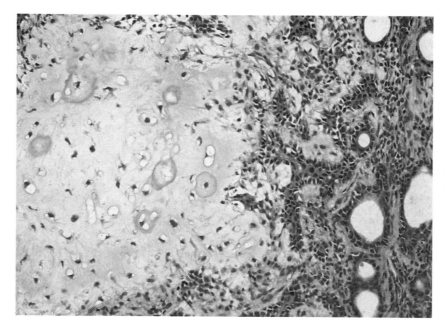

Figure 4-8
MIXED TUMOR
This prototypic mixed tumor has closely associated epithelial islands and ductal structures, and shows cartilaginous differentiation.

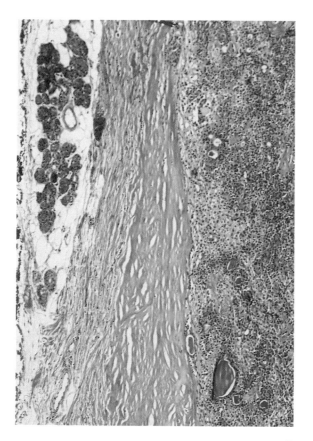 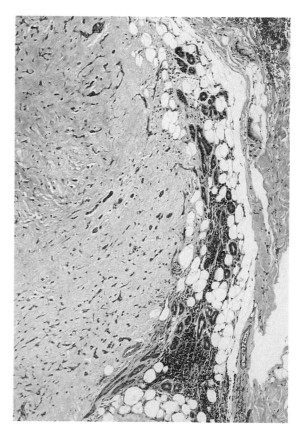

Figure 4-9
VARIATION OF ENCAPSULATION IN MIXED TUMORS
Left: Some mixed tumors have a thick and somewhat hyalinized capsule separating the tumor from the gland.
Right: Note the close proximity of this prominently myxoid tumor to normal ducts but the lack of infiltration by individual cells or tumor islands beyond the tumor-gland interface.

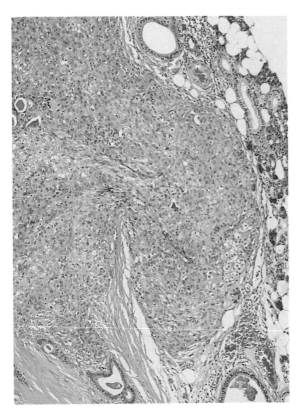

Figure 4-10
MIXED TUMOR WITH CAPSULAR PENETRATION
Tongue of mixed tumor is seen extending through the capsule (right) and contacts peripheral parenchymal tissue.

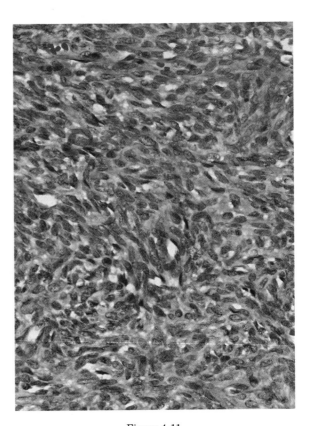

Figure 4-11
MIXED TUMOR
Hypercellular area of spindle and ovoid cells forms interlacing fascicles.

Distinctive epithelial cell types that comprise mixed tumors include spindle, clear, squamous, basaloid, cuboidal, plasmacytoid, oncocytoid, mucous, and sebaceous (figs. 4-11, 4-12). The various cell types are often closely associated with one another and transition from one type to another is common. Squamous differentiation is frequently abrupt and in discrete islands that are seemingly superimposed on sheets of less distinctive epithelial cells (fig. 4-13). Spindle and plasmacytoid cells often appear to be in transition from one form to the other (fig. 4-14). The nuclear features of all cell types are uniformly bland, nucleoli are small or absent, and mitoses are few. Exceptions are those tumors that have been previously manipulated by biopsy or fine-needle aspiration. Occasionally, these tumors reveal an infarct in which scattered viable epithelial cells within the necrotic tissue demon-strate atypical cytomorphology (fig. 4-15). Although spontaneous central necrosis in a mixed tumor has been reported (46), its presence in the absence of previous surgical manipulation suggests malignant transformation and warrants review of additional sections. Rarely, tumor cells are seen within vascular spaces (fig. 4-16), presumably due to surgical manipulation. This feature has not been correlated with a greater likelihood of metastasis (90).

An infinite number of architectural configurations occur; they vary within each tumor and from one tumor to another. Frequently, anastomosing trabeculae of epithelial cells have occasional well-formed ductal or tubular structures and are closely associated with an interposed stromal component. The epithelium may instead form broad, solid sheets (fig. 4-17). Small cystic structures are often lined by squamous epithelium and contain

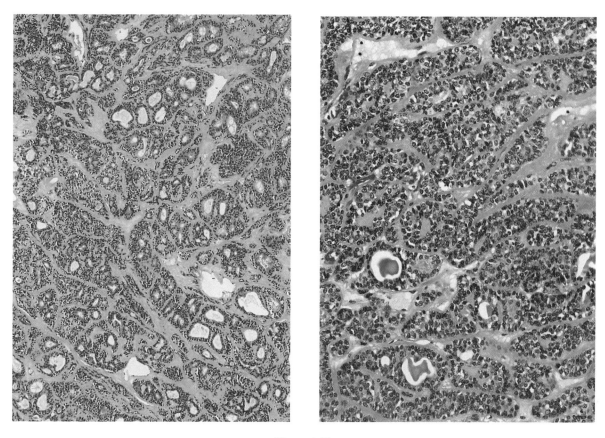

Figure 4-12
MIXED TUMOR
Some tumors with tubular or solid structures composed of round to ovoid basaloid cells may resemble either adenoid cystic carcinoma (left) or basal cell adenoma (right).

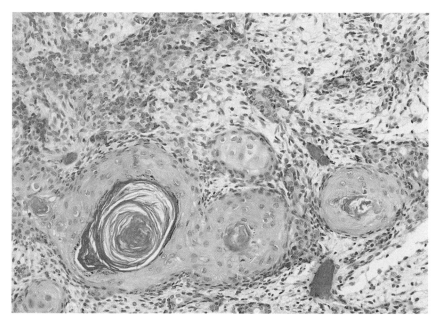

Figure 4-13
MIXED TUMOR
WITH SQUAMOUS
DIFFERENTIATION
Islands of well-differentiated squamous cells with a small, keratin-filled cyst are surrounded by more typical myxoid zones.

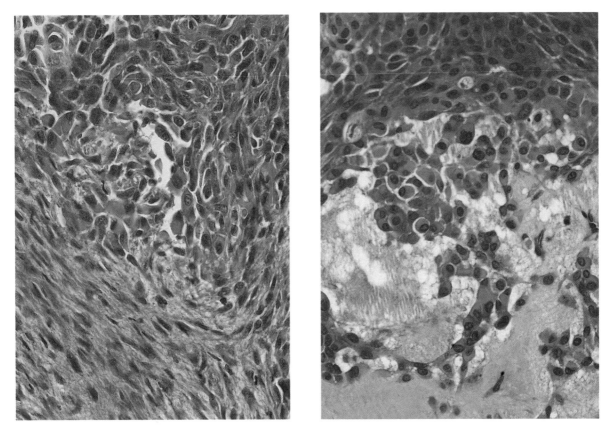

Figure 4-14
MIXED TUMOR

Left: This tumor has distinct zones of spindle and plasmacytoid cells; the interface is a transitional area of one type to the other.

Right: Individual cells appear to float in abundant mucinous material. The plasmacytoid cells lack the perinuclear clearing that is characteristic of plasma cells.

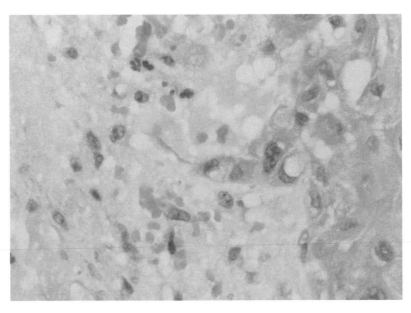

Figure 4-15
INFARCTED MIXED TUMOR

Contained within this largely ne-crotic and unrecognizable zone of mixed tumor are scattered, viable and atypi-cal neoplastic epithelial cells.

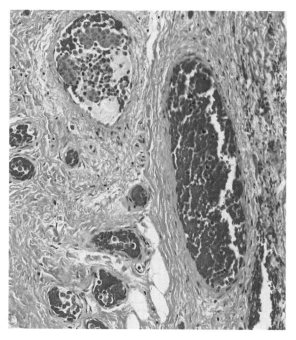

Figure 4-16
INTRAVASCULAR MIXED TUMOR
An isolated cluster of neoplastic cells is evident within an endothelial-lined space. This was an incidental finding in an otherwise unremarkable mixed tumor.

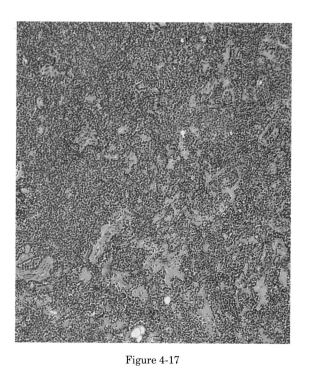

Figure 4-17
CELLULAR MIXED TUMOR
This mixed tumor has sheets of basaloid cells with little intervening stroma.

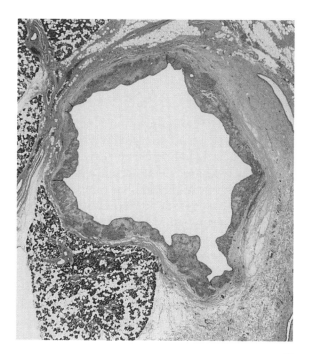

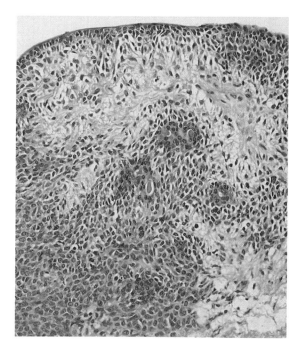

Figure 4-18
CYSTIC MIXED TUMOR
Presumably, cystic degeneration in this mixed tumor resulted in the formation of a large central space (left) that has a rim composed of elements typical of solid mixed tumors (right).

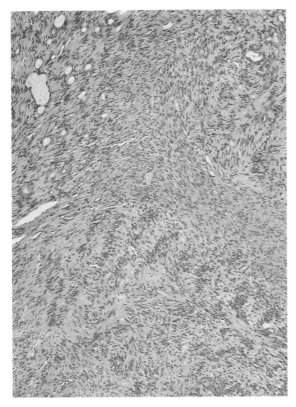

Figure 4-19
SCHWANNOMA-LIKE AREA IN MIXED TUMOR
This mixed tumor has a prominent spindle cell component that focally demonstrates palisading of nuclei around amorphous material; this resembles the Verocay bodies characteristic of schwannomas.

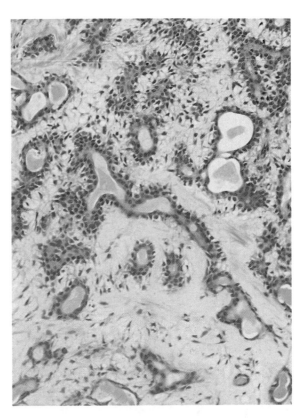

Figure 4-20
MIXED TUMOR
The focal arrangement of dark luminal cells surrounded by clear cells simulates the biphasic growth characteristic of epithelial-myoepithelial carcinoma.

keratin, and occasionally narrow bands of tumor surround large cystic spaces (fig. 4-18). The mesenchymal-like stromal component accumulates between and around the epithelial elements and often isolates individual epithelial islands and trabecular structures as well as individual epithelial cells. Spindle cells form fibrous-like interlacing fascicles and, rarely, demonstrate schwannoma-like palisading of nuclei (fig. 4-19).

Ductal structures in mixed tumors are usually randomly scattered and more numerous in richly epithelial than "mesenchymal" areas. In some cases they are large and have distinct lumens whereas in others the lumens are small and ill-defined. The lumens are variously lined by cuboidal or columnar epithelium that is itself sometimes surrounded by a layer of larger clear, spindle, or stellate cells. These two elements

together mimic the organization of normal ducts or the biphasic structures characteristic of epithelial-myoepithelial carcinoma (fig. 4-20).

Myxoid, hyaline, chondroid, and osseous areas constitute the mesenchymal-like component. The myxoid or myxochondroid areas (fig. 4-21) are rich in heparan sulfate (71). Amorphous to slightly fibrillar eosinophilic hyaline stroma may be sparsely distributed between epithelial cells or dominate large epithelium-poor areas (fig. 4-22). Cartilaginous zones result from the accumulation of myxohyaline material around individual cells, and only rarely resemble mature hyaline cartilage. Bone is relatively rare but may occasionally be a dominant feature (fig. 4-23). Surprisingly, bone morphogenetic protein has been found in a high percentage of mixed tumors (47). Amorphous "stromal" material encircled by

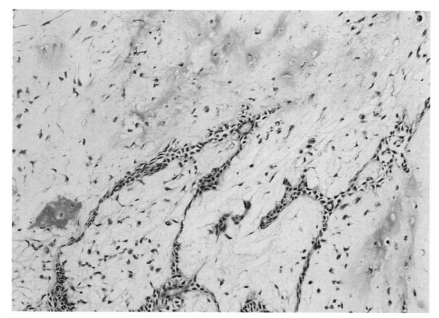

Figure 4-21
MYXOCHONDROID
MIXED TUMOR
Myxochondroid area contains anastomosing strands of epithelial cells. Several small ducts are present within these strands.

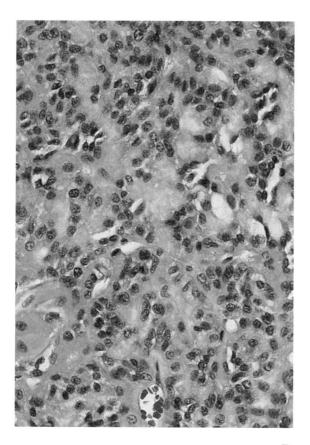

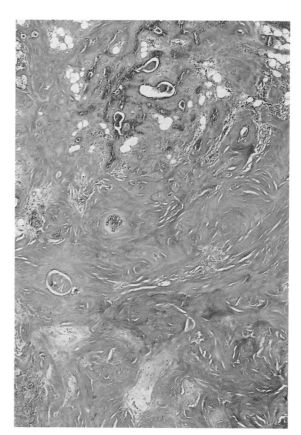

Figure 4-22
MIXED TUMOR
Deposits of amorphous hyaline material may be limited to small intercellular deposits (left) or have a fibrotic or desmoplastic appearance that comprises a large proportion of the tumor (right). On the right there is evidence of early dystrophic calcification.

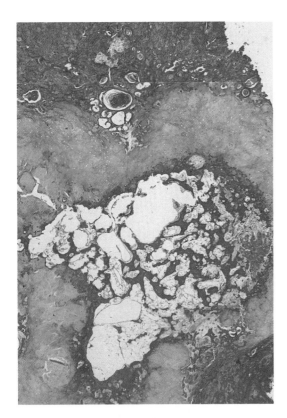 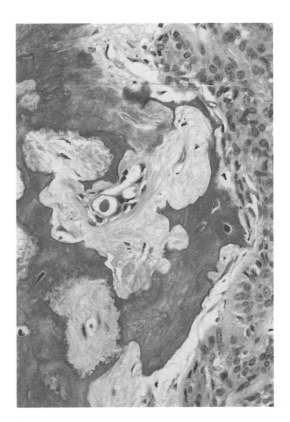

Figure 4-23
PROMINENT OSSEOUS DIFFERENTIATION IN MIXED TUMOR
Left: This tumor is centrally composed of bone with a peripheral rim of pale-staining cartilage.
Right: Higher magnification shows woven bone trabeculae in close association with neoplastic epithelium.

narrow strands of epithelial cells may simulate the tubular type of adenoid cystic carcinoma. Similarly, small, basaloid cells in a lattice arrangement can mimic cribriform adenoid cystic carcinoma. These patterns are typically limited to small foci but if they are more pronounced additional sampling for characteristic zones of mixed tumor may be indicated. Small to medium ovoid cells with darkly staining nuclei and vague peripheral palisading may resemble basal cell adenoma cells.

Crystalloids are more often present in mixed tumors than in any other salivary gland neoplasm: their incidence varies from 1.5 to 21 percent (8,9,62,82). Among AFIP cases, the frequency has been toward the lower end of that range. Three types of crystalloids have been described. The most common type is composed of eosinophilic, needle-shaped fibers radially arranged around a small circular space that sometimes contains a few connective tissue cells or a capillary. These are nonrefractile, collagenous crystalloids that stain bright blue with Masson's trichrome and red with the van Gieson method (8). Routine formalin fixation and processing may diminish evidence of their presence (40). A second type of crystalloid is composed of radially arranged, "petal-shaped," blunt-ended clusters of eosinophilic tubular structures (fig. 4-24). These are so-called tyrosine-rich crystalloids because they react with Millon's reagent. They are refractile with light microscopy and do not stain for collagen. Some contain more arginine than tyrosine (9,84). It has been suggested that they result from the precipitation on stromal collagen of products secreted by neoplastic myoepithelial cells (38). The third type of crystalloid resembles oxalate crystals (23).

Recurrent mixed tumors, as would be expected from the gross appearance, often form multiple, separate nodules within remaining salivary gland, periparotid tissues, dermis, or scar tissue that develop following the initial surgery (fig. 4-25) (69).

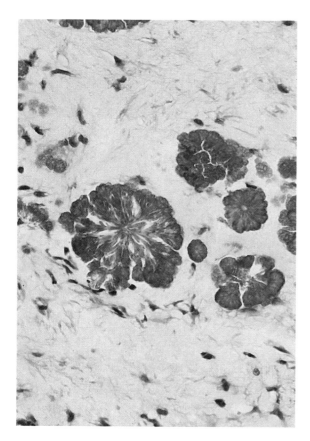

Figure 4-24
CRYSTALLOIDS IN MIXED TUMOR
Dark, hematoxyphilic, tyrosine-rich crystalloids are scattered throughout a myxoid area in this tumor. A large rosette of crystals with the characteristic radially arranged, blunt-ended structures is evident.

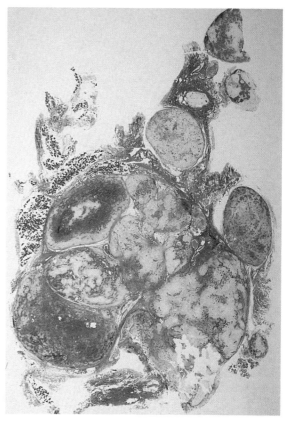

Figure 4-25
RECURRENT MIXED TUMOR
There are numerous pale-staining, myxoid, recurrent tumor nodules in parotid tissue and periparotid fat. This tumor recurred 2 years after the initial treatment.

Ultrastructural and Immunohistochemical Findings. Ultrastructurally, the principal proliferating tumor cells are structurally modified myoepithelial cells that have basal lamina, small microvilli, and well-developed desmosomes. Squamous differentiation is often prominent among these cells, but they rarely resemble normal myoepithelial cells, particularly in areas of matrix accumulation (fig. 4-26). They are mixed with neoplastic luminal epithelial cells and infrequent acinar cells. The organization of these cells often mimics that of the normal salivary gland duct in which peripheral myoepithelial cells are attached to centrally situated luminal cells by tonofilament-associated desmosomes (15,16,26). Some cells in chondroid areas resemble chondrocytes within an electron-lucent lacuna and contain compact glycogen clusters (15).

Evidence that the "mesenchymal" cells are modified myoepithelial cells includes the variable presence of tonofilaments and microfilaments within their cytoplasm, linear densities of the plasma membrane, pinocytotic vesicles, and remnants of basement membrane (26,57). The extracellular spaces often contain elastic fibers (16,18,19). Elastic fibers are usually seen close to the neoplastic myoepithelial-like cells and all stages of elastogenesis are present (18,60).

The normal myoepithelial cell is typically immunoreactive for antibodies to cytokeratin and smooth muscle actin, and variably immunoreactive for glial fibrillary acidic protein (GFAP), vimentin, and S-100 protein. GFAP reactivity is usually limited to myxoid areas and absent in cellular tumors. In mixed tumors, many cell types are reactive with cytokeratin, including those in

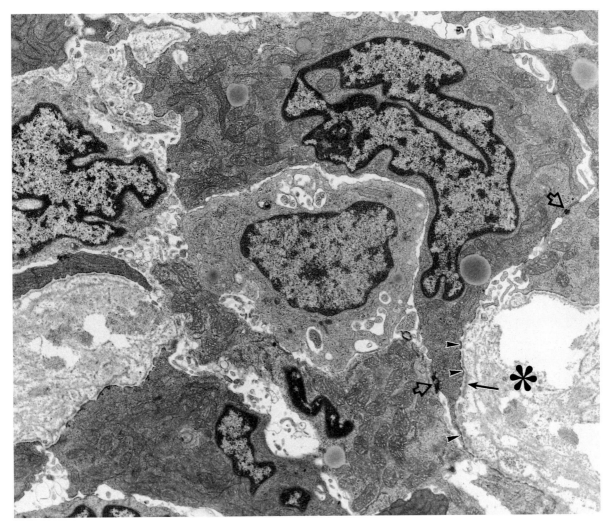

Figure 4-26
MIXED TUMOR

Ultrastructurally, the cytoplasm of an irregularly shaped epithelial cell borders a microcystic space (asterisk) that is partly lined by basal lamina (arrow) and filled with a "stromal" product. The lining also demonstrates linear plasma membrane densities (arrowheads). Several desmosomes (open arrows), microvilli, and numerous mitochondria are apparent (X3,000).

stromal-rich areas. Smooth muscle actin usually reacts strongly with periductal and spindle cells, but is variably reactive in other cell types and usually nonreactive in plasmacytoid cells (fig. 4-27). S-100 protein is seen in all cell types in epithelial and stromal regions. However, because this protein is not usually demonstrable in normal myoepithelium (13), its presence in neoplastic salivary gland cells does not necessarily indicate myoepithelial differentiation. Vimentin is seen to a lesser degree (56,57).

Other Special Techniques. Cytogenetic studies have shown that many mixed tumors demonstrate clonal chromosomal abnormalities (4–7,49,78). Three cytogenetic subtypes have been described: normal karyotypes; rearrangement of chromosome 8, band q12; and rearrangement of chromosome 12 in the q13-15 region. Patients whose tumors show the 8q12 abnormality are younger than those with other tumor subtypes and these tumors are less likely to have a histologic predominance of a mesenchymal-like component. These subtypes show a geographically related incidence (5–7). Thus far there is no definitive evidence of a correlation between the cytogenetic features and the likelihood of recurrence or malignant transformation.

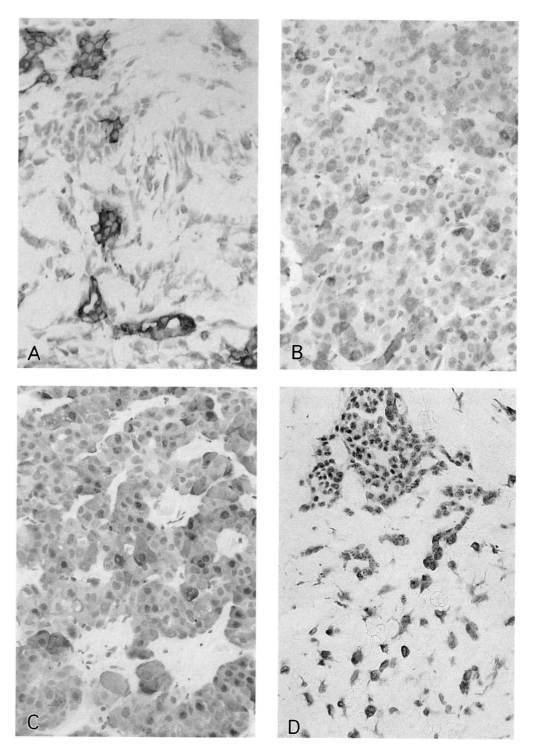

Figure 4-27
IMMUNOREACTIVITY OF MIXED TUMOR

A: Cytokeratin immunoreactivity is typically stronger and less variable in the clusters of duct-like epithelial cells than in the spindled "stromal" cells.

B: Reactivity for smooth muscle actin is constantly seen in spindle cells but also may be seen in the larger, more polygonal cells.

C: S-100 protein immunoreactivity is variable but may be found in all cell types.

D: Glial fibrillary acidic protein is more intense and consistently seen in the myxoid element in contrast to the ductal epithelium. (Avidin-biotin peroxidase stain)

Studies of argyrophilic nucleolar organizer regions (AgNORs) in mixed tumors indicate a greater proliferative activity in the solid cellular regions compared with the myxoid or chondroid areas (31,45). Data on a limited number of cases also suggest that there is a higher AgNOR count in the carcinomatous element of carcinoma ex mixed tumor than in benign mixed tumors (52,85). Analysis of DNA content by flow cytometric analysis indicates mixed tumors are usually diploid, as are some carcinomas ex mixed tumor (90). Martin and associates (50) found a wide range of S-phase percent values in benign and malignant tumors without a statistical difference between them. They also observed aneuploidy and increased proliferative activity using p105 in benign mixed tumors. The significance of the expression of p53 protein and c-*myc* and *ras* p21 tumor-suppressor oncogenes in both benign mixed tumor and carcinoma ex mixed tumor is unclear at this time (21,54,65).

Differential Diagnosis. Most mixed tumors have the characteristic mixture of epithelial and mesenchymal-like features that permit unequivocal identification. A common problem in diagnosis is caused by small, fragmented tissue samples that lack an interface between neoplastic cells and surrounding tissues. In these cases a wide variety of neoplasms are often considered. If such a biopsy has chondroid or myxoid foci and a ductal element, an appropriate interpretation would be "suggestive of a mixed tumor." Since other benign and malignant salivary gland tumors, such as canalicular adenoma and polymorphous low-grade adenocarcinoma, contain duct-like structures and myxoid or edematous areas, caution in definitive diagnosis is advised. Correlation with the clinical presentation may help, but review of additional tissue is often necessary.

Distinguishing salivary gland mixed tumor from dermal mixed tumor (chondroid syringoma) may be difficult if not impossible. This dilemma occurs most often in specimens from the upper lip (fig. 4-28). The presence of salivary gland tissue adjacent to the tumor and the clinical presentation of a mucosal rather than dermal protuberance lend some support to a salivary origin. Mixed tumors of both origins show similar immunoreactivity.

At the AFIP, immunohistochemical studies have not been particularly helpful in separating mixed tumors from other types of salivary gland

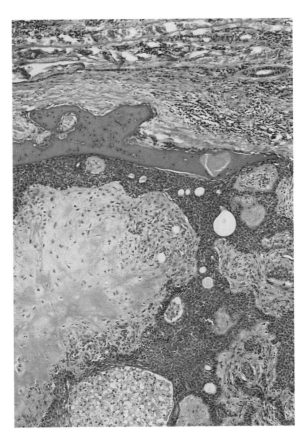

Figure 4-28
MIXED TUMOR OF SKIN
Similarity to mixed tumor of the salivary gland is evident in this tumor of the skin from the upper lip. Because of the proximity of skin and buccal mucosa, it may also be difficult to determine the origin of lesions in the cheek.

tumors because of similar immunoreactivity of neoplastic cells among many types of benign and malignant salivary gland tumors, despite claims to the contrary (66,80). While coexpression of cytokeratin and smooth muscle actin support myoepithelial differentiation, other tumor types have a myoepithelial element that is similarly immunoreactive. Neoplastic cells of other tumors, such as adenoid cystic carcinoma, also react with anti-GFAP which limits its value for identifying mixed tumor.

Occasionally, mixed tumors appear to be composed exclusively of myxoid, chondroid, or osseous tissue, and mesenchymal neoplasms such as myxoma, myxoid lipoma, myxoid neurofibroma, osteoma, or osteochondroma are considered in the differential diagnosis. Review of multiple sections of mixed tumors nearly always reveals

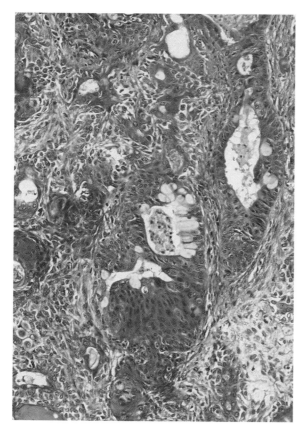

Figure 4-29
MIXED TUMOR WITH FOCUS
RESEMBLING MUCOEPIDERMOID CARCINOMA

The cystic growth and admixture of mucous, epidermoid, and "intermediate" cells make this single focus suggestive of mucoepidermoid carcinoma. Recognition of the limited, focal presence of these features and typical features of mixed tumor elsewhere is critical to proper interpretation.

an epithelial component, but immunohistochemical analysis for cytokeratin reactivity can assist this search and help confirm the diagnosis.

Foci of squamous differentiation and mucous cells in mixed tumors occasionally resemble mucoepidermoid carcinoma (fig. 4-29). However, mucoepidermoid carcinoma is focally infiltrative, lacks myxochondroid elements, is usually cystic, and usually lacks the discrete epidermoid islands with focal keratinization. In the minor salivary glands, polymorphous low-grade adenocarcinoma (PLGA) is also considered in the differential diagnosis because it is generally circumscribed, has uniform bland cytomorphology, and often contains myxoid areas. In contradistinction to mixed tumor, PLGA frequently shows perineural growth; infiltrates adjacent fibrous

connective tissue, fat, and salivary parenchyma; and forms small tubular structures or single-file cords of tumor cells at the periphery (see section, Polymorphous Low-Grade Adenocarcinoma).

Neoplastic tissue within or extending through the fibrous capsule causes concern for malignant transformation. However, in the absence of abnormal cytomorphologic features, capsular involvement is an acceptable feature in benign mixed tumor. On the other hand, morphologic atypia, such as enlarged, pleomorphic or hyperchromatic nuclei and frequent or abnormal mitoses, is indicative of carcinomatous transformation. At the AFIP, tumors with mild or focally limited cytologic atypia (fig. 4-30) are designated as atypical mixed tumor and indicate an increased likelihood of malignant transformation if the tumor should recur. Hypercellularity is acceptable if abnormal cytomorphologic features, including a high mitotic rate, are absent (70). When prominent abnormal cytologic features are confined within the capsule, the terms *intracapsular carcinoma, carcinoma in situ,* or *noninvasive carcinoma ex mixed tumor* are appropriate (see section, Carcinoma Ex Mixed Tumor) (86). Absence of a capsule that allows tumor to directly abut parenchymal tissue but has a well-delineated periphery is acceptable in mixed tumors in the absence of cytologic abnormalities. However, penetration of parenchyma by individual tumor cells or by clusters of tumor cells indicates malignancy. Recurrent mixed tumors often have multiple foci of tumor within the normal gland parenchyma, but these foci are usually discrete and circumscribed, and without cytologic atypia.

Clinical Behavior and Treatment. There is agreement that enucleation of mixed tumors of the parotid, defined as opening the capsule of the tumor followed by surgical removal or aspiration of its contents, leads to a high recurrence rate (22,24,59,83). Similarly, surgical exposure of the tumor or tumor capsule risks spillage and dramatically increases the risk of recurrence. Furthermore, it is difficult to treat the multiple foci of recurrent mixed tumors (63), and the risk of malignant degeneration increases with time (see Carcinoma Ex Mixed Tumor). However, controversy remains over whether superficial (lateral) parotidectomy or extracapsular dissection (lumpectomy) with a margin of normal tissue is the best option for both controlling the tumor and minimizing surgical complications. Recent studies

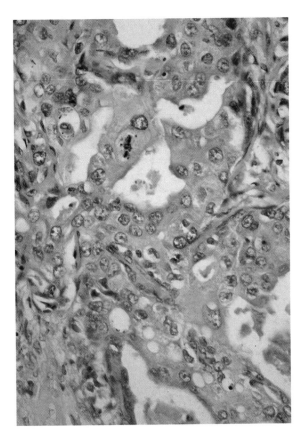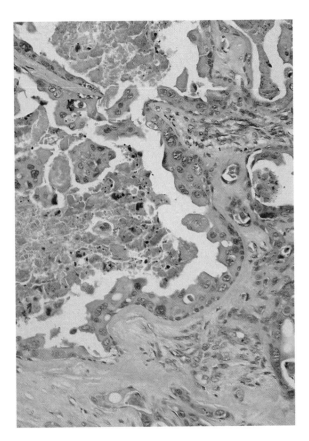

Figure 4-30
ATYPICAL MIXED TUMOR

Substantial atypical features are present in one area of this mixed tumor.
Left: Pleomorphic and hyperchromatic enlarged nuclei, and prominent nucleoli are evident in this field.
Right: This area reveals necrotic debris within the lumens of the irregular neoplastic ductal structures.

evaluating the efficacy of these techniques, both with facial nerve preservation, show similar recurrence rates in the range of 0 to 8 percent (11,29,32,36,37,39,51,53,67,81,91,93). Donovan and Conley (22) have suggested that while superficial parotidectomy is conceptualized as an en bloc resection, more often than not in specimens obtained with that procedure, tumor extends to or closely approximates the surgical margins. Conservative parotidectomy does not ensure complete excision (35). Three-dimensional reconstructions of whole organ sections made from parotidectomy specimens have shown that mixed tumors often have irregular projections from the tumor surface, incomplete capsules, and focal absence of a covering of parenchymal tissue (44). These studies emphasize that with either procedure great care is needed to prevent surgical compromise of the tumor margin.

Among other complications of parotid surgery are Frey's syndrome (gustatory sweating) and temporary or permanent damage to branches of the facial nerve, especially the marginal mandibular branch (58). Some investigators believe that compared to extracapsular dissection, superficial parotidectomy unnecessarily increases the risks of damage to the fine branches of the facial nerve as they leave the anterior and superior borders of the gland (32,53). Several investigators have found that the risk of developing Frey's syndrome and facial nerve damage are greater with superficial parotidectomy than with extracapsular dissection (51,68,91). A procedure for performing a conservative parotidectomy that may lower the incidence of Frey's syndrome has been described (94).

Recurrence of mixed tumors predisposes patients to an increased risk of facial nerve injury because of the need for additional surgery. Furthermore, recurrent mixed tumors typically are associated with scar tissue that may be adhesive to the facial nerve, complicating dissection. Total parotidectomy and excision of the scar tissue with preservation of the facial nerve are recommended for recurrent tumor (42,48,59,61,72,77). Some investigators emphasize that this aggressive approach is indicated because of the increased difficulty in removing additional recurrences that might require en bloc parotidectomy (59,61). Because many recurrent mixed tumors of the parotid are discovered more than 5 years after the initial surgery (42,79,88), follow-up should continue well beyond that period.

The risks associated with the use of radiotherapy contraindicate its routine use for primary mixed tumors (88), although some investigators find it useful in the treatment of selected recurrent mixed tumors (20,72).

Treatment of mixed tumors of the submandibular gland consists of complete resection of the gland (89). Mixed tumors of the minor glands seem to have little propensity for recurrence. Chau and Radden (10), in a study of 27 cases with follow-up, found no recurrences even though many of the tumors had been treated by excisional biopsy. Complete excision with a rim of normal tissue is recommended.

MYOEPITHELIOMA

Definition. Myoepithelioma is a benign tumor composed of sheets and islands of various proportions of spindle, plasmacytoid, epithelioid, and clear cells that exhibit myoepithelial but not ductal differentiation. These tumors sometimes have abundant, acellular, mucoid or hyalinized stroma but lack chondroid and myxochondroid foci.

Myoepithelioma probably represents one end of the spectrum of mixed tumor and has a similar, if not identical, biologic behavior. Criteria for distinguishing mixed tumors with a predominance of myoepithelial cells from myoepitheliomas are relatively subjective. Some investigators (99) stipulate that no more than 5 to 10 percent of a microscopic section of myoepithelioma be comprised of ducts whereas others (105) suggest that no more than one or more ducts for every medium- to high-power field (X200 to 400) or no more than one small cluster of ducts is acceptable. Primarily for simplicity and reproducibility, this Fascicle

accepts as myoepithelioma only those tumors that do not demonstrate duct formation. While distinction between mixed tumor and myoepithelioma is primarily academic and not critical to patient management, awareness of this entity helps prevent its misdiagnosis as malignant epithelial and mesenchymal neoplasms.

Designation of tumors comprised primarily of plasmacytoid (hyaline) cells as myoepithelioma is controversial (95,105). Based on a study of a small number of plasmacytoid and spindle cell tumors, Franquemont and Mills (103) argue that such tumors are better designated as plasmacytoid adenomas because of the lack of ultrastructural and immunohistochemical evidence of myogenous differentiation. Dardick and colleagues (99,101,102) have noted that even normal myoepithelial cells exhibit a range of filament expression and that the modified neoplastic myoepithelial cell shows a broad range of differentiation, rarely with the fully differentiated characteristics of normal myoepithelium. In support of this view, some formalin-fixed spindle cell myoepitheliomas also lack demonstrable myogenous immunoreactivity. As a possible explanation for this dilemma, it has been suggested that the tumor cells in myoepithelioma may be the neoplastic counterpart of duct basal cells in some cases, more typical myoepithelial cells in others, or a mixture of the two cell types in still others (96). In this Fascicle, tumors of plasmacytoid epithelial cells are accepted as myoepitheliomas, but more study is needed in this area.

General Features. Using the relatively strict definition stated, myoepitheliomas represent 1.5 percent of all salivary gland tumors from both major and minor salivary gland sites in the AFIP files reviewed since 1985. They represent 2.2 and 5.7 percent of all benign major and minor salivary gland tumors, respectively. Men and women are affected with equal frequency. The age range of civilian patients in these files is 9 to 85, with an average of 44 years. Similar to mixed tumor but unlike most other salivary gland tumors, the peak age of occurrence is in the third decade of life. The two most common sites of occurrence are the parotid gland (40 percent) and the hard and soft palates (21 percent), but all salivary gland sites have been affected. In either the major or minor salivary gland, myoepitheliomas present as asymptomatic masses (110).

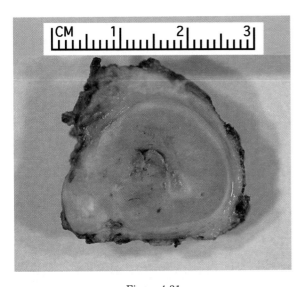

Figure 4-31
MYOEPITHELIOMA
This parotid tumor is generally well circumscribed but shows a nodular extension (lower left) into the surgical margin.

Gross and Microscopic Findings. Grossly, myoepitheliomas are well circumscribed and have a solid, tan or yellow-tan glistening cut surface (fig. 4-31) (105). Microscopically, they often have a fibrous capsule that varies in thickness (fig. 4-32). The AFIP and other investigators have noted that some heterogeneity of the cellular composition and architecture is usually evident within individual tumors, but the architectural growth pattern of each tumor often appears to be largely dependent on the predominant cell type (96,105,108). Tumors composed principally of spindle-shaped cells are often compactly arranged in single or multiple nodules. Interlacing fascicles of these cells are often more suggestive of fibrous than epithelial tissue. Tumors are hypercellular and have limited myxoid or mucoid stroma (fig. 4-33) but often have scattered clusters of epithelioid and clear cells with occasional microcystic spaces (fig. 4-34). Sometimes, amorphous hyaline material accumulates

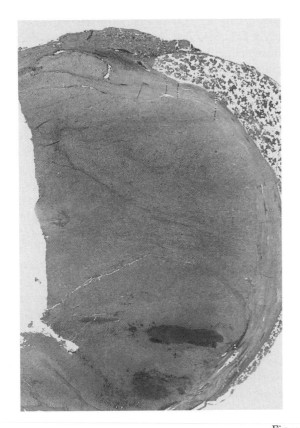

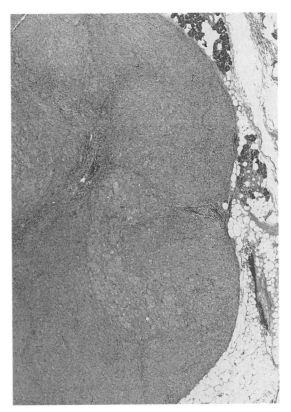

Figure 4-32
MYOEPITHELIOMA
Left: A thick, fibrous capsule separates this tumor from the rim of parotid tissue present at the right of the illustration.
Right: This tumor is in direct contact with surrounding parenchyma and intraglandular fat.

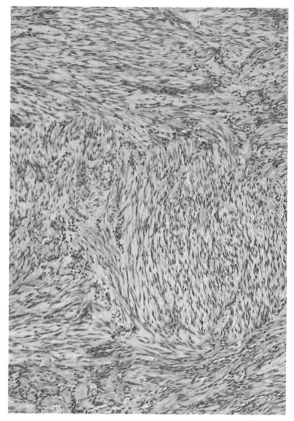

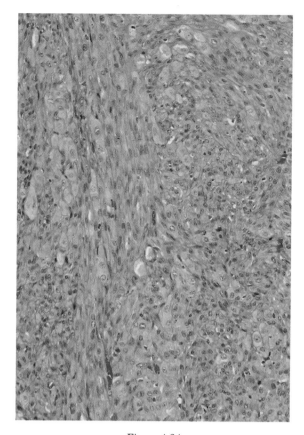

Figure 4-33
MYOEPITHELIOMA, SPINDLE CELL VARIANT
Interlacing fascicles of spindle cells suggest a mesenchymal rather than epithelial neoplasm. This variant is characterized by cellular, compactly arranged, interwoven collections of spindle cells that usually have limited intercellular stroma.

Figure 4-34
MYOEPITHELIOMA, SPINDLE CELL VARIANT
This predominantly spindle cell tumor focally is composed of polygonal epithelioid cells, some of which have faintly eosinophilic or clear cytoplasm.

between islands or cords of tumor cells (fig. 4-35). In many cases a few clusters of epithelial cells within a large sheet of spindle cells are the only obvious evidence of the epithelial nature of the tumor. The spindle cells have centrally located, fusiform, often vesicular nuclei with blunt or tapered ends and inconspicuous nucleoli. The cytoplasm is eosinophilic and finely granular, but the cell borders are poorly defined except in areas that exhibit widened intercellular spaces. Sometimes the spindle cells are outnumbered by smaller, round to ovoid cells that are admixed with cells that have slightly elongated fusiform nuclei (fig. 4-36). The clear cells contain glycogen and comprise a small proportion of most tumors but in some tumors they are prominent and associated with microcystic spaces (fig. 4-37). In some areas epithelioid cells, which are larger

ovoid or polygonal cells, predominate (fig. 4-38); in other areas the spindle cells are admixed with plasmacytoid cells, and there often appears to be transformation from one cell type to the other (fig. 4-39). Foci of oncocytes may also be present.

In some tumors there is a predominance of epithelioid cells; these tumors often have a paucity of spindle and plasmacytoid cells. Occasionally, there are narrow interconnected cords that are surrounded by abundant mucoid, relatively acellular stroma. Dardick et al. (96) have designated this tumor variant as the *reticular type of myoepithelioma* and have noted that the stroma may become somewhat hyalinized. More solid cellular areas may be present. Because these tumors share features with the tubulotrabecular variant of basal cell adenoma, distinction between the two can be difficult (fig. 4-40).

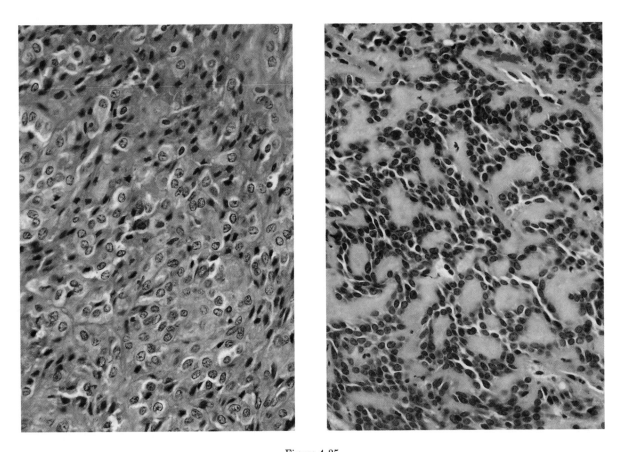

Figure 4-35
MYOEPITHELIOMA
These two different examples show focal variation in the amount and distribution of intercellular hyaline deposition.

Figure 4-36
MYOEPITHELIOMA
Compactly arranged cells with round, ovoid, and fusiform nuclei and very limited cytoplasm characterize this tumor.

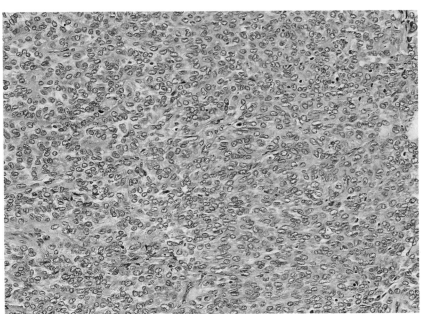

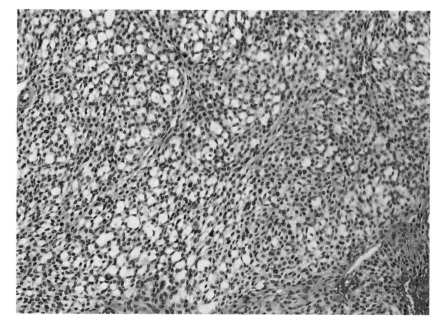

Figure 4-37
MYOEPITHELIOMA
This example is dominated by numerous microcystic spaces and clear cells.

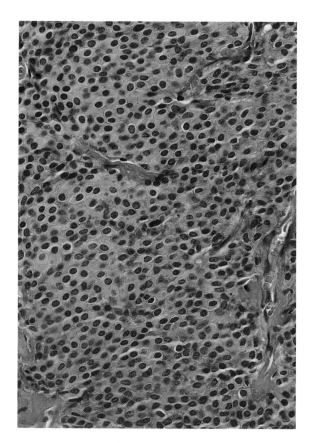
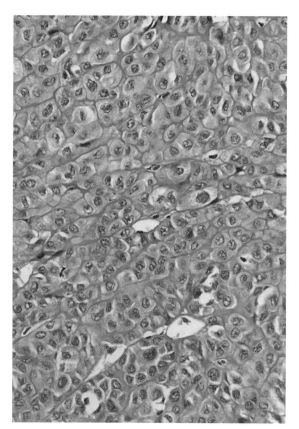

Figure 4-38
MYOEPITHELIOMA
Sheets of epithelioid cells are present in these two examples. The cell borders are well delineated in both. The example on the right shows a cord-like arrangement of large cells that have abundant cytoplasm, suggesting oncocytic change.

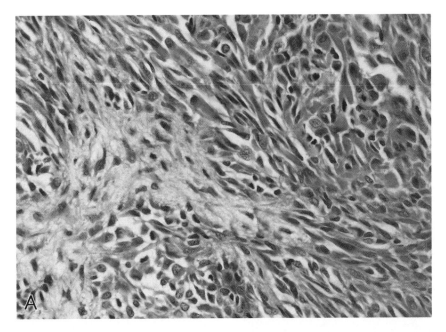

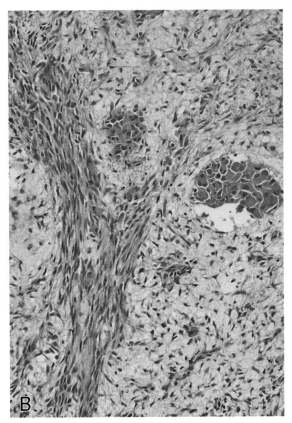

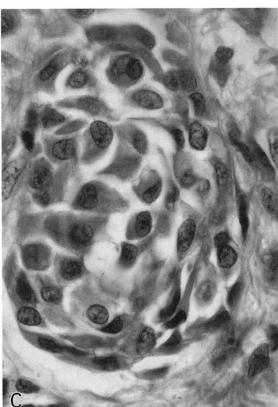

Figure 4-39

MYOEPITHELIOMA WITH SPINDLE AND PLASMACYTOID CELLS

A: Many areas of this tumor have an admixture of spindle and plasmacytoid cells. It appears there is progressive transformation from one cell type to the other, a feature also seen in mixed tumors.

B: Plasmacytoid cells are seen both as discrete islands and within the spindle cell focus.

C: Higher magnification reveals a nest of cells with uniform, ovoid, eccentrically placed nuclei admixed with several spindle cells.

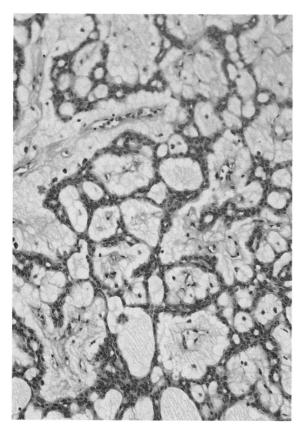

Figure 4-40
SO-CALLED RETICULAR VARIANT
OF MYOEPITHELIOMA

In this example, ramifying cords of polygonal and basaloid cells are surrounded by ample mucoid stroma. More solid tumor growth was evident elsewhere.

Plasmacytoid cells can vastly outnumber other cell types. This occurs more often in the palate than the parotid gland. Typically, multiple small islands of plasmacytoid tumor cells lie in abundant, loosely collagenous or hematoxyphilic mucoid stroma (fig. 4-41). The cells appear less cohesive than other cell types. Individual cells are usually evident. The cells are round to ovoid; have abundant, eosinophilic, "hyaline" cytoplasm; eccentrically placed nuclei that are slightly pyknotic; and small nucleoli.

Immunohistochemical Findings. Normal myoepithelium is often immunoreactive with antibodies to cytokeratin and muscle-specific actin. Desmin has not been demonstrated (107). Of the keratin filaments, cytokeratin 14 is expressed most consistently (99). Immunoreactivity with S-100 protein is limited to rare myoepithelial cells,

often in glands that are in close proximity to an inflammatory process or a neoplasm. Dardick and colleagues (98) have shown that the S-100 protein immunoreactivity of the tissue surrounding acini results from the antibody reacting with unmyelinated nerves rather than myoepithelial cells. Glial fibrillary acidic protein (GFAP) is expressed only in occasional normal myoepithelial cells of tissue adjacent to a neoplasm or inflammation.

The neoplastic cells of myoepitheliomas consistently demonstrate cytokeratin immunoreactivity, although reactivity of the spindle cells is variable. There is considerable variation of tumor cell expression of muscle-specific actin, presumably because the tumor cells vary in their degree of differentiation (97). At the AFIP, the spindle cells of all architectural forms of myoepithelioma react strongly for muscle-specific actin, the epithelioid cells react sporadically, and plasmacytoid and clear cells are generally nonreactive. Immunoreactivity for S-100 protein is usually strong, whereas it is more variable for vimentin and GFAP (fig. 4-42) (96,103).

Ultrastructural Findings. The neoplastic spindle cells of myoepitheliomas often contain microfilaments with dense bodies, intermediate filaments, tonofilaments, micropinocytotic vesicles, basal lamina, and desmosomes (fig. 4-43) (99,100,108,109). The intercellular spaces are frequently widened and contain stroma rich in proteoglycans and elastic fibers. Microglandular lumina with microvilli occur that are not appreciated on light microscopy (99). The fine structure of the plasmacytoid cells is similar to their counterparts in mixed tumors (99). The cytoplasm is typically packed with haphazardly arranged intermediate filaments. Although microfilaments with dense bodies are normally lacking, at least one investigation has shown the presence of microfilaments within a larger accumulation of intermediate filaments (106). The epithelioid cells often contain limited numbers of filaments, many polyribosomes, and some glycogen (99).

Differential Diagnosis. Myoepitheliomas may be mistaken for a variety of benign and malignant epithelial and mesenchymal tumors (108). Myoepitheliomas composed of a variety of spindle-shaped, epithelioid, and plasmacytoid cells and focally abundant mucoid stroma are likely to be interpreted as mixed tumors. The lack

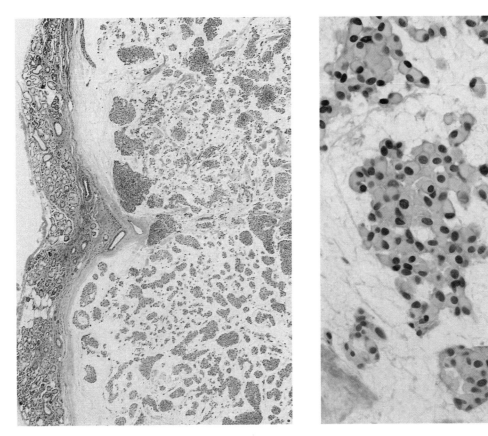

Figure 4-41
MYOEPITHELIOMA, PLASMACYTOID VARIANT

Left: A well-delineated proliferation of small islands, clusters, and individual cells lie in a richly mucoid stroma.

Right: Higher magnification shows a homogeneous population of plasmacytoid cells comprising the cellular component of this tumor.

Figure 4-42
IMMUNOHISTOCHEMICAL
PROFILE OF
MYOEPITHELIOMA

A: Characteristically strong, diffuse immunoreactivity for cytokeratin is seen in these polygonal cells. In contrast, the reactivity of spindle cells is often more variable.

B: Some variability in smooth muscle actin reactivity is evident in this case.

C: Anti-S-100 protein highlights nearly all cells of a different tumor.

D,E: The majority of cells in this cluster of plasmacytoid cells are reactive for both vimentin and glial fibrillary acidic protein.

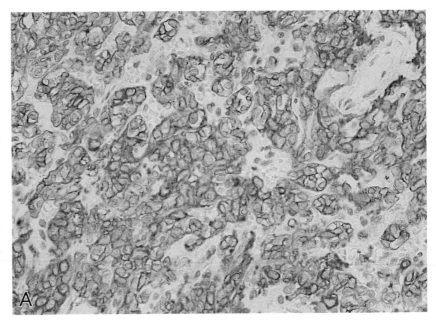

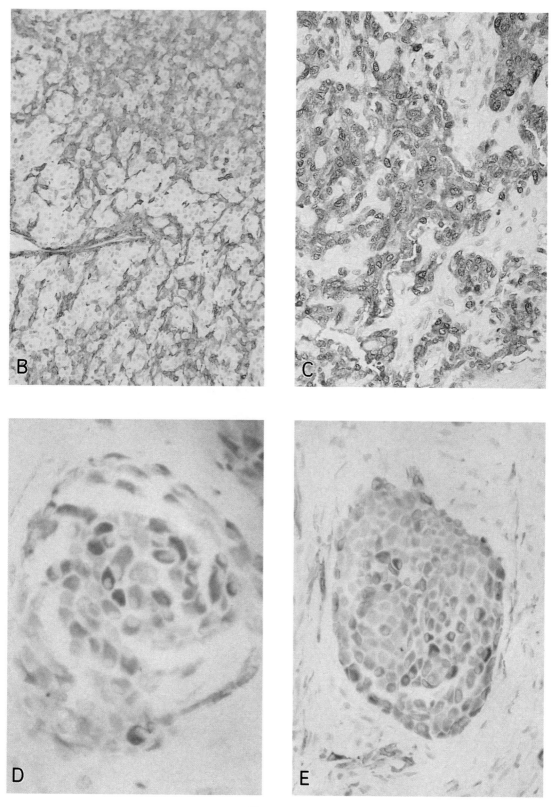

Figure 4-42
IMMUNOHISTOCHEMICAL PROFILE OF MYOEPITHELIOMA (continued)

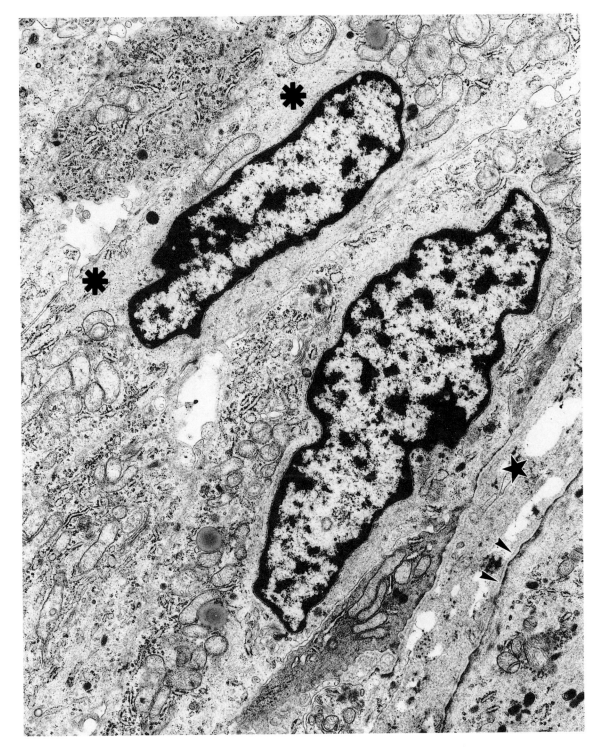

Figure 4-43
MYOEPITHELIOMA, SPINDLE CELL TYPE

The cytoplasm of the spindle cell on the top contains more intermediate filaments (asterisks) but fewer organelles than the cell below it. Proteoglycans occupy the widened intercellular space (star) bordered on either side by membranes highlighted by subplasmalemmal densities. A narrow external basal lamina is evident focally (arrowheads) (X4,600). (Courtesy of Dr. Irving Dardick, Toronto, Canada.)

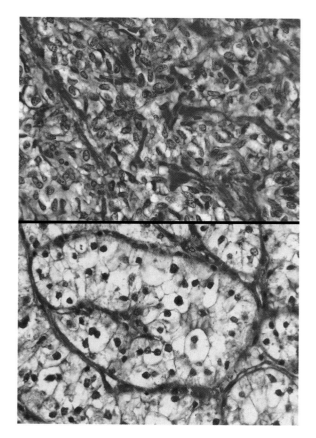

Figure 4-44
MYOEPITHELIOMA WITH
PREDOMINANCE OF CLEAR CELLS
The myoepithelioma on the top shows a vaguely organoid growth pattern and many clear cells. Organoid growth is much more distinct in the metastatic renal cell carcinoma on the bottom, which also showed greater vascularity. In some cases, however, the differences are more subtle and require clinical evaluation of the patient to rule out renal disease.

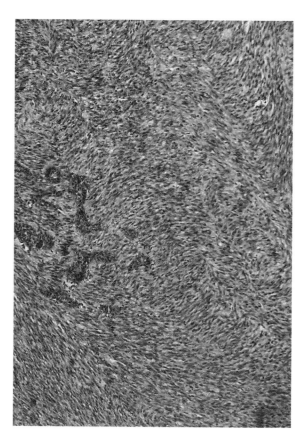

Figure 4-45
MYOEPITHELIOMA
A hypercellular, spindle cell myoepithelioma that demonstrated distinct focal epithelial differentiation. Islands of epithelium are usually found in small groups rather than as isolated individual structures.

of ductal differentiation and absence of chondromyxoid or chondroid foci support interpretation as myoepithelioma. Solid cellular myoepitheliomas, especially those that contain scattered clear cells, must be distinguished from adenocarcinoma. Lack of infiltrative growth and presence of cells with uniform nuclei support a benign interpretation, as does lack of features of specific forms of adenocarcinoma that often contain numerous clear cells, such as mucoepidermoid carcinoma and epithelial-myoepithelial carcinoma.

Spindle cell myoepitheliomas must be distinguished from nerve sheath tumors, fibrous histiocytoma, nodular fasciitis, synovial sarcoma, leiomyoma and leiomyosarcoma, and hemangiopericytoma. An organoid arrangement of epithe-

lioid cells in a tumor removed from the "neck" needs to be differentiated from paraganglioma. Immunohistochemical studies that include antineuron-specific enolase can be of help. A predominance of clear cells suggests metastatic renal cell carcinoma (fig. 4-44). Spindle and epithelioid cell myoepitheliomas suggest biphasic synovial sarcoma (fig. 4-45). The spindle and epithelial elements in both tumors are usually immunoreactive for cytokeratin. However, synovial sarcoma may demonstrate nuclear abnormalities and increased mitotic activity, formation of pseudoglandular or cleft-like spaces by the epithelial element, and, most importantly, infiltrative growth. Strong diffuse immunoreactivity of the tumor cells for cytokeratin, however, should help rule out other mesenchymal considerations. Leiomyoma, leiomyosarcoma, nodular fasciitis, and myoepithelioma are all immunoreactive for smooth muscle actin so only cytokeratin reactivity helps discriminate between them. Separation from spindle cell carcinoma, possibly arising in a mixed tumor, must be based on the lack of nuclear abnormalities and the absence of infiltrative growth in myoepitheliomas.

The hyaline cells in plasmacytoid myoepithelioma do not have the perinuclear clearing of tumor cells in plasmacytoma. The latter are not clustered within a myxoid stroma. Furthermore, the hyaline cells of myoepithelioma are immunoreactive for cytokeratin but not for immunoglobulin light chains.

Separation of myoepithelioma from myoepithelial carcinoma is based primarily on the infiltrative growth of the carcinoma (see Myoepithelial Carcinoma).

Treatment and Prognosis. Myoepitheliomas are less likely to recur than mixed tumors. In a series of 16 cases with follow-up that ranged from 1 month to 7 years, one recurrence was observed (108). The initial tumor had been removed in fragments 7 years earlier. At least one other recurrence has been reported (104). As with mixed tumors, surgical excision that ensures tumor-free margins is indicated (see Mixed Tumor).

WARTHIN'S TUMOR (PAPILLARY CYSTADENOMA LYMPHOMATOSUM)

Definition. Warthin's tumor is an adenoma in which bilayered columnar and basaloid oncocytic epithelia form multiple cysts that have numerous papillations; it is accompanied by a proliferation of follicle-containing lymphoid tissue. This tumor occurs almost exclusively in the parotid gland. The term papillary cystadenoma lymphomatosum is descriptively accurate and synonymous with the eponymic term, Warthin's tumor. Adenolymphoma is a term that could be misinterpreted for a lymphoid malignancy.

General Features. Warthin's tumor is the second most common benign parotid salivary gland tumor and accounts for between 4 to 11.2 percent of all salivary gland tumors in several large studies (139,140,202). In cases seen at the AFIP since 1985, it comprises about 3.5 percent of all epithelial tumors, 5.3 percent of all parotid tumors, and 10.4 percent of benign parotid tumors. Except for mixed tumor, it occurs at least

three times more frequently than all other specific types of adenomas. The frequency of Warthin's tumor as a proportion of all benign parotid salivary gland tumors has been reported to be 9.1 percent in Greece (175), 13.6 percent in a study of primarily American patients (202), 15 percent in Canada (145), over 16 percent in England (140,141) and China (172), and above 27 percent in one region of Denmark (193). It has been suggested that the relatively low incidence of Warthin's tumor in blacks, and the relatively higher number of blacks in the American population, may account for the lower incidence in American studies (141). In a report from Malawi no examples were seen (205), and in a Jamaican study Warthin's tumor represented only 3.7 percent of all benign and malignant salivary gland tumors (198). However, there are studies of Americans in which the incidence among benign parotid tumors was as high as 29 and 34 percent (177,184).

In AFIP data, Warthin's tumor has an unusually low frequency among black patients: only 2.5 percent occurred in a black civilian population, representing 7.4 percent of all patients of known race. In comparison, 8.1 percent of mixed tumors occurred in blacks. Of the nearly 1,100 black patients with primary benign and malignant salivary gland tumors in the AFIP files, only 12 (1.1 percent) had Warthin tumors (138). In one study, the observed frequency among black Americans was twenty times less than expected (135).

Nearly all Warthin tumors occur in the parotid gland or periparotid region. Most involve the tail of the gland, but about 10 percent occur in the deep lobe (170). The AFIP and others have found that tumors initially thought to have arisen in the submandibular gland arose instead in the anterior tail of the parotid or in periparotid lymph nodes (135,141). Rare examples have been reported in sites other than the parotid gland (114, 143,147,155,169,170).

Several pathogenetic theories for Warthin's tumor have been suggested. The very basis of this lesion as neoplastic has been challenged by the suggestion that it represents a metaplastic process with a secondary lymphoid reaction (112, 189). The most popular concept, however, is that it is a neoplasm that develops from heterotopic salivary ducts present within preexisting intraparotid or paraparotid lymphoid tissue (111). Its predilection for the parotid gland supports this proposal.

Unlike other salivary glands, the parotid normally contains lymphoid tissue in the form of either small intraglandular lymph nodes or small unorganized collections of lymphoid cells. Serial sections of the gland have revealed an average of 20 intraparotid lymph nodes (144) (see Normal Glands). Salivary gland tissue is often seen within lymph nodes, and this tissue occasionally gives rise to neoplasms, such as mixed tumor and mucoepidermoid carcinoma. Several studies have shown that as much as 8 percent of Warthin tumors occur in periparotid lymph nodes and that these are often found incidentally following neck dissection for an unrelated malignancy (120,135,200).

An alternative view is that Warthin's tumor is an epithelial neoplasm that incites a lymphocytic response. In support of this proposal is the finding that several other benign and malignant salivary gland tumors are occasionally similarly accompanied by a prominent tumor-associated lymphoid proliferation (113). The characteristic bilayered epithelial proliferation of Warthin's tumor occasionally occurs with only limited lymphoid tissue or there may be an abundant lymphoid element that unquestionably is not a lymph node. This suggests a dependent relationship between the two elements rather than coincidental intranodal occurrence. Cytogenetic abnormalities of the epithelial component have also been described (122, 173,174). An antigen-induced response is plausible (159,160) and perhaps is related to the increased incidence of these tumors in tobacco users.

Multicentric occurrence, synchronous or metachronous and unilateral or bilateral, is seen more often with Warthin's tumor than any other salivary gland tumor (152). About 12 percent of patients develop more than one tumor (135,170). In one series, as many as six separate tumor foci were reported in a single patient, and in about one quarter of the patients with multicentric tumors, the tumors were synchronous and bilateral (170). Overall, Warthin tumors are bilateral in 5 to 7.5 percent of patients (137,141,171,197).

Studies have shown a male to female ratio of 26 to 1 (172), 10 to 1 (146), and 5 to 1 (127). Recent studies claim a markedly reduced male predilection of between 1.1 to 1 and 1.6 to 1 (137,141,163, 170,184); this ratio is 1.2 to 1 among civilian patients at the AFIP. The apparent change in male predilection may be related to the etiologic role of tobacco smoking in the development of these tumors. Recent evidence strongly suggests that the increasing relative incidence of Warthin's tumor in women parallels their increased smoking (184,211) and incidence of pulmonary carcinoma (170). Compared to nonsmokers, smokers have eight times the risk of developing Warthin's tumor (168), and patients with Warthin's tumor are much heavier smokers than patients who develop mixed tumors (125). This knowledge may also explain a high incidence among certain patient populations that typically are heavy smokers (179).

In the AFIP material, the average patient age is 62 years and is nearly identical for both the civilian and military populations. Less than 6 percent of Warthin tumors occurred before the age of 40 years whereas over 60 percent occurred between the ages of 50 and 79 years. The average age of men and women is nearly identical, with a range of 29 to 88 years. This mean is similar to that in another study of American patients (135) but slightly younger than patients from the British Salivary Gland Tumor Panel (141).

Clinical Features. Most Warthin tumors present as a painless, sometimes fluctuant, swelling in the lower portion of the parotid gland. The tumors are normally 2 to 4 cm in diameter but they may achieve considerable size (209). Fluctuation sometimes suggests abscess or other inflammatory disorder. It has been suggested that rapid increase in size of a few tumors results from leakage of fluid into surrounding tissues and retrograde infection from the oral cavity through Stenson's duct (126). The constellation of acute onset of pain and a sudden increase in size has been referred to as the *papillary cystadenoma lymphomatosum syndrome* (118). According to Eveson and Cawson (141), the average duration of the tumor is 21 months, but over 40 percent are present less than 6 months. These investigators also note that pain, varying from mild to severe, is experienced by about 9 percent of patients. Ipsilateral ear symptoms, including earache, tinnitus, and deafness, also occur. Rarely, facial paralysis results from associated inflammation and fibrosis (133,190). Infection causes the tumor's borders to be indefinite when examined with magnetic resonance imaging (182).

Warthin's tumor has the ability to concentrate sodium pertechnetate (^{99m}Tc), making it amenable to scintigraphic examination (126,157,161,201,

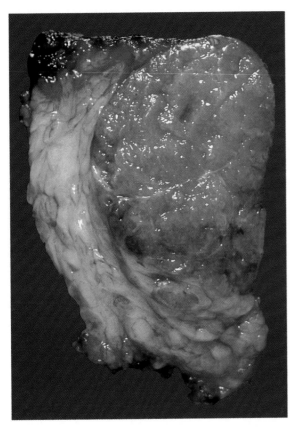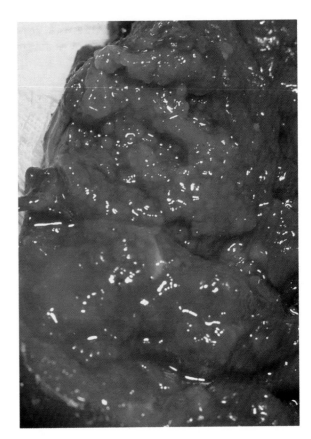

Figure 4-46
WARTHIN'S TUMOR

Left: This well-circumscribed bisected Warthin's tumor of the parotid gland is partially surrounded by a rim of salivary gland and fat. (Courtesy of Anatomic Pathology, Walter Reed Army Medical Center, Washington, DC.)

Right: Closer examination of a different tumor reveals several irregular cystic spaces that have small, papillary luminal excrescences and supporting lymphoid-rich stroma.

208). The uptake of ^{99m}Tc in Warthin tumors is greater than in normal gland and causes the tumor to appear as a "hot" lesion. In a study by Ishikawa and Ishii (161), mixed tumors and other benign and malignant salivary gland tumors showed no radionuclide uptake or, less often, the same uptake as normal gland. In contrast, Warthin tumors retain the radionuclide after stimulation with ascorbic acid. However, the peripheral region of most salivary gland tumors also retain radioactivity. Oncocytoma also has the ability to concentrate ^{99m}Tc, so this method of imaging, while highly suggestive of Warthin's tumor, is not pathognomonic.

Normal salivary glands and Warthin tumors also concentrate radioactive iodine, which is an important consideration in scintigraphy for metastatic thyroid carcinoma (124,183,199).

Gross Findings. Warthin's tumor is usually spherical to ovoid and nearly always well circumscribed unless secondarily inflamed. The cut surface of the tumor reveals a variable number of cysts that exude clear, mucoid, or brown fluid, or caseous semisolid debris (207). The cysts vary from small slit-like spaces to those that are several centimeters and occupy a considerable proportion of the entire lesion (fig. 4-46). The lining of the cysts have small, knob-like excrescences that represent the papillary epithelial proliferation supported by lymphoid tissue. The intercystic areas are composed of small tan to white nodular foci and, occasionally, contain focal hemorrhage. When the tumor has been fixed, the coagulated contents of the cysts have a rubbery consistency. Parotidectomy specimens should be examined thoroughly for separate tumor foci.

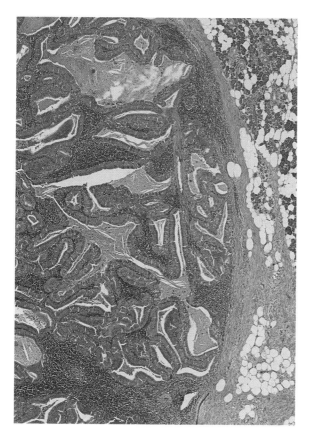

Figure 4-47
WARTHIN'S TUMOR

A thin capsule separates this tumor from the surrounding parotid tissue. The typical bilayered oncocytic epithelium lines numerous fluid-containing cystic spaces and has closely associated foci of lymphoid tissue. There are no features in this case to suggest the tumor occurred in a lymph node.

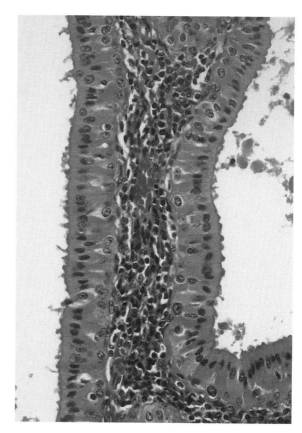

Figure 4-48
BILAYERED ONCOCYTIC EPITHELIUM

The luminal columnar cells are uniformly orientated and have palisaded and slightly hyperchromatic nuclei. The basal cells appear less numerous, have round to ovoid nuclei with small but distinct nucleoli, and have ill-defined cytoplasmic borders.

Microscopic Findings. The term papillary cystadenoma lymphomatosum is a descriptively accurate designator for this tumor. The tumor is characterized by cystic spaces lined by a papillary proliferation of bilayered oncocytic epithelium whose supporting stroma is composed largely of lymphoid tissue. Warthin tumors have thin capsules and are usually sharply demarcated from surrounding parenchyma (fig. 4-47). If the tumor occurs in a lymph node, there should be a capsule, subcapsular sinus, paracortical or medullary areas, and afferent and efferent lymphatics. The inner aspect of the capsular sinus has an endothelial lining.

The luminal epithelium is composed of tall columnar cells that often show palisading of their ovoid nuclei, which are in the centers or apical ends of the cells (fig. 4-48). In many cases the bilayered epithelium is focally disrupted by round to ovoid cells that are several layers thick and sometimes contain scattered mucous cells (fig. 4-49). The cytoplasm is finely granular and brightly eosinophilic but in some cases there is variation in its staining intensity. The cytoplasmic borders are easily delineated. The granularity is due to abundant mitochondria, which may be verified with use of the phosphotungstic acid–hematoxylin stain or electron microscopy. The luminal surface of these cells demonstrates apocrine-like secretions in the form of small protuberances, and cilia have been reported (141). The lumens typically contain secretions that are admixed with cellular debris and, sometimes, laminated bodies that resemble corpora amylacea (fig. 4-50) (132,141).

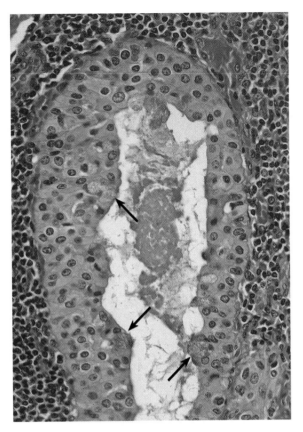

Figure 4-49
SQUAMOUS AND MUCOUS METAPLASIA
OF LINING EPITHELIUM
Scattered mucous cells (arrows) are evident within the thickened epithelium that has lost its characteristic bilayered, columnar appearance. Many of the polygonal cells have a squamous appearance and sharply demarcated cytoplasmic borders.

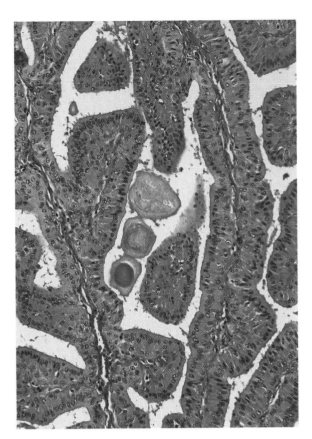

Figure 4-50
INTRACYSTIC CALCIFICATIONS
The cysts of some Warthin tumors contain calcified structures that often have a laminated appearance. In this example it appears that there is progressive inspissation and condensation of the three small pools of fluid, possibly indicating the mechanism for the formation of the calcifications.

Beneath and between the columnar cells are less obvious, smaller basaloid cells. They often are triangular, but occasionally have fusiform nuclei arranged perpendicular to the long axis of the tall columnar cells. These cells may appear contiguous for short distances but are more haphazardly arranged than the luminal cells. Their cytoplasm has a fine granularity that is similar to that of the columnar cells, but it is much less abundant and its borders are less distinct.

The epithelium forms variably sized and shaped papillae that project into the luminal spaces. Fibrovascular connective tissue supports the epithelial papillations, but often this tissue is obscured by the dense lymphoid element that is composed of small uniform lymphocytes (fig. 4-51). In over half of the tumors, well-formed germinal centers and mantle zones are present. Mast cells are often scattered throughout the lymphoid stroma and plasma cells are usually present.

The proportion of the epithelial and lymphoid components varies among different tumors and within the same tumor (fig. 4-52), and is dependent on whether or not nodal tissue is evident (fig. 4-53). In order to emphasize these variations, some investigators subclassify Warthin's tumor into *typical* (epithelial component of 50 percent), *stroma-poor* (epithelial component of 70 to 80 percent), *stroma-rich* (epithelial component of 20 to 30 percent, and *metaplastic* forms (197). These investigators found that 77 percent of Warthin tumors were typical, 14 percent stroma-poor, 2 percent stroma-rich, and 8 percent metaplastic.

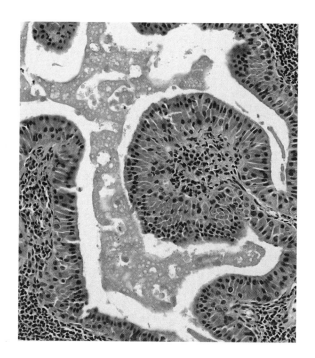
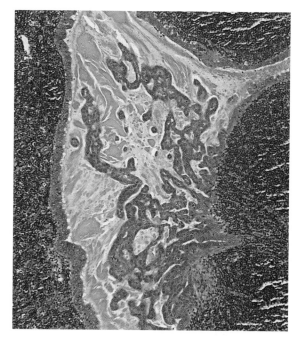

Figure 4-51
PAPILLARY GROWTH
Left: The intraluminal papilla has a covering of characteristic bilayered epithelium and is supported by lymphoid stroma.
The abundant intraluminal secretions show artifactual shrinkage.
Right: Slightly more complex papillae are seen.

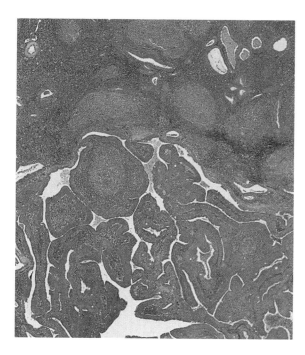
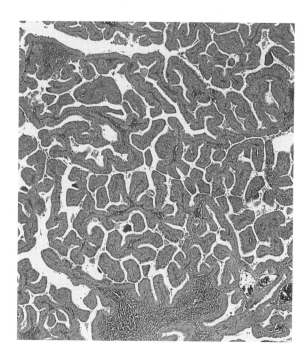

Figure 4-52
VARIATION IN PROPORTION OF LYMPHOID STROMA
Left: This Warthin's tumor reveals a predominance of lymphoid stroma in one portion and a paucity of it in another. In both
areas follicles with germinal centers are evident.
Right: This tumor had abundant lymphoid tissue in some peripheral areas, but in most areas the tissue was limited to
small focal collections, as seen in this illustration.

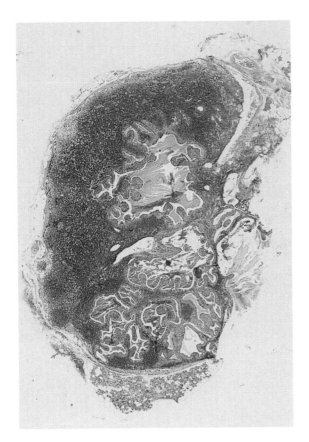
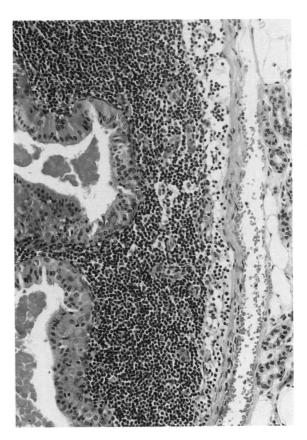

Figure 4-53
INTRANODAL WARTHIN'S TUMOR
Left: This tumor appeared to have developed within a lymph node.
Right: In some portions a capsule and subcapsular sinus that was partially lined by endothelium were evident.

Other variations from the characteristic microscopic features are numerous and involve both the epithelial and lymphoid components. Focal squamous metaplasia of the epithelium may be evident. The epithelial lining of the cystic structures may demonstrate focal oncocytosis characterized by replacement of the bilayered columnar lining with nodular collections of closely packed oncocytes, which may also be seen in adjacent parotid gland. Most striking are tumors that exhibit necrosis, squamous and mucous metaplasia, fibrosis, and acute and chronic inflammation. The typical epithelial and stromal features are sometimes obscured by these secondary changes (fig. 4-54) and result in the need to examine additional sections of the specimen. In some cases most or all of the tumor is infarcted (fig. 4-55), which is sometimes secondary to fine-needle aspiration and can be associated clinically with facial weakness (164,188). Focally prominent granulomatous inflammation may be associated with Langhans type giant cells or with cholesterol granulomas (142). The cytologic and architectural atypia of the metaplastic changes occasionally simulate squamous cell or mucoepidermoid carcinoma (203), but there is a lack of frank cytomorphologically malignant changes and infiltrative growth (fig. 4-56).

In rare cases carcinoma may arise from the epithelial component of Warthin's tumor. The most common type of carcinoma ex Warthin tumor at the AFIP and in published studies is squamous cell carcinoma (115,117,130,178,186), but mucoepidermoid carcinoma (149), oncocytic adenocarcinoma (119,204), undifferentiated carcinomas (121,165,185), and other forms (187, 191,192) have been reported. Of the cases reported, one third metastasized to regional nodes,

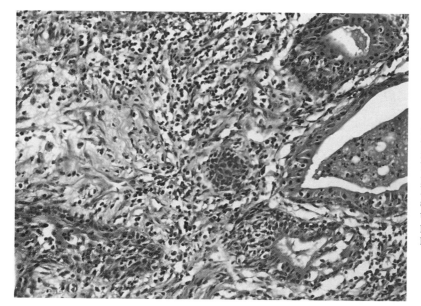

Figure 4-54
WARTHIN'S TUMOR WITH
INFLAMMATORY CHANGES

Chronic inflammation in this case resulted in loss of many diagnostic features. In this field the epithelium has focally retained its oncocytic appearance but also shows squamous metaplasia and proliferation of small solid epithelial islands. Mild fibrosis and edema of the stroma as well as an inflammatory infiltrate, including eosinophils, have replaced much of the characteristic lymphoid element.

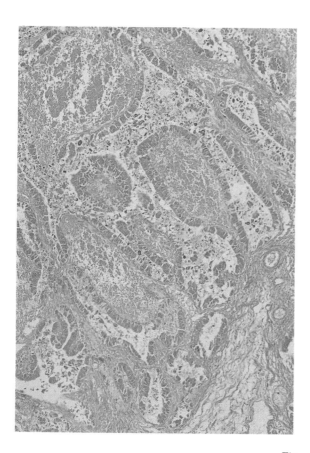

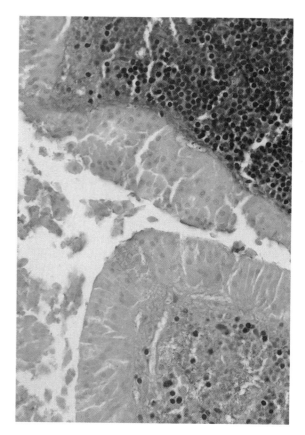

Figure 4-55
INFARCTED WARTHIN'S TUMOR

Left: While only vaguely evident, the characteristic architectural epithelial features are maintained in this area of an otherwise completely necrotic and unrecognizable lesion. The lymphoid component is also necrotic.

Right: Higher magnification of a different example shows that necrotic epithelium is associated with both viable and necrotic lymphoid tissue.

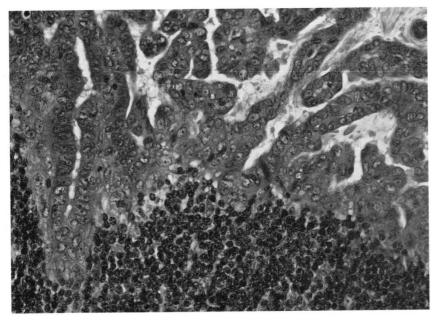

Figure 4-56
ATYPICAL EPITHELIUM
IN WARTHIN'S TUMOR
The epithelial component in this Warthin's tumor focally reveals enlarged, somewhat variable nuclei with prominent nucleoli and relatively disorganized papillary growth.

and a single case had distant metastasis (165, 204). Occasionally, microscopic sections fortuitously show atypical lining epithelium that indicates malignant transformation (fig. 4-57). More often, in patients with a carcinoma adjacent to a Warthin's tumor, the lack of definitive evidence of malignant transformation of the benign tumor leads to consideration that the carcinoma represents a coexistent second neoplasm or metastatic disease. Multiple sections may reveal the area of transformation.

Equally rare are those instances in which malignant lymphoma comprises a portion of the lymphoid element of a Warthin's tumor. The lymphomatous infiltrate is recognized by its striking monomorphic appearance and distortion of the characteristic epithelial and lymphoid architecture (fig. 4-58). As in other sites, immunohistologic or gene rearrangement studies provide confirmatory evidence for the diagnosis (116,123,128,153, 154,180,181). Some patients have involvement of other sites at the time of diagnosis (180), but in a minority of cases the staging results support a primary origin in Warthin's tumor (151,154,181). Even in some of these studies, however, nodal lymphoma was discovered less than 1 year following parotidectomy. As with any malignant lymphoma that presents first in the parotid gland (see Malignant Lymphoma), the patient must be evaluated for involvement of other sites.

Immunohistochemical and Ultrastructural Findings. The immunoreactivities of luminal and basal epithelia are not identical: the cytokeratin polypeptide complement of the two cell populations differ (131), and the neoplastic cells react differently for carcinoembryonic antigen, secretory component, and lactoferrin (195). Neither type of epithelium is reactive for vimentin, GFAP, or polyclonal S-100 protein (131,195). Reactivity with monoclonal anti-S-100 protein, principally S-100-alpha, has been noted (158).

Electron microscopy reveals that both the luminal and basal cells have an abundance of mitochondria, but the basal cells appear more electron dense (fig. 4-59) (131,162). The basal cells have more prominent tonofilament bundles and more numerous desmosomal attachments to both other basal cells and the overlying luminal cells.

Immunohistochemical studies have been performed in an attempt to determine whether the lymphoid stroma represents normal lymph node, a reaction to neoplastic epithelium, a typical immune response of exocrine glands, or a combination of these. Unfortunately, these studies have shown conflicting results. Some investigators have concluded that the stroma is composed predominantly of T cells with scattered polyclonal B cells, suggesting normal nodal tissue with reactive lymphoid areas (134). Other studies have concluded that the lymphoid element essentially represents

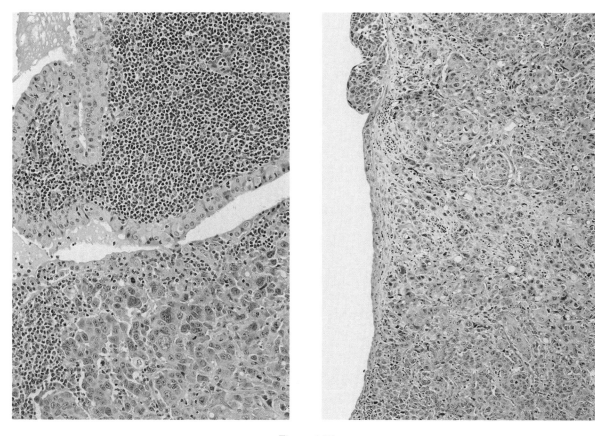

Figure 4-57
SQUAMOUS CELL CARCINOMA IN WARTHIN'S TUMOR
Left: Warthin's tumor has characteristic epithelial and lymphoid components but, in addition, has an associated squamous cell carcinoma.
Right: In some areas the carcinoma was covered by lining epithelium that demonstrated atypical proliferative activity, although unequivocal malignant transformation was not found.

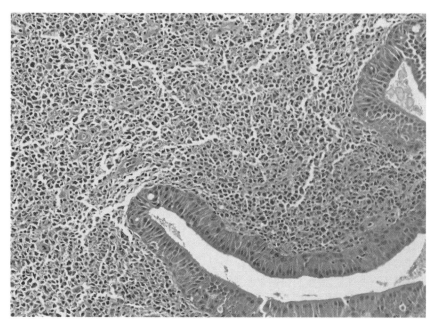

Figure 4-58
MALIGNANT LYMPHOMA
IN WARTHIN'S TUMOR
The lymphoid stroma in this Warthin's tumor has been replaced by a monomorphic lymphomatous infiltrate. The characteristic bilayered appearance of the epithelium is maintained.

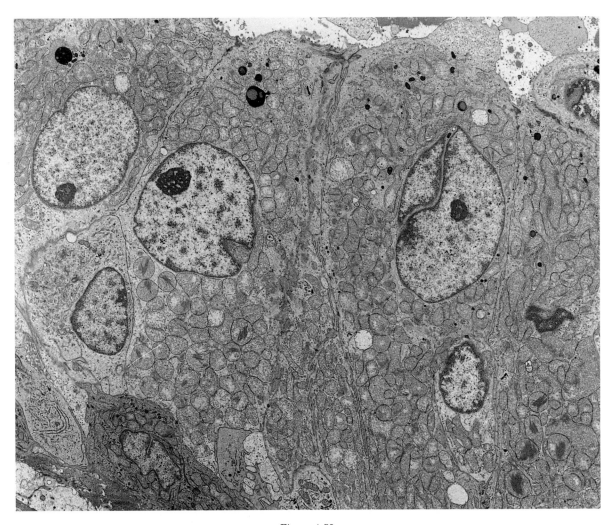

Figure 4-59
ULTRASTRUCTURE OF EPITHELIUM IN WARTHIN'S TUMOR
The cytoplasm of the tall columnar cells that line the lumen, seen at the top, and the flattened basal cell (lower left) is packed with mitochondria. The basal cells often show increased electron density. (Courtesy of Dr. Irving Dardick, Toronto, Canada.)

a reactive lymphoid proliferation, perhaps in response to, or modulated by, the epithelium (129, 194,196,206). The finding that more immunoglobulin-producing cells contain IgG than IgA supports an immune response of lymphoid tissue rather than a secretory immune response of an exocrine gland (166,167,176), but those who have demonstrated a predominance of IgA-containing plasma cells contend that the lymphoid stroma represents an exaggerated, antigen-independent, secretory immune response (159,210). The presence of follicular dendritic cells has led to speculation that they have an important immunologic role in Warthin's tumor (176).

Differential Diagnosis. The epithelial and lymphoid elements are so characteristic in typical examples of Warthin's tumor that other lesions are not usually considered in the differential diagnosis. It is helpful to recognize that Warthin's tumor often demonstrates focal variations, such as oncocytic hyperplasia and squamous metaplasia, and shows a widely variable proportion of epithelial and lymphoid components. Difficulty occurs when: 1) other salivary gland lesions have a papillary oncocytic epithelial component; 2) Warthin tumors show severe secondary reactive changes; and 3) other epithelial lesions have abundant lymphoid tissue associated

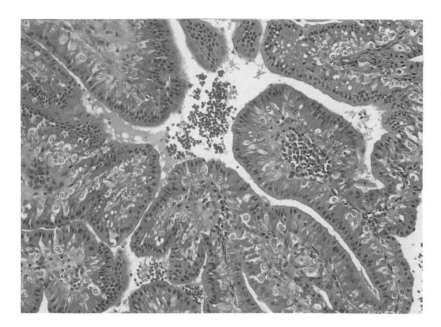

Figure 4-60
PAPILLARY ONCOCYTIC
CYSTADENOMA
The epithelium in this rare
form of cystadenoma closely mimics that of Warthin's tumor but
lacks the accompanying lymphoid
proliferation. A small collection of
chronic inflammatory cells is seen
within a papilla.

with them. Diagnostic errors would most likely result in significant therapeutic consequences in the last situation.

The salivary gland tumor whose epithelial component is cytologically and architecturally most similar to Warthin's tumor is the occasional cystadenoma composed of papillary oncocytic epithelium. Unlike Warthin's tumor, papillary oncocytic cystadenoma usually arises from minor glands rather than the parotid, and lacks a well-organized lymphoid element (fig. 4-60).

Infarcted and necrotic Warthin tumors that are accompanied by fibrosis and squamous and mucinous metaplasia need to be distinguished from squamous cell or mucoepidermoid carcinoma. Recognition of the outlines of necrotic intracystic papillae formed by tall columnar and basal cells can be diagnostic. Minimal cytomorphologic atypia may be present, but the strands and islands of metaplastic epithelium fail to infiltrate adjacent parenchyma.

In addition to Warthin's tumor, parotid lesions that have a prominent lymphoid element and cystic configuration include lymphoepithelial cysts, acquired immunodeficiency syndrome (AIDS)–related lymphadenopathy with multiple cysts, lymphadenoma, metastatic carcinoma, and tumor-associated lymphoid proliferation in mucoepidermoid carcinoma, acinic cell adenocarcinoma, and cystadenocarcinoma (113). The epithelium of these lesions does not show the characteristic bilayered epithelium of Warthin's tumor. Parotid duct cysts sometimes demonstrate papillary epithelial proliferation and focal sialadenitis but not the dense lymphoid stroma of Warthin's tumor. An abundant lymphoid response in any benign or malignant salivary gland may obscure their characteristic features and complicate interpretation (fig. 4-61).

Treatment. Studies of Warthin's tumor have reported recurrence rates as high as 12 to 25 percent (148,150), but most recent studies indicate a rate of 2 percent or less (136,137,141,156, 197). Some recurrences probably represent multifocal occurrence rather than true recurrence. Because of the propensity of Warthin's tumor to develop multifocal lesions, wide surgical exposure and careful inspection and palpation of parotid gland and periparotid tissues is recommended (170). Concern for multifocal tumor has even led some investigators to recommend total parotidectomy (150). In order to reduce the risk of facial nerve paralysis and Frey's syndrome, other investigators recommend enucleation in cases in which the diagnosis is known preoperatively and the location is amenable to such a procedure (137,156). Using this approach, these investigators report that less than 2 percent of tumors recur.

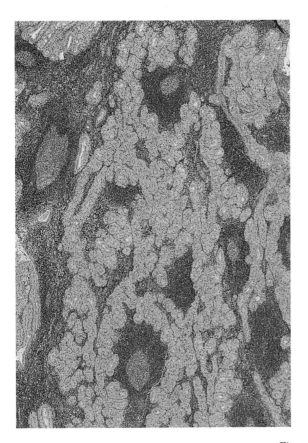 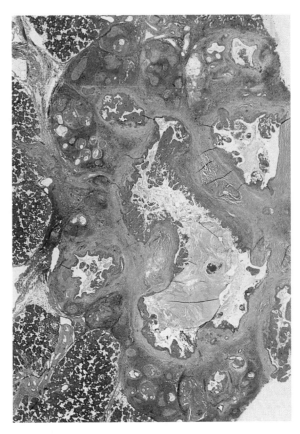

Figure 4-61

SALIVARY GLAND TUMORS WITH TUMOR-ASSOCIATED LYMPHOID PROLIFERATION

Left: This oncocytoma shows a considerable lymphoid element. The typical solid growth of oncocytoma is seen with some of the numerous neoplastic nests having small lumens. Papillary cystic growth is not evident in this tumor.

Right: Papillary cystic growth is obvious in this mucoepidermoid carcinoma which has a substantial peripheral lymphoid response. The cystic structures are lined by epidermoid, mucous, and intermediate-type cells rather than the bilayered oncocytic epithelium of Warthin's tumor.

BASAL CELL ADENOMA

Definition. Basal cell adenoma is a benign epithelial neoplasm with a uniform, monomorphous histologic appearance that is dominated by basaloid cells and is without the myxochondroid tissue characteristic of mixed tumor. The arrangement of the tumor cells is categorized as solid, trabecular, tubular, or membranous or dermal analogue type.

Confusion and disagreement about the terminology and the spectrum of tumors that properly belong within this group of tumors has existed since their designation by Kleinsasser and Klein in 1967 (240). Other terms that have been associated with this group of tumors include *tubular adenoma, trabecular adenoma, dermal analogue tumor, canalicular adenoma, basaloid adenoma, clear cell adenoma,* and *monomorphic adenoma.* The term monomorphic adenoma was originally proposed as a general category to encompass all varieties of salivary gland adenomas other than mixed tumors (pleomorphic adenomas) (232). Unfortunately, many published investigations of monomorphic adenomas have not adequately identified the various histologic types within this heterogeneous group so that conclusions about the clinicopathologic parameters of each type are not possible from these reports (218,228,229,238, 245,250,257,258,265,266). This amalgamation of various histopathologic types of adenoma is probably a result of the 1972 World Health Organization (WHO) monograph on the histologic typing of salivary gland tumors (263) in which there were two categories of adenoma: pleomorphic and monomorphic. Within the category of monomorphic adenoma, the WHO monograph listed Warthin's tumor, oncocytoma, and "other types." Without clear definitions of the "other" types, many pathologists began using the term monomorphic adenoma as a specific diagnostic entity. The more recent WHO monograph (256) on the classification of salivary gland tumors, published in late 1991, no longer uses monomorphic adenoma as a diagnostic category. Instead, it classifies a variety of specific types of adenomas, including basal cell adenoma.

Adding further confusion to our understanding of basal cell adenoma, some investigators lump basaloid and canalicular types of tumors into a single category of basal cell adenoma (216, 230,242,247,267), while others segregate these tumors into basal cell adenoma and canalicular adenoma (221,232,241). This Fascicle conforms to the WHO's preference and segregates these two entities (256). A comparison of the data presented below with that in the section on canalicular adenoma indicates different site predilections as well as different histopathologic features for these two adenoma types.

Despite some confusion about the nosology of these tumors, it should be remembered that these are benign adenomas, and whether they are called monomorphic adenoma, basal cell adenoma, canalicular adenoma, or another term, therapy is essentially the same.

General Features. As just described, previous disparity in the classification and reporting of basal cell adenomas in the literature makes it difficult to derive meaningful data. An incidence of 2 percent of all primary salivary gland tumors is often cited (227). Maurizi et al. (246) had an incidence of about 4 percent in a series reported from Italy. In a report on the Japanese experience, Nagao et al. (249) reported the incidence of basal cell adenomas as 7.5 percent among parotid gland neoplasms, while Takahashi et al. (262) found an incidence of 1.0 percent among intraoral minor salivary gland tumors. In a series of 426 intraoral salivary gland tumors in the United States, Waldron et al. (267) found 13 (3 percent) basal cell type adenomas. However, they also identified 7 tumors with overlapping basal cell and canalicular features. In the files of the British Salivary Gland Tumour Panel, Eveson and Cawson (229)

found that 11 percent of intraoral tumors were monomorphic adenomas, but they provided no breakdown of the various histologic types. A South African study (238) reported similar results but, again, without identifying the specific types of monomorphic adenoma. In the registry of salivary gland tumors at the AFIP, basal cell adenomas, excluding canalicular adenomas, comprise 1.5 percent of all epithelial salivary gland neoplasms and 2.4 percent of all benign epithelial tumors.

Although several reports state that a large portion of monomorphic adenomas or basal cell adenomas occur in the upper lip, most of these tumors are canalicular adenomas (229,230,242, 247,267). When canalicular adenoma is distinguished from basal cell adenoma, the parotid gland is the dominant site of occurrence of the basal cell adenoma (216). In the AFIP's data, over 75 percent occur in the parotid gland while 5 percent arise in the submandibular gland. The upper lip is the most common intraoral location, but only about 6 percent develop in this site.

Basal cell adenomas are tumors of adults: the only case recorded in the AFIP files in a child occurred in an infant. In retrospect, this tumor would be more appropriately classified as the newly defined sialoblastoma (see section on Sialoblastoma). Seifert et al. (255) also reported a virtual absence of monomorphic adenomas in children in the Salivary Gland Register at the University of Hamburg, Germany. The mean age of patients is 58 years, with a small peak incidence in the seventh decade of life, which is an older population than patients with mixed tumors. There is about a 2 to 1 predominance of women over men at the AFIP when the male bias of military patients is eliminated. Batsakis and Brannon (214), in a series that included cases from the AFIP files, and others (216,244) have commented on the marked predominance of men among patients with the membranous type of basal cell adenoma (dermal analogue tumor; see discussion below) as compared with other types of basal cell adenomas, but recent experience at the AFIP has shown an equal distribution among men and women for this subtype of basal cell adenoma.

There is a notable histologic similarity between dermal eccrine tumors (eccrine spiradenoma and cylindroma) and basal cell adenomas, and a diathesis of skin eccrine tumors and basal cell adenomas of the parotid gland has been observed in many patients by several investigators (214, 215,231,233,236,237,244,253,254) and at the AFIP. One report documents bilateral basal cell adenomas of the parotid glands in a patient with the diathesis who had several family members with similar skin tumors (270). Most of the basal cell adenomas associated with the diathesis have been of the membranous type, and most of the skin tumors have been dermal cylindromas. Because of the histologic similarity to and synchronous occurrence with dermal cylindromas, Batsakis and Brannon (214) designated the parotid tumors *dermal analogue tumors,* although Headington et al. (236) who were the first to describe the diathesis, used the term *membranous basal cell adenoma.* In addition, trichoepitheliomas, spiradenomas, trichilemmomas, and basal cell epitheliomas have been reported in patients with the diathesis (233,236,253,254).

Clinical Features. Typical of most types of adenoma of the salivary glands, the signs and symptoms commonly associated with basal cell adenoma are few. Swelling is the most constant finding. Like mixed tumors, most basal cell adenomas are single, well-defined nodules at presentation; the membranous type is an exception as many are multifocal. The tumors are usually firm to hard although an occasional tumor is cystic and more compressible. The tumors are usually movable by palpation unless they are located in the hard palate.

Gross Findings. With the exception of some of the membranous type basal cell adenomas that are multinodular or multifocal, these tumors are typically sharply circumscribed, and most are less than 3.0 cm in diameter at the time of excision (fig. 4-62), although much larger tumors have been excised. In the parotid gland, their most common location, they are usually in the superficial portion of the lateral lobe, and a well-defined capsule is usually evident. In fact, some surgeons have mistaken these tumors for lymph nodes. Intraoral tumors are also well circumscribed, but encapsulation is less often grossly apparent. The color of the cut surface is usually uniform and gray-white, tan-white, pink-red, or brown. The texture is also usually homogeneous, but some tumors are cystic.

Microscopic Findings. For several years following the initial description of this category of tumors by Kleinsasser and Klein (240), many

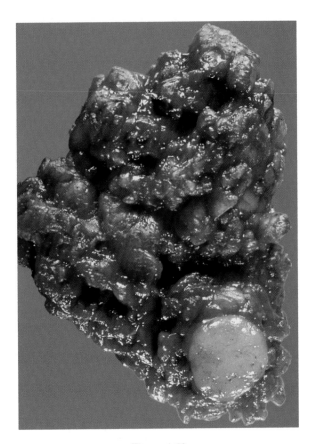

Figure 4-62
BASAL CELL ADENOMA
This gross specimen of the superficial (lateral) lobe of the parotid gland shows a basal cell adenoma near the inferior pole that is a well-circumscribed mass.

reviewers erroneously interpreted the "monomorphous" appearance to indicate isomorphism of the epithelial cell type and absence of myoepithelial differentiation (213,217,219,220,227, 264,269). More recent evaluations, including electron microscopic and immunohistochemical studies, have shown that basal, ductal, and myoepithelial cell differentiation occurs to variable degrees in basal cell adenomas just as in most other types of salivary gland tumors (212,223, 225,239,252,259–261,268,270). The monomorphous character of these tumors is a result of more or less uniform, monotonous growth patterns with an absence of the myxochondroid type tissue of mixed tumors. In contrast to other types of so-called monomorphic adenomas, basal cell adenomas have a predominance of basaloid cells. It is convenient to use the term basaloid cell in terms of routine light microscopy because it

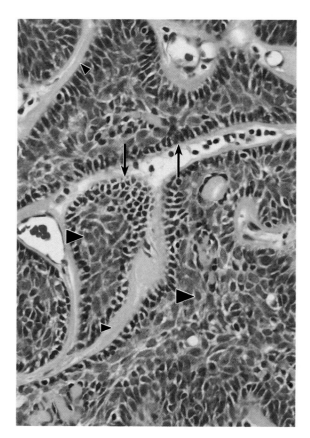

Figure 4-63
BASAL CELL ADENOMA, MEMBRANOUS TYPE
The tumor is composed of cells of two morphologic forms. Some cells, which are mostly located toward the periphery of the epithelial islands, have small, very basophilic nuclei and scant cytoplasm and impart a deeply basophilic (dark) appearance to the tissue in which they are aggregated (arrows). More numerous are larger cells with large, pale-staining nuclei (large arrowheads). Eosinophilic hyaline material is adjacent to the tumor islands (small arrowheads).

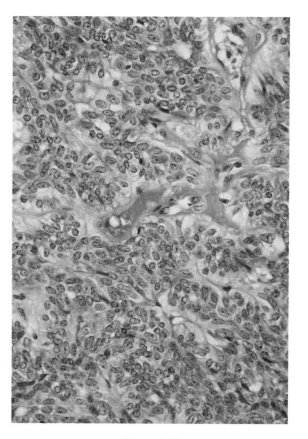

Figure 4-64
BASAL CELL ADENOMA
This field from a solid and trabecular tumor is composed exclusively of larger, lighter staining basaloid cells, some of which have one or two small basophilic nucleoli.

avoids having to determine whether particular cells are actually basal cells, myoepithelial cells, or ductal cells, which can often be difficult in these tumors without special studies such as electron microscopy or immunohistochemistry.

In basal cell adenoma the basaloid cells frequently have two morphologic appearances: dark cells and light cells (fig. 4-63). Both types are typically uniform small cells with pale eosinophilic to amphophilic cytoplasm, indistinct cell borders, and round to oval nuclei. The dark cells have less cytoplasm and more basophilic nuclei than the light cells, and thus give the tissue a more basophilic appearance when they occur in aggregates. The nuclei of the larger light cells are pale baso-

philic, and some contain one or more small basophilic nucleoli (fig. 4-64). The light cells usually predominate, and the dark cells are often clustered near the peripheral stromal interface of the epithelial nests. In many tumors, there is palisading of the nuclei of the epithelial cells along the stromal interface (fig. 4-65).

While basaloid cells predominate, cuboidal ductal cells that surround small lumens are evident in most basal cell adenomas (fig. 4-66). They are most conspicuous in the tubular subtype (see below).

Kleinsasser and Klein (240) described solid, trabecular, and tubular patterns for basal cell adenomas, and with the addition of the subsequently identified membranous type these are still appropriate conceptualizations for the microscopic growth characteristics. Any single tumor may have more than one of these growth

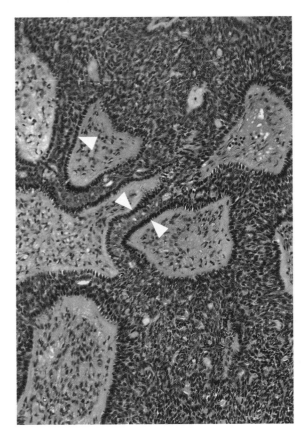

Figure 4-65
BASAL CELL ADENOMA
The palisading of the nuclei of epithelial cells along the stromal interface (arrowheads) is especially prominent in this solid type basal cell adenoma.

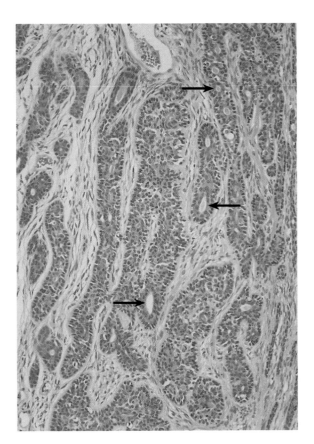

Figure 4-66
BASAL CELL ADENOMA
Several small duct lumens (arrows) that are bordered by cuboidal ductal cells are evident among the basaloid cells in this basal cell adenoma.

patterns, but most basal cell adenomas can be subtyped into one of these categories based on the predominant pattern. Except for the membranous type, identification of the specific subtype is for recognition purposes only and does not imply any predicable biologic behavior (see Behavior and Treatment below).

A solid pattern is characterized by varying sized and shaped aggregates of epithelial tumor cells that are separated from adjacent aggregates by varying amounts of stromal tissue. The tumor cells are arranged as large sheets or nodules; small, closely approximated nodules; separated, small nodules (an insular appearance); or irregular-shaped, sometimes anastomosing, broad bands (fig. 4-67). Within sheets or large aggregates of basaloid cells, foci of epidermoid-appearing cells can sometimes be found. These foci tend to be circular and can be described as squamous whorls

or "eddies." Occasionally, these squamous eddies are even keratinized (fig. 4-67A). The stroma associated with the solid type is usually moderately dense to very dense collagenous tissue.

The trabecular type is evinced by an interlacing network of narrow bands of basaloid cells. Palisading of the epithelial nuclei along the stromal interface is evident less frequently than in the solid type, and small dark cells are typically fewer (fig. 4-68). The bands of basaloid cells are punctuated by a few or many small cysts or ductal lumens in some tumors (fig. 4-69). Because of this, some investigators have preferred to consider the trabecular and tubular types as one tubulotrabecular type (216). The stroma in these tumors is often less densely collagenous than in the solid type and is sometimes very loose with only a few thin strands of collagen (fig. 4-69). This pattern most closely resembles canalicular adenoma and is one reason

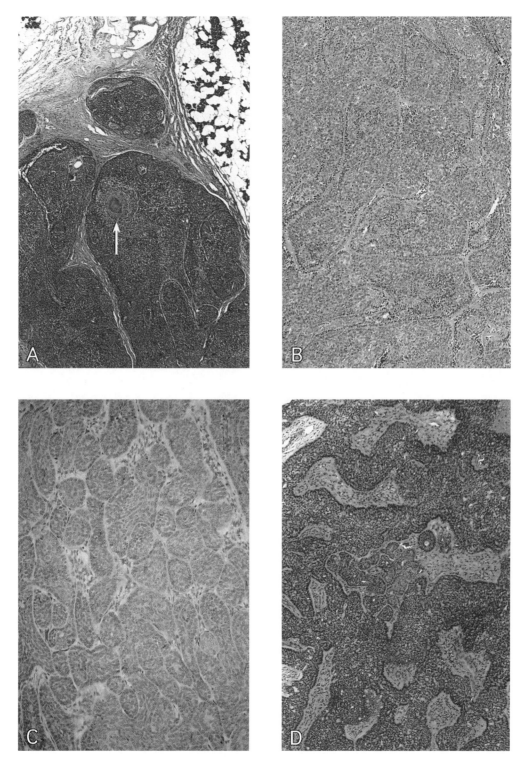

Figure 4-67
BASAL CELL ADENOMAS, SOLID TYPE

In the so-called solid type of basal cell adenoma the basaloid epithelial cells form large irregular-shaped sheets (A); smaller, closely apposed, varying sized nests (B); small, slightly separated nodules in an insular pattern (C); or irregular, thick, anastomosing bands (D). In A, areas of apparent epidermoid differentiation are recognized as focal whorls or "eddies" of squamous cells (arrow).

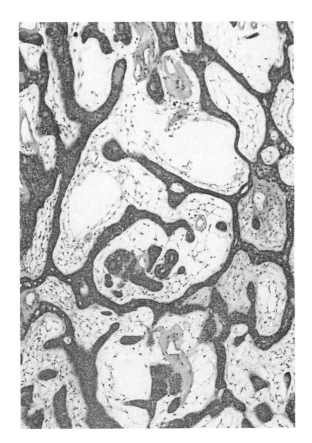 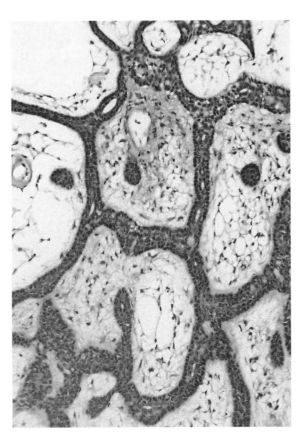

Figure 4-68
BASAL CELL ADENOMA, TRABECULAR TYPE

Left: Narrow, anastomosing cords of uniform basaloid epithelial cells are evident in this low-magnification photomicrograph.

Right: At higher magnification the interconnecting cords of basaloid cells are uniform, and some peripheral palisading of epithelial cell nuclei is evident.

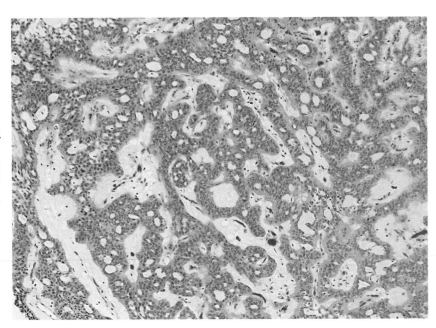

Figure 4-69
BASAL CELL ADENOMA,
TRABECULAR TYPE

Many small lumens are evident within the trabecular cords of basaloid cells in this tumor. This microscopic growth pattern has been termed tubulotrabecular. In contrast to the solid and membranous patterns, the stroma associated with the trabecular pattern is often loose, scantily collagenous tissue.

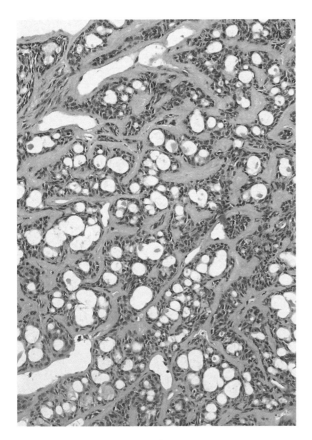

Figure 4-70
BASAL CELL ADENOMA, TUBULAR TYPE
Many small lumens that are lined by ductal or basaloid cells characterize the tubular pattern. One to several layers of basaloid cells are arranged peripheral to the lumens.

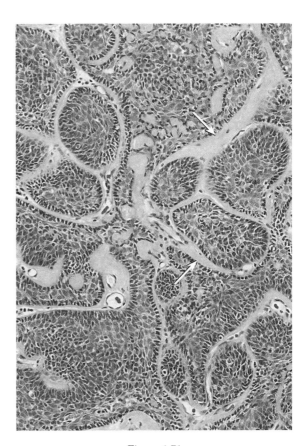

Figure 4-71
BASAL CELL ADENOMA, MEMBRANOUS TYPE
Conspicuous hyaline membranes of basal lamina (arrows) surround and separate irregular-shaped nests of basaloid cells.

why some authors prefer to include canalicular adenoma as a subtype of basal cell adenoma. However, the predominant cell and growth morphology, as well as certain clinical features, are distinct enough to consider canalicular adenoma separate from basal cell adenoma (see Canalicular Adenoma).

Duct cell differentiation is most prominent in the tubular type, which is the least common type of basal cell adenoma. Lumens are often bordered by cuboidal ductal cells, and peripheral to the ductal cells are one to several layers of basaloid cells (fig. 4-70). These epithelial aggregations are sometimes tightly arranged with little intervening stroma.

The most characteristic feature of the membranous type basal cell adenoma, or dermal analogue tumor, is the production of a conspicuous amount of basal lamina that is recognized as an eosinophilic, PAS-positive hyaline material. This hyaline material forms thick bands at the periphery of the basaloid cell islands (figs. 4-63, 4-71). The pattern of closely aggregated nests of tumor cells surrounded by hyaline has been described as "jigsaw puzzle"-like. In addition, small droplets of hyaline material, which sometimes appear to coalesce, often are present intercellularly within the tumor aggregates (fig. 4-72). However, this hyaline material is not pathognomonic of membranous basal cell adenoma. Occasional foci of hyaline can be observed in some solid types of basal cell adenoma, and the PAS stain can sometimes highlight thin bands of hyaline at the periphery of tumor nests that are inconspicuous with hematoxylin and eosin stain (fig. 4-73). The stroma associated with membranous basal cell adenoma is usually densely collagenous. Diathesis of membranous basal cell

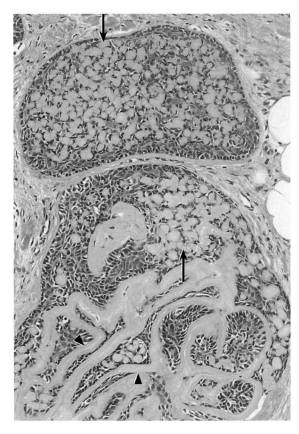

Figure 4-72
BASAL CELL ADENOMA, MEMBRANOUS TYPE
In addition to the prominent linear hyaline membranes (arrowheads) around tumor nests, multiple, small, round, intercellular hyaline droplets (arrows) are present within the epithelial islands.

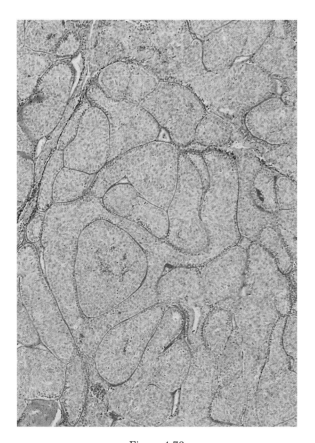

Figure 4-73
BASAL CELL ADENOMA, SOLID TYPE
Periodic acid–Schiff stain highlights the thin layer of basal lamina material around tumor cell nests that was relatively inconspicuous with hematoxylin and eosin stain.

adenoma and dermal cylindroma has been noted, and these two tumors are histologically similar (fig. 4-74).

For most basal cell adenomas, low magnification microscopic examination generally confirms the clinical and gross examination finding of a circumscribed and encapsulated tumor in the parotid gland (fig. 4-75). The membranous subtype is an exception and is frequently multinodular; however, other patterns of basal cell adenoma are occasionally multifocal (fig. 4-76). This multifocal growth should not be misinterpreted as malignant behavior (216); however, there are basaloid tumors that demonstrate invasive growth and other characteristics that indicate a more aggressive behavior (see Basal Cell Adenocarcinoma). Cystic degeneration within basal cell adenomas varies from none to, rarely, marked (fig. 4-77).

Immunohistochemical and Electron Microscopic Findings. Immunohistochemical staining of formalin-fixed and paraffin-embedded tissue sections of basal cell adenoma is quite variable from one tumor to another (fig. 4-78), and different investigators have obtained varying results (235,251,252,261,268). Cytokeratin is demonstrable in nearly all tumors, but the number of reactive cells varies from few to many. Similarly, immunoreactivity to S-100 protein, smooth muscle actin (SMA), and vimentin can be demonstrated in most basal cell adenomas but is typically localized to the peripheral tumor cells adjacent to the connective tissue stroma (222, 235,251,268). SMA and vimentin are considered indicative of myoepithelial differentiation. Morinaga et al. (248) have reported focal reactivity for myosin. Williams et al. (268) have even

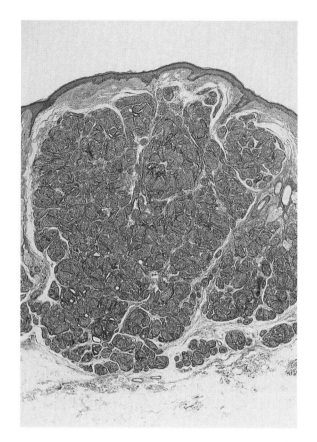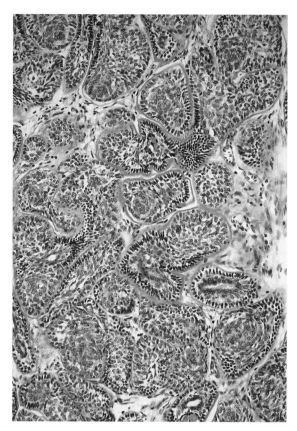

Figure 4-74
DERMAL CYLINDROMA
This scalp tumor bears a remarkable resemblance to membranous basal cell adenoma of the parotid at both low (left) and high (right) magnification. A basal cell adenoma of the parotid occurred synchronously with this scalp cylindroma.

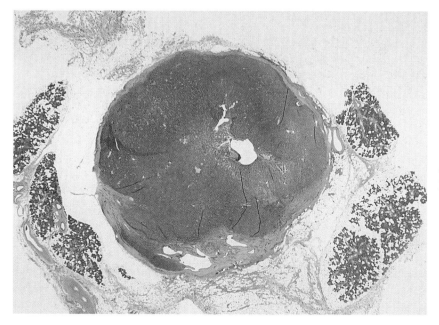

Figure 4-75
BASAL CELL ADENOMA,
SOLID TYPE

A fibrous capsule is evident around this well-circumscribed, solid type basal cell adenoma of the parotid gland.

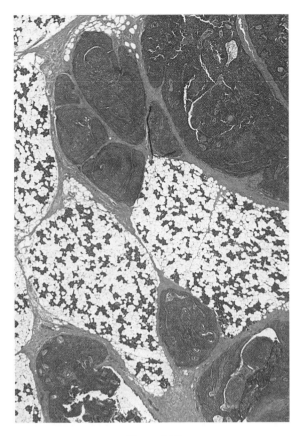

Figure 4-76
BASAL CELL ADENOMA, SOLID TYPE
Multinodular growth is evident in this solid type basal cell adenoma of the parotid, which did not contain any of the hyalinized membranes or droplets indicative of membranous basal cell adenoma.

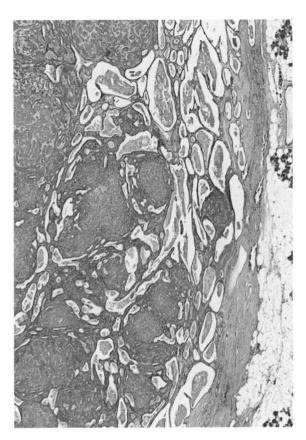

Figure 4-77
CYSTIC CHANGE IN BASAL CELL ADENOMA
Numerous variable-sized cystic spaces are present in the subcapsular region of this solid type basal cell adenoma of the parotid gland.

found rare, faint staining for glial fibrillary acidic protein (GFAP), a tumor marker most often associated with mixed tumors; others have not seen this (234,251,270). Carcinoembryonic antigen and epithelial membrane antigen reactivity is mostly confined to luminal cells (252, 261,268). Dardick et al. (222) described some tubulotrabecular basal cell adenomas with S-100 protein immunoreactivity of spindled "stromal" cells (fig. 4-79) that they interpreted as myoepithelial cells with electron microscopy. Unlike the myoepithelial cells in other neoplasms, studies at the AFIP have found that these spindled stromal cells were unreactive for cytokeratin, SMA, and GFAP.

Ultrastructural studies have also confirmed ductal, myoepithelial, and basal cell differentiation (fig. 4-80) (212,224,225,254). The ductal

cells border lumens and have microvilli, tight junctions, and desmosomes, and some even have a few secretory granules. The basal cells have moderate rough endoplasmic reticulum, a few vesicles, and several mitochondria, and the modified myoepithelial cells typically have abundant cytoplasmic microfilaments, plasmalemmal extensions, and desmosomes. Basal lamina is associated with myoepithelial and basal type cells.

Differential Diagnosis. Mixed tumor, adenoid cystic carcinoma, and basal cell adenocarcinoma are the principal tumor entities to be differentiated from basal cell adenoma of salivary gland. The similarity to dermal eccrine tumors already has been noted, but the site of the tumor should resolve the dermal versus salivary origin question in most cases. A preference to separate canalicular adenoma from basal cell adenoma

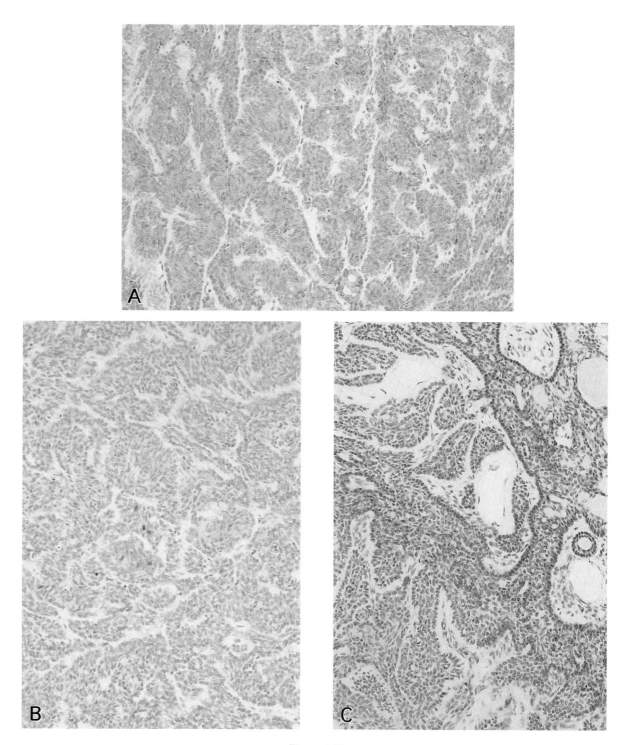

Figure 4-78
IMMUNOHISTOCHEMICAL STAINING OF BASAL CELL ADENOMA

A: Immunostaining for cytokeratin is diffuse in the basaloid cells, but in other tumors cytokeratin may only stain a portion of the tumor cells.

B: The immunoreactivity for S-100 protein can be quite variable in basal cell adenomas, even within different areas of the same tumor. In this field about 25 to 50 percent of the tumor cells are immunostained.

C: Immunostaining for smooth muscle actin in salivary gland tumors is considered indicative of myoepithelial differentiation. In this basal cell adenoma most of the immunostained cells are along the periphery adjacent to the stroma of the neoplasm. (Avidin-biotin peroxidase stain)

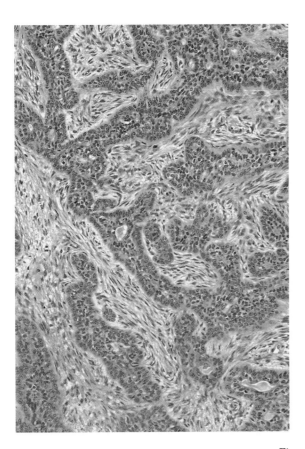 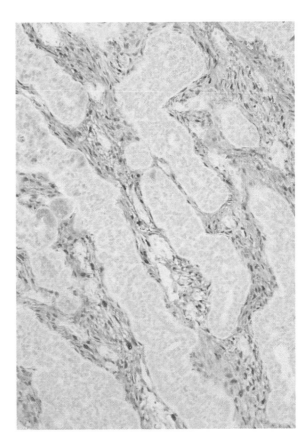

Figure 4-79
BASAL CELL ADENOMA WITH SPINDLED STROMA

Left: In this unusual basal cell adenoma the stromal tissue between the trabeculae of basaloid cells is very cellular and the cells are spindle shaped.

Right: Immunohistochemical staining for S-100 protein shows strong reactivity in the spindled stromal cells. (Avidin-biotin peroxidase stain)

also has been noted, and the reader should refer to the section on Canalicular Adenoma for a more detailed discussion. In brief, basal cell adenoma occurs predominately in the parotid gland and canalicular adenoma occurs predominantly in the upper lip. Histologically, canalicular adenoma is dominated by low columnar cells rather than basaloid cells. The columnar cells are arranged in branching and anastomosing cords of double cell rows that frequently separate to form single cell-lined cystic structures of varying diameters. The supporting stroma is very finely fibrillar and in many cases almost invisible with routine light microscopy (fig. 4-81).

The chondromyxoid tissue of mixed tumors readily distinguishes them from basal cell adenomas, but a few mixed tumors are markedly cellular with minimal amounts of chondromyxoid tissue. A thorough examination of multiple sections for chondromyxoid tissue is often fruitful. In addition, plasmacytoid and spindled cells help distinguish cellular mixed tumors from basal cell adenomas; these abluminal cells appear to form a continuum around the ductal elements that blends into the "stroma." In basal cell adenomas the boundaries between the epithelial tumor cells and the stroma is usually quite distinct and abrupt. Although the use of immunohistochemistry to distinguish one type of salivary gland tumor from another is fraught with pitfalls, significant immunoreactivity for GFAP favors mixed tumor; sparse or absent GFAP reactivity is not helpful (see Mixed Tumor).

Cytomorphologically, the cribriform pattern that is common in adenoid cystic carcinoma is rare in basal cell adenoma (224,249) and, when present,

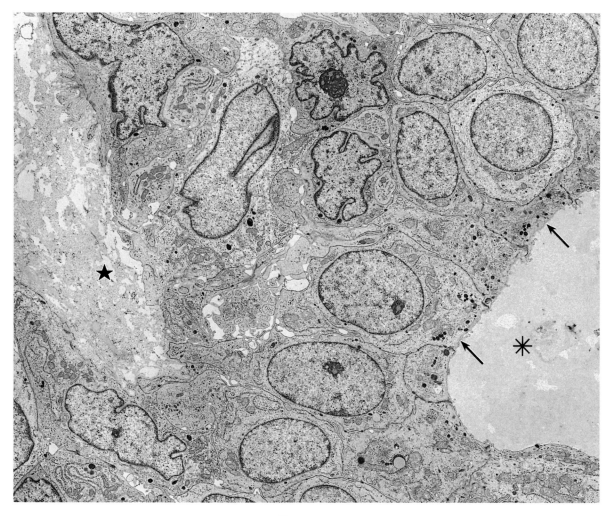

Figure 4-80
BASAL CELL ADENOMA
Electron micrograph shows that ductal cells (arrows) bordering a lumen (asterisk) have tight junctions, microvilli, and a few secretory granules. Abundant basal lamina material (star) is associated with basal or modified myoepithelial cells (X4,600). (Courtesy of Dr. Irving Dardick, Toronto, Canada.)

is accompanied by more typical solid or trabecular growth patterns. Unlike adenoid cystic carcinomas, basal cell adenomas are composed of eosinophilic cells with smooth ovoid to round nuclei and lack cells with pale to clear cytoplasm and irregular angular-shaped nuclei (fig. 4-82). In addition to cytologic differences, infiltration and perineural invasion help distinguish adenoid cystic carcinoma from basal cell adenoma (see Adenoid Cystic Carcinoma). Basal cell adenocarcinoma is the malignant counterpart to basal cell adenoma, and its distinction from basal cell adenoma is primarily based upon growth features

indicative of more aggressive behavior (see Basal Cell Adenocarcinoma). These features include infiltration of parotid parenchyma (as distinct from multifocal growth) and adjacent tissues such as fat, muscle, skin, and bone, and perineural and vascular invasion. A mitotic count greater than 3 per 10-high power fields is also suggestive of malignancy although a lower count is not pathognomonic of a benign lesion.

Prognosis and Treatment. The prognosis is good. Except for the membranous type, the recurrence rate is so low as to be almost nonexistent, especially when conservatively but adequately

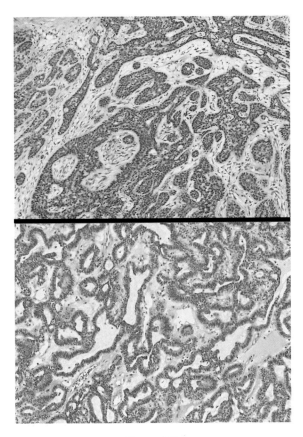

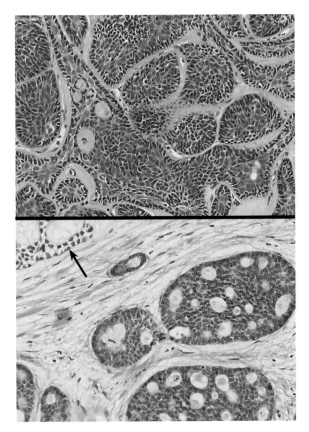

Figure 4-81
BASAL CELL ADENOMA
VERSUS CANALICULAR ADENOMA

Usually, basal cell adenoma (top) has wider, more cellular epithelial trabeculae than canalicular adenoma (bottom), and the stroma is more collagenous. In canalicular adenoma the epithelial cells are more columnar than basaloid.

Figure 4-82
BASAL CELL ADENOMA
VERSUS ADENOID CYSTIC CARCINOMA

Basal cell adenoma (top) usually lacks the cribriform pattern of adenoid cystic carcinoma (bottom). In adenoid cystic carcinoma, cells with clear cytoplasm and dark, angular nuclei (arrow) are usually evident.

excised. This usually means partial parotidectomy, submandibular glandectomy, partial sublingual glandectomy, or excision with a rim of normal intraoral tissue for tumors in these respective sites.

In contrast to the other subtypes of basal cell adenoma, the recurrence rate for the membranous subtype has been reported to be 25 percent, which is probably because of its tendency to be multifocal and unencapsulated (216). The high recurrence rate, resemblance to dermal cylindroma, and association with the skin-salivary diathesis has led some investigators to suggest, perhaps with justification, that the membranous type of basal cell adenoma should be classified separately from other basal cell adenomas (216).

Membranous basal cell adenomas that arose in periparotid lymph nodes and lymphoepithelial cyst of the parotid have been reported (226,244).

Malignant transformation of benign basal cell adenoma, akin to carcinoma arising in mixed tumor (carcinoma ex mixed tumor), has been reported (216,243). In fact, Batsakis et al. (216) have cited a transformation rate of 28 percent for membranous basal cell adenomas, which is considerably higher than for mixed tumors, and about 4 percent for other types of basal cell adenomas. Due to the bland cytologic features of many basal cell adenocarcinomas, it is very difficult to determine whether an invasive basal cell tumor arose within a preexisting benign basal cell tumor or de novo.

CANALICULAR ADENOMA

Definition. Canalicular adenoma is a benign neoplasm that is predominantly composed of branching and interconnecting cords of single and double cell–thick rows of columnar epithelium in a very loose stroma. It has a remarkable predilection for occurrence in the upper lip.

As discussed in the section on basal cell adenoma, there is some disagreement among investigators about whether canalicular adenoma should be identified as a distinct tumor type or within the histologic spectrum of basal cell adenoma (273,276,277,282,290,294). Among investigators who favor inclusion within the basal cell adenoma group, some identify canalicular adenoma as a distinct variant while others do not (271,281,290,294). In addition, some investigators have included canalicular adenomas among reviews of so-called monomorphic adenomas without distinguishing them within this heterogenous group of salivary adenomas that share in common the absence of mesenchymal-like, myxochondroid tissue characteristic of mixed tumor (pleomorphic adenoma)(274,279,280,284, 286,288,289,291,293,296–299).

In agreement with the updated classification of salivary gland tumors of the WHO (295), this Fascicle identifies canalicular adenoma as distinct from other adenomas, including basal cell adenoma, because it has unique clinical and histologic features. It is recognized that distinction from basal cell adenoma or other monomorphic adenomas has little therapeutic significance, but recognition of this tumor as distinct from more aggressive neoplasms with which it has been confused, such as adenoid cystic carcinoma, has major therapeutic implications.

General Features. The historical discord on terminology and classification makes it difficult to extract meaningful data from the literature for this group of tumors. Perhaps the agreement between this Fascicle and the WHO classification will make this easier in the future.

Data from the AFIP files show that canalicular adenoma constitutes about 1 percent of salivary gland neoplasms. Only two developed in the major salivary glands, and they comprised about 4 percent of all minor salivary gland tumors, which is about 8 percent of the benign tumors of minor salivary gland origin. Surprisingly, in a report of their experience in China, Ma and Yu (287) classified no tumors as canalicular adenoma, basal cell adenoma, or monomorphic adenoma among 243 minor salivary gland tumors. In their study of 426 tumors of minor salivary glands, Waldron et al. (300) reported 26 (6 percent) canalicular adenomas, but 7 additional tumors had features that overlapped with those of basal cell adenoma.

Nearly three quarters of canalicular adenomas at the AFIP have occurred in the upper lip; this preference for the lip is specific to the upper lip since only 2.6 percent occurred in the lower lip. This can be compared to the nearly 45 percent of all tumors of minor salivary glands that occur in the palate. It also contrasts with the occurrence of basal cell adenoma, which develops in the major salivary glands in over 80 percent of cases and in the upper lip in only 5.4 percent of cases. The predilection of canalicular adenoma for the upper lip probably accounts for observations that the upper lip is the most common site for basal cell adenoma and monomorphic adenoma by investigators who place canalicular adenoma within one of these latter categories (271, 280,281,286,288,291). Mixed tumor is the only salivary gland tumor that occurs in the upper lip more often than canalicular adenoma. The buccal mucosa is the second most frequent site for canalicular adenoma (13.5 percent), and most of these tumors are located in close proximity to the upper lip. Batsakis et al. (272) found 4 canalicular adenomas in the parotid in a study of 96 monomorphic adenomas of the major salivary glands.

In AFIP data, women outnumber men by a ratio of about 1.8 to 1, although in an earlier AFIP study that was not corrected for the military bias, Nelson and Jacoway (292) reported a slight predominance of men. In a report of basal cell adenomas of the upper lip, which probably were mostly canalicular adenomas, Fantasia and Neville (281) also had a 1.8 to 1 ratio of women to men; Daley et al. (277) reported a female predominance in their series as well. Like basal cell adenomas, canalicular adenomas are tumors of adults with a peak incidence in the seventh decade of life. They are distinctly uncommon in patients under 50 years old. The average age of patients based on AFIP cases is 65 years; the youngest patient was 34 years old.

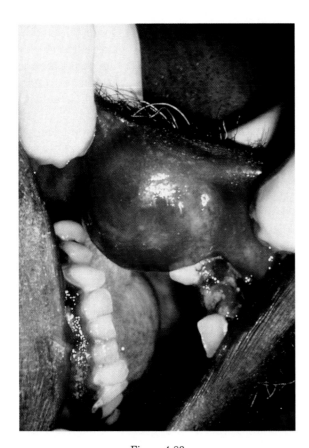

Figure 4-83
CANALICULAR ADENOMA
The upper lip is the site for over 70 percent of canalicular adenomas.

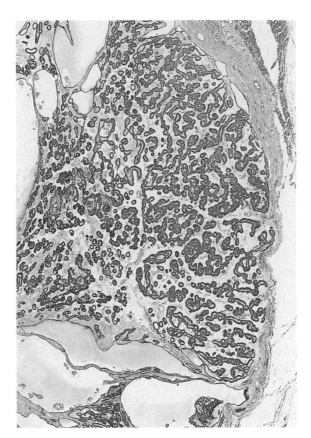

Figure 4-84
CANALICULAR ADENOMA
Small, residual ducts of salivary gland tissue are adjacent to the fibrous capsule that extends along the right portion of this photomicrograph of canalicular adenoma. Cystic dilatation of the canalicular epithelium is evident on the top and bottom.

Clinical Features. Excluding rare parotid tumors, canalicular adenomas develop as slowly enlarging, movable, compressible nodules in the mucosa (fig. 4-83). There are usually no symptoms associated with the swellings. Tumors located superficially beneath the mucosal epithelium sometimes produce a slightly bluish coloration to the otherwise pink mucosa. The multifocal occurrence of canalicular adenomas in the upper lip and buccal mucosa have been noted by several investigators (276,285,290,291). Tumor durations of months to many years have been described.

Gross Findings. Typically, canalicular adenomas are well-circumscribed, light yellow to tan to brown nodules that range from 0.5 to 2.0 cm in diameter. Tumors larger than 3 cm are rare. The majority of tumors are single nodules, but multinodular or multifocal tumors occur. As

much as 22 percent of tumors were reported to be multifocal in one series (276), but that incidence is probably high. They are usually, but not always, encapsulated. The cut surface is often homogeneous but usually reveals many small cysts and a gelatinous or mucoid texture.

Microscopic Findings. The microscopic features confirm the gross findings in most cases. The tumors are usually well-circumscribed and encapsulated nodules (fig. 4-84), but partially encapsulated or unencapsulated tumors are not rare (fig. 4-85). Multifocal tumors occasionally occur, and some of these foci are microscopic and are not clinically evident (fig. 4-86).

In contrast to basal cell adenomas and several other types of salivary gland tumors that have several different microscopic growth patterns, canalicular adenomas are relatively consistent

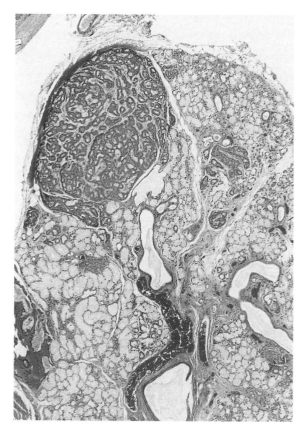

Figure 4-85
UNENCAPSULATED CANALICULAR ADENOMA
This small tumor from the upper lip has no capsule. Its size may indicate that a capsule had not had an opportunity to form, but occasionally larger tumors are only partially encapsulated as well.

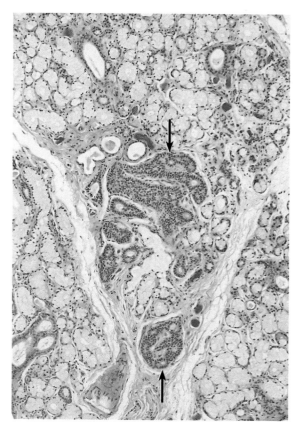

Figure 4-86
MULTIFOCAL CANALICULAR ADENOMA
Small microscopic foci (arrows) of adenomatous tissue that may be an incipient stage of canalicular adenoma are located in a salivary gland lobule adjacent to the larger canalicular adenoma shown in figure 4-85.

in appearance from tumor to tumor. Variation in appearance is mostly due to differences in cellular density and extent of microcyst formation while the basic morphologic structure is similar in all tumors (fig. 4-87).

This basic structure is created by double rows of columnar epithelial cells that form branching and interconnecting cords in a very loose stroma. The proximity of the two rows of cells to one another varies along the course of the cords of epithelium (fig. 4-88). For short distances they can be closely apposed so that they abut to form a tight double row. On either side of this abutment the rows of cells slightly separate to produce narrow channels (the canaliculi for which the term canalicular adenoma was adopted). These canaliculi can branch and interconnect to form a dense to loose meshwork of epithelium.

This alternating abutment and separation of the rows of columnar cells along the canaliculi has been referred to as beading (fig. 4-89) (277). At irregular intervals, the strands of cells that form the canaliculi can separate more widely to produce small cysts. Some of the cystic formations can be markedly dilated, and some are even visible during examination of the gross specimen (fig. 4-90). Some strands of epithelium are cut in cross section and appear as isolated, small ducts or cysts without connection to adjacent epithelium (fig. 4-88).

The epithelial cells that form cords and canaliculi vary from cuboidal to tall columnar, but the majority are typically short columnar cells. The cytoplasm is amphophilic to eosinophilic, and the nuclei are round to elliptical with uniform to lightly stippled, basophilic chromatin.

97

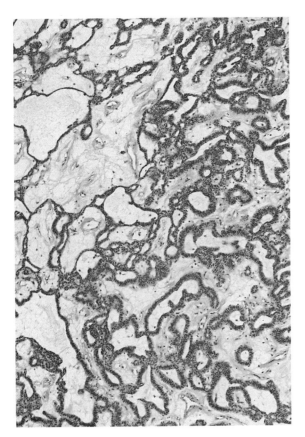 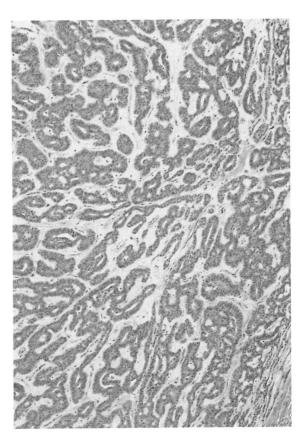

Figure 4-87
CANALICULAR ADENOMAS
Two different canalicular adenomas shown at the same medium magnification (left and right) have differences in the density of the epithelium and dilatation of the canaliculi, but the same morphologic structure is common to both.

Figure 4-88
CANALICULAR ADENOMA
Cords of double rows of columnar cells branch and interconnect. The luminal space between the rows is variable in size. Some of the cords are cut in cross section and appear as isolated tubules (arrows). The stroma has few cells and little collagen.

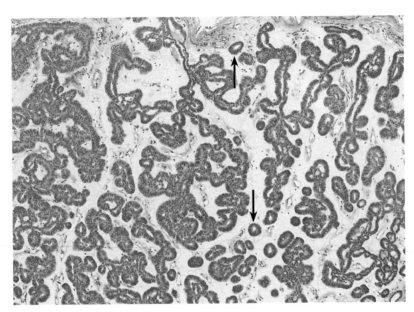

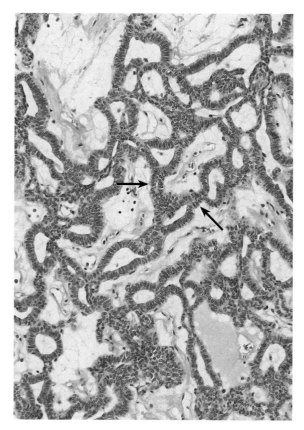

Figure 4-89
"BEADING" IN CANALICULAR ADENOMA
Double rows of epithelial cells are alternatingly closely apposed (arrows) and slightly separated for short distances to roughly produce a "beads on a string" appearance. Areas of the loose, sparsely collagenous stroma are frequently surrounded by epithelial cells and contain many small blood vessels.

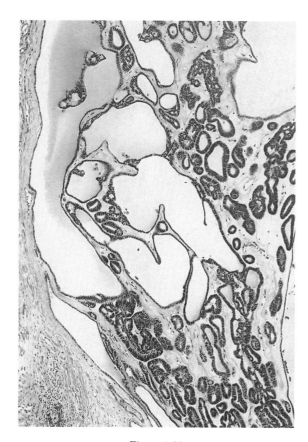

Figure 4-90
CYST FORMATION IN CANALICULAR ADENOMA
Cystic dilatation in the canalicular structures is prominent in this illustration but is variable from one area of a tumor to another and from tumor to tumor.

The nuclei are uniform in size and shape, with little or no pleomorphism or pleochromatism. Mitotic figures are absent or rare (fig. 4-91).

In some tumors, foci of basaloid-appearing cells can be found between rows of columnar cells. The number of these foci in a tumor can vary from few to many. In some tumors these foci appear to be portions of canaliculi cut en face; in other tumors, the number of basaloid cells in some foci is too many to simply represent a plane of section along the surface of some canaliculi (fig. 4-92).

The stroma associated with canalicular adenoma is also very characteristic and consistent from one tumor to another. It is a very loose, lightly fibrillar collagenous tissue with few fibroblasts. In some tumors, the stroma is nearly invisible with low-magnification microscopic examination and

the epithelium appears to be "floating in air." In other tumors, the ground substance, principally hyaluronic acid, is more evident. Within the stroma, which is frequently divided into isolated segments by cords of epithelium, are many scattered small capillaries. The capillaries often have an eosinophilic cuff that is probably basal lamina and collagen (figs. 4-87–4-89, 4-91).

There is little information on the immunohistochemistry of canalicular adenomas. Zarbo et al. (301) found that all 15 canalicular adenomas in their study were reactive for S-100 protein. Of the canalicular adenomas studied at the AFIP with immunohistochemistry on paraffin tissue sections, nearly all of the tumor cells were immunoreactive for cytokeratin and many were reactive for S-100 protein (fig. 4-93). Generally,

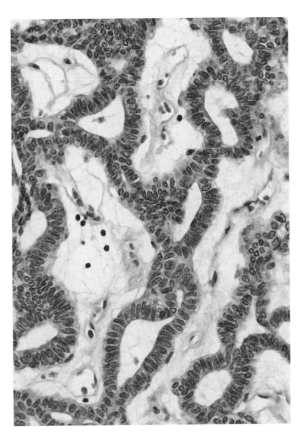

Figure 4-91
COLUMNAR CELLS IN CANALICULAR ADENOMA
This high-magnification photomicrograph shows that the cords of epithelium are composed of rows of columnar cells that alternately abut and separate and branch to form the canaliculi. The stroma is very loose and faintly stained with few cells but several small capillaries.

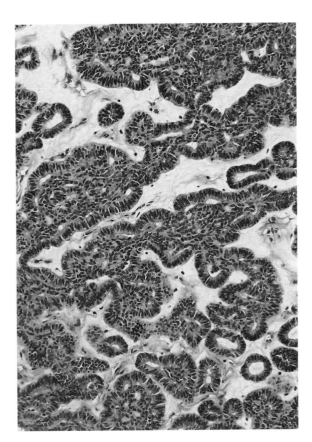

Figure 4-92
BASALOID CELLS IN CANALICULAR ADENOMA
Between some of the rows of columnar cells in this canalicular adenoma are many smaller, poorly demarcated basaloid cells.

none of the tumor cells were reactive with anti-smooth muscle actin (SMA), and very focal reactivity for glial fibrillary acidic protein (GFAP) was found in one tumor. SMA is considered a marker of myoepithelial differentiation in salivary gland tumors, and GFAP is often found in myoepithelial cells of mixed tumors. The implication is that there is little or no myoepithelial differentiation in canalicular adenomas. Electron microscopic examination seems to confirm this impression (275,277,278,283). Columnar cells extend from a luminal surface to basement membrane without intervening basaloid or myoepithelial cells between the columnar cells and basement membrane. Between some of the luminal cells are short columnar cells that do not extend to the luminal surface. The boundary

between adjacent cells is fairly straight, without much interdigitation. The luminal surfaces of the cells have a few microvilli, and occasional cells have a few secretory granules.

Differential Diagnosis. Basal cell adenoma and adenoid cystic carcinoma are the principal considerations in the differential diagnosis. Distinguishing canalicular adenoma from basal cell adenoma has little therapeutic significance, but distinction from adenoid cystic carcinoma has important prognostic and therapeutic implications.

Foci of basaloid cells in some canalicular adenomas is the reason some investigators consider canalicular adenoma to be a variant of basal cell adenoma, and perhaps justifying their argument is the observation that occasional tumors have a high percentage of basaloid type cells. On the

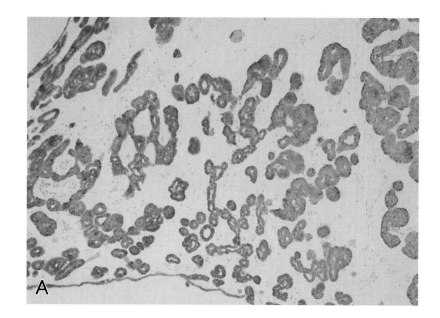

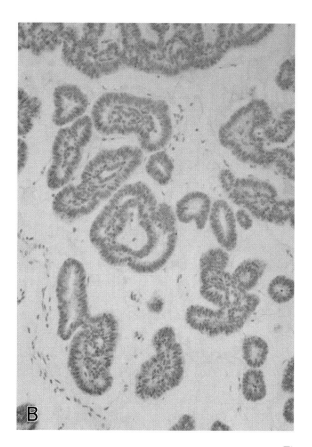

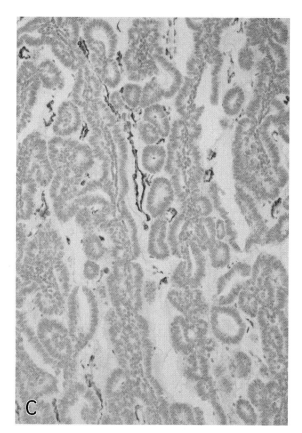

Figure 4-93
IMMUNOHISTOCHEMISTRY OF CANALICULAR ADENOMA
A: A cocktail of monoclonal anti-cytokeratin antibodies reacts diffusely and uniformly with the cords of epithelial cells.
B: Anti-S-100 protein antibody reacts with most of the epithelial cells.
C: Anti-smooth muscle actin monoclonal antibody does not react with the epithelial cells, but highlights the many small blood vessels in an otherwise almost acellular stroma. (Avidin-biotin peroxidase stain)

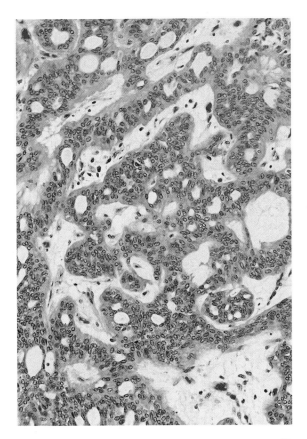 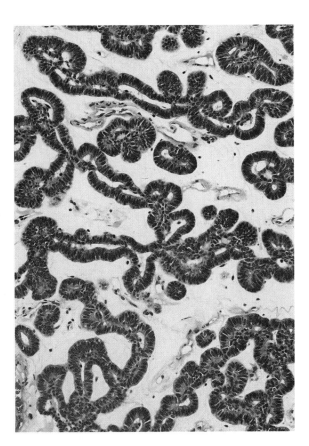

Figure 4-94
BASAL CELL ADENOMA VERSUS CANALICULAR ADENOMA
Left: Tubulotrabecular basal cell adenoma is composed of small basaloid cells with foci of low cuboidal cells around lumens.
Right: This can be contrasted with the rows of columnar cells that form the branching canaliculi of canalicular adenoma.

other hand, with rare exceptions, tumors composed of columnar cells and canaliculi appear limited to the minor salivary glands, predominantly the upper lip. Foci of these columnar cells and canaliculi are not observed in basaloid cell adenomas of the parotid gland, the predominant site of occurrence of basal cell adenomas. Perhaps canalicular adenoma represents a site-specific morphologic variation of basal cell adenoma, but its features are so characteristic and unique that it seems preferable to identify canalicular adenoma separately. In practical terms, the debate over canalicular adenoma and basal cell adenoma is unresolvable at this time and relatively unimportant. Canalicular adenoma is frequently identified as the tubulotrabecular pattern of basal cell adenoma. However, tubulotrabecular basal cell adenoma lacks the peripheral rows and branching canaliculi of co-

lumnar cells that are characteristic of canalicular adenoma, and the "beading" phenomenon is not present (fig. 4-94). The ductal or cystic spaces in basal cell adenoma are lined by cuboidal cells or basaloid cells (see Basal Cell Adenoma).

The cribriform-tubular pattern of adenoid cystic carcinoma (see Adenoid Cystic Carcinoma) may be confused with canalicular adenoma. Both often have thin interconnecting cords of epithelial cells that segregate islands of stromal tissue, which frequently appears acellular. However, the infiltrative destructive growth of adenoid cystic carcinoma is usually readily distinguished from the circumscribed, and usually encapsulated, pattern of canalicular adenoma. Occasionally, however, small adenoid cystic carcinomas appear quite circumscribed, and the occasional multifocal canalicular adenoma presents an initial impression of infiltration. Yet, subtle but important differences in the epithelium and stroma distinguish canalicular adenoma from adenoid cystic carcinoma. Adenoid cystic carcinoma lacks the rows of columnar cells of canalicular adenoma. The basaloid cells of adenoid cystic carcinoma frequently have pale to clear cytoplasm with indistinct cell boundaries and irregular-shaped nuclei. The stroma in the pseudocystic, or cylindromatous, spaces of adenoid cystic carcinoma contains basophilic glycosaminoglycans or eosinophilic basal lamina. Capillaries are nearly always absent in these cylindromatous stromal areas. In contrast, capillaries are easily found in the poorly staining stroma of canalicular adenomas. Dense collagenous tissue typically surrounds the nests or aggregates of epithelial cells in adenoid cystic carcinomas while dense collagenous tissue is usually only found in the capsular region of canalicular adenomas.

Prognosis and Treatment. The prognosis for canalicular adenoma is excellent. Recurrence is uncommon even though many of these tumors have been treated by "lumpectomy" (276,277,281 292,294). In cases with a recurrence, there is always a question as to whether the excised tumor recurred or whether another adenoma developed from a small adenomatous focus of a multifocal lesion. Local excision is appropriate therapy.

ONCOCYTOMA

Definition. Oncocytomas are rare benign epithelial neoplasms composed of oncocytes, which are large cells with granular eosinophilic cytoplasm containing excessive and atypical mitochondria. Since the normal striated duct cells of salivary gland contain many mitochondria relative to other cell types, a large number of cytoplasmic mitochondria is insufficient by itself to define an oncocyte. Identified criteria for salivary gland oncocytes include: 1) appearance after maturity of the salivary gland; 2) a high level of oxidative activity; 3) an unusually large number of mitochondria; and 4) absence of specialized features of normal cells, such as brush borders and basal enfolding (310–313). An estimated 60 percent of the cytoplasmic volume is occupied by mitochondria in salivary oncocytes (304,305,311). Oncocytic cells have been identified in many organs but most frequently in sali-

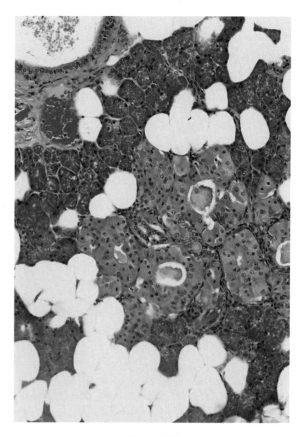

Figure 4-95
ONCOCYTIC METAPLASIA
Several eosinophilic oncocytic cells are situated around a striated duct and adjacent to unremarkable, normal serous acinar cells of the parotid gland.

vary gland, thyroid gland, parathyroid gland, pulmonary tree, and kidney (305).

Oncocytic cells in salivary glands occur in varying numbers and growth patterns, and the distinction between oncocytic hyperplasia and neoplasia is problematic and controversial. Fortunately, the distinction significantly influences prognosis and treatment only in the very rare case of malignant oncocytic neoplasia (see Oncocytic Carcinoma). The occurrence of oncocytic cells in salivary glands can be categorized as *oncocytic metaplasia, nodular* or *diffuse oncocytosis,* and *oncocytoma.*

Oncocytic metaplasia is the transformation of ductal and acinar epithelium to oncocytes (fig. 4-95). Oncocytes in the salivary glands are uncommon in persons under the age of 50 years, but the percentage of the population with focal oncocytic metaplasia increases thereafter until

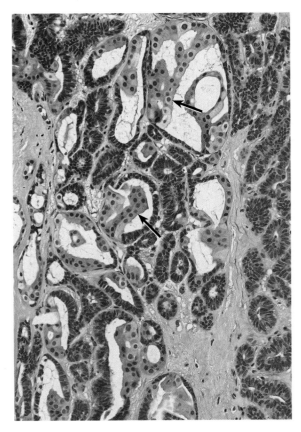

Figure 4-96
ONCOCYTIC METAPLASIA
IN CANALICULAR ADENOMA
Small foci of oncocytic cells (arrows) are apparent in a
canalicular adenoma that was excised from buccal mucosa.

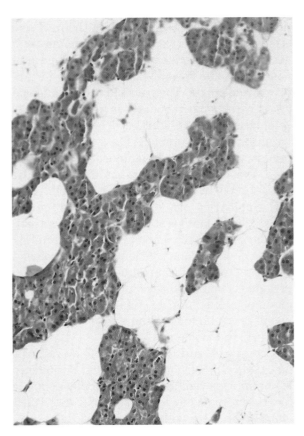

Figure 4-97
DIFFUSE ONCOCYTOSIS
Nearly all of the parenchymal tissue from an enlarged
parotid gland that was removed from a 73-year-old woman
manifested the illustrated oncocytic metaplasia. The ratio
of parenchymal tissue to adipose tissue is decreased.

nearly universal in the population over 70 years
of age (305,310). Whether oncocytic metaplasia is
the result of an internal cellular derangement or
a response to the extracellular microenvironment
remains controversial (303,305,311). Oncocytic
metaplasia occasionally occurs in tumor cells of
salivary gland neoplasms other than oncocytoma. This is most frequently observed in mixed
tumors and mucoepidermoid carcinomas, but
has been seen in nearly every type of salivary
gland neoplasm (fig. 4-96).

Oncocytosis is the accumulation and proliferation of oncocytes in the salivary glands. Rarely,
nearly the entire parotid gland parenchyma is
replaced by oncocytes (*diffuse oncocytosis*) (fig.
4-97) (319,328), but typically multiple foci are observed. These foci produce microscopic and macroscopic nodules that have been termed *nodular*

oncocytic hyperplasia or *nodular oncocytosis* (fig.
4-98) (311,319,323). The distinction between a
large nodule in nodular oncocytic hyperplasia
and oncocytoma, the putative benign neoplasm of
oncocytes, is subtle and perhaps semantic.
Brandwein and Huvos (303) defined oncocytoma
as a single nodule and nodular oncocytic hyperplasia as two or more distinct tumor nodules.
Hartwick and Batsakis (311) stated that hyperplastic nodules are less organized and circumscribed than oncocytoma, are lobular rather than
lobar, and do not present as a single dominant
nodule. Palmer et al. (319) had similar criteria
but also stated that oncocytomas had at least a
partial fibrous capsule while nodules of oncocytic
hyperplasia were unencapsulated and mostly
composed of clear cells. In general, oncocytoma is
a nodule of oncocytes that is clinically detectable,

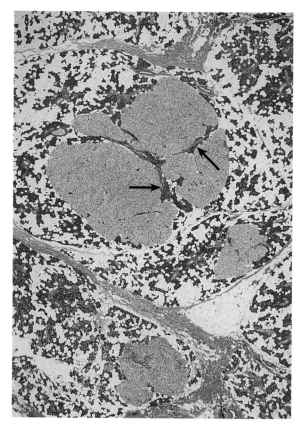

Figure 4-98
NODULAR ONCOCYTIC HYPERPLASIA
Several nodules of oncocytes of varying size and shape are situated in the parotid tissue. They are not encapsulated and appear to have encompassed normal, darker staining serous acinar tissue (arrows). Many of the oncocytes have partially clear cytoplasm, which accounts for the pale eosinophilic appearance.

is circumscribed and demarcated from surrounding salivary gland parenchyma by at least an incomplete fibrous capsule, and is significantly larger than other nodules of oncocytic cells that are present in the gland. However, since the distinction between oncocytoma and nodular oncocytic hyperplasia is often subtle, both conditions are included in this discussion.

Light and electron microscopy shows that the epithelial cells in Warthin's tumor are oncocytic. But because of the distinctive papillary cystic architecture and lymphoid stroma, Warthin's tumor is classified separately from oncocytoma. Still, a relationship between the two entities is evinced by focal nodular proliferations of oncocytes in some Warthin tumors and focal cyst

formation with lymphoid cells in rare oncocytomas. Uncommonly, tumors dominated by a cystic and papillary architecture appear to be composed of oncocytic cells. Some investigators have classified these tumors, which occur mostly in the minor salivary glands, as oncocytomas (306,320), but in this Fascicle these tumors are classified as oncocytic cystadenomas (see Cystadenoma).

General Features. Many of the large surveys of salivary gland neoplasms do not specifically identify oncocytomas, and they may be included within a category of "monomorphic adenoma." In other surveys, oncocytomas constitute between 0 and 3 percent of salivary gland neoplasms; the average is just under 1 percent (309,316,319,324,326,327,329). At the AFIP since 1985, oncocytomas have comprised about 2 percent of all salivary gland epithelial neoplasms and about 3.5 percent of parotid gland tumors. The parotid gland is the predominant site of occurrence, and about 85 to 90 percent occur in this site (303,319). Most of the remainder occur in the submandibular gland, and oncocytomas in the minor salivary glands are rare. Waldron et al. (330) found none among 426 minor salivary gland tumors. Regezi et al. (320) reported 2 oncocytomas among 238 minor gland tumors, but the description suggests that one was an oncocytic cystadenoma. Likewise, the 1 oncocytoma in 189 minor gland tumors reported by Chaudhry et al. (306) was probably an oncocytic cystadenoma. Damm et al. (307) reported one solid oncocytoma of minor gland origin and found only four other well-documented cases in the literature. Among 72 recent oncocytomas in the AFIP files, 2 were from intraoral salivary glands.

Oncocytomas are rare in patients younger than 50 years: less than 6 percent of the oncocytomas in the AFIP files since 1985 occurred in patients less than 50 years old; the youngest patient was 39 years old. The peak incidence is in the seventh to ninth decades of life. A similar experience is reported by other investigators (305,310,311,319). Many investigators have reported an equal predilection for men and women (302,303,310,319), although the data of the AFIP and others indicate a slight female predominance among patients (305). Among patients with clear cell dominant oncocytomas, there is a marked female predilection (308).

Etiologic factors in salivary gland neoplasia have rarely been identified. An increased incidence of salivary gland neoplasms has been associated with exposure of the head and neck region to ionizing radiation, but most of the associated neoplasms have been malignancies (318,321,322, 325,331) (see General Considerations). Brandwein and Huvos (303) reported that 9 of 44 oncocytomas they followed occurred in patients with a history of radiation exposure prior to discovery of the tumors. These oncocytomas occurred, on average, in much younger patients than those without a history of radiation exposure.

Clinical Features. Swelling is the only complaint of patients in nearly all cases of oncocytoma; rarely, pain is associated with these tumors. The duration of tumor before surgery is a few weeks to 20 years, but less than 2 years is typical (319). The swellings are single or multiple nodules. In glands affected by diffuse nodular oncocytic hyperplasia, a generalized enlargement of the parotid gland is usually noted.

Brandwein and Huvos (303) estimated that bilateral parotid gland or submandibular gland disease, synchronous or metachronous, occurs in at least 7 percent of patients. Five of 13 patients with oncocytomas reported by Blanck et al. (302) had bilateral parotid tumors. The tumors in many patients with bilateral disease could probably be categorized as multinodular oncocytic hyperplasia; but, as previously stated, the distinction from neoplastic oncocytoma is sometimes obscure.

Gross Findings. In most cases a single, encapsulated or well-circumscribed, tan to red-brown nodule is evident within the resected salivary gland tissue by macroscopic examination. In some cases additional nodules of varying size are also observed. Occasionally, one or more cysts are present within the tumor nodules. The tumors range in size from 1 to 7 cm, but 3 to 4 cm is typical.

Microscopic Findings. With light microscopic examination oncocytes are usually characterized by abundant, strongly eosinophilic, finely granular cytoplasm. Still, the intensity of the eosinophilia varies, and "light" and "dark" stained cells often can be observed (fig. 4-99). The cells contain a single round nucleus with dispersed chromatin and, frequently, a noticeable nucleolus. The cell boundaries are usually distinct. The cells are relatively large and about one to two times the size of normal acinar cells.

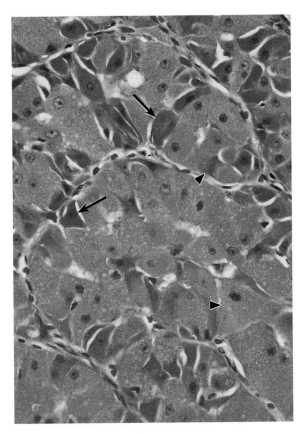

Figure 4-99
ONCOCYTE
Large polygonal cells have prominent, granular eosinophilic cytoplasm and centrally placed nuclei with dispersed chromatin and nucleoli, usually single. The intensity of cytoplasmic staining is variable, and darker (arrows) and lighter (arrowheads) cells can be identified.

Some variability in cellular and nuclear size is acceptable and has no prognostic significance, but mitotic figures are rare. Ultrastructurally, the most conspicuous feature is abundant cytoplasmic mitochondria, which account for the light microscopic eosinophilia. The mitochondria sometimes nearly fill the entire cytoplasmic compartment, but a volume of about 60 percent is typical (fig. 4-100) (304). The mitochondria vary in shape from round to elongated to irregular. Desmosomal cell attachments are usually evident. Some oncocytes border glandular lumens, and in such cases tight junctions and microvilli are observed. Concordant with the light microscopic appearance, round nuclei have dispersed chromatin and nucleoli.

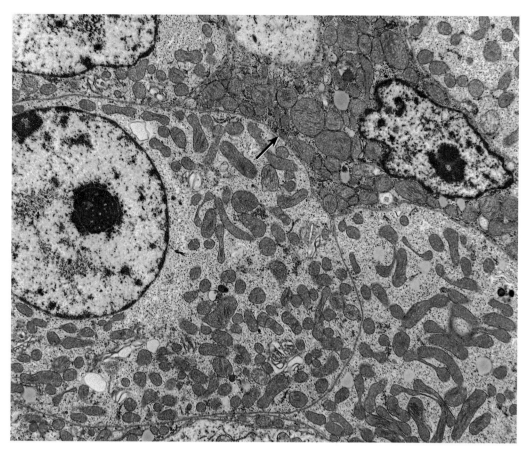

Figure 4-100
ULTRASTRUCTURE OF ONCOCYTES
In the dark cell (arrow) mitochondria are tightly packed together and occupy nearly all the cytoplasmic area. In the adjacent lighter cells mitochondria are still numerous but less dense. No specialized cell junctions are evident in this field. The nucleus in the light cell is almost symmetrically round while the nucleus in the dark cell is slightly irregular. Nucleoli are evident in both nuclei (X9,600). (Courtesy of Dr. Irving Dardick, Toronto, Canada.)

Oncocytoma typically occurs as a single mass of neoplastic oncocytes (fig. 4-101) but sometimes presents as a dominant mass in a setting of multinodular oncocytic hyperplasia. The distinction between hyperplasia and neoplasia is less than definitive. One criterion has been the presence or absence of fibrous encapsulation, which is often minimal: oncocytoma is encapsulated while oncocytic hyperplasia is not (fig. 4-102). However, even this criterion is subject to interpretation, as illustrated by examples of multinodular oncocytic proliferations with fibrous capsules (fig. 4-103). It is not a critical issue.

The oncocytes in oncocytomas typically are arranged in a organoid pattern of tightly packed clusters that are separated and surrounded by thin, inconspicuous capillaries and strands of fibrovascular stroma (fig. 4-104). Small lumens are often apparent in the centers of the clusters. In other tumors, the oncocytes are arranged in short serpentine cords separated by fibrovascular stroma (fig. 4-105). Most tumors are solid masses, but occasional tumors contain one or more microcysts or macrocysts (fig. 4-106). Some of these cysts have an associated lymphoid infiltrate and resembled Warthin's tumor (fig. 4-107). Conversely, Warthin tumors sometimes contain foci of nodular oncocytic hyperplasia (fig. 4-108), so there is possibly some loose relationship between these two oncocytic lesions. While squamous metaplasia is a common finding in Warthin's tumor, it is rare in oncocytomas, but has been observed in some oncocytomas at the AFIP that had been aspirated by fine needle prior to excision (fig. 4-109).

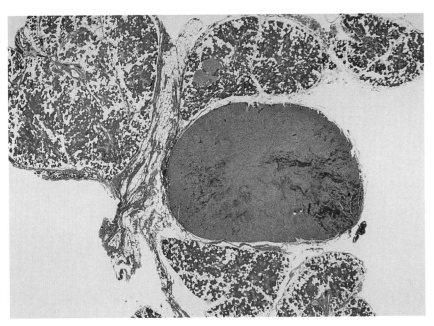

Figure 4-101
ONCOCYTOMA

A well-circumscribed and demarcated nodule of oncocytes is larger than some of the lobules of normal parotid gland that are adjacent to it.

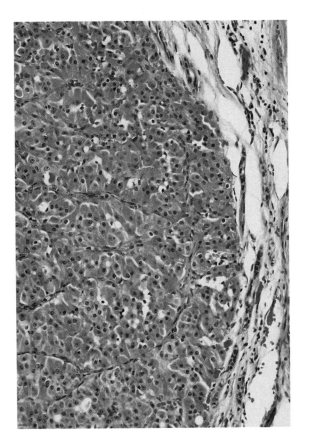

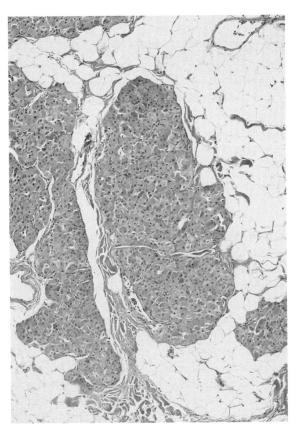

Figure 4-102
ONCOCYTOMA AND NODULAR ONCOCYTIC HYPERPLASIA

Left: Moderately dense fibrous tissue with a few inflammatory cells forms a capsule along the surface of an oncocytoma.

Right: Small nodules of oncocytes are unencapsulated and irregular shaped. While one or more of these nodules might continue to enlarge in the manner of a benign neoplasm, at this stage they are best classified as nodular hyperplasia.

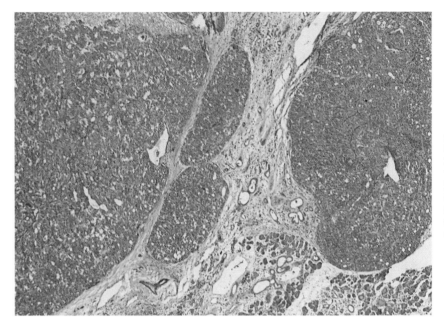

Figure 4-103
MULTINODULAR
ONCOCYTOMA
This low-magnification photograph shows several varying sized nodules of oncocytes in a dense fibrous stroma. Normal parotid tissue is present in the lower right portion of the field. The large size and the fibrous tissue capsule suggest that it is appropriate to classify these oncocytic nodules as oncocytomas.

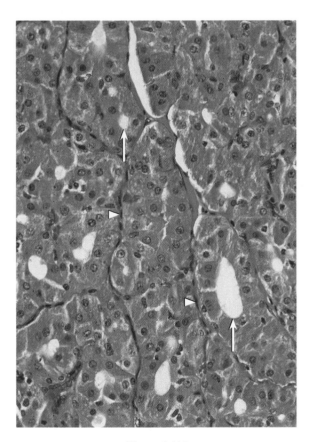

Figure 4-104
ONCOCYTOMA
Very thin capillaries (arrowheads) separate organoid clusters of oncocytes. Small but varying sized lumens are evident within some of the clusters (arrows).

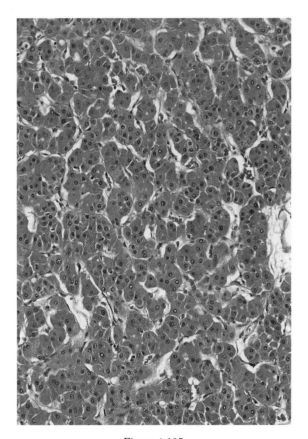

Figure 4-105
ONCOCYTOMA
The fibrovascular stroma is more visible in this oncocytoma in which the oncocytes appear to form cords in a hepatic-like arrangement.

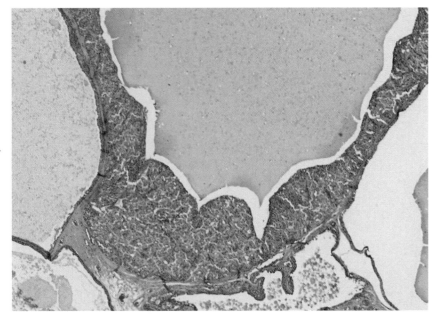

Figure 4-106
CYSTIC ONCOCYTOMA
Several cysts are lined by a layer
of oncocytes of varying thickness.

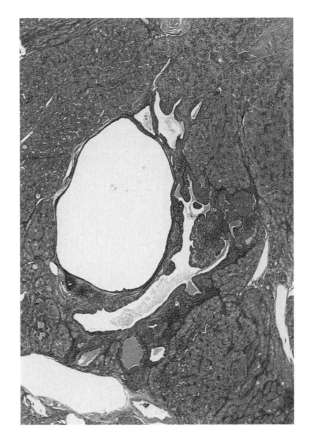

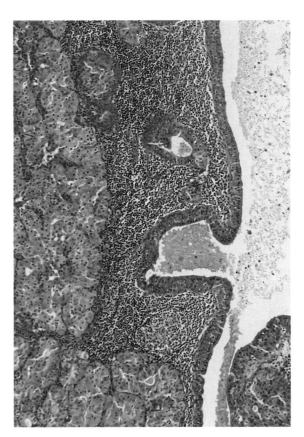

Figure 4-107
CYSTIC ONCOCYTOMA WITH LYMPHOID INFILTRATE

Left: This low-magnification photograph shows a focal cystic region in an otherwise solid oncocytoma.

Right: Higher magnification reveals the cysts are lined by columnar oncocytes and a lymphoid infiltrate, which together resemble Warthin's tumor.

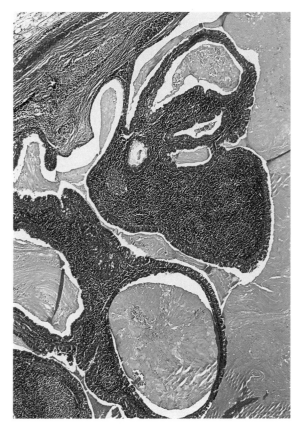 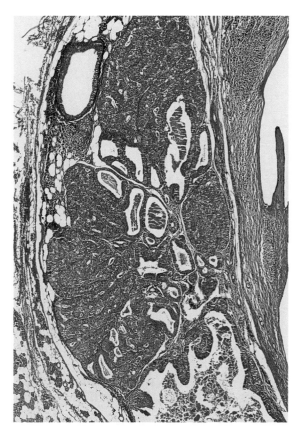

Figure 4-108
WARTHIN'S TUMOR WITH NODULAR ONCOCYTIC PROLIFERATION
The interrelationship of oncocytoma and Warthin's tumor (left) is accentuated by this nodule of oncocytic proliferation in the tumor capsule (right).

Oncocytes are cells with prominent eosinophilic cytoplasm, but, paradoxically, clear cells dominate some lesions (fig. 4-110). Clear cells have been noted to be particularly common in multinodular oncocytic hyperplasia (figs. 4-98, 4-111) (302,303,319). Clear cell oncocytomas have the same organoid architectural arrangement as conventional oncocytomas. The clear cytoplasm is due to the accumulation of cytoplasmic glycogen in the oncocytes, which can be demonstrated by staining with PAS before and after tissue digestion with diastase (fig. 4-112). Conventional eosinophilic oncocytes sometimes can be found in the midst of nodules of clear cells and help confirm the diagnosis (fig. 4-113).

Although electron microscopic evidence of mitochondrial proliferation is the best evidence for oncocytic differentiation, ultrastructural examination is usually unnecessary to establish a diagnosis of oncocytoma in the salivary glands. Well-demarcated masses of organoid clusters of large polyhedral cells with prominent eosinophilic cytoplasm and uniform round nuclei are sufficiently characteristic to be diagnostic. In addition, phosphotungstic acid–hematoxylin (PTAH) staining, although not consistently reliable, is often useful for identifying oncocytes because this stain has an affinity for mitochondria (fig. 4-114) (303, 305). Brandwein and Huvos (303) recommend a 48-hour incubation rather than routine overnight incubation for PTAH staining of mitochondria. Normal striated ducts in adjacent salivary gland tissue can be useful as an internal control for the PTAH stain.

Differential Diagnosis. For the most part, recognition of oncocytoma is uncomplicated, but oncocytic metaplasia in other salivary gland neoplasms as well as clear cell neoplasms are considered in the differential diagnosis.

111

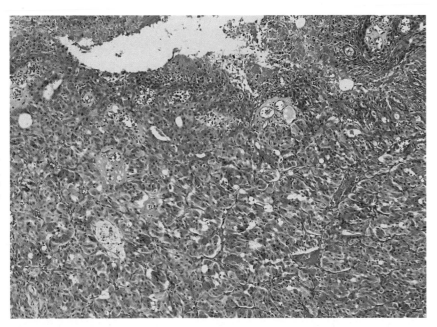

Figure 4-109
SQUAMOUS METAPLASIA
IN ONCOCYTOMA
Stratified squamous epithelium (top) lines a cystic area in an oncocytoma that had undergone fine-needle aspiration a week before it was excised.

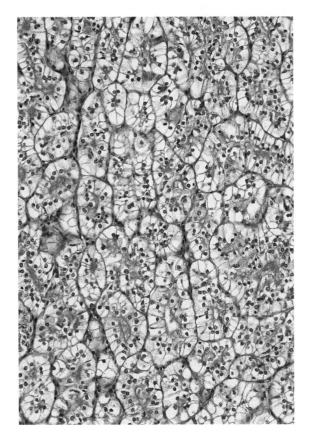

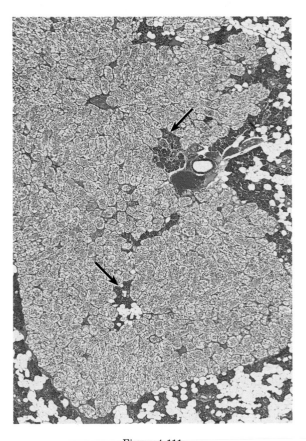

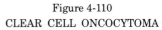

Figure 4-110
CLEAR CELL ONCOCYTOMA

A typical organoid architecture and cellular morphology are evident in this clear cell variant of oncocytoma. While most of the cytoplasmic compartments are clear, some eosinophilic cytoplasm is evident along the periphery of some cells.

Figure 4-111
CLEAR CELL NODULAR ONCOCYTIC HYPERPLASIA

An unencapsulated, irregular-shaped mass of mostly clear staining oncocytes has entrapped foci of normal-staining serous acini (arrows) in the parotid gland.

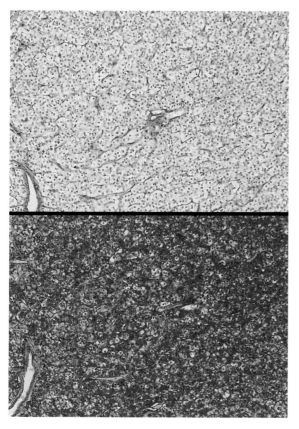

Figure 4-112
GLYCOGEN IN CLEAR CELL ONCOCYTOMA
PAS staining of a clear cell oncocytoma with (top) and without (bottom) prior diastase digestion of the tissue demonstrates abundant intracellular glycogen.

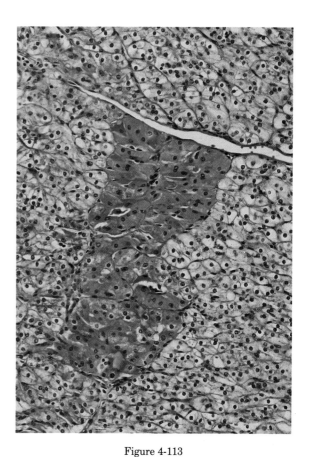

Figure 4-113
CLEAR CELL ONCOCYTOMA
A focus of typical eosinophilic oncocytes is present within a mass of pale- to clear-staining oncocytes from a parotid gland oncocytoma.

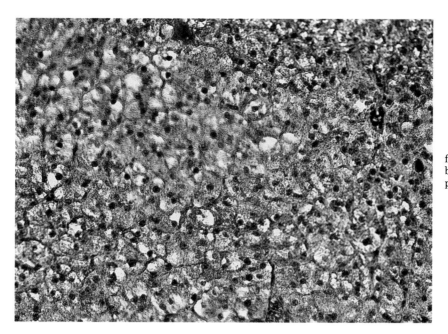

Figure 4-114
PTAH STAINING OF ONCOCYTOMA
PTAH is often helpful in confirming oncocytic differentiation because the mitochondria stain to produce a granular blue cytoplasm.

Mixed tumor and mucoepidermoid carcinoma are the two salivary gland neoplasms that most frequently demonstrate oncocytic metaplasia (see sections on Mixed Tumor and Mucoepidermoid Carcinoma). Oncocytomas lack the pleomorphic architectural patterns, myxochondroid tissue, and proliferation of noncohesive myoepithelial type cells that typify mixed tumors. Mucous cell differentiation, which is demonstrated with mucicarmine stain and is requisite for a diagnosis of mucoepidermoid carcinoma, is rare in oncocytoma. While squamous metaplasia is occasionally present in oncocytomas, the organoid architectural pattern of oncocytomas is uncharacteristic of mucoepidermoid carcinoma.

Clear cell neoplasms that need to be distinguished from clear cell oncocytoma include clear cell mucoepidermoid carcinoma, clear cell adenocarcinoma, epithelial-myoepithelial carcinoma, clear cell acinic cell adenocarcinoma, and metastatic renal cell carcinoma. All of these tumors are malignant and usually demonstrate an infiltrative growth pattern, which distinguishes them from oncocytomas, including those with multinodular growth. Still, in smaller malignant neoplasms infiltrative growth is not always evident. Clear cell mucoepidermoid carcinoma is never completely composed of clear cells and can be differentiated by the features noted in the paragraph above as well as the negative reaction of the clear cells with PTAH. Both clear cell adenocarcinomas and clear cell oncocytomas often contain demonstrable glycogen, but clear cell adenocarcinomas are unreactive with PTAH (see Clear Cell Adenocarcinoma). The characteristic bicellular arrangement of epithelial-myoepithelial carcinoma, with ductal cells surrounded by clear staining myoepithelial cells, is not present in clear cell oncocytoma. Multinodular oncocytic hyperplasia and oncocytomas with clear cells have been mistaken for acinic cell adenocarcinomas (317). The microcystic, papillary cystic, and follicular growth patterns of acinic cell adenocarcinoma are not manifest in oncocytomas. The clear cells in acinic cell adenocarcinomas are negative for glycogen and are not hematoxylinophilic with PTAH stain. Intracytoplasmic diastase-resistant, PAS-positive granules are sometimes evident in a few cells of oncocytomas, but they are less marked than in acinar differentiated cells of acinic cell adenocarcinoma (see

Acinic Cell Adenocarcinoma). Although rare, metastatic renal cell carcinoma in the salivary gland may be the most difficult entity to differentiate from clear cell oncocytoma on the basis of histopathologic features (see Metastatic Disease). Both tumors have an organoid architectural pattern, contain glycogen, and stain with PTAH. In addition to infiltrative growth, prominent vascularity is commonly present in renal cell carcinomas and absent in oncocytomas. Cellular and nuclear pleomorphism is usually more extensive in renal cell carcinoma. Clinical evaluation of the patient for a primary kidney tumor is prudent if any doubt persists about a diagnosis of clear cell oncocytoma.

Prognosis and Treatment. Reported recurrence rates for oncocytomas have ranged from 0 to 30 percent (302,303,305,307,310,319). Brandwein and Huvos (303) reported that 4 of 39 patients had recurrences and that 3 of these 4 patients had multifocal primary tumors. Recurrences have developed 0.5 to 13 years after initial diagnosis. Importantly, neither nuclear pleomorphism nor local tumor infiltration have been independently correlated with a more aggressive or malignant biologic course (303) (see Oncocytic Carcinoma). Multifocal tumor growth and incomplete excision appear to be factors in the incidence of recurrence. In a review of malignant oncocytomas reported in the literature, Gray et al. (310) identified a group of six oncocytic tumors that they considered more aggressive than typical oncocytomas but not malignant. Local infiltration of capsule or adjacent tissues, scattered mitotic figures, and focal cellular pleomorphism were the reasons the original authors had considered them malignant. Interestingly, four of these tumors developed either in the seromucous glands of the nasal mucosa or in the palate. This contrasts with the four intraoral oncocytomas reviewed by Damm et al. (307), which did not recur or grow aggressively.

Excision is the principal modality of therapy for primary and recurrent tumors. Radiation has been used in some cases (302), but Lidang Jensen (315) reported malignant transformation in radiated multinodular oncocytic hyperplasia 15 years after radiation therapy. Kosuda et al. (314) recommended radioiodine therapy after finding reduction in tumor volume of an oncocytoma in a patient treated with therapeutic doses of ^{131}I.

CYSTADENOMA

Definition. Cystadenoma is a rare benign epithelial tumor characterized by predominantly unicystic or multicystic growth; there is focal intraluminal papillary proliferation of the lining epithelium. Neoplastic duct-like structures are also occasionally present.

This neoplasm is probably underestimated in the literature because it has been interpreted as an intraductal hyperplastic, rather than neoplastic, process (333,334,346) and its terminology has been inconsistent. This precludes meaningful comparative analysis of the literature. Supporting the neoplastic nature of cystadenomas are their occasional large size and capacity to displace and compress normal tissues. Morphologically similar lesions occur in many other anatomic sites and are recognized as neoplastic. A malignant counterpart (cystadenocarcinoma) occurs in these sites as well as in the salivary glands (332). Cystadenoma has been classified as a nonspecific form of monomorphic adenoma (344) and as cystic duct adenoma (341). It has been proposed that cystadenoma or papillary cystadenoma represents Warthin's tumor without lymphoid stroma, but the constellation of histopathologic features does not support this (339,340).

General Features. The frequency of occurrence of cystadenoma in the AFIP files reviewed since 1985 is 4.1 percent of all benign epithelial tumors. It is relatively more frequent among benign tumors in the minor than major glands (7.0 versus 3.1 percent, respectively). Its frequency is slightly less than that of oncocytoma and canalicular adenoma. In comparison, Waldron et al. (345) found that cystadenoma represented 8.1 percent of the 245 benign minor gland tumors in their series. There is nearly a 2 to 1 female predominance in AFIP cases and women outnumbered men 3 to 1 in one series (345). The average age of patients with cystadenoma at the time of diagnosis is about 57 years; the youngest and oldest patients are 12 and 89 years, respectively. Cystadenoma rarely occurs before the age of 20 years. About 45 percent of all tumors occur in the parotid gland, and 7 percent occur in the submandibular gland. Compared to AFIP data, parotid lesions are rare in the literature and this observation may relate to differences in diagnostic criteria (343). More than half of all minor gland cystadenomas at the AFIP occurred in the lips and buccal mucosa, a distribution similar to that reported by Waldron et al. (345). This distribution in minor glands is unusual when compared to other salivary gland tumors, which are much more common in the palatal area.

Clinical Features. Cystadenomas of the major glands typically present as slowly enlarging, asymptomatic masses that may be slightly compressible (332). In oral mucosa, these tumors sometimes produce smooth-surfaced nodules that resemble mucoceles. In the minor glands cystadenomas are nearly always less than 1 cm in greatest dimension (332).

Gross and Microscopic Findings. Cut sections reveal multiple small cystic spaces or, occasionally, a single large space, surrounded by lobules of salivary gland or connective tissue. Intraluminal intracystic folds are evident in some tumors but are usually less prominent than those seen in Warthin's tumor. Microscopically, cystadenomas are often well circumscribed but capsular tissue is variable from one tumor to the next and within a single tumor. In one series only 25 percent showed evidence of a distinct fibrous capsule (345). Small foci of tumor may be evident within the connective tissue wall. In some cases the interface of tumor with surrounding tissues is irregular, and the multifocal neoplastic structures suggest infiltrative growth.

The number and size of the cystic structures are also variable among different tumors (fig. 4-115). Single large "cysts" invariably reveal luminal papillary growth. Waldron et al. (345) reported that 20 percent of their cases were unilocular. The individual cystic structures are separated by limited, dense fibrous stroma or completely lack intervening stroma (fig. 4-115A,B). The lumens usually contain eosinophilic or lightly hematoxyphilic fluid that is focally inspissated and contains scattered epithelial and inflammatory cells. Many cases have small duct-like structures that presumably develop into larger cysts (fig. 4-116). Rarely, psammoma-like calcifications (fig. 4-117) or crystalloids are present within the luminal secretions. The epithelium lining these structures is most often cuboidal or columnar (fig. 4-118), but mucous and oncocytic cells are sometimes present focally and can even predominate occasionally (337). Infrequently, the cysts and duct-like structures are

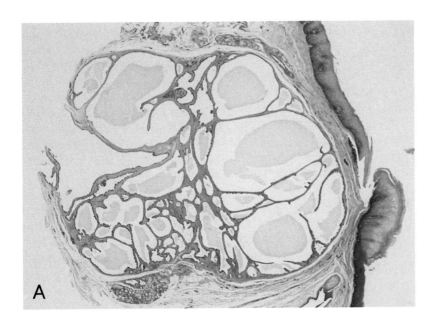

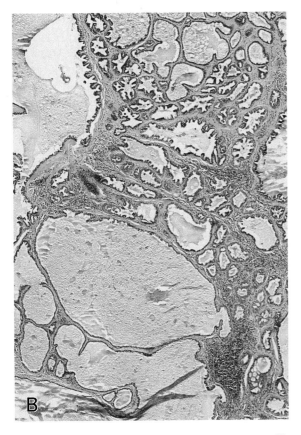

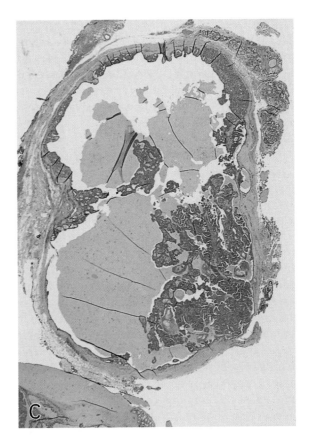

Figure 4-115
CYSTADENOMA

Cystadenomas are composed of several large cystic spaces with limited intraluminal growth (A), numerous small and medium-sized spaces (B), or a single large space (C). Papillary proliferation of the lining epithelium varies from absent to prominent in any of these types. All three examples are well circumscribed but encapsulation is variable. In A it is evident that the tumor is clearly demarcated from the minor glands by a thin rim of fibrous connective tissue.

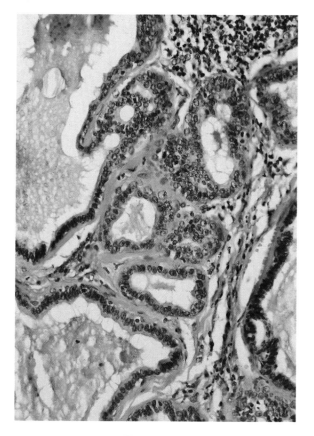

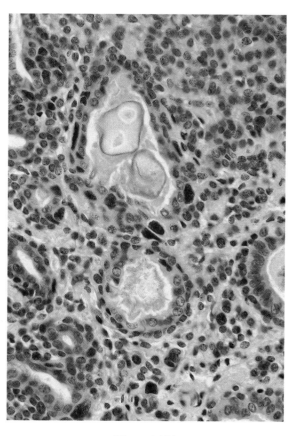

Figure 4-116
DUCT-LIKE STRUCTURES
Several well-formed, intercystic neoplastic ducts are lined by cuboidal epithelium. Focal proliferation of the lining epithelium appears to result in the development of additional ductal structures.

Figure 4-117
CALCIFICATIONS IN CYSTADENOMA
Laminated calcifications are numerous within the lumens of many of the cysts and ductal structures in this case.

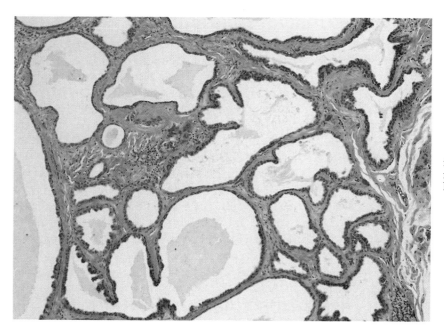

Figure 4-118
CYSTADENOMA
The columnar and cuboidal epithelial lining in this case has a relatively uniform thickness and limited papillary growth.

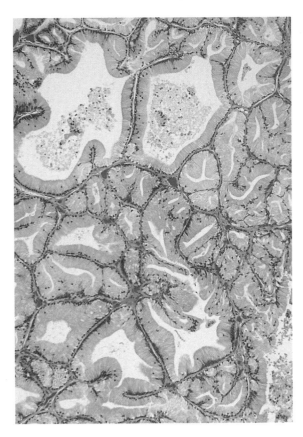

Figure 4-119
CYSTADENOMA, MUCOUS CELL TYPE
The small cysts and duct-like structures in this case are formed entirely of mucous cells. The tall columnar cells have small, basally situated nuclei.

formed exclusively of mucous cells (fig. 4-119). Oncocytic cells, when present, are normally haphazardly arranged, but the AFIP has reviewed several cases in which they were bilayered and resembled the epithelium of Warthin's tumor (fig. 4-120). About 15 percent of the cases in the AFIP files showed some oncocytic change, but in one series nearly three quarters did so (345). Squamous epithelium may be present focally but rarely predominates (fig. 4-121). The nuclei of all cell types are uniformly bland and mitotic figures are extremely rare.

The lining epithelium typically varies in thickness and configuration from uniformly thin to markedly thickened to ramifying papillary projections with central cores of connective tissue. About two thirds of cases have intraluminal papillary growth. Solid rather than cystic tumor growth is limited but occurs as thickenings of the cyst lining, intraluminal papillary structures, and occasional

small islands situated between larger cysts. Extraluminal sheet-like growth is not characteristic of cystadenoma. Patchy collections of lymphocytes are often evident. In rare cases melanin is present in some of the epithelial cells (332,336).

Differential Diagnosis. Distinction between cystadenoma and ductal ectasia with focal epithelial proliferation, which often occurs secondary to duct blockage, is occasionally difficult (335). Normally, fibrosis, acinar atrophy, squamous metaplasia, chronic inflammation, and a convoluted lining epithelium with periductal hyalinization are present in obstructive disease (fig. 4-122). The submandibular gland is the most frequently and severely involved site. The number of closely associated cystic structures and degree of intraluminal epithelial proliferation are usually much greater in cystadenomas. Ectatic ducts and cysts secondary to obstruction are more widely spaced than comparable structures in cystadenoma, and occasionally they track to an obvious duct.

Unlike Warthin's tumor, a large proportion of cystadenomas arise in salivary glands other than the parotid. Warthin's tumor has a striking lymphoid stroma and has a characteristic bilayered oncocytic epithelium. In cystadenoma that has oncocytic epithelium (so-called papillary oncocytic cystadenoma) the epithelium is usually not bilayered, focally may have other types of epithelium admixed with the oncocytic cells, and, although patchy inflammatory infiltrates may be present, a diffuse and dense lymphoid stroma with germinal centers is not evident.

Some reported cases of cystadenoma represent intraductal papilloma (338,343). The two lesions share some features, but unlike cystadenomas, intraductal papillomas are always unicystic because they occur in a dilated salivary gland duct. The intraluminal papillary fronds in papilloma are more numerous and complex than those of papillary cystadenoma and are entirely contained by the single cystic structure (see Intraductal Papilloma).

In some cases, the difference between low-grade cystadenocarcinoma and cystadenoma is subtle. Only a minority of cystadenomas have a distinct fibrous capsule and both lack obvious cytomorphologic abnormalities. Distinction between them depends on the identification of frank invasion of salivary gland parenchyma or connective tissue in cystadenocarcinoma. Step sections are recommended for equivocal cases.

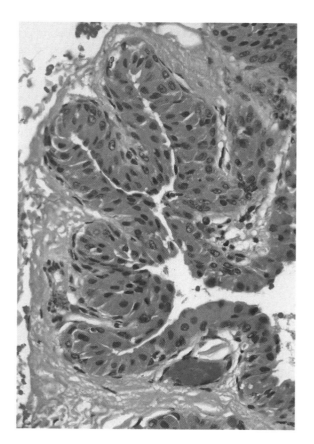
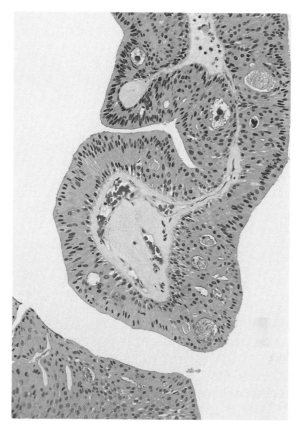

Figure 4-120
ONCOCYTIC EPITHELIUM IN CYSTADENOMA
The example on the left shows somewhat variable and unorganized oncocytic cells, an appearance that is much more common than the bilayered appearance evident on the right. Both types are often designated papillary oncocytic cystadenoma when the oncocytic epithelium predominates.

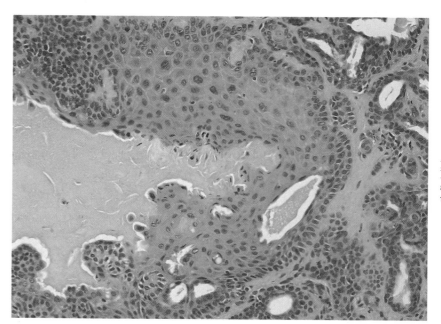

Figure 4-121
SQUAMOUS METAPLASIA
Squamous epithelium comprises a small proportion of the lining epithelium in this case. In some lesions its presence appears to be secondary to inflammation.

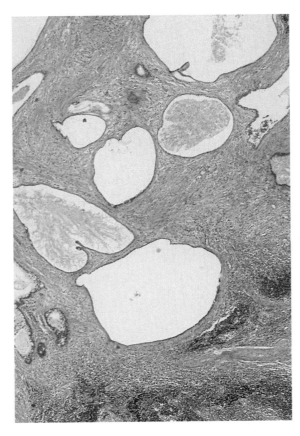

Figure 4-122
DUCTAL ECTASIA SECONDARY TO OBSTRUCTION

Numerous ectatic ducts are widely spaced by prominent fibrotic tissue that has dense collections of chronic inflammatory cells. In addition to the inflammation and fibrosis, an inflammatory rather than neoplastic process is suggested by the uniform thickness of the lining epithelium and the lack of focal epithelial proliferation.

Similar to cystadenoma, some low-grade mucoepidermoid carcinomas are prominently cystic, demonstrate papillary growth, are partly circumscribed, and are composed of several similar cell types. The most important distinguishing criterion is the noncystic epithelial proliferation in mucoepidermoid carcinoma. The epithelium lining the cystic structures is often markedly thickened. Papillae, if present, are irregular and more complex than those seen in cystadenoma, and extraluminal solid islands of tumor are often evident. The cellular proliferation is more varied than in cystadenoma and often reveals combinations of epidermoid, mucous, and smaller intermediate or basaloid cells. In rare mucoepidermoid carcinomas that are composed almost exclusively of mucous cells, the cells and the structures they form are more irregular than those found in cystadenoma, and they infiltrate surrounding tissues (see Mucoepidermoid Carcinoma).

Polycystic disease is a rare developmental malformation of the duct system (342). It is distinguished from cystadenoma by its more diffuse involvement of the parotid lobules, focal apocrine-like lining epithelium, and presence of spheroliths within the luminal spaces.

Treatment and Prognosis. Data from case reports and small series of cystadenomas over the past two decades and at the AFIP indicate that this tumor is unlikely to recur (336,338, 343). Conservative but complete surgical removal is recommended.

DUCTAL PAPILLOMAS

A papillary histomorphologic architecture is a common component of several types of salivary gland neoplasm, including Warthin tumors, cystadenomas, cystadenocarcinomas, acinic cell adenocarcinomas, mucoepidermoid carcinomas, and polymorphous low-grade adenocarcinomas. In addition, there is a group of rare benign adenomas of ductal epithelium whose principal architectural feature is papillary growth, yet they are distinct, both clinically and morphologically, from these other more common types. On the basis of cell type, morphology, and location along the salivary gland duct unit, these so-called ductal papillomas have been categorized into three subtypes: intraductal papilloma, inverted ductal papilloma, and sialadenoma papilliferum (354,371).

These three types of ductal papilloma have been defined in the updated WHO classification of salivary gland tumors (371), but terminology has been confusing in previous literature. For example, the intraductal papilloma reported by Castigliano and Gold (350) is consistent with sialadenoma papilliferum, which had not been described at the time of their report, but some reports of sialadenoma papilliferum (353,361,366,367) do not fulfill the clinicopathologic criteria for that diagnosis established by Abrams and Finck (348). Some of the papillary cystadenomas reported by Kerpel et al. (364), Sher (372), and Goldman (360) appear to be consistent with the definition of intraductal papilloma. The rarity of ductal papillomas and inconsistent terminology have caused problems with assessment and interpretation of these tumors.

Intraductal Papilloma

Definition. Intraductal papilloma is a luminal papillary proliferation that causes unicystic dilatation of a duct.

Intraductal papilloma and papillary cystadenoma have several features in common, and some investigators include tumors with features of intraductal papilloma within their spectrum of cystadenoma (364,372,375). Whether intraductal papilloma is distinct from papillary cystadenoma is debatable; however, generally, cystadenomas are multicystic structures while intraductal papillomas are unicystic. Intraductal papilloma distends a duct lumen with an exuberant papillary proliferation of ductal epithelium, which typically appears to emanate from a portion of the cyst wall. In contrast, rare unicystic cystadenomas are characterized by folds and excrescence of ductal epithelium at multiple foci along the wall of the cyst's lumen (see Cystadenoma).

General Features. Intraductal papillomas have been infrequently reported (347,363) and rarely categorized in surveys of large series of salivary gland neoplasms (354,355). Waldron et al. (375) reported 4 unicystic cystadenomas among 426 minor salivary gland tumors, but it is not known if any of these had features of intraductal papilloma. Among a survey of 103 salivary gland tumors of the lip, Neville et al. (368) reported 1 intraductal papilloma. The histologic features of the intraductal papillomas reported by Castigliano and Gold (350) and King and Hill (365) are more consistent with sialadenoma papilliferum and epithelial-myoepithelial carcinoma, respectively.

Since 1985, 4 intraductal papillomas have been identified among nearly 3,100 epithelial salivary gland tumors reviewed at the AFIP. Including the few comparable cases reported in the literature (347,363,368,372), all tumors, with the exception of one tumor in the parotid gland, involved excretory ducts of intraoral minor salivary glands. The oral sites were palate (3 cases), lip (2 cases), buccal mucosa (1 case), and ventral tongue (1 case). Five of the eight patients were male. Patient age ranged from 40 to 70 years, with a median age of 58 years. The tumors presented as asymptomatic submucosal swellings.

Pathologic Findings. Grossly, intraductal papillomas are well-circumscribed, unilocular, submucosal cystic structures that range in size

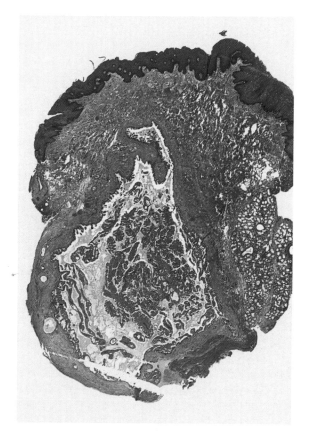

Figure 4-123
INTRADUCTAL PAPILLOMA

Cyst in the submucosa of the lower lip contains multiple irregular fragments of epithelium and pale-staining mucinous material. The upper portion of the cyst lumen appears to be contiguous with a dilated duct. At the far right are lobules of minor salivary gland tissue.

from 0.5 to 2.0 cm. The lumens are partially or completely filled with a friable tissue that extends from the wall. Microscopically, a fortuitous plane of section reveals that the cyst is in continuity with an interlobular or excretory duct of salivary gland tissue (fig. 4-123). Typically, the lumen of the cyst contains an extensive papillary tissue proliferation characterized by numerous intricately branching fronds (fig. 4-124). In many planes of section the papillary tissue appears not to be in continuity with the wall of the cyst, but in one or more foci the papillary epithelial proliferation is continuous with the lining epithelium of the cystic duct. The papillary proliferations are composed of ductal epithelium supported by thin cores of fibrovascular tissue. The epithelium is generally a uniform single or

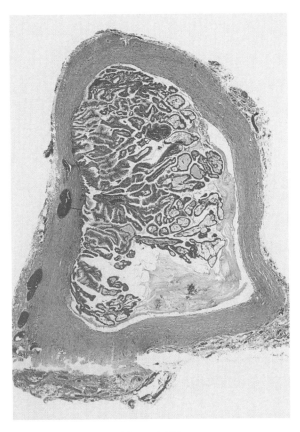

Figure 4-124
INTRADUCTAL PAPILLOMA

The cystic structure has a thick fibrous tissue wall, and the lumen contains a branching, papillary epithelial proliferation that extends from the lateral portion of the cyst wall and nearly fills the lumen. Some of the papillary epithelial proliferation appears to be floating in the lumen in this plane of section.

double layer. From one tumor to another the character of the epithelium can vary from low cuboidal to tall columnar and from eosinophilic to goblet cell-like mucocytes (fig. 4-125). Mitotic figures are absent or scarce, and little cytologic atypia is evident. The luminal surface of the cyst wall is usually covered by the same ductal epithelium as the papillary fronds, but in two tumors it was markedly attenuated. Dense fibrous tissue of 1 to 2 mm usually forms the wall of the cyst and contains scattered to moderately dense inflammatory cells.

Differential Diagnosis. The morphologic distinction of intraductal papilloma from papillary cystadenoma is noted in the definition. Inverted ductal papilloma shares some morphologic features with intraductal papilloma, and the pathogenesis of the two lesions is probably sim-

ilar. However, the cellular composition and specific location within the salivary duct differentiate these two types of ductal papilloma (see Inverted Ductal Papilloma below). Salivary duct blockage due to sialoliths or other factors often causes duct dilatation, and the ductal epithelium proximal to the blockage often demonstrates focal hyperplasia (356). The duct dilatation is usually less than that produced by intraductal papillomas, and the epithelial hyperplasia is much less extensive and lacks the complex papillary architecture. Rarely, low-grade mucoepidermoid carcinoma and acinic cell adenocarcinoma occur as unicystic lesions with foci of luminal epithelial proliferation along the cyst walls. The complex papillary architecture of intraductal papilloma is absent. These neoplasms are correctly identified by the characteristic epidermoid, intermediate, clear and mucous cell proliferation or acinar cell differentiation in mucoepidermoid carcinoma and acinic cell adenocarcinoma, respectively.

Prognosis and Treatment. Intraductal papillomas are not known to recur and are treated by simple excision.

Inverted Ductal Papilloma

Definition. Inverted ductal papilloma is a luminal papillary proliferation that arises at the junction of a salivary gland duct and the oral mucosal surface epithelium and expands as a nodular mass into the lamina propria. Conforming to the character of the normal ductal epithelium at this junction, the proliferation is predominantly of basal epidermoid cells and fewer columnar type duct cells. This salivary gland tumor has several features that are similar to the inverted papilloma of sinonasal tract mucosa (362), but the growth potential is significantly different.

General Features. At the time of preparation of this text only 13 documented cases of inverted ductal papilloma of salivary gland had been reported (349,352,376,377). This excludes the parotid gland tumor reported by Gardiner et al. (359), which did not fulfill the parameters described by White et al. (376) and described below. Since by definition inverted ductal papilloma occurs at the junction of ductal and mucosal epithelia, it does not occur within the parotid or submandibular glands. Like other rare tumors, it has not been included in most general surveys

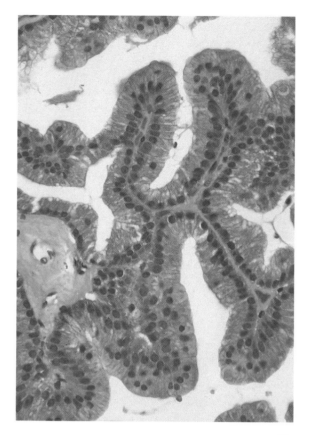 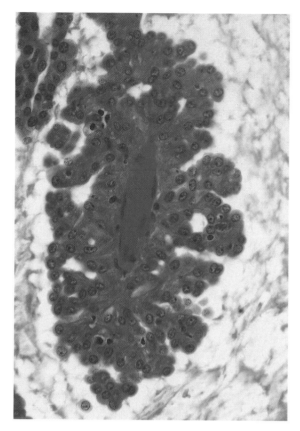

Figure 4-125
INTRADUCTAL PAPILLOMA
Thin cores of fibrovascular tissue support the elaborate papillary proliferation observed within the lumen.
Left: The epithelium in this intraductal papilloma is a single cell layer of tall columnar cells with eosinophilic cytoplasm and basally oriented nuclei. The cells are very uniform.
Right: The epithelium from another intraductal papilloma is cuboidal and forms a layer one to three cells thick around an engorged capillary.

of salivary gland neoplasia. Regezi et al. (369) counted 4 inverted ductal papillomas among 238 minor salivary gland neoplasms they reviewed, but Waldron et al. (375) did not identify any among 426 minor salivary gland tumors. Since 1985, four cases have been accessioned into the files of the AFIP.

Among the 13 reported and 4 AFIP cases the sites of involvement were lip (8 cases), buccal mucosa/mandibular vestibule (7 cases), floor of mouth (1 case), and soft palate (1 case). There was no sex predilection, and the patients ranged in age from 32 to 66 years (mean age, 50 years). The lesions presented as 1.0 to 1.5 cm, asymptomatic mucosal swellings. A pit, indention, or crater in the mucosal surface overlying the swelling has been described in some cases, and fluid could be expressed from these pores (358,

376,377). They are generally described as slow growing lesions with durations before treatment of several months to a year.

Pathologic Findings. Microscopic examination of inverted ductal papilloma at low magnification reveals a well-demarcated, rounded epithelial tumor mass with a broad, relatively smooth interface with the fibrous tissue of the lamina propria (fig. 4-126) Depending upon the plane of section, the tumor is located just beneath the mucosal epithelium or is in continuity with the surface epithelium. In those sections that show continuity with the mucosal surface, the mucosal epithelium focally inverts to form a lip that borders a pit or crater that connects to the lumen of the tumor mass, and the mucosal epithelium at the site of inversion is continuous with the tumor epithelium (fig. 4-127). The size of the mucosal pore

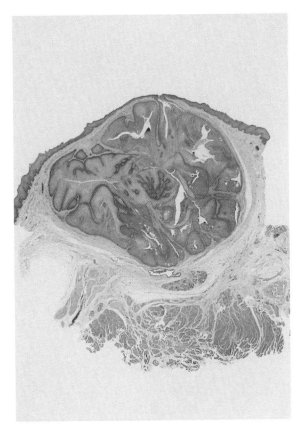

Figure 4-126
INVERTED DUCTAL PAPILLOMA
A well-circumscribed, partly cystic, epithelial tumor is located in the lamina propria above the skeletal muscle and just beneath the mucosal epithelium of the lower lip.

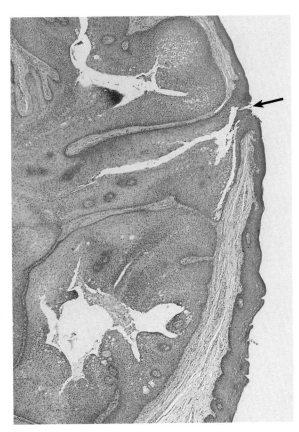

Figure 4-127
INVERTED DUCTAL PAPILLOMA
The mucosal epithelium of the lip inverts to form a small pore (arrow). The epithelium of this pore is continuous with the tumor epithelial proliferation.

varies from a tiny pit to an opening of 1 to 2 mm (fig. 4-128). The tumor is composed of large, often bulbous, papillary epithelial proliferations that occupy most of the lumen of the lesion. The visual impression is that the papillary epithelial proliferation has filled the lumen of a salivary gland duct and expanded outwardly into the lamina propria (figs. 4-126, 4-128). The tumor appears to have pushed rather than infiltrated into the lamina propria. Although the tumor develops in the extraglandular excretory duct, lobules of salivary gland tissue are frequently observed along the periphery of the tumor mass (fig. 4-128).

Most of the neoplastic epithelium is epidermoid, with features similar to the basal one third of the mucosal stratified squamous epithelium. The epithelial cells are uniform, and there are few or no cytologic features of malignancy, such

as mitotic figures and cellular and nuclear pleomorphism. The luminal surface of many of the papillary epithelial proliferations is covered by a columnar epithelium similar to the ductal epithelium of the normal excretory duct of the salivary gland (fig. 4-129). Within the columnar epithelial layer or the subjacent epidermoid cells are often small aggregates or individual mucocytes with pale basophilic cytoplasm that stains with mucicarmine, PAS, and Alcian blue.

Differential Diagnosis. Inverted ductal papilloma has histopathologic features that are similar to those of inverted papilloma of the sinonasal tract. The papillary growth, extension into the lamina propria, and cellular composition are quite similar, except that the surface layer of columnar epithelium of the sinonasal papilloma is often ciliated (fig. 4-130). On the other hand,

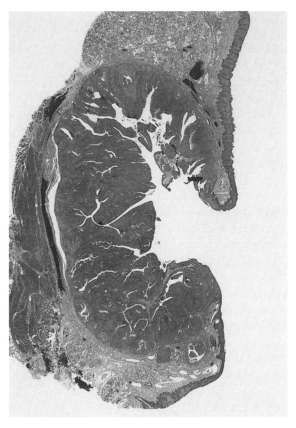

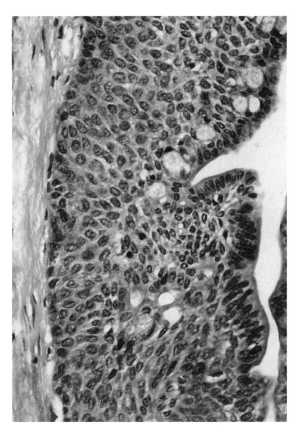

Figure 4-128
INVERTED DUCTAL PAPILLOMA
This inverted ductal papilloma of the lower lip has a small crater-like opening at the mucosal surface. The mucosal opening is continuous with the lumen of the ductal papilloma. Lobules of minor salivary gland tissue are present at the top and bottom, and skeletal muscle is evident at the base.

Figure 4-129
INVERTED DUCTAL PAPILLOMA
Most of the epithelial cells are basaloid squamous cells, but the luminal surface in this section is lined by columnar duct-type epithelial cells that overlie the epidermoid cells. Several pale-staining cells within the epithelium are mucocytes.

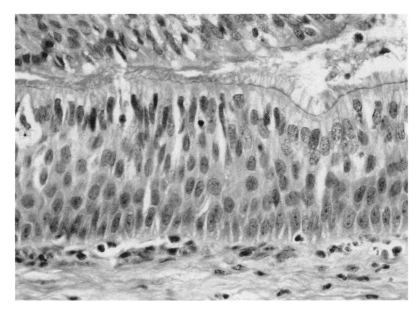

Figure 4-130
INVERTED
SINONASAL PAPILLOMA
This section of the epithelium from a papilloma of the nasal cavity shows a five- to six-cell layer of epidermoid type cells and a surface layer of ciliated columnar cells.

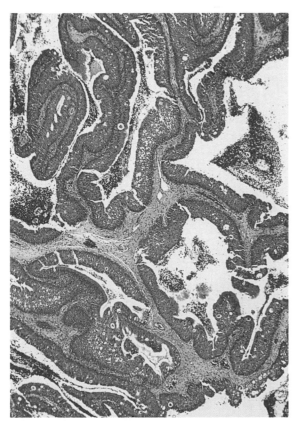

Figure 4-131
INVERTED SINONASAL PAPILLOMA
The sinonasal papilloma is not a discrete mass and can involve extensive areas of sinonasal mucosa, which sometimes makes it difficult to excise.

there are important differences between these two tumors. The inverted ductal papilloma is a small and confined nodular mass that is easily excised. The more common inverted sinonasal papilloma often involves extensive areas of mucosa, can be difficult to surgically eradicate, and has a significant recurrence rate (fig. 4-131). Malignant transformation occurs in sinonasal papillomas but is not known to occur in inverted ductal papillomas of salivary gland. Epidermoid, mucous, and ductal cells are characteristic of both inverted ductal papilloma and mucoepidermoid carcinoma. Unlike the limited and confined growth of inverted ductal papilloma, mucoepidermoid carcinoma is typically a multicystic, multinodular, and infiltrative neoplasm that rarely is dominated by a papillary growth pattern.

Treatment and Prognosis. Inverted ductal papillomas are treated by local excision and are not known to recur.

Sialadenoma Papilliferum

Definition. Sialadenoma papilliferum is an exophytic papillary proliferation that involves mucosal surface epithelium or epidermis and salivary duct epithelium.

General Features. Sialadenoma papilliferum was first reported as an entity in 1969 by Abrams and Finck (348), but a tumor with the features of sialadenoma papilliferum had been reported in 1954 by Castigliano and Gold (350) as an intraductal papilloma. It is unique among salivary gland neoplasms because it manifests as an exophytic papillary excrescence of the mucosa rather than as a submucosal or intraglandular mass. Clinically, it is usually described and diagnosed as a mucosal squamous papilloma. Although there are more reports in the literature of sialadenoma papilliferum than inverted ductal papilloma or intraductal papilloma, it is an uncommon salivary gland neoplasm. Twenty-nine acceptable cases had been reported at the time of preparation of this text (350,351,369,374). Waldron et al. (375) had 5 cases in their survey of 426 minor salivary gland tumors, and Regezi et al. (369) found 2 among 238 minor salivary gland tumors. The AFIP has only recorded 2 cases among over 1,000 minor salivary gland tumors accessioned since 1985. Confusion about the criteria for diagnosis has existed since some reported cases (353,361,366,367) did not fulfill the parameters described by Abrams and Finck (348) and lacked an exophytic surface component or proliferative ductal component. Solomon et al. (373) reported an intriguing case of a large, exophytic, papillary neoplasm of the soft palate that initially had features of mucosal papilloma but recurrences had features of a glandular component. The glandular component, however, was formed by ciliated pseudostratified epithelium more suggestive of respiratory epithelium. The tumor metastasized to a submandibular lymph node, and the authors suggested that this tumor may have been a malignant sialadenoma papilliferum. No other reported cases of sialadenoma papilliferum have had these features or behavior, and the diagnosis of sialadenoma papilliferum for this tumor remains questionable.

The hard or soft palate has been the site of occurrence of 85 percent of the tumors. In fact, the junction of the hard and soft palate is a frequently noted site. The buccal mucosa, mandibular retromolar pad, tonsillar pillar, and lip are other intraoral sites. Only one tumor involved a major salivary gland, the parotid gland tumor described in the original report by Abrams and Finck (348). This tumor was also remarkable for its large size (7.5 cm) because most lesions are less than 1 cm in diameter. It also involved the epidermis of the skin overlying the parotid gland rather than the oral mucosal epithelium, which has been involved by all other tumors. All patients have been adults who ranged in age from 32 to 87 years (mean age, 62 years). Masi et al. (367) reported a sialadenoma papilliferum of the adenoids in a 2-year-old child, but the site and composition of this lesion indicate it was probably not a sialadenoma papilliferum. There is only a slight male predilection. The tumors are generally asymptomatic. The duration of the lesions before treatment is usually several months, but durations of 10 years have been reported (348,374).

Pathologic Findings. Grossly, sialadenoma papilliferum is a well-circumscribed, round to oval excrescence of the mucosal surface. The surface texture is pebbly, verrucoid, or papillary. The base of the lesion is broad or pedunculated. Cut section shows that papillae extend from about 0.1 to 1.0 cm above the level of the surrounding mucosa. At the base of the lesion a nodular mass extends 0.1 to 0.5 cm below the level of the mucosal surface, and small cystic spaces are sometimes visible.

At low magnification, the initial microscopic impression typically suggests squamous papilloma since papillary stalks of fibrovascular tissue covered with acanthotic and parakeratotic stratified squamous epithelium extend above the level of adjacent mucosa (fig. 4-132). Further inspection discloses a glandular proliferation immediately subjacent to the papillary mucosa (fig. 4-133). The glandular component is composed of multiple rounded cysts or elongated and dilated duct-like structures that have proliferated in the lamina propria. There is no capsule around this glandular proliferation, which is only moderately well circumscribed (fig. 4-134). The glandular structures usually have irregular luminal contours due to folds and papillae of the epithelial linings. The duct-type epithelium is typically a double layer composed of luminal columnar cells and basal cuboidal or flattened cells (fig. 4-135).

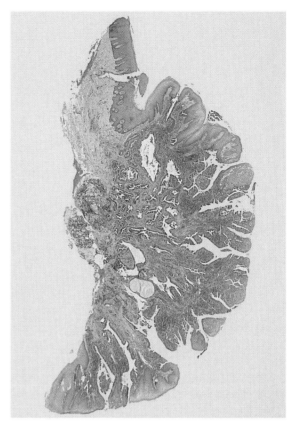

Figure 4-132
SIALADENOMA PAPILLIFERUM
Multiple papillary extensions of the mucosa above the level of the adjacent palatal mucosa are more indicative of an oral squamous papilloma than most types of salivary gland neoplasms except sialadenoma papilliferum.

The eosinophilic cytoplasm and conformation of these cells are typical of interlobular and excretory duct epithelia. Mucocytes are occasionally evident among the ductal cells. Branching ductal structures extend from the glandular proliferation toward the mucosal surface and are contiguous with many of the clefts between the surface papillary projections (fig. 4-136). Toward the base of many of the interpapillary clefts a transition from stratified squamous epithelium to ductal epithelium is observed (fig. 4-137). A modest to intense inflammatory infiltrate is usually evident in the lamina propria of the mucosal papilla, and within the stroma of the glandular proliferation. At the junction with the papillary tumor, the normal mucosal epithelium is often acanthotic, with elongated rete pegs. The mucosal stratified squamous epithelium is continuous with the epithelium of the stalk of pedunculated tumors.

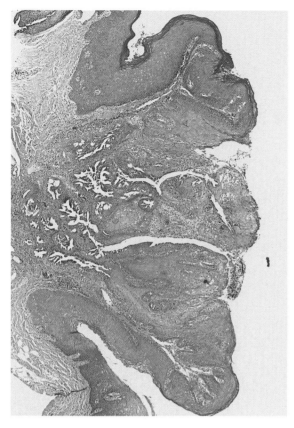

Figure 4-133
SIALADENOMA PAPILLIFERUM
Irregularly contoured, elongated and rounded clear spaces beneath the raised surface of this sialadenoma papilliferum represent ductal proliferation.

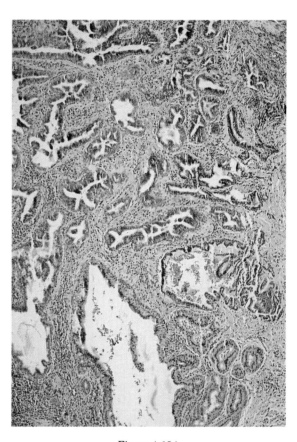

Figure 4-134
SIALADENOMA PAPILLIFERUM
The absence of a capsule and poor circumscription of this proliferation of irregular ductal structures at the base of a palatal sialadenoma papilliferum may incorrectly suggest more aggressive behavior.

Figure 4-135
SIALADENOMA
PAPILLIFERUM
The dilated ductal structures have many folds and papillae that give them irregular lumens. The epithelium that lines the lumens is typically a two cell–thick layer of eosinophilic columnar cells covering short basaloid cells. The stroma contains an infiltrate of plasma cells and lymphocytes.

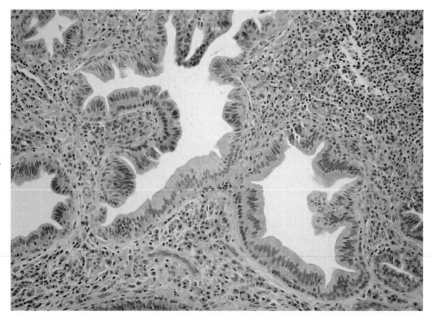

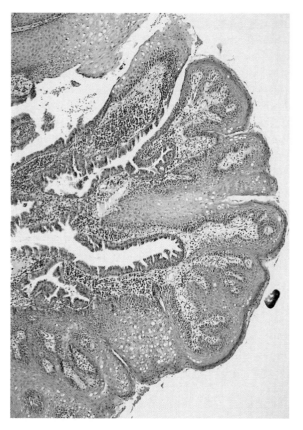

Figure 4-136
SIALADENOMA PAPILLIFERUM
Branching ductal structures extend into the papillary mucosa, and their lumens are frequently contiguous with clefts of the mucosal papillae.

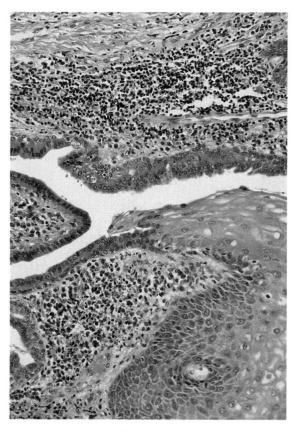

Figure 4-137
SIALADENOMA PAPILLIFERUM
An abrupt transition from stratified squamous epithelium that covers the mucosal papillae to columnar epithelium that lines branching ducts is evident at the base of an interpapillary cleft.

Electron microscopic study of a sialadenoma papilliferum by Fantasia et al. (357) showed that the ductal cells had numerous mitochondria, desmosomal attachments, junctional complexes, cytoplasmic filaments parallel to the long axis of the cells, and apical-oriented nuclei. Along the basilar surface was a well-defined lamina. The cells at the tips of the papillary projections had features typical of squamous epithelial cells, such as desmosomal attachments and bundles of tonofilaments.

Differential Diagnosis. Squamous papilloma is the entity that most closely resembles sialadenoma papilliferum, both clinically and histopathologically. The glandular proliferation and ductal epithelium found in transition from the superficial squamous epithelium distinguishes sialadenoma papilliferum from the common squamous papilloma.

A papillary configuration and epidermoid, ductal, and mucous cells are features of both sialadenoma papilliferum and inverted ductal papilloma. Likewise, both these tumors occur at the junction of glandular ducts with the mucosal epithelium. Inverted ductal papilloma is endophytic while sialadenoma papilliferum is exophytic. Inverted ductal papilloma lacks the proliferation of ductal structures present in sialadenoma papilliferum.

Some cellular and morphologic features of sialadenoma papilliferum are similar to mucoepidermoid carcinoma, including squamous, mucous, and ductal cell types; cystic glandular structures; and absence of encapsulation. The unique exophytic papillomatous architecture of sialadenoma papilliferum readily differentiates it. In addition, the organization and relationship of the epidermoid, mucous, and ductal epithelium in sialadenoma papilliferum is quite different from that of mucoepidermoid carcinoma: in sialadenoma papilliferum there is a progression from squamous epithelium at the surface to ductal epithelium to glandular proliferation at the base of the lesion; in mucoepidermoid carcinoma all of these cellular elements are intermingled.

Treatment and Prognosis. Other than the uncharacteristic and questionable sialadenoma papilliferum reported by Solomon et al. (373), only the palatal tumor reported by Rennie et al. (370) is known to have recurred following local excision. The recurrent tumor was again treated by local excision and had not recurred after a year.

SEBACEOUS ADENOMA AND SEBACEOUS LYMPHADENOMA

Sebaceous glands are commonly found in normal oral mucosa (383), and in about 10 percent of normal parotid glands and 6 percent of submandibular glands (389). They may be found in major glands that are involved by inflammatory, cystic, or neoplastic disease (379,389,390). Sebaceous glandular elements have also been seen in intraparatoid and periparotid lymph nodes (379,388,389). The morphology and lipid composition of these sebaceous glands, at least in the parotid gland, are identical to cutaneous sebaceous glands (392). Despite the frequent occurrence of sebaceous glands in salivary tissue, tumors that demonstrate sebaceous differentiation are exceptionally rare and comprise less than 0.2 percent of all benign and malignant salivary gland tumors.

Sebaceous Adenoma

Definition. Sebaceous adenoma is a rare, benign, encapsulated epithelial tumor composed of cells that form solid, variably shaped islands and cysts, both showing focal sebaceous differentiation.

General Features. Cases from the AFIP reviewed since 1985, showed sebaceous adenomas represent about 0.7 percent of all adenomas of the major salivary glands. A recent review of the literature (379) observed that the mean age of patients with these neoplasms is 58 years, with

a range of 22 to 90 years. More men than woman are affected, with a ratio of 1.6 to 1. Of the 21 cases reported for which the site of occurrence was known, 12 involved the parotid gland and 2 were in the submandibular gland. Four cases from the buccal mucosa and three from the posterior mandibular mucosa have been reported. Because sebaceous glands are commonly found in oral mucosa and these may give rise to adenoma (381,383), it is difficult to confirm a salivary origin in tumors from minor gland sites. The size has varied from 0.4 to 3.0 cm. Duration has varied from 2 months to 15 years. Most patients were asymptomatic and noted a firm to hard, slowly growing mass in the involved site.

Gross and Microscopic Findings. Grossly, sebaceous adenomas are usually sharply circumscribed. They may be focally cystic and vary in color from grayish white to yellowish gray (379, 386). Microscopically, they are at least partially encapsulated (fig. 4-138) but cystic areas in particular may have an irregular interface with surrounding tissues without a well-defined capsule (fig. 4-139). Numerous nests and islands of tumor cells are surrounded by fibrous stroma, which may be focally hyalinized. The tumor cells are often predominantly squamous with only focal sebaceous differentiation but in some cases many of the epithelial nests are largely sebaceous (fig. 4-140). As noted, some cases show the formation of small, closely associated ductal or cyst-like proliferations instead of the solid islands of tumor cells (fig. 4-141). These structures are lined by cells that reveal both squamous and sebaceous differentiation in variable proportions (fig. 4-142). Scattered mucus-containing cells may be seen among the lining cells but sebaceous cells are themselves negative for mucin. A foreign body reaction or collections of histiocytes (fig. 4-143) are seen in some cases (386). Occasionally, these tumors are composed of solid sheets of oncocytic cells, presumably representing metaplasia (379,382,386,387).

Treatment and Prognosis. Follow-up information is available for 13 patients over a period that ranges from 3 months to 16 years (mean of 4.5 years) (379). No recurrences have been recorded. Treatment has consisted of total excision of the tumor, parotidectomy, or total submandibulectomy.

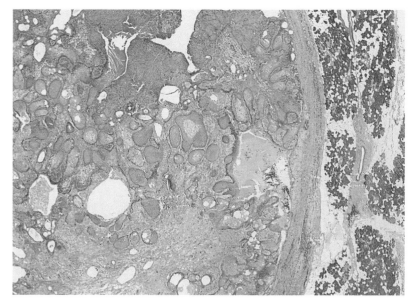

Figure 4-138
SEBACEOUS ADENOMA
Distinct capsular tissue clearly delineates the tumor from the surrounding parotid gland tissue.

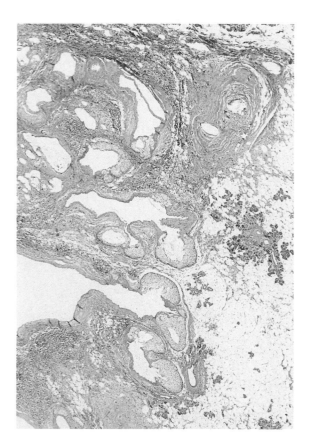
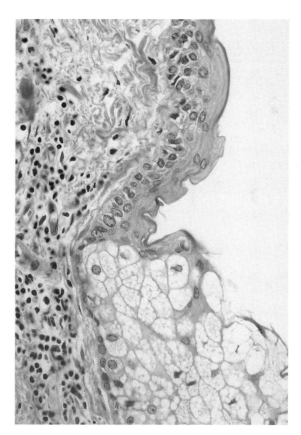

Figure 4-139
CYSTIC SEBACEOUS ADENOMA

In this sebaceous adenoma cystic rather than solid growth predominates. The unencapsulated neoplastic tissue has an irregular interface and directly contacts adjacent salivary gland.

Left: The marked replacement of glandular parenchyma by fat is explained by the advanced age of the patient.

Right: Squamous and sebaceous differentiation are sharply demarcated in the lining epithelium.

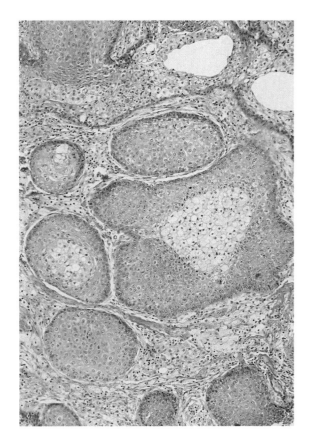
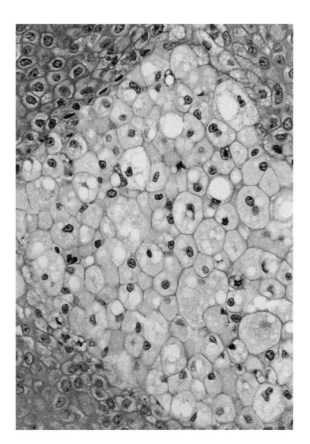

Figure 4-140
SEBACEOUS ADENOMA

Left: In many cases numerous solid islands are seen that vary in size and are composed primarily of squamous cells. Centrally, some of the islands demonstrate sebaceous differentiation.

Right: At higher magnification the sebaceous nature of the central focus of cells and sebaceous features in several of the cells in the adjacent squamous areas are evident.

Figure 4-141
SEBACEOUS ADENOMA

In this example many cystic and duct-like structures are surrounded by dense fibrous stroma. Sebaceous differentiation is lacking or subtle in many areas but obvious in others.

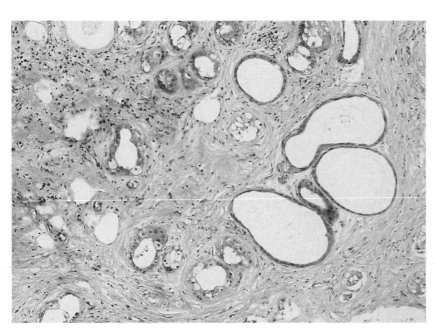

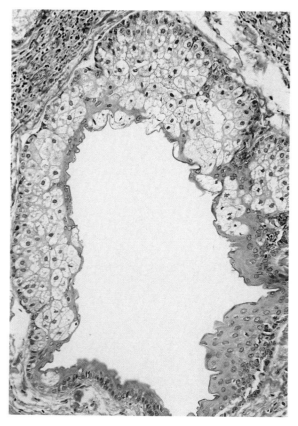

Figure 4-142
CYSTIC SEBACEOUS ADENOMA
This lesion was characterized by the presence of numerous cystic structures. The prominent sebaceous element appears to be considerably more proliferative than the squamous component.

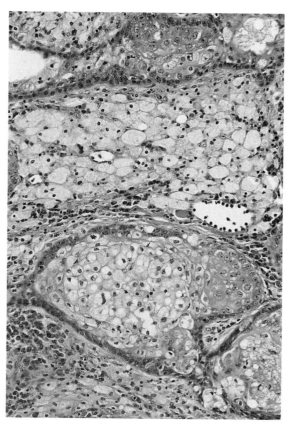

Figure 4-143
HISTIOCYTES IN
SEBACEOUS ADENOMA
A large focus of foamy histiocytes is seen between islands of sebaceous and squamous cells. Scattered inflammatory cells are also evident.

Sebaceous Lymphadenoma

Definition. Sebaceous lymphadenoma is a rare benign tumor that is composed of irregular, proliferating nests and islands of epithelium, including solid and gland-like sebaceous elements, surrounded by lymphoid stroma.

General Features. Sebaceous lymphadenoma represents about 0.1 percent (13 of 9,253) of all adenomas in the AFIP files. A recent review of 39 cases (379) showed that about three quarters were diagnosed when the patients were between the ages of 50 and 80 years, with a range of 25 to 89 years. Men and women were affected nearly equally. Of the tumors with known site of occurrence, 36 (92 percent) were in the parotid gland or in the area of the gland, and 1 occurred in the anterior midline of the neck. Duration

ranged from less than a month to 18 years. Most patients noted a progressively enlarging, painless mass. One example associated with Warthin's tumor has been reported (384).

The nature of the lymphoid tissue in this lesion is controversial, and closely parallels the controversy that surrounds the lymphoid element found in Warthin's tumor. The WHO monograph on the histologic typing of salivary gland tumors (391) points out that the similarity of sebaceous lymphadenoma to Warthin's tumor suggests the tumor may arise from salivary duct inclusions within a parotid lymph node, with sebaceous rather than oncocytic metaplasia. As observed elsewhere (see Warthin's Tumor), there are examples of Warthin's tumor in which there is no evidence of existing or previously existing nodal structure. Although there are fewer cases

133

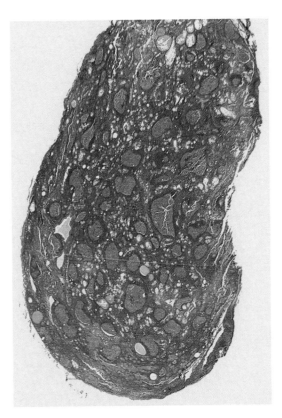
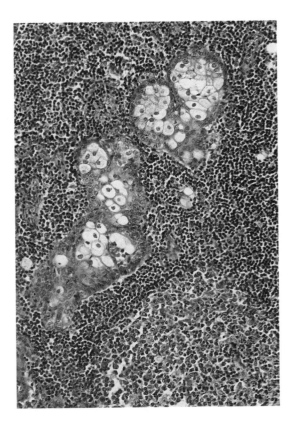

Figure 4-144
SEBACEOUS LYMPHADENOMA
Left: This well-circumscribed mass is composed of numerous germinal centers between which are many small proliferating epithelial islands.
Right: Sebaceous differentiation within many of the islands becomes evident at higher magnification.

of sebaceous lymphadenoma available for study, we have seen examples in which the lymphoid component does not appear to represent nodal tissue. It may be that the lymphoid element represents a secondary, reactive response to the epithelial proliferation, as seen in various other parotid gland tumors. We have referred to this phenomenon as tumor-associated lymphoid proliferation (378).

Gross and Microscopic Findings. The gross appearance has been reported as solid to multicystic (379,387) and yellow to yellow-white (380,386). Sebum-filled spaces may be observed (392). Sebaceous lymphadenomas may have a well-developed capsule but just as often are partially, or occasionally, completely unencapsulated. When unencapsulated the tumor demonstrates a well-circumscribed periphery that pushes against adjacent parenchyma and connective tissue in an expansive rather than infil-

trative manner (fig. 4-144). The tumor typically consists of numerous islands, duct-like structures, and small to medium sized cysts composed of squamous, cuboidal, columnar, and sebaceous cells (fig. 4-145). Oncocytic change may be evident. Gnepp and Sporck (388) reported a case that was grossly unilocular and may have represented a lymphoepithelial cyst that demonstrated sebaceous differentiation. They nonetheless referred to this case as cystic sebaceous lymphadenoma. The lining of the cysts consists of variable proportions of squamous, columnar, and sebaceous cells; it is often focally thickened or develops small intraluminal nodular excrescences (fig. 4-146). Many of the lumina contain secretions. The lymphoid stroma is uniformly dense between the epithelial elements but exocytosis is not usually evident. The presence of lymphoid follicles is variable and may be numerous, with well-formed and prominent mantle zones, few

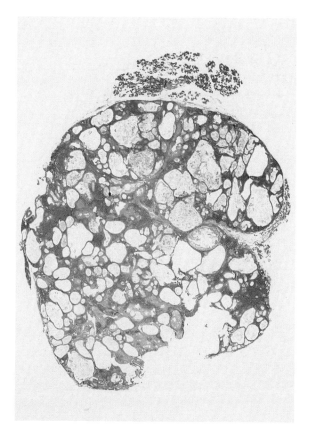

Figure 4-145
CYSTIC SEBACEOUS LYMPHADENOMA
Just as with sebaceous adenoma, cystic growth may predominate in sebaceous lymphadenoma. A small amount of parotid gland tissue is seen at the top.

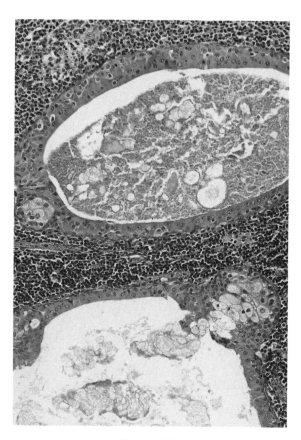

Figure 4-146
SEBACEOUS LYMPHADENOMA
Higher magnification of the previous case shows that sebaceous differentiation was limited to small focal areas in the lining of the neoplastic cysts.

and ill-defined mantle zones, or no mantle zones. Foci showing foreign body giant cell reaction may be seen (379).

Treatment and Prognosis. Treatment has varied from parotidectomy in 10 patients, local excision in 13, and enucleation in 2 (379). Of 22 cases with available follow-up information, only 1 recurred and the initial surgical procedure used in that case is not known (379,385).

Lymphadenoma That Lacks Sebaceous Differentiation. Occasionally a tumor is removed from the parotid gland that is similar to sebaceous lymphadenoma in all respects except that the epithelium fails to show sebaceous differentiation. This tumor may have either solid or cystic epithelial islands (fig. 4-147) or a combination of the two, but even serial sectioning fails to reveal any sebaceous elements. Awareness of this lesion is important to avoid misinter-

preting it as metastatic adenocarcinoma. While most pathologists are aware of sebaceous lymphadenomas, when confronted with a specimen that has epithelial islands (that lack sebaceous differentiation) scattered haphazardly through a collection of lymphocytes, metastatic disease may become a diagnostic consideration. The epithelium in lymphadenoma is morphologically bland and does not infiltrate connective tissue or parenchyma (fig. 4-148). As with sebaceous lymphadenoma, the epithelium lining the cystic spaces may focally contain mucous cells (fig. 4-149). Compared to a mucoepidermoid carcinoma that shows a tumor-associated lymphoid response, the islands, cysts, and ducts in lymphadenomas show an even rather than haphazard distribution and demonstrate less variation in size and shape. Furthermore, the lining epithelium in the cysts does not show papillary growth or extensive,

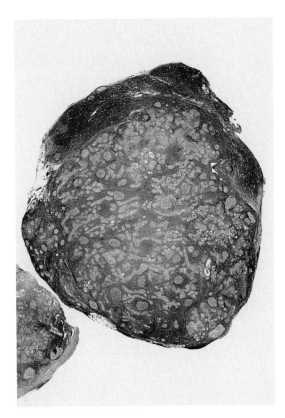 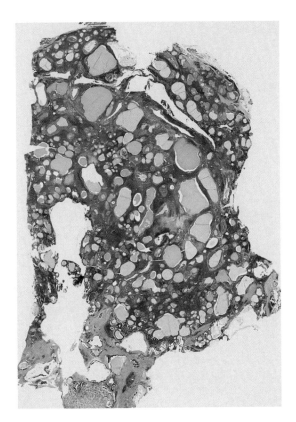

Figure 4-147
LYMPHADENOMA

The epithelium may proliferate as small solid islands and duct-like structures (left), as small to medium-sized cysts (right), or as a combination of the two.

poorly organized intraluminal proliferation, and does not include clear and intermediate cells. In the few cases in the AFIP files, lymphoid follicles have been numerous. We are not aware of a recurrence of this lesion but have seen too few cases to be confident of its behavior.

SIALOBLASTOMA

Definition. Sialoblastoma is a rare, congenital or perinatal, aggressive and potentially low-grade malignant, basaloid salivary gland neoplasm that occurs in the major salivary glands.

In a thorough review of this lesion by Hsueh and Gonzalez-Crussi (400) it was noted that tumors with many morphologically and clinically similar features have been reported under a variety of names. The initial cases were reported as *embryomas* by Vawter and Tefft (407), but these same two cases were later reported as *congenital carcinomas* (402). Other terms have

included *congenital basal cell adenoma* (394,397,401,403,406), *adenoid cystic carcinoma* (398), *hybrid basal cell adenoma-adenoid cystic carcinoma* (404), and *low-grade basaloid adenocarcinoma* (393). The term sialoblastoma was first used by Taylor (405) and is currently the term preferred by many other investigators and this Fascicle (395,399,400).

Although the rarity of this tumor makes comparison of photomicrographs of reported cases difficult, Hsueh and Gonzalez-Crussi (400) reported that the cases share features that warrant their recognition as a specific entity. Nonetheless, some histologic variability has been noted among these cases. For instance, acinar, squamous, and sebaceous differentiation have been described in individual cases but are not observed in most cases (399,403,405). Furthermore, variation in cytomorphologic atypia, mitotic rate, necrosis, and frank infiltration among these tumors suggest they may not all be identical (397,400,404).

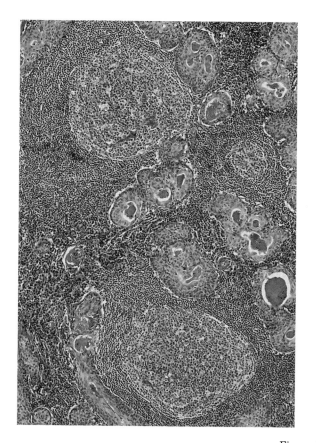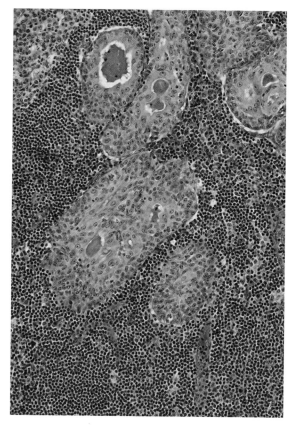

Figure 4-148
LYMPHADENOMA

Left: Solid squamous islands and duct-like structures are seen within dense lymphocytic stroma that shows several well-developed lymphoid follicles.

Right: On higher magnification the squamous epithelium demonstrates uniformly bland cytomorphologic nuclear features.

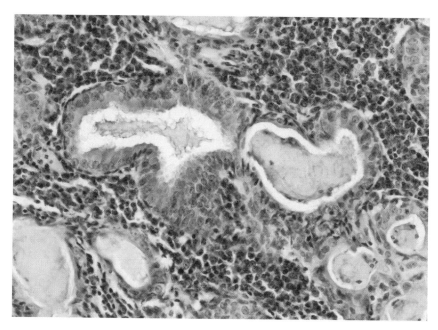

Figure 4-149
LYMPHADENOMA

Some of the cells lining the neoplastic ducts often contain mucin, as seen in this case. (Mucicarmine stain)

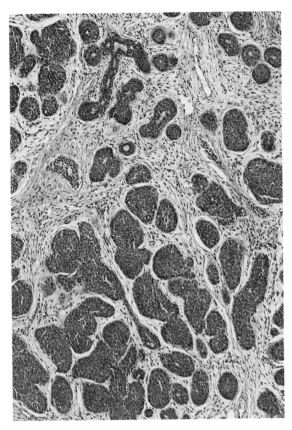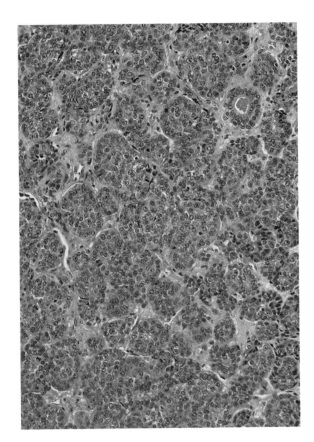

Figure 4-150
SIALOBLASTOMA
Characteristic of two different sialoblastomas are the individual nests of basaloid epithelium with focal ductal proliferation. The nests on the left are more widely scattered than on the right.

Batsakis and Frankenthaler (395) have suggested separating these tumors into benign and malignant types. Their criteria for malignancy include invasion of nerves or vascular spaces, necrosis, and cytologic atypia beyond that expected for embryonic epithelium. These criteria seem reasonable based on their correlation with behavior in the limited number of cases reported thus far.

Clinical Features. Most sialoblastomas present at birth, or shortly thereafter, as a mass over the angle of the mandible. They have ranged in size from 1.5 cm in greatest dimension to as large as 15 cm. The latter was a lesion that complicated delivery (400,404,405). In contrast to other examples, the tumor in one infant was first noted as a swelling at the age of 2 years and 7 months (393). In nearly all cases the tumor is asymptomatic, but one infant had facial paralysis at birth that was associated with a "bump" under the right ear (404). There is no gender predilection among the

reported cases. Over 75 percent have involved the parotid gland, and the remainder involved the submandibular gland. The mass is usually firm and nodular and may sometimes be fixed to underlying structures and overlying skin (405).

Gross and Microscopic Findings. Macroscopically, the tumors appear at least partially encapsulated, well circumscribed, and lobulated, but are difficult to distinguish from surrounding salivary parenchyma (403–405,407). The cut surface is gray, tan, or tan-yellow; firm; and usually solid rather than semicystic. Central hemorrhage and necrosis occur (402,405).

Microscopically, sialoblastoma is comprised of numerous small, individual and solid hypercellular islands of primitive basaloid cells (fig. 4-150) separated by fibrous or fibromyxomatous stroma (fig. 4-151). Many areas resemble the primitive basaloid epithelium seen in sebaceous adenoma and, as previously noted, focal sebaceous

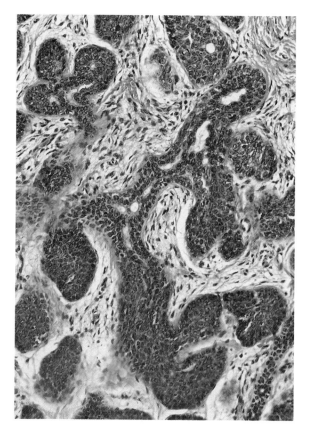

Figure 4-151
SIALOBLASTOMA
High magnification shows separation of the epithelial islands, including budding ductal epithelium, by fibromyxoid connective tissue.

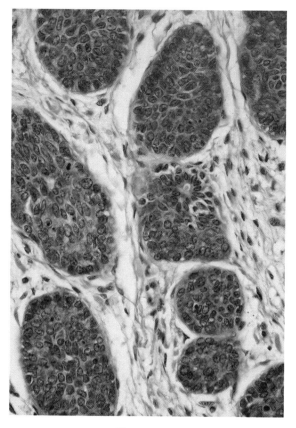

Figure 4-152
SIALOBLASTOMA
There is vague palisading of the peripheral layer of cells in some islands. The small ductal structure (center) contains a small amount of secretory product in its lumen.

differentiation has been described (403) (see Sebaceous Adenoma). The peripheral layer of cells in some tumors demonstrates palisading of their nuclei (fig. 4-152). In some areas the islands are separated from one another only by thin fibrovascular septa resulting in the formation of large, solid sheets of tumor (fig. 4-153). Small ducts lined by cuboidal or low columnar cells that form distinct lumina are evident within some of the epithelial islands. The lumina commonly contain a basophilic secretory product. The proliferation of ductal and solid islands of epithelia mimic the developing fetal salivary gland (see Normal Anatomy).

Much of the tumor is well circumscribed but often focally extends into surrounding tissues (fig. 4-154). The facial nerve is sometimes infiltrated by tumor, and necrosis may be evident (404,405). A tumor that metastasized to a lymph node 2 months after treatment initially extensively involved the nerve and had foci of necrosis (404).

The tumor cells have large, round to ovoid vesicular nuclei and abundant eosinophilic cytoplasm with indistinct cell borders (fig. 4-155). In some cases the more solid areas of tumor have cells with an increased nuclear/cytoplasmic ratio, and the nuclei have large basophilic nucleoli. The number of mitoses is variable but are occasionally numerous. Atypical mitoses are not seen. Cribriform spaces are evident focally in some tumors. Calcifications have also been reported (400,407).

Immunohistochemical Findings. Anticytokeratin consistently highlights the ductal cells (400,405) but is only sporadically immunoreactive with the cells that form the solid tumor nests (fig. 4-156). Anti-smooth muscle actin stains

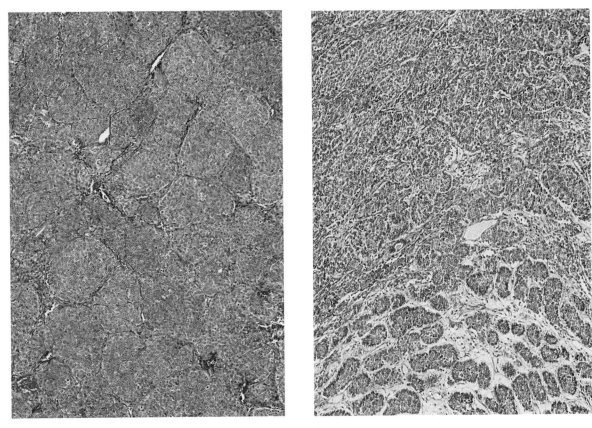

Figure 4-153
SIALOBLASTOMA
Left: This example is characterized by solid growth with limited stromal tissue.
Right: A different example is composed of both solid tumor areas (top) and multiple, distinct individual islands (bottom).

Figure 4-154
SIALOBLASTOMA
Although the interface of this tumor with surrounding tissues was clearly demarcated in some areas, here it is irregular and reveals infiltrative tumor islands. Several residual ducts are evident.

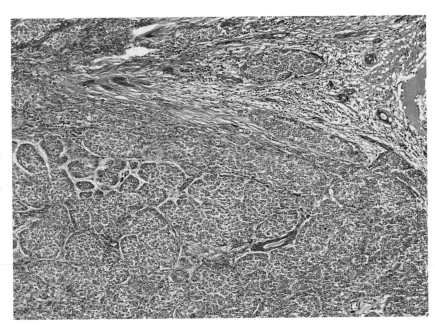

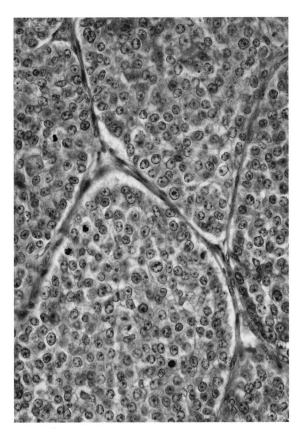

Figure 4-155
SIALOBLASTOMA

Thin septa of fibrovascular tissue separate islands composed of cells with large, vesicular nuclei. The nuclei have prominent single or multiple nucleoli. Several mitotic figures are evident.

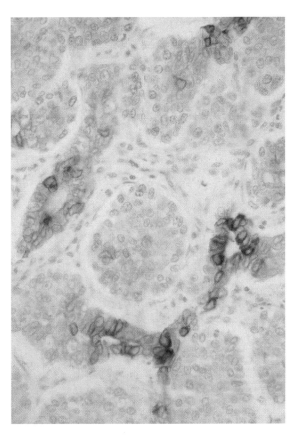

Figure 4-156
SIALOBLASTOMA

The ductal component is strongly immunoreactive for cytokeratin whereas the solid areas are variably reactive.

many of the abluminal cells, particularly those at the periphery of the tumor nests (fig. 4-157), and, in addition to the electron microscopic features, has led to speculation that the cells surrounding the ductal cells are of myoepithelial origin (400,405). Anti-S-100 protein immunoreactivity occurs in both the ductal and surrounding epithelia and often has strong nuclear staining. GFAP reactivity has not been seen (400). The immunoreactivity of sialoblastomas with antibodies to cytokeratin, smooth muscle actin, and S-100 protein is similar to that of basal cell adenomas and basal cell adenocarcinomas (408).

Ultrastructural Findings. The ductal and surrounding neoplastic cells are connected by cell junctions (400,404). Some of the cells forming the solid nests have well-developed endoplasmic reticulum and free ribosomes, and are surrounded

by basement lamina (400). Microvilli and apical electron-dense secretory granules are seen in some ductal cells (404). Numerous free ribosomes and limited development of endoplasmic reticulum in the nonductal cells indicate their embryonic quality (404). Hsueh and Gonzalez-Crussi (400) have described spindled, peripheral myoepithelial cells that have intracytoplasmic thin filaments and small subplasmalemmal densities.

Differential Diagnosis. As suggested by the terms applied to sialoblastoma in many reports, other diagnostic considerations are predominantly basaloid tumors, most frequently basal cell adenoma. In contrast to basal cell adenoma, sialoblastoma is composed of more primitive cells that have less peripheral palisading of nuclei, demonstrate significant cytomorphologic atypia, often have much greater mitotic activity,

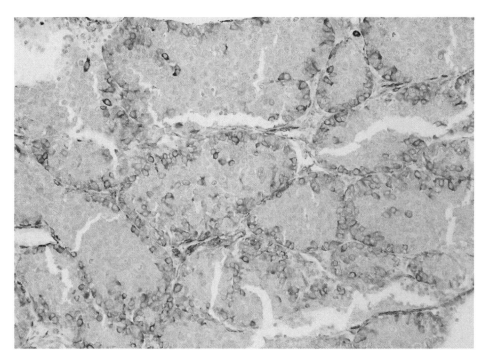

Figure 4-157
SIALOBLASTOMA
Immunoreactivity for smooth muscle actin is most pronounced at the periphery of the neoplastic islands and is absent or extremely weak in the ductal cells.

and often infiltrate surrounding tissues. Basal cell adenoma is rare in patients less than 20 years of age. Similarly, occurrence of other basaloid neoplasms, such as adenoid cystic carcinoma or basal cell adenocarcinoma, is extremely rare in the first decade of life.

Treatment and Prognosis. The extremely limited collective experience with this lesion precludes definitive conclusions regarding its biologic behavior or appropriate treatment but does suggest the tumor is aggressive and potentially malignant. Of the 15 reported tumors, 4 recurred and 3 of these recurred multiple times (393,396–405). Recurrences occurred several months to 1.5 years after excision. One patient with four recurrences had persistent inoperable tumor at 43 months of age because of extension into the skull (405). Another patient had metastasis to a

regional lymph node at 8 months of age that was confirmed by fine-needle aspiration (404). The metastasis was treated with adriamycin, which resulted in disappearance of the enlarged mid-jugular node, followed by neck dissection, which revealed no evidence of disease. At 4.5 years of age the child appeared to be free of disease. Distant metastases have not yet been reported.

Hsueh and Gonzalez-Crussi (400) have emphasized that enucleation is inadequate even if the tumor initially appears well circumscribed. They conclude that surgical excision with tumor-free margins is crucial to successful therapy. While chemotherapy appears to have been successful in the previously mentioned case, the efficacy of both chemotherapy and radiotherapy, used in several other cases, is difficult to assess (402–404,407).

REFERENCES

Mixed Tumor

1. Allison RS, van der Waal I, Snow GB. Parapharyngeal tumours: a review of 23 cases. Clin Otolaryngol 1989; 14:199–203.

2. Blevins NH, Jackler RK, Kaplan MJ, Boles R. Facial paralysis due to benign parotid tumors. Arch Otolaryngol Head Neck Surg 1992;118:427–30.

3. Breitenecker G, Wepner F. A pleomorphic adenoma (so-called mixed tumor) in the wall of a dentigerous cyst. Oral Surg Oral Med Oral Pathol 1973;36:63–71.

4. Bullerdiek J, Bschen C, Bartnitzke S. Aberrations of chromosome 8 in mixed salivary gland tumors—cytogenetic findings in seven cases. Cancer Genet Cytogenet 1987;24:205–12.

5. Bullerdiek J, Chilla R, Haubrich J, Meyer K, Bartnitzke S. A causal relationship between chromosomal rearrangements and the genesis of salivary gland pleomorphic adenomas. Arch Otorhinolaryngol 1988;245:244–9.

6. Bullerdiek J, Takla G, Bartnitzke S, Brandt G, Chilla R, Haubrich J. Relationship of cytogenetic subtypes of salivary gland pleomorphic adenomas with patient age and histologic type. Cancer 1989;64:876–80.

7. Bullerdiek J, Wobst G, Meyer-Bolte K, et al. Cytogenetic subtyping of 220 salivary gland pleomorphic adenomas: correlation to occurrence, histological subtype, and in vitro cellular behavior. Cancer Genet Cytogenet 1993;65:27–31.

8. Campbell WG Jr, Priest RE, Weathers DR. Characterization of two types of crystalloids in pleomorphic adenomas of minor salivary glands. A light-microscopic, electron-microscopic, and histochemical study. Am J Pathol 1985;118:194–202.

9. Chaplin AJ, Darke P, Patel S. Tyrosine-rich crystals in pleomorphic adenomas of parotid glands. J Oral Pathol 1983;12:342–6.

10. Chau MN, Radden BG. A clinical-pathological study of 53 intra-oral pleomorphic adenomas. Int J Oral Maxillofac Surg 1989;18:158–62.

11. Dallera P, Marchetti C, Campobassi A. Local capsular dissection of parotid pleomorphic adenomas. Int J Oral Maxillofac Surg 1993;22:154–7.

12. Dardick I, Ostrynski VL, Ekem JK, Leung R, Burford-Mason AP. Immunohistochemical and ultrastructural correlates of muscle-actin expression in pleomorphic adenomas and myoepitheliomas based on comparison of formalin and methanol fixation. Virchows Arch [A] 1992;421:95–104.

13. Dardick I, Stratis M, Parks WR, DeNardi FG, Kahn HJ. S-100 protein antibodies do not label normal salivary gland myoepithelium. Histogenetic implications for salivary gland tumors. Am J Surg Pathol 1991;138:619–28.

14. Dardick I, van Nostrand AW. Myoepithelial cells in salivary gland tumors—revisited. Head Neck Surg 1985;7:395–408.

15. Dardick I, van Nostrand AW, Jeans MT, Rippstein P, Edwards V. Pleomorphic adenoma, I: ultrastructural organization of epithelial regions. Hum Pathol 1983;14:780–97.

16. Dardick I, van Nostrand AW, Jeans MT, Rippstein P, Edwards V. Pleomorphic adenoma, II: ultrastructural organization of stromal regions. Hum Pathol 1983;14:798–809.

17. Dardick I, van Nostrand AW, Phillips MJ. Histogenesis of salivary gland pleomorphic adenoma (mixed tumor) with an evaluation of the role of the myoepithelial cell. Hum Pathol 1982;13:62–75.

18. David R, Buchner A. Elastosis in benign and malignant salivary gland tumors. A histochemical and ultrastructural study. Cancer 1980;45:2301–10.

19. David R, Buchner A. Tannic acid-glutaraldehyde fixative and pleomorphic adenomas of the salivary gland: an ultrastructural study. J Oral Pathol 1982;11:26–38.

20. Dawson AK. Radiation therapy in recurrent pleomorphic adenoma of the parotid. Int J Radiat Oncol Biol Phys 1989;16:819–21.

21. Deguchi H, Hamano H, Hayashi Y. c-myc, ras p21 and p53 expression in pleomorphic adenoma and its malignant form of the human salivary glands. Acta Pathol Jpn 1993;43:413–22.

22. Donovan DT, Conley JJ. Capsular significance in parotid tumor surgery: reality and myths of lateral lobectomy. Laryngoscope 1984;94:324–9.

23. Dyke PC, Hajdu SI, Strong EW, Erlandson RA, Fleisher M. Mixed tumor of parotid containing calcium oxalate crystals. Arch Pathol 1971;91:89–92.

24. Dykun RJ, Deitel M, Borowy ZJ, Jackson S. Treatment of parotid neoplasms. Can J Surg 1980;23:14–9.

25. Eneroth CM. Salivary gland tumors in the parotid gland, submandibular gland, and the palate region. Cancer 1971;27:1415–8.

26. Erlandson RA, Cardon-Cardo C, Higgins PJ. Histogenesis of benign pleomorphic adenoma (mixed tumor) of the major salivary glands. An ultrastructural and immunohistochemical study. Am J Surg Pathol 1984;8:803–20.

27. Eveson JW, Cawson RA. Salivary gland tumours. A review of 2410 cases with particular reference to histological types, site, age and sex distribution. J Pathol 1985;146:51–8.

28. Eveson JW, Cawson RA. Tumours of the minor (oropharyngeal) salivary glands: a demographic study of 336 cases. J Oral Pathol 1985;14:500–9.

29. Federspil PA, Federspil P, Schatzle W. Pleomorphe parotisadenome und ihre rezidive. HNO 1994;42:28–35.

30. Fitzpatrick PJ, Black KM. Salivary gland tumors. J Otolaryngol 1985;14:296–300.

31. Fujita S, Takahashi H, Okabe H. Proliferative activity in normal salivary gland and pleomorphic adenoma. A study by argyrophilic nucleolar organizer region (AgNOR) staining. Acta Pathol Jpn 1992;42:573–8.

32. Gleave EN, Whittaker JS, Nicholson A. Salivary tumours—experience over thirty years. Clin Otolaryngol 1979;4:247–57.

33. Gnepp DR, Schroeder W, Heffner D. Synchronous tumors arising in a single major salivary gland. Cancer 1989;63:1219–24.

34. Goodwin WJ Jr, Chandler JR. Transoral excision of lateral pharyngeal space tumors presenting intraorally. Laryngoscope 1988;98:266–9.

35. Gunn A, Parrott NR. Parotid tumours: a review of parotid tumour surgery in the Northern Regional Health Authority of the United Kingdom 1978–1982. Br J Surg 1988;75:1144–6.

36. Hancock BD. Pleomorphic adenomas of the parotid: removal without rupture. Ann R Coll Surg Engl 1987;69:293–5.

37. Hardingham M. Complications of superficial parotidectomy versus extracapsular lumpectomy in the treatment of benign parotid lesions [Letter]. J R Coll Surg Edinb 1993;38:180–1.

38. Harris BR, Shipkey F. Tyrosine-rich crystalloids in neoplasms and tissues of the head and neck. Arch Pathol Lab Med 1986;110:709–12.

39. Hickman RE, Cawson RA, Duffy SW. The prognosis of specific types of salivary gland tumors. Cancer 1984;54:1620–4.

40. Humphrey PA, Ingram P, Tucker A, Shelburne JD. Crystalloids in salivary gland pleomorphic adenomas. Arch Pathol Lab Med 1989;113:390–3.

41. Isacsson G, Shear M. Intraoral salivary gland tumors: a retrospective study of 201 cases. J Oral Pathol 1983;12:57–62.

42. Jackson SR, Roland NJ, Clarke RW, Jones AS. Recurrent pleomorphic adenoma. J Laryngol Otol 1993;107:546–9.

43. Lack EE, Upton MP. Histopathologic review of salivary gland tumors in childhood. Arch Otolaryngol Head Neck Surg 1988;114:898–906.

44. Lam KH, Wei WI, Ho HC, Ho CM. Whole organ sectioning of mixed parotid tumors. Am J Surg 1990;160:377–81.

45. Landini G. Nucleolar organizing regions (NORs) in pleomorphic adenomas of the salivary glands. J Oral Pathol Med 1990;19:257–60.

46. Layfield LJ, Reznicek M, Lowe M, Bottles K. Spontaneous infarction of a parotid gland pleomorphic adenoma. Report of a case with cytologic and radiographic overlap with a primary salivary gland malignancy. Acta Cytol 1992;36:381–6.

47. Lianjia Y, Yan J, Hitoshi N, Shinichiro S, Akihide K, Masahiko M. An immunohistochemical study of bone morphogenetic protein in pleomorphic adenoma of the salivary gland. Virchows Arch [A] 1993;422:439–43.

48. Maran AG, Mackenzie IJ, Stanley RE. Recurrent pleomorphic adenomas of the parotid gland. Arch Otolaryngol Head Neck Surg 1984;110:167–71.

49. Mark J, Dahlenfors R. Cytogenetical observations in 100 human benign pleomorphic adenomas: specificity of the chromosomal aberrations and their relationship to sites of localized oncogenes. Anticancer Res 1986;6:299–308.

50. Martin AR, Mantravadi J, Kotylo PK, Mullins R, Walker S, Roth LM. Proliferative activity and aneuploidy in pleomorphic adenomas of the salivary glands. Arch Pathol Lab Med 1994;118:252–9.

51. Martis C. Parotid benign tumors: comments on surgical treatment of 263 cases. Int J Oral Surg 1983;12:211–20.

52. Matsumura K, Sasaki K, Tsuji T, Shinozaki F. The nucleolar organizer regions associated protein (AgNORs) in salivary gland tumors. Int J Oral Maxillofac Surg 1989;18:76–8.

53. Maynard JD. Management of pleomorphic adenoma of the parotid. Br J Surg 1988;75:305–8.

54. Milasin J, Pujic N, Dedovic N, et al. H-ras gene mutations in salivary gland pleomorphic adenomas. Int J Oral Maxillofac Surg 1993;22:359–61.

55. Miller AS, Winnick M. Salivary gland inclusion in the anterior mandible. Report of a case with a review of the literature on aberrant salivary gland tissue and neoplasms. Oral Surg Oral Med Oral Pathol 1971;31:790–7.

56. Mori M, Ninomiya T, Okada Y, Tsukitani K. Myoepitheliomas and myoepithelial adenomas of salivary gland origin. Immunohistochemical evaluation of filament proteins, S-100 alpha and beta, glial fibrillary acidic proteins, neuron-specific enolase, and lactoferrin. Pathol Res Pract 1989;184:168–78.

57. Morinaga S, Nakajima T, Shimosato Y. Normal and neoplastic myoepithelial cells in salivary glands: an immunohistochemical study. Hum Pathol 1987;18:1218–26.

58. Mra Z, Komisar A, Blaugrund SM. Functional facial nerve weakness after surgery for benign parotid tumors: a multivariate statistical analysis. Head Neck 1993;15:147–52.

59. Myssiorek D, Ruah CB, Hybels RL. Recurrent pleomorphic adenomas of the parotid gland. Head Neck 1990;12:332–6.

60. Nikai H, Ogawa I, Ijuhin N, Yamasaki A, Takata T, Elbardaie A. Ultrastructural cytochemical demonstration of elastin in the matrix of salivary gland tumors. Acta Pathol Jpn 1983;33:1171–81.

61. Niparko JK, Beauchamp ML, Krause CJ, Baker SR, Work WP. Surgical treatment of recurrent pleomorphic adenoma of the parotid gland. Arch Otolaryngol Head Neck Surg 1986;112:1180–4.

62. Nochomovitz LE, Kahn LB. Tyrosine crystals in pleomorphic adenomas of the salivary gland. Arch Pathol 1974;97:141–2.

63. O'Dwyer PJ, Farrar WB, Finkelmeier WR, McCabe DP, James AG. Facial nerve sacrifice and tumor recurrence in primary and recurrent benign parotid tumors. Am J Surg 1986;152:442–5.

64. O'Dwyer TP, Gullane PJ, Dardick I. A pseudo-malignant Warthin's tumor presenting with facial nerve paralysis. J Otolaryngol 1990;19:353–7.

65. Okutsu S, Takeda A, Suzuki T, et al. Expression of ras-P21 and ras gene alteration in pleomorphic adenomas. J Nihon Univ Sch Dent 1993;35:200–3.

66. Ostrzega N, Cheng L, Layfield L. Glial fibrillary acid protein immunoreactivity in fine-needle aspiration of salivary gland lesions: a useful adjunct for the differential diagnosis of salivary gland neoplasms. Diagn Cytopathol 1989;5:145–9.

67. Owen ER, Banerjee AK, Kissin M, Kark AE. Complications of parotid surgery: the need for selectivity. Br J Surg 1989;76:1034–5.

68. Prichard AJ, Barton RP, Narula AA. Complications of superficial parotidectomy versus extracapsular lumpectomy in the treatment of benign parotid lesions. J R Coll Surg Edinb 1992;37:155–8.

69. Rice DH. Surgery of the salivary glands. Trenton: CV Mosby, 1982:92–7.

70. Ryan RE Jr, DeSanto LW, Weiland LH, Devine KD, Beahrs OH. Cellular mixed tumors of the salivary glands. Arch Otolaryngol Head Neck Surg 1978;104:451–3.

71. Saku T, Cheng J, Okabe H, Koyama Z. Immunolocalization of basement membrane molecules in the stroma of salivary gland pleomorphic adenoma. J Oral Pathol Med 1990;19:208–14.

72. Samson MJ, Metson R, Wang CC, Montgomery WW. Preservation of the facial nerve in the management of recurrent pleomorphic adenoma. Laryngoscope 1991;101:1060–2.

73. Seifert G, Langrock I, Donath K. Pathomorphologische subklassifikation der pleomorphen spreichel-drüsenadenome. Analyse von 310 parotisadenomen. HNO 1976;24:415–26.

74. Seifert G, Miehlke A, Haubrich J, Chilla R. Diseases of the salivary glands: diagnosis, pathology, treatment, facial nerve surgery. Stuttgart: Georg Thieme Verlag, 1986:182–93.

75. Seifert G, Miehlke A, Haubrich J, Chilla R. Diseases of the salivary glands: diagnosis, pathology, treament, facial nerve surgery. Stuttgart: Georg Thieme Verlag, 1986:171.

76. Spiro RH. Salivary neoplasms: overview of a 35-year experience with 2,807 patients. Head Neck Surg 1986;8:177–84.

77. Stanley RE, Mackenzie IJ, Maran AG. The surgical approach to recurrent pleomorphic adenoma of the parotid gland. Ann Acad Med Singapore 1984;13:91–5.

78. Stenman G, Sahlin P, Mark J, Landys D. Structural alterations of the c-mos locus in benign pleomorphic adenomas with chromosome abnormalities of 8q12. Oncogene 1991;6:1105–8.

79. Stevens KL, Hobsley M. The treatment of pleomorphic adenomas by formal parotidectomy. Br J Surg 1982;69:1–3.

80. Takahashi M, Kumai M, Kamito T, Uehara M, Unno T. Clinico-pathological findings of recurrent pleomorphic adenomas of the parotid gland [Abstract]. Nippon Jibiinkoka Gakkai Kaiho 1991;94:489–94.

81. Takahashi M, Tsuda N, Tezuka F, Okabe H. Immuno-histochemical localization of carcinoembryonic antigen in carcinoma in pleomorphic adenoma of salivary gland: use in the diagnosis of benign and malignant lesions. Tohoku J Exp Med 1986;149:329–40.

82. Thomas K, Hutt MS. Tyrosine crystals in salivary gland tumours. J Clin Pathol 1981;34:1003–5.

83. Touquet R, Mackenzie IJ, Carruth JA. Management of the parotid pleomorphic adenoma, the problem of exposing tumour tissue at operation. The logical pursuit of treatment policies. Br J Oral Maxillofac Surg 1990;28:404–8.

84. Valente PT, Hoober JK, Phillips SJ. Tyrosine-rich crystalloids in pleomorphic adenoma: SEM findings and partial biochemical characterization. Ultrastruct Pathol 1988;12:613–20.

85. van Heerden WF, Raubenheimer EJ. Evaluation of the nucleolar organizer region associated proteins in minor salivary gland tumors. J Oral Pathol Med 1991;20:291–5.

86. Waldron CA. Mixed tumor (pleomorphic adenoma) and myoepithelioma. In: Ellis GL, Auclair PL, Gnepp DR, eds. Surgical pathology of the salivary glands. Philadelphia: WB Saunders, 1991:165–186.

87. Waldron CA, el-Mofty SK, Gnepp DR. Tumors of the intraoral minor salivary glands: a demographic and histologic study of 426 cases. Oral Surg Oral Med Oral Pathol 1988;66:323–33.

88. Watkin GT, Hobsley M. Influence of local surgery and radiotherapy on the natural history of pleomorphic adenomas. Br J Surg 1986;73:74–6.

89. Weber RS, Byers RM, Petit B, Wolf P, Ang K, Luna M. Submandibular gland tumors. Adverse histologic factors and therapeutic implications. Arch Otolaryngol Head Neck Surg 1990;116:1055–60.

90. Wenig BM, Hitchcock CL, Ellis GL, Gnepp DR. Metastasizing mixed tumor of salivary glands. A clinicopathologic and flow cytometric analysis. Am J Surg Pathol 1992;16:845–58.

91. Wennmo C, Spandow O, Emgård P, Krouthën B. Pleomorphic adenomas of the parotid gland: superficial parotidectomy or limited excision? J Laryngol Otol 1988;102:603–5.

92. Woods JE, Chong GC, Beahrs OH. Experience with 1,360 primary parotid tumors. Am J Surg 1975;130:460–2.

93. Yamashita T, Tomoda K, Kumazawa T. The usefulness of partial parotidectomy for benign parotid gland tumors. A retrospective study of 306 cases. Acta Otolaryngol Suppl (Stockh) 1993;500:113–6.

94. Yu LT, Hamilton R. Frey's syndrome: prevention with conservative parotidectomy and superficial musculo-aponeurotic system preservation. Ann Plast Surg 1992;29:217–22.

Myoepithelioma

95. Buchner A, David R, Hansen LS. Hyaline cells in pleomorphic adenoma of salivary gland origin. Oral Surg Oral Med Oral Pathol 1981;52:506–12.

96. Dardick I, Cavell S, Boivin M, et al. Salivary gland myoepithelioma variants. Histological, ultrastructural, and immunocytological features. Virchows Arch [A] 1989;416:25–42.

97. Dardick I, Ostrynski VL, Ekem JK, Leung R, Burford-Mason AP. Immunohistochemical and ultrastructural correlates of muscle-actin expression in pleomorphic adenomas and myoepitheliomas based on comparison of formalin and methanol fixation. Virchows Arch [A] 1992;421:95–104.

98. Dardick I, Stratis M, Parks WR, DeNardi FG, Kahn HJ. S-100 protein antibodies do not label normal salivary gland myoepithelium. Histogenetic implications for salivary gland tumors. Am J Surg Pathol 1991;138:619–28.

99. Dardick I, Thomas MJ, van Nostrand AW. Myoepithelioma—new concepts of histology and classification:

a light and electron microscopic study. Ultrastruct Pathol 1989;13:187–224.

100. Dardick I, van Nostrand AW. Myoepithelial cells in salivary gland tumors—revisited. Head Neck Surg 1985;7:395–408.

101. Dardick I, van Nostrand AW, Jeans MT, Rippstein P, Edwards V. Pleomorphic adenoma, I: ultrastructural organization of "epithelial" regions. Hum Pathol 1983; 14:780–97.

102. Dardick I, van Nostrand AW, Phillips MJ. Histogenesis of salivary gland pleomorphic adenoma (mixed tumor) with an evaluation of the role of the myoepithelial cell. Hum Pathol 1982;13:62–75.

103. Franquemont DW, Mills SE. Plasmacytoid monomorphic adenoma of salivary glands. Absence of myogenous differentiation and comparison to spindle cell myoepithelioma. Am J Surg Pathol 1993;17:146–53.

104. Leifer C, Miller AS, Putong PB, Harwick RD. Myoepithelioma of the parotid gland. Arch Pathol 1974;98:312–9.

105. Lomax-Smith JD, Azzopardi JG. The hyaline cell: a distinctive feature of mixed salivary tumors. Histopathology 1978;2:77–92.
106. Nikai H, el-Bardaie AM, Takata T, Ogawa I, Ijuhin N. Histologic evaluation of myoepithelial participation in salivary gland tumors. Int J Oral Maxillofac Surg 1986;15:597–605.
107. Redman RS. Myoepithelium of salivary glands. Microsc Res Tech 1994;27:25–45.
108. Sciubba JJ, Brannon RB. Myoepithelioma of salivary glands: report of 23 cases. Cancer 1982;49:562–72.
109. Sciubba JJ, Foldstein BH. Myoepithelioma. Review of the literature and report of a case with ultrastructural confirmation. Oral Surg Oral Med Oral Pathol 1976;42:328–38.
110. Waldron CA. Mixed tumor (pleomorphic adenoma) and myoepithelioma. In: Ellis GL, Auclair PL, Gnepp DR, eds. Surgical pathology of the salivary glands. Philadelphia: WB Saunders, 1991:165–186.

Warthin's Tumor

111. Albrecht D, Arzt L. Beitrge zur Frage der Gewebsverirrung. Papillre Cystadenome in Lymphdrsen. Frankfurt Z Pathol 1910;4:47–69.
112. Allegra SR. Warthin's tumor: a hypersensitivity disease? Ultrastructural, light, and immunofluorescent study. Hum Pathol 1971;2:403–20.
113. Auclair PL. Tumor-associated lymphoid proliferation in the parotid gland. A potential diagnostic pitfall. Oral Surg Oral Med Oral Pathol 1994;77:19–26.
114. Baden E, Pierce M, Selman AJ, Roberts TW, Doyle JL. Intraoral papillary cystadenoma lymphomatosum. J Oral Surg 1976;34:533–41.
115. Baker M, Yuzon D, Baker BH. Squamous cell carcinoma arising in benign adenolymphoma (Warthin's tumor) of the parotid gland. J Surg Oncol 1980;15:7–10.
116. Banik S, Howell JS, Wright DH. Non-Hodgkin's lymphoma arising in adenolymphoma—a report of two cases. J Pathol 1985;146:167–77.
117. Batsakis JG, Sneige N, el-Naggar AK. Fine-needle aspiration of salivary glands: its utility and tissue effects. Ann Otol Rhinol Laryngol 1992;101:185–8.
118. Baugh RF, McClatchey KD. Papillary cystadenoma lymphomatosum syndrome. J Otolaryngol 1986;15:166–8.
119. Bengoechea O, Sanchez F, Larrnaga B, Martonez-Peñuela JM. Oncocytic adenocarcinoma arising in Warthin's tumor. Pathol Res Pract 1989;185:907–11.
120. Bernier JL, Bhaskar SN. Lymphoepithelial lesions of salivary glands. Histogenesis and classification based on 186 cases. Cancer 1958;11:1156–79.
121. Brown L, Aparicio SP. Malignant Warthin's tumor: an ultrastructural study. J Clin Pathol 1984;37:170–5.
122. Bullerdiek J, Haubrich J, Meyer K, Bartnitzke S. Translocation t(11;19)(q21;p13.1) as the sole chromosome abnormality in a cystadenolymphoma (Warthin's tumor) of the parotid gland. Cancer Genet Cytogenet 1988;35:129–32.
123. Bunker ML, Locker J. Warthin's tumor with malignant lymphoma. DNA analysis of paraffin-embedded tissue. Am J Clin Pathol 1989;91:341–4.
124. Burt RW. Accumulation of ^{123}I in a Warthin's tumor. Clin Nucl Med 1978;3:155–6.
125. Cadier M, Watkin G, Hobsley M. Smoking predisposes to parotid adenolymphoma. Br J Surg 1992;79:928–30.
126. Chapnik JS. The controversy of Warthin's tumor. Laryngoscope 1983;93:695–716.
127. Chaudhry AP, Gorlin R. Papillary cystadenoma lymphomatosum (adenolymphoma): a review of the literature. Am J Surg 1958;95:923–31.
128. Colby TV, Dorfman RF. Malignant lymphomas involving the salivary glands. Pathol Annu 1979;14 [Pt 2]:307–24.
129. Cossman J, Deegan MJ, Batsakis JG. Warthin's tumor: B-lymphocytes within the lymphoid infiltrate. Arch Pathol Lab Med 1977;101:354–6.
130. Damjanov I, Sneff EM, Delerme AN. Squamous cell carcinoma arising in Warthin's tumor of the parotid gland. A light, electron microscopic, and immunohistochemical study. Oral Surg Oral Med Oral Pathol 1983;55:286–90.
131. Dardick I, Claude A, Parks WR, et al. Warthin's tumor: an ultrastructural and immunohistochemical study of basilar epithelium. Ultrastruct Pathol 1988;12:419–32.
132. David R, Buchner A. Corpora amylacea in adenolymphoma (Warthin's tumor). Am J Clin Pathol 1978;69:173–5.
133. DeLozier HL, Spinella MJ, Johnson GD. Facial nerve paralysis with benign parotid masses. Ann Otol Rhinol Laryngol 1989;98:644–7.
134. Diamond LW, Braylan RC. Cell surface markers on lymphoid cells from Warthin's tumor. Cancer 1979;44:580–3.
135. Dietert SE. Papillary cystadenoma lymphomatosum (Warthin's tumor) in patients in a general hospital over a 24-year period. Am J Clin Pathol 1975;63:866–75.
136. Dykun RJ, Deitel M, Borowy ZJ, Jackson S. Treatment of parotid neoplasms. Can J Surg 1980;23:14–9.
137. Ebbs SR, Webb AJ. Adenolymphoma of the parotid: aetiology, diagnosis and treatment. Br J Surg 1986;73:627–30.
138. Ellis GL, Auclair PL. Classification of salivary gland neoplasms. In: Ellis GL, Auclair PL, Gnepp DR, eds. Surgical pathology of the salivary glands. Philadelphia: WB Saunders, 1991:129–134.
139. Eneroth CM. Salivary gland tumors in the parotid gland, submandibular gland, and the palate region. Cancer 1971;27:1415–8.
140. Eveson JW, Cawson RA. Infarcted (infected) adenolymphomas. A clinicopathological study of 20 cases. Clin Otolaryngol 1989;14:205–10.
141. Eveson JW, Cawson RA. Salivary gland tumours. A review of 2410 cases with particular reference to histological types, site, age and sex distribution. J Pathol 1985;146:51–8.
142. Eveson JW, Cawson RA. Warthin's tumor (cystadenolymphoma) of salivary glands. A clinicopathologic investigation of 278 cases. Oral Surg Oral Med Oral Pathol 1986;61:256–62.
143. Fantasia JE, Miller AS. Papillary cystadenoma lymphomatosum arising in minor salivary glands. Oral Surg Oral Med Oral Pathol 1981;52:411–6.

144. Feind CR. The head and neck. In: Haagensen CD, Feind CR, Herter FP, eds. The lymphatics in cancer. 10th ed. Philadelphia: WB Saunders, 1972:63–4.

145. Fitzpatrick PJ, Black KM. Salivary gland tumors. J Otolaryngol 1985;14:296–300.

146. Foote FW Jr, Frazell EL. Tumors of the major salivary glands. Cancer 1953;6:1065–133.

147. Foulsham CK II, Johnson GS, Snyder GG III, Carpenter RJ III, Shafi NQ. Immunohistopathology of papillary cystadenoma lymphomatosum (Warthin's tumor). Ann Clin Lab Sci 1984;14:47–63.

148. Frazell EL. Clinical aspects of tumors of the major salivary glands. Cancer 1954;7:637–59.

149. Gadient SE, Kalfayan B. Mucoepidermoid carcinoma arising within a Warthin's tumor. Oral Surg Oral Med Oral Pathol 1975;40:391–8.

150. Gant TD, Hovey LM, Williams C. Surgical management of parotid gland tumors. Ann Plast Surg 1981;6:389–92.

151. Giardini R, Mastore M. Follicular non-Hodgkin's lymphoma in adenolymphoma: report of a case. Tumori 1990;76:212–5.

152. Gnepp DR, Schroeder W, Heffner D. Synchronous tumors arising in a single major salivary gland. Cancer 1989;63:1219–24.

153. Griesser GH, Hansmann ML, Bogman MJ, Pielsticker K, Lennert K. Germinal center derived malignant lymphoma in cystadenolymphoma. Virchows Arch [A] 1986;408:491–6.

154. Hall G, Tesluk H, Baron S. Lymphoma arising in an adenolymphoma. Hum Pathol 1985;16:424–7.

155. Hart MN, Andrews JL. Papillary cystadenoma lymphomatosum arising in the oral cavity. Oral Surg Oral Med Oral Pathol 1968;26:588–91.

156. Heller KS, Attie JN. Treatment of Warthin's tumor by enucleation. Am J Surg 1988;156:294–6.

157. Higashi T, Murahashi H, Ikuta H, Mori Y, Watanabe Y. Identification of Warthin's tumor with technetium-99m pertechnetate. Clin Nucl Med 1987;12:796–800.

158. Hosaka M, Orito T, Horike H, Okada Y, Mori M. Heterogeneous expression of S-100 protein subunits alpha and beta in cystadenolymphomas of salivary glands. Acta Histochem 1989;86:15–21.

159. Hsu SM, Hsu PL, Nayak RN. Warthin's tumor: an immunohistochemical study of its lymphoid stroma. Hum Pathol 1981;12:251–7.

160. Hsu SM, Raine L. Warthin's tumor—epithelial cell differences. Am J Clin Pathol 1982;77:78–82.

161. Ishikawa H, Ishii Y. Evaluation of salivary gland tumors with 99mTc-pertechnetate. J Oral Maxillofac Surg 1993;

162. Kataoka R, Hyo Y, Hoshiya T, Miyahara H, Matsunaga T. Ultrastructural study of mitochondria in oncocytes. Ultrastruct Pathol 1991;15:231–9.

163. Kennedy TL. Warthin's tumor: a review indicating no male predominance. Laryngoscope 1983;93:889–91.

164. Kern SB. Necrosis of a Warthin's tumor following fine needle aspiration. Acta Cytol 1988;32:207–8.

165. Kessler E, Koznizky IL, Schindel J. Malignant Warthin's tumor. Oral Surg Oral Med Oral Pathol 1977;43:111–5.

166. Korsrud FR, Brandtzaeg P. Immunohistochemical characterization of cellular immunoglobulins and epi-thelial marker antigens in Warthin's tumor. Hum Pathol 1984;15:361–7.

167. Korsrud FR, Brandtzaeg P. Immunohistochemical studies on the epithelial and lymphoid components of Warthin's tumour. Acta Otolaryngol Suppl (Stockh) 1979;360:221–4.

168. Kotwall CA. Smoking as an etiologic factor in the development of Warthin's tumor of the parotid gland. Am J Surg 1992;164:646–7.

169. Kukreja HK, Jain HK. Adenolymphoma of submandibular salivary gland. J Laryngol Otol 1971;85:1201–3.

170. Lamelas J, Terry JH Jr, Alfonso AE. Warthin's tumor: multicentricity and increasing incidence in women. Am J Surg 1987;154:347–51.

171. Lefor AT, Ord RA. Multiple synchronous bilateral Warthin's tumors of the parotid glands with pleomorphic adenoma. Case report and review of the literature. Oral Surg Oral Med Oral Pathol 1993;76:319–24.

172. Li WY, Liu HC. Histopathological study of neoplasms of the salivary glands, a review of 657 cases. Chin Med J 1987;39:231–46.

173. Mark J, Dahlenfors R, Stenman G, Nordquist A. A human adenolymphoma showing the chromosomal aberrations del (7)(p12p14-15) and t(11;19)(q21;p12-13). Anticancer Res 1989;9:1565–6.

174. Mark J, Dahlenfors R, Stenman G, Nordquist A. Chromosomal patterns in Warthin's tumor. A second type of human benign salivary gland neoplasm. Cancer Genet Cytogenet 1990;46:35–9.

175. Martis C. Parotid benign tumors: comments on surgical treatment of 263 cases. Int J Oral Surg 1983;12:211–20.

176. Masuda A. Immunohistochemical study of Warthin's tumour with special regard to the germinal centre. Histol Histopathol 1988;3:81–91.

177. Matteson SR, Cutler LS, Herman PA. Warthin's tumor. Report of a case and survey of 205 salivary neoplasms. Oral Surg Oral Med Oral Pathol 1976;41:129–34.

178. McClatchey KD, Appelblatt NH, Langin JL. Carcinoma in papillary cytadenoma lymphomatosum (Warthin's tumor). Laryngoscope 1982;92:98–9.

179. McQuarrie DG, Winter L. Papillary cystadenoma lymphomatosum. An unusual incidence. Arch Surg 1966;93:511–6.

180. Medeiros LJ, Rizzi R, Lardelli P, Jaffe ES. Malignant lymphoma involving a Warthin's tumor: a case with immunophenotypic and gene rearrangement analysis. Hum Pathol 1990;21:974–7.

181. Miller R, Yanagihara ET, Dubrow AA, Lukes RJ. Malignant lymphoma in the Warthin's tumor. Report of a case. Cancer 1982;50:2948–50.

182. Minami M, Tanioka H, Oyama K, et al. Warthin tumor of the parotid gland: MR-pathologic correlation. AJNR Am J Neuroradiol 1993;14:209–14.

183. Moinuddin M, Rockett JF. Warthin's tumor and the I-123 scan [Letter]. J Nucl Med 1980;21:898–0.

184. Monk JS Jr, Church JS. Warthin's tumor. A high incidence and no sex predominance in central Pennsylvania. Arch Otolaryngol Head Neck Surg 1992;118:477–8.

185. Moosavi H, Ryan C, Schwartz S, Donnelly JA. Malignant adenolymphoma. Hum Pathol 1980;11:80–3.

186. Morrison GA, Shaw HJ. Squamous carcinoma arising within a Warthin's tumour of the parotid gland. J Laryngol Otol 1988;102:1189–91.

187. Nakashima N, Goto K, Takeuchi J. Malignant papillary cystadenoma lymphomatosum. Light and electron microscopic study. Virchows Arch [A] 1983;399:207–19.

188. Newman L, Loukota RA, Bradley PF. An infarcted Warthin's tumour presenting with facial weakness. Br J Oral Maxillofac Surg 1993;31:311–2.

189. Noyek AM, Pritzker KP, Greyson ND, Blackstein M, Chapnik JS, Shapiro BJ. Familial Warthin's tumor. 1. Its synchronous occurrence in mother and son. 2. Its association with cystic oncocytic metaplasia of the larynx. J Otolaryngol 1980;9:90–6.

190. O'Dwyer TP, Gullane PJ, Dardick I. A pseudo-malignant Warthin's tumor presenting with facial nerve paralysis. J Otolaryngol 1990;19:353–7.

191. Onder T, Tiwari RM, van der Waal I, Snow GB. Malignant adenolymphoma of the parotid gland: report of carcinomatous transformation. J Laryngol Otol 1990;104:656–61.

192. Podlesák T, Doleckovó V, Sibl O. Malignancy of a cystadenolymphoma of the parotid gland. Eur Arch Otorhinolaryngol 1992;249:233–5.

193. Poulsen P, Jorgensen K, Grontved A. Benign and malignant neoplasms of the parotid gland: incidence and histology in the Danish county of Funen. Laryngoscope 1987;97:102–4.

194. Ruco LP, Rosati S, Remotti D, Modesti A, Vitolo D, Baroni CD. Immunohistology of adenolymphoma (Warthin's tumour): evidence for a role of vascularization in the organization of the lympho-epithelial structure. Histopathology 1987;11:557–65.

195. Segami N, Fukuda M, Manabe T. Immunohistological study of the epithelial components of Warthin's tumor. Int J Oral Maxillofac Surg 1989;18:133–7.

196. Segatto O, Giacomini P, Santoro L, Perrino A, Natali PG. Lymphoid stroma of Warthin's tumor: phenotypic analogies with gut-associated lymphoid tissue. Clin Immunol Immunopathol 1985;34:39–47.

197. Seifert G, Bull HG, Donath K. Histologic subclassification of the cystadenolymphoma of the parotid gland. Analysis of 275 cases. Virchows Arch [A] 1980;388:13–38.

198. Shah D, Williams E, Brooks SE. Warthin's tumour in Jamaica. Incidence, electron microscopy and immunoenzyme studies. West Indian Med J 1990;39:225–32.

199. Siddiqui AR, Weisberger EC. Possible explanation of appearance of Warthin's tumor on I-123 and Tc-99m-pertechnetate scans. Clin Nucl Med 1981;6:258–60.

200. Snyderman C, Johnson JT, Barnes EL. Extraparotid Warthin's tumor. Otolaryngol Head Neck Surg 1986;94:169–75.

201. Sostre S, Medina L, de Arellano GR. The various scintigraphic patterns of Warthin's tumor. Clin Nucl Med 1987;12:620–6.

202. Spiro RH. Salivary neoplasms: overview of a 35-year experience with 2,807 patients. Head Neck Surg 1986;8:177–84.

203. Taxy JB. Necrotizing squamous/mucinous metaplasia in oncocytic salivary gland tumors. A potential diagnostic problem. Am J Clin Pathol 1992;97:40–5.

204. Therkildsen MH, Christensen N, Andersen LJ, Larsen S, Katholm M. Malignant Warthin's tumour: a case study. Histopathology 1992;21:167–71.

205. Thomas KM, Hutt MS, Borgstein J. Salivary gland tumors in Malawi. Cancer 1980;46:2328–34.

206. Tubbs RR, Sheibani K, Weiss RA, Lee V, Sebek BA, Valenzuela R. Immunohistochemistry of Warthin's tumor. Am J Clin Pathol 1980;74:795–7.

207. Warnock GR. Papillary cystadenoma lymphomatosum (Warthin's tumor). In: Ellis GL, Auclair PL, Gnepp DR, eds. Surgical pathology of the salivary glands. Philadelphia: WB Saunders, 1991:187–201.

208. Weinstein GS, Harvey RT, Zimmer W, Ter S, Alavi A. Technetium-99m pertechnetate salivary gland imaging: its role in the diagnosis of Warthin's tumor [clinical conference]. J Nucl Med 1994;35:179–83.

209. White RR, Arm RN, Randall P. A large Warthin's tumor of the parotid. Case report. Plast Reconstr Surg 1978;61:452–4.

210. Yamamoto H, Caselitz J, Seifert G. Cystadenolymphoma: an immunohistochemical study with special reference to IgE and mast cells. Pathol Res Pract 1985;180:364–8.

211. Yoo GH, Eisele DW, Askin FB, Driben JS, Johns ME. Warthin's tumor: a 40-year experience at The Johns Hopkins Hospital. Laryngoscope 1994;104:799–803.

Basal Cell Adenoma

212. Abiko Y, Shimono M, Hashimoto S, et al. Ultrastructure of basal cell adenoma in the parotid gland. Bull Tokyo Dent Coll 1989;30:145–53.

213. Batsakis JG. Basal cell adenoma of the parotid gland. Cancer 1972;29:226–30.

214. Batsakis JG, Brannon RB. Dermal analogue tumours of major salivary glands. J Laryngol Otol 1981;95:155–64.

215. Batsakis JG, Brannon RB, Sciubba JJ. Monomorphic adenomas of major salivary glands: a histologic study of 96 tumours. Clin Otolaryngol 1981;6:129–43.

216. Batsakis JG, Luna MA, el-Naggar AK. Basaloid monomorphic adenomas. Ann Otol Rhinol Laryngol 1991;100:687–90.

217. Bernacki EG, Batsakis JG, Johns ME. Basal cell adenoma. Distinctive tumor of salivary glands. Arch Otolaryngol 1974;99:84–7.

218. Chau MN, Radden BG. Intra-oral salivary gland neoplasms: a retrospective study of 98 cases. J Oral Pathol 1986;15:339–42.

219. Chilla R, Casjens R, Eysholdt U, Droese M. Maligne speicheldrusentumoren. Der einfluss von histologie und lokalisation auf die prognose. HNO 1983;31:286–90.

220. Christ TF, Crocker D. Basal cell adenoma of minor salivary gland origin. Cancer 1972;30:214–9.

221. Daley TD, Gardner DG, Smout MS. Canalicular adenoma: not a basal cell adenoma. Oral Surg Oral Med Oral Pathol 1984;57:181–8.

222. Dardick I, Daley TD, van Nostrand AW. Basal cell adenoma with myoepithelial cell-derived "stroma": a new major salivary gland tumor entity. Head Neck Surg 1986;8:257–67.

223. Dardick I, Kahn HJ, van Nostrand AW, Baumal R. Salivary gland monomorphic adenoma. Ultrastructural, immunoperoxidase, and histogenetic aspects. Am J Pathol 1984;115:334–48.

224. Dardick I, Lytwyn A, Bourne AJ, Byard RW. Trabecular and solid-cribriform types of basal cell adenoma. A morphologic study of two cases of an unusual variant of monomorphic adenoma. Oral Surg Oral Med Oral Pathol 1992;73:75–83.

225. Dardick I, van Nostrand AW. Myoepithelial cells in salivary gland tumors—revisited. Head Neck Surg 1985;7:395–408.

226. Evans CS, Goldman RL. Dermal analogue tumor arising in a lymphoepithelial cyst of the parotid gland. Arch Pathol Lab Med 1986;110:561–2.

227. Evans RW, Cruickshank AH. Epithelial tumours of the salivary glands. Philadelphia: WB Saunders, 1970:58–76.

228. Eveson JW, Cawson RA. Salivary gland tumours. A review of 2410 cases with particular reference to histological types, site, age and sex distribution. J Pathol 1985;146:51–8.

229. Eveson JW, Cawson RA. Tumours of the minor (oropharyngeal) salivary glands: a demographic study of 336 cases. J Oral Pathol 1985;14:500–9.

230. Fantasia JE, Neville BW. Basal cell adenomas of the minor salivary glands. A clinicopathologic study of seventeen new cases and a review of the literature. Oral Surg Oral Med Oral Pathol 1980;50:433–40.

231. Ferrandiz C, Campo E, Baumann E. Dermal cylindromas (turban tumour) and eccrine spiradenomas in a patient with membranous basal cell adenoma of the parotid gland. J Cutan Pathol 1985;12:72–9.

232. Gardner DG, Daley TD. The use of the terms monomorphic adenoma, basal cell adenoma, and canalicular adenoma as applied to salivary gland tumors. Oral Surg Oral Med Oral Pathol 1983;56:608–15.

233. Gerber JE, Descalzi ME. Eccrine spiradenoma and dermal cylindroma. J Cutan Pathol 1983;10:73–8.

234. Gupta RK, Naran S, Dowle C, Simpson JS. Coexpression of vimentin, cytokeratin and S-100 in monomorphic adenoma of salivary gland; value of marker studies in the differential diagnosis of salivary gland tumours. Cytopathology 1992;3:303–9.

235. Hamano H, Abiko Y, Hashimoto S, et al. Immunohistochemical study of basal cell adenoma in the parotid gland. Bull Tokyo Dent Coll 1990;31:23–31.

236. Headington JT, Batsakis JG, Beals TF, Campbell TE, Simmons JL, Stone WD. Membranous basal cell adenoma of parotid gland, dermal cylindromas, and trichoepitheliomas. Comparative histochemistry and ultrastructure. Cancer 1977;39:2460–9.

237. Herbst EW, Utz W. Multifocal dermal-type basal cell adenomas of parotid glands with co-existing dermal cylindromas. Virchows Arch [A] 1984;403:95–102.

238. Isacsson G, Shear M. Intraoral salivary gland tumors: a retrospective study of 201 cases. J Oral Pathol 1983;12:57–62.

239. Jao W, Keh PC, Swerdlow MA. Ultrastructure of the basal cell adenoma of parotid gland. Cancer 1976;37:1322–33.

240. Kleinsasser O, Klein HJ. Basalzelladenome der speidheldrüsen. Arch Klin Exp Ohren Nasen Kehlkopfheilkd 1967;189:302–16.

241. Kratochvil FJ. Canalicular adenoma and basal cell adenoma. In: Ellis GL, Auclair PL, Gnepp DR, eds. Surgical pathology of the salivary glands. Philadelphia: WB Saunders, 1991:202–24.

242. Levine J, Krutchkoff DJ, Eisenberg E. Monomorphic adenoma of minor salivary glands: a reappraisal and report of nine new cases. J Oral Surg 1981;39:101–7.

243. Luna MA, Batsakis JG, Tortoledo ME, del Junco GW. Carcinomas ex monomorphic adenoma of salivary glands. J Laryngol Otol 1989;103:756–9.

244. Luna MA, Tortoledo ME, Allen M. Salivary dermal analogue tumors arising in lymph nodes. Cancer 1987;59:1165–9.

245. Main JH, Orr JA, McGurk FM, McComb RJ, Mock D. Salivary gland tumors: review of 643 cases. J Oral Pathol 1976;5:88–102.

246. Maurizi M, Salvinelli F, Capelli A, Carbone A. Monomorphic adenomas of the major salivary glands: clinicopathological study of 44 cases. J Laryngol Otol 1990;104:790–6.

247. Mintz GA, Abrams AM, Melrose RJ. Monomorphic adenomas of the major and minor salivary glands. Report of twenty-one cases and review of the literature. Oral Surg Oral Med Oral Pathol 1982;53:375–86.

248. Morinaga S, Nakajima T, Shimosato Y. Normal and neoplastic myoepithelial cells in salivary glands: an immunohistochemical study. Hum Pathol 1987;18:1218–26.

249. Nagao K, Matsuzaki O, Saiga H, et al. Histopathologic studies of basal cell adenoma of the parotid gland. Cancer 1982;50:736–45.

250. Neville BW, Damm DD, Weir JC, Fantasia JE. Labial salivary gland tumors. Cancer 1988;61:2113–6.

251. Nishimura T, Furukawa M, Kawahara E, Miwa A. Differential diagnosis of pleomorphic adenoma by immunohistochemical means. J Laryngol Otol 1991;105:1057–60.

252. Ogawa I, Nikai H, Takata T, Miyauchi M, Ito H, Ijuhin N. The cellular composition of basal cell adenoma of the parotid gland: an immunohistochemical analysis. Oral Surg Oral Med Oral Pathol 1990;70:619–26.

253. Reingold IM, Keasbey LE, Graham JH. Multicentric dermal-type cylindromas of the parotid glands in a patient with florid turban tumor. Cancer 1977;40:1702–10.

254. Schmidt KT, Ma A, Goldberg R, Medenica M. Multiple adnexal tumors and a parotid basal cell adenoma. J Am Acad Dermatol 1991;25:960–4.

255. Seifert G, Okabe H, Caselitz J. Epithelial salivary gland tumors in children and adolescents. Analysis of 80 cases (Salivary Gland Register 1965-1984). ORL J Otorhinolaryngol Relat Spec 1986;48:137–49.

256. Seifert G, Sobin LH. Histological typing of salivary gland tumours. World Health Organization international histological classification of tumours. 2nd ed. New York: Springer-Verlag, 1991.

257. Sharkey FE. Systematic evaluation of the World Health Organization classification of salivary gland tumors: a clinicopathologic study of 366 cases. Am J Clin Pathol 1977;67:272–8.

258. Spiro RH. Salivary neoplasms: overview of a 35-year experience with 2,807 patients. Head Neck Surg 1986;8:177–84.

259. Suzuki K. Basal cell adenoma with acinic differentiation. Acta Pathol Jpn 1982;32:1085–92.

260. Suzuki K, Mori I, Masawa N, Ooneda G. A case report of basal cell adenoma showing elastic fiber (elastin-basement membrane complex) formation of the submandibular gland. Acta Pathol Jpn 1980;30:275–83.

261. Takahashi H, Fujita S, Okabe H, Tsuda N, Tezuka F. Immunohistochemical characterization of basal cell adenomas of the salivary gland. Pathol Res Pract 1991;187:145–56.

262. Takahashi H, Fujita S, Tsuda N, Tezuka F, Okabe H. Intraoral minor salivary gland tumors: a demographic and histologic study of 200 cases. Tohoku J Exp Med 1990;161:111–28.

263. Thackray AC, Sobin LH. Histological typing of salivary gland tumours. International histological classification of tumours No. 7. Geneva: World Health Organization, 1972.

264. Thawley SE, Ward SP, Ogura JH. Basal cell adenoma of the salivary glands. Laryngoscope 1974;84:1756–65.

265. Theron EJ, Middlecote BD. Tumours of the salivary glands. The Bloemfontein experience. S Afr J Surg 1984;22:237–42.

266. Thomas KM, Hutt MS, Borgstein J. Salivary gland tumors in Malawi. Cancer 1980;46:2328–34.

267. Waldron CA, el-Mofty SK, Gnepp DR. Tumors of the intraoral minor salivary glands: a demographic and histologic study of 426 cases. Oral Surg Oral Med Oral Pathol 1988;66:323–33.

268. Williams SB, Ellis GL, Auclair PL. Immunohistochemical analysis of basal cell adenocarcinoma. Oral Surg Oral Med Oral Pathol 1993;75:64–9.

269. Youngberg G, Rao MS. Ultrastructural features of monomorphic adenoma of the parotid gland. Oral Surg Oral Med Oral Pathol 1979;47:458–61.

270. Zarbo RJ, Ricci A Jr, Kowalczyk PD, Cartun RW, Knibbs DR. Intranasal dermal analogue tumor (membranous basal cell adenoma). Ultrastructure and immunohistochemistry. Arch Otolaryngol 1985;111:333–7.

Canalicular Adenoma

271. Anderson JH, Provencher RF, McKean TW. Basal cell adenoma: review of the literature and report of case. J Oral Surg 1980;38:844–6.

272. Batsakis JG, Brannon RB, Sciubba JJ. Monomorphic adenomas of major salivary glands: a histologic study of 96 tumours. Clin Otolaryngol 1981;6:129–43.

273. Batsakis JG, Luna MA, el-Naggar AK. Basaloid monomorphic adenomas. Ann Otol Rhinol Laryngol 1991;100:687–90.

274. Chau MN, Radden BG. Intra-oral salivary gland neoplasms: a retrospective study of 98 cases. J Oral Pathol 1986;15:339–42.

275. Chen SY, Miller AS. Canalicular adenoma of the upper lip: an electron microscopic study. Cancer 1980;46:552–6.

276. Daley TD. The canalicular adenoma: considerations on differential diagnosis and treatment. J Oral Maxillofac Surg 1984;42:728–30.

277. Daley TD, Gardner DG, Smout MS. Canalicular adenoma: not a basal cell adenoma. Oral Surg Oral Med Oral Pathol 1984;57:181–8.

278. Dardick I, Kahn HJ, van Nostrand AW, Baumal R. Salivary gland monomorphic adenoma. Ultrastructural, immunoperoxidase, and histogenetic aspects. Am J Pathol 1984;115:334–48.

279. Eveson JW, Cawson RA. Salivary gland tumours. A review of 2410 cases with particular reference to histological types, site, age and sex distribution. J Pathol 1985;146:51–8.

280. Eveson JW, Cawson RA. Tumours of the minor (oropharyngeal) salivary glands: a demographic study of 336 cases. J Oral Pathol 1985;14:500–9.

281. Fantasia JE, Neville BW. Basal cell adenomas of the minor salivary glands. A clinicopathologic study of seventeen new cases and a review of the literature. Oral Surg Oral Med Oral Pathol 1980;50:433–40.

282. Gardner DG, Daley TD. The use of the terms monomorphic adenoma, basal cell adenoma, and canalicular adenoma as applied to salivary gland tumors. Oral Surg Oral Med Oral Pathol 1983;56:608–15.

283. Guccion JG, Redman RS. Canalicular adenoma of the buccal mucosa. An ultrastructural and histochemical study. Oral Surg Oral Med Oral Pathol 1986;61:173–8.

284. Isacsson G, Shear M. Intraoral salivary gland tumors: a retrospective study of 201 cases. J Oral Pathol 1983;12:57–62.

285. Khullar SM, Best PV. Adenomatosis of minor salivary glands. Report of a case. Oral Surg Oral Med Oral Pathol 1992;74:783–7.

286. Levine J, Krutchkoff DJ, Eisenberg E. Monomorphic adenoma of minor salivary glands: a reappraisal and report of nine new cases. J Oral Surg 1981;39:101–7.

287. Ma DQ, Yu GY. Tumours of the minor salivary glands. A clinicopathologic study of 243 cases. Acta Otolaryngol (Stockh) 1987;103:325–31.

288. Mader CL, Nelson JF. Monomorphic adenoma of the minor salivary glands. J Am Dent Assoc 1981;102:657–9.

289. Main JH, Orr JA, McGurk FM, McComb RJ, Mock D. Salivary gland tumors: review of 643 cases. J Oral Pathol 1976;5:88–102.

290. Mair IW, Stalsberg H. Basal cell adenomatosis of minor salivary glands of the upper lip. Arch Otorhinolaryngol 1988;245:191–5.

291. Mintz GA, Abrams AM, Melrose RJ. Monomorphic adenomas of the major and minor salivary glands. Report of twenty-one cases and review of the literature. Oral Surg Oral Med Oral Pathol 1982;53:375–86.

292. Nelson JF, Jacoway JR. Monomorphic adenoma (canalicular type). Report of 29 cases. Cancer 1973;31:1511–3.

293. Neville BW, Damm DD, Weir JC, Fantasia JE. Labial salivary gland tumors. Cancer 1988;61:2113–6.

294. Pogrel MA. The intraoral basal cell adenoma. J Craniomaxillofac Surg 1987;15:372–5.

295. Seifert G, Sobin LH. Histological typing of salivary gland tumours. World Health Organization international histological classification of tumours. 2nd ed. New York: Springer-Verlag, 1991.

296. Sharkey FE. Systematic evaluation of the World Health Organization classification of salivary gland tumors: a clinicopathologic study of 366 cases. Am J Clin Pathol 1977;67:272–8.

297. Spiro RH. Salivary neoplasms: overview of a 35-year experience with 2,807 patients. Head Neck Surg 1986;8:177–84.

298. Theron EJ, Middlecote BD. Tumours of the salivary glands. The Bloemfontein experience. S Afr J Surg 1984;22:237–42.

299. Thomas KM, Hutt MS, Borgstein J. Salivary gland tumors in Malawi. Cancer 1980;46:2328–34.

300. Waldron CA, el-Mofty SK, Gnepp DR. Tumors of the intraoral minor salivary glands: a demographic and histologic study of 426 cases. Oral Surg Oral Med Oral Pathol 1988;66:323–33.

301. Zarbo RJ, Regezi JA, Batsakis JG. S-100 protein in salivary gland tumors: an immunohistochemical study of 129 cases. Head Neck Surg 1986;8:268–75.

Oncocytoma

302. Blanck C, Eneroth CM, Jakobsson PA. Oncocytoma of the parotid gland: neoplasm or nodular hyperplasia? Cancer 1970;25:919–25.

303. Brandwein MS, Huvos AG. Oncocytic tumors of major salivary glands. A study of 68 cases with follow-up of 44 patients. Am J Surg Pathol 1991;15:514–28.

304. Carlsöö B, Domeij S, Helander HF. A quantitative ultrastructural study of a parotid oncocytoma. Arch Pathol Lab Med 1979;103:471–4.

305. Chang A, Harawi SJ. Oncocytes, oncocytosis, and oncocytic tumors. Pathol Annu 1992;27 [Pt 1]:263–304.

306. Chaudhry AP, Labay GR, Yamane GM, Jacobs MS, Cutler LS, Watkins KV. Clinico-pathologic and histogenetic study of 189 intraoral minor salivary gland tumors. J Oral Med 1984;39:58–78.

307. Damm DD, White DK, Geissler RH Jr, Drummond JF, Henry BB. Benign solid oncocytoma of intraoral minor salivary glands. Oral Surg Oral Med Oral Pathol 1989;67:84–6.

308. Ellis GL. Clear cell oncocytoma of salivary gland. Hum Pathol 1988;19:862–7.

309. Eveson JW, Cawson RA. Salivary gland tumours. A review of 2410 cases with particular reference to histological types, site, age and sex distribution. J Pathol 1985;146:51–8.

310. Gray SR, Cornog JL Jr, Seo IS. Oncocytic neoplasms of salivary glands: a report of fifteen cases including two malignant oncocytomas. Cancer 1976;38:1306–17.

311. Hartwick RW, Batsakis JG. Non-Warthin's tumor oncocytic lesions. Ann Otol Rhinol Laryngol 1990;99:674–7.

312. Johns ME, Batsakis JG, Short CD. Oncocytic and oncocytoid tumors of the salivary glands. Laryngoscope 1973;83:1940–52.

313. Johns ME, Regezi JA, Batsakis JG. Oncocytic neoplasms of salivary glands: an ultrastructural study. Laryngoscope 1977;87:862–71.

314. Kosuda S, Ishikawa M, Tamura K, Mukai M, Kubo A, Hashimoto S. Iodine-131 therapy for parotid oncocytoma. J Nucl Med 1988;29:1126–9.

315. Lidang Jensen M. Multifocal adenomatous oncocytic hyperplasia in parotid glands with metastatic deposits or primary malignant transformation? Pathol Res Pract 1989;185:514–21.

316. Main JH, Orr JA, McGurk FM, McComb RJ, Mock D. Salivary gland tumors: review of 643 cases. J Oral Pathol 1976;5:88–102.

317. Nelson DW, Nichols RD, Fine G. Bilateral acinous cell tumors of the parotid gland. Laryngoscope 1978;88:1935–41.

318. Palmer JA, Mustard RA, Simpson WJ. Irradiation as an etiologic factor in tumours of the thyroid, parathyroid and salivary glands. Can J Surg 1980;23:39–42.

319. Palmer TJ, Gleeson MJ, Eveson JW, Cawson RA. Oncocytic adenomas and oncocytic hyperplasia of salivary glands: a clinicopathological study of 26 cases. Histopathology 1990;16:487–93.

320. Regezi JA, Lloyd RV, Zarbo RJ, McClatchey KD. Minor salivary gland tumors. A histologic and immunohistochemical study. Cancer 1985;55:108–15.

321. Scanlon EF, Sener SF. Head and neck neoplasia following irradiation for benign conditions. Head Neck Surg 1981;4:139–45.

322. Schneider AB, Shore-Freedman E, Ryo UY, Bekerman C, Favus M, Pinsky S. Radiation-induced tumors of the head and neck following childhood irradiation. Prospective studies. Medicine (Baltimore) 1985;64:1–15.

323. Schwartz IS, Feldman M. Diffuse multinodular oncocytoma ("oncocytosis") of the parotid gland. Cancer 1969;23:636–40.

324. Seifert G, Miehlke A, Haubrich J, Chilla R. Diseases of the salivary glands: pathology, diagnosis, treatment, facial nerve surgery. New York: Georg Thieme Verlag, 1986:171.

325. Sener SF, Scanlon EF. Irradiation induced salivary gland neoplasia. Ann Surg 1980;191:304–6.

326. Sharkey FE. Systematic evaluation of the World Health Organization classification of salivary gland tumors: a clinicopathologic study of 366 cases. Am J Clin Pathol 1977;67:272–8.

327. Spiro RH. Salivary neoplasms: overview of a 35-year experience with 2,807 patients. Head Neck Surg 1986;8:177–84.

328. Takeda Y. Diffuse hyperplastic oncocytosis of the parotid gland. Int J Oral Maxillofac Surg 1986;15:765–8.

329. Theron EJ, Middlecote BD. Tumours of the salivary glands. The Bloemfontein experience. S Afr J Surg 1984;22:237–42.

330. Waldron CA, el-Mofty SK, Gnepp DR. Tumors of the intraoral minor salivary glands: a demographic and histologic study of 426 cases. Oral Surg Oral Med Oral Pathol 1988;66:323–33.

331. Walker MJ, Chaudhuri PK, Wood DC, Das Gupta TK. Radiation-induced parotid cancer. Arch Surg 1981;116:329–31.

Cystadenoma

332. Auclair PL, Ellis GL, Gnepp DR. Other benign epithelial neoplasms. In: Ellis GL, Auclair PL, Gnepp DR, eds. Surgical pathology of the salivary glands. Philadelphia: WB Saunders, 1991:252–68.

333. Chaudhry AP, Labay GR, Yamane GM, Jacobs MS, Cutler LS, Watkins KV. Clinico-pathologic and histogenetic study of 189 intraoral minor salivary gland tumors. J Oral Med 1984;39:58–78.

334. Evans RW, Cruickshank AH. Epithelial tumours of the salivary glands. Philadelphia: WB Saunders, 1970.

335. Eversole LR, Sabes WR. Minor salivary gland duct changes due to obstruction. Arch Otolaryngol Head Neck Surg 1971;94:19–24.

336. Goldman RL. Melanogenic papillary cystadenoma of the soft palate. Am J Clin Pathol 1967;48:49–52.

337. Greene GW, Lipani C, Woytash JJ, Meenaghan MA. Seromucous cystadenoma of the oral cavity. J Oral Maxillofac Surg 1984;42:48–53.

338. Kerpel SM, Freedman PD, Lumerman H. The papillary cystadenoma of minor salivary gland origin. Oral Surg Oral Med Oral Pathol 1978;46:820–6.

339. Krogdahl AS, Bretlau P, Hastrup N. Multiple tumours of the parotid gland. J Laryngol Otol 1983;97:1035–7.

340. Kuhn AJ. Cystadenoma of the parotid gland and larynx. Arch Otolaryngol Head Neck Surg 1961;73:404–6.

341. Seifert G, Miehlke A, Haubrich J, Chilla R. Diseases of the salivary glands: diagnosis, pathology, treament, facial nerve surgery. Stuttgart: Georg Thieme Verlag, 1986:182–93.

342. Seifert G, Thomsen S, Donath K. Bilateral dysgenetic parotid glands. Morphological analysis and differential diagnosis of a rare disease of the salivary glands. Virchows Arch [A] 1981;390:273–88.

343. Sher L. The papillary cystadenoma of salivary gland origin. Diastema 1982;10:37–41.

344. Thackray AC, Lucas RB. Tumors of the major salivary glands. Atlas of Tumor Pathology, 2nd Series, Fascicle 10. Washington, D.C.: Armed Forces Institute of Pathology, 1974:60.

345. Waldron CA, el-Mofty SK, Gnepp DR. Tumors of the intraoral minor salivary glands: a demographic and histologic study of 426 cases. Oral Surg Oral Med Oral Pathol 1988;66:323–33.

346. Wilson DF, MacEntee MI. Papillary cystadenoma of minor salivary gland orgin. Oral Surg Oral Med Oral Pathol 1974;915:918.

Ductal Papilloma

347. Abbey LM. Solitary intraductal papilloma of the minor salivary glands. Oral Surg Oral Med Oral Pathol 1975;40:135–40.

348. Abrams AM, Finck FM. Sialadenoma papilliferum. A previously unreported salivary gland tumor. Cancer 1969;24:1057–63.

349. Batsakis JG. Oral monomorphic adenomas. Ann Otol Rhinol Laryngol 1991;100:348–50.

350. Castigliano SG, Gold L. Intraductal papilloma of the hard palate. Case report of a minor salivary gland. Oral Surg Oral Med Oral Pathol 1954;7:232–8.

351. Chan KW, Ng WL, Lau WF. Sialadenoma papilliferum. Pathology 1985;17:119–22.

352. Clark DB, Priddy RW, Swanson AE. Oral inverted ductal papilloma. Oral Surg Oral Med Oral Pathol 1990;69:487–90.

353. Crocker DJ, Christ TF, Cavalaris CJ. Sialadenoma papilliferum: report of case. J Oral Surg 1972;30:520–1.

354. Ellis GL, Auclair PL. Ductal papillomas. In: Ellis GL, Auclair PL, Gnepp DR, eds. Surgical pathology of the salivary glands. Philadelphia: WB Saunders, 1991:238–51.

355. Ellis GL, Gnepp DR. Unusual salivary gland tumors. In: Gnepp DR, ed. Pathology of the head and neck. New York: Churchill Livingstone, 1988:585–661.

356. Eversole LR, Sabes WR. Minor salivary gland duct changes due to obstruction. Arch Otolaryngol 1971; 94:19–24.

357. Fantasia JE, Nocco CE, Lally ET. Ultrastructure of sialadenoma papilliferum. Arch Pathol Lab Med 1986;110:523–7.

358. Franklin CD, Ong TK. Ductal papilloma of the minor salivary gland. Histopathology 1991;19:180–2.

359. Gardiner GW, Briant TD, Sheman L. Inverted ductal papilloma of the parotid gland. J Otolaryngol 1984;13:23–6.

360. Goldman RL. Melanogenic papillary cystadenoma of the soft palate. Am J Clin Pathol 1967;48:49–52.

361. Grushka M, Podoshin L, Boss JH, Fradis M. Sialadenoma papilliferum of the parotid gland. Laryngoscope 1984;94:231–3.

362. Hyams VJ, Batsakis JG, Michaels L. Tumors of the upper respiratory tract and ear. Atlas of Tumor Pathology, 2nd Series, Fascicle 25. Washington, D. C.: Armed Forces Institute of Pathology, 1986:34–44.

363. Ishikawa T, Imada S, Ijuhin N. Intraductal papilloma of the anterior lingual salivary gland. Case report and immunohistochemical study. Int J Oral Maxillofac Surg 1993;22:116–7.

364. Kerpel SM, Freedman PD, Lumerman H. The papillary cystadenoma of minor salivary gland origin. Oral Surg Oral Med Oral Pathol 1978;46:820–6.

365. King PH, Hill J. Intraduct papilloma of parotid gland. J Clin Pathol 1993;46:175–6.

366. Kronenberg J, Horowitz A, Leventon G. Sialadenoma papilliferum of the parotid gland. J Laryngol Otol 1989;103:1089–90.

367. Masi JD, Hoang KG, Sawyer R. Sialadenoma papilliferum of the adenoids in a 2-year-old child. Arch Pathol Lab Med 1986;110:558–60.

368. Neville BW, Damm DD, Weir JC, Fantasia JE. Labial salivary gland tumors. Cancer 1988;61:2113–6.

369. Regezi JA, Lloyd RV, Zarbo RJ, McClatchey KD. Minor salivary gland tumors. A histologic and immunohistochemical study. Cancer 1985;55:108–15.

370. Rennie JS, MacDonald DG, Critchlow HA. Sialadenoma papilliferum. A case report and review of the literature. Int J Oral Surg 1984;13:452–4.

371. Seifert G, Sobin LH. Histological typing of salivary gland tumours. World Health Organization international histological classification of tumours. 2nd ed. New York: Springer-Verlag, 1991.

372. Sher L. The papillary cystadenoma of salivary gland origin. Diastema 1982;10:37–41.

373. Solomon MP, Rosen Y, Alfonso A. Intraoral papillary squamous cell tumor of the soft palate with features of sialadenoma papilliferum–? malignant sialadenoma papilliferum. Cancer 1978;42:1859–69.

374. van der Wal JE, van der Waal I. The rare sialadenoma papilliferum. Report of a case and review of the literature. Int J Oral Maxillofac Surg 1992;21:104–6.

375. Waldron CA, el-Mofty SK, Gnepp DR. Tumors of the intraoral minor salivary glands: a demographic and histologic study of 426 cases. Oral Surg Oral Med Oral Pathol 1988;66:323–33.

376. White DK, Miller AS, McDaniel RK, Rothman BN. Inverted ductal papilloma: a distinctive lesion of minor salivary gland. Cancer 1982;49:519–24.

377. Wilson DF, Robinson BW. Oral inverted ductal papilloma. Oral Surg Oral Med Oral Pathol 1984;57:520–3.

Sebaceous Adenoma and Sebaceous Lymphadenoma

378. Auclair PL. Tumor-associated lymphoid proliferation in the parotid gland: a potential diagnostic pitfall. Oral Surg Oral Med Oral Pathol 1994;77:19–26.
379. Auclair PL, Ellis GL, Gnepp DR. Other benign epithelial neoplasms. In: Ellis GL, Auclair PL, Gnepp DR, eds. Surgical pathology of the salivary glands. Philadelphia: WB Saunders, 1991:252–68.
380. Baratz M, Loewenthal M, Rozin M. Sebaceous lymphadenoma of the parotid gland. Arch Pathol Lab Med 1976;100:269–70.
381. Batsakis JG, Littler ER, Leahy MS. Sebaceous cell lesions of the head and neck. Arch Otolaryngol Head Neck Surg 1972;95:151–7.
382. Cameron WR, Stenram U. Adenoma of parotid gland with sebaceous and oncocytic features. Cancer 1979;43:1429–33.
383. Daley TD. Intraoral sebaceous hyperplasia. Diagnostic criteria. Oral Surg Oral Med Oral Pathol 1993;75:343–7.
384. Dreyer T, Battmann A, Silberzahn J, Glanz H, Schulz A. Unusual differentiation of a combination tumor of the parotid gland. A case report. Pathol Res Pract 1993;189:577–81.

385. Foote FW Jr, Frazell EL. Tumors of the major salivary glands. Cancer 1953;6:1065–133.
386. Gnepp DR. Sebaceous neoplasms of salivary gland origin: a review. Pathol Annu 1983;18 (Pt. 1):71–102.
387. Gnepp DR, Brannon R. Sebaceous neoplasms of salivary gland origin. Report of 21 cases. Cancer 1984;53:2155–70.
388. Gnepp DR, Sporck FT. Benign lymphoepithelial parotid cyst with sebaceous differentiation—cystic sebaceous lymphadenoma. Am J Clin Pathol 1980;74:683–7.
389. Linhartová A. Sebaceous glands in salivary gland tissue. Arch Pathol 1974;98:320–4.
390. Mesa-Chavez L. Sebaceous glands in normal and neoplastic parotid glands in respect to the origin of tumors of the salivary glands. Am J Pathol 1949;25:627–45.
391. Seifert G, Sobin LH. Histological typing of salivary gland tumours. World Health Organization international histological classification of tumours. 2nd ed. New York: Springer-Verlag, 1991.
392. Tschen JA, McGavran MH. Sebaceous lymphadenoma: ultrastructural observations and lipid analysis. Cancer 1979;44:1388–92.

Sialoblastoma

393. Adkins GF. Low grade basaloid adenocarcinoma of salivary gland in childhood—the so-called hybrid basal cell adenoma—adenoid cystic carcinoma. Pathology 1990;22:187–90.
394. Batsakis JG, Brannon RB, Sciubba JJ. Monomorphic adenomas of major salivary glands: a histologic study of 96 tumours. Clin Otolaryngol 1981;6:129–43.
395. Batsakis JG, Frankenthaler R. Embryoma (sialoblastoma) of salivary glands. Ann Otol Rhinol Laryngol 1992;101:958–60.
396. Batsakis JG, Mackay B, Ryka AF, Seifert RW. Perinatal salivary gland tumours (embryomas). J Laryngol Otol 1988;102:1007–11.
397. Canalis RF, Mok MW, Fishman SM, Hemenway WG. Congenital basal cell adenoma of the submandibular gland. Arch Otolaryngol Head Neck Surg 1980;106:284–6.
398. Danzinger H. Adenoid cystic carcinoma of the submaxillary gland in an 8 month old infant. Can Med Assoc J 1964;91:759–61.
399. Harris MD, McKeever P, Robertson JM. Congenital tumours of the salivary gland: a case report and review. Histopathology 1990;17:155–7.
400. Hsueh C, Gonzalez-Crussi F. Sialoblastoma: a case report and review of the literature on congenital epithelial tumors of salivary gland origin. [Published erratum appears in Pediatr Pathol 1992 Jul-Aug;12(4):631]. Pediatr Pathol 1992;12:205–14.
401. Krolls SO, Trodahl JN, Boyers RC. Salivary gland lesions in children. A survey of 430 cases. Cancer 1972;30:459–69.
402. Lack EE, Upton MP. Histopathologic review of salivary gland tumors in childhood. Arch Otolaryngol Head Neck Surg 1988;114:898–906.
403. Roth A, Micheau C. Embryoma (or embryonal tumor) of the parotid gland: report of two cases. Pediatr Pathol 1986;5:9–15.
404. Simpson PR, Rutledge JC, Schaefer SD, Anderson RC. Congenital hybrid basal cell adenoma—adenoid cystic carcinoma of the salivary gland. Pediatr Pathol 1986;6:199–208.
405. Taylor GP. Congenital epithelial tumor of the parotid-sialoblastoma. Pediatr Pathol 1988;8:447–52.
406. Thackray AC, Lucas RB. Tumors of the major salivary glands. Atlas of Tumor Pathology, 2nd Series, Fascicle 10. Washington, D.C.: Armed Forces Institute of Pathology, 1974:125–6.
407. Vawter GF, Tefft M. Congenital tumors of the parotid gland. Arch Pathol 1966;82:242–5.
408. Williams SB, Ellis GL, Auclair PL. Immunohistochemical analysis of basal cell adenocarcinoma. Oral Surg Oral Med Oral Pathol 1993;75:64–9.

5

MALIGNANT EPITHELIAL TUMORS

MUCOEPIDERMOID CARCINOMA

Definition. Mucoepidermoid carcinoma is a malignant epithelial tumor that is composed of varying proportions of mucous, epidermoid, intermediate, columnar, and clear cells, and often demonstrates prominent cystic growth. On the basis of morphologic and cytologic features it is divided into low-, intermediate-, and high-grade types. With the recognition that even the low-grade neoplasms may metastasize, the term mucoepidermoid tumor is considered inappropriate.

General Features. Among cases reviewed at the Armed Forces Institute of Pathology (AFIP) since 1985, mucoepidermoid carcinoma is the most common malignant salivary gland tumor. It is encountered as often as the three next most common specific salivary gland malignancies combined: acinic cell adenocarcinoma, polymorphous low-grade adenocarcinoma, and adenoid cystic carcinoma. It represents 15.5 percent of the benign and malignant tumors at all sites, 29 percent of the malignant tumors originating in both major and minor glands, and 22 and 41 percent of the malignant tumors in the major and minor glands, respectively. These frequencies are comparable to those published from two large treatment centers in the United States (71, 73,75), and to those from many other countries including Brazil (58), West Germany (65), China (54,91), India (10), South Africa (45), Canada (31), and France (18). In the United Kingdom, however, mucoepidermoid carcinoma represents just over 2 percent of all salivary gland tumors at all sites and is the fifth most common type of malignant tumor; this suggests a geographic-related variable (30). There are also studies of the minor and submandibular glands from the United States and Japan in which the frequency of adenoid cystic carcinoma was greater than that of mucoepidermoid carcinoma (46,64,78).

Prior exposure to ionizing radiation appears to substantially increase the risk of developing malignant salivary gland tumors in the major glands, particularly mucoepidermoid carcinoma. In a study of 57 patients who had previous irradiation and later developed a salivary malignancy, Spitz

and Batsakis (75) found that the tumor type in 44 percent was mucoepidermoid carcinoma. The latent period between irradiation to the head and neck and tumor development was 7 to 32 years, suggesting a need for long-term follow-up of previously irradiated patients (51,75).

Of site-specific tumors, about 53 percent of mucoepidermoid carcinomas occur in the major glands: 45, 7, and 1 percent occur in the parotid, submandibular, and sublingual glands, respectively; 21 percent originate from the minor glands of the palate; and 19 percent occur, in decreasing frequency, in the buccal mucosa, upper and lower lips, retromolar region, and tongue. Although most types of salivary gland tumors occur much more frequently in the upper than lower lip, among AFIP cases mucoepidermoid carcinoma occurs three times more frequently in the lower lip. In a study of 103 salivary gland tumors of the lips, Neville and colleagues (59) found 13 mucoepidermoid carcinomas in the lower lip but none in the upper lip.

Occurrence of mucoepidermoid carcinoma in the first decade of life is unusual, but 7 percent occur in the second decade. Between the third through the seventh decades there is a relatively uniform frequency of 10 to 18 percent. The only other salivary gland tumor with a comparable age distribution is acinic cell adenocarcinoma (6). The mean age of all civilian patients in the AFIP Registry is 47 years, and the range is from 8 to 92 years. Patients with tumors of the hard and soft palates are about 7 years younger than the average while those with tumors in the lower lip, floor of the mouth, and base of tongue are 8 to 12 years older than the average. Of patients with mucoepidermoid carcinomas of the hard palate, 41 percent are less than 30 years and over 58 percent are under 40 years of age. In contrast, less than 9 percent of patients with tumors located in the lower lip, floor of mouth, or base of tongue are under the age of 30 years.

Mucoepidermoid carcinoma has a predilection for women (60.2 percent) similar to that for salivary gland tumors in general (6). Women outnumber men in all large published studies (1,26,57,58,60,73).

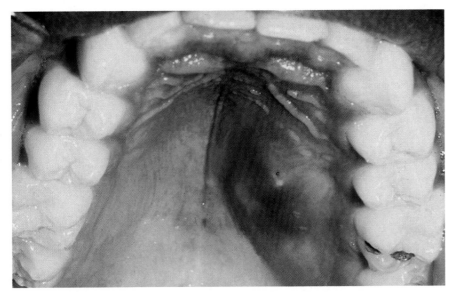

Figure 5-1
MUCOEPIDERMOID
CARCINOMA OF PALATE
These tumors frequently are slightly raised, fluctuant, bluish discolorations of the palatal mucosa that are clinically thought to represent mucous escape reactions.

Rarely, mucoepidermoid carcinoma may be associated with benign salivary gland tumors such as mixed tumors, Warthin's tumor, and oncocytoma. Other combinations of unilateral synchronous and metachronous occurrences have been reported (36).

Clinical Features. In the parotid and submandibular glands these tumors typically present as solitary, painless masses in the preauricular and submandibular regions. AFIP data on 234 patients showed the average known tumor duration for mucoepidermoid carcinomas of the major glands was 1.5 years. More than half the patients were aware of their tumors for 6 months or less, but 34 patients first noticed a swelling more than 3 years before diagnosis; the interval was more than 25 years for 3 patients. Other investigators have also reported tumor durations of 20 years and longer (1,42,58,73). Two thirds of patients are asymptomatic. Symptoms include tenderness, pain, drainage from the ipsilateral ear, dysphagia, trismus, and facial paralysis. About 7 percent of patients experience a rapid increase in size of their tumors following a period of quiescence.

The clinical appearance of mucoepidermoid carcinoma of the minor glands varies considerably. These tumors often masquerade as benign neoplastic and inflammatory conditions. Many lesions, especially of the palate, are fluctuant, bluish, smooth-surfaced swellings that resemble mucoceles (fig. 5-1). Others have a magenta color that suggests a vascular or melanin-containing lesion. Some discharge fluid through a small mucosal opening, resembling draining dental abscesses. Rarely, they have a granular or even papillary surface. At the AFIP, about 40 percent of patients are symptomatic (7). Symptoms include dysphagia, pain, paresthesia, numbness of teeth, ulceration, or hemorrhage. Radiographs of palatal lesions occasionally show erosion of underlying bone.

Gross Findings. Macroscopically, mucoepidermoid carcinomas are occasionally circumscribed and at least partially encapsulated, although these two features are not typical of most tumors and are lacking altogether in high-grade tumors (73). The cut surface is usually firm, gray, tan-yellow, or pink, and lobulated. Cysts are often seen, but their size and prominence varies. The cysts frequently contain viscid mucoid material that is blood-tinged or hemorrhagic. In AFIP cases, the tumor size has varied from less than 1 cm to over 12 cm in the major glands and as large as 5 cm in the minor glands.

Microscopic Findings. The term mucoepidermoid carcinoma was suggested as a contraction of the phrase "mixed epidermoid and mucus-secreting carcinoma" (76) used in an early report of this tumor (22). Both terms emphasize mucous and epidermoid cells (fig. 5-2) but other cell types, such as the frequently predominant intermediate cell and the less conspicuous clear and columnar cells, also are important in mucoepidermoid carcinomas.

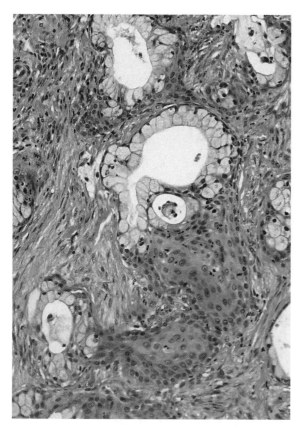

Figure 5-2
MUCOUS AND EPIDERMOID CELLS
The close association of mucous and epidermoid cells is characteristic of mucoepidermoid carcinoma but often not as distinctly seen as in this example.

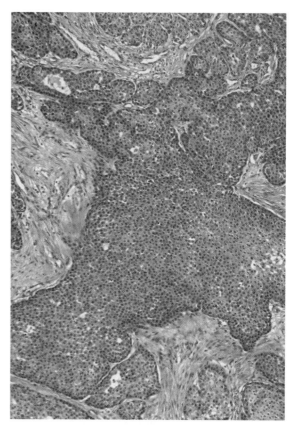

Figure 5-3
INTERMEDIATE CELLS
Solid sheets and islands of intermediate cells dominate this tumor. The neoplastic epithelium is surrounded by dense connective tissue, a feature that may help distinguish it from other tumors.

In most tumors, intermediate cells outnumber the other cell types. The term "intermediate" was originally used for cells whose size and appearance were between basal cells and the larger polygonal epidermoid cells (76). Today, however, most investigators include the smaller basal cells in this term. Thus, intermediate cells range from cells slightly larger than lymphocytes (fig. 5-3) with little cytoplasm to cells two or three times larger. The larger forms are round to ovoid (fig. 5-4). In many tumors there appears to be a transition from small intermediate (basal) to larger intermediate to polygonal and epidermoid forms. In the original description of mucoepidermoid carcinomas, this cellular transition was referred to as "epidermoid metaplasia" (76). The smaller basaloid forms have been referred to as "maternal cells" because of proposed trans-

formation to the larger forms, which further differentiate into epidermoid, mucous, and clear cells (66). Most of the enlargement from small basal cells can be attributed to increased cytoplasm; in larger cells the nuclei become slightly larger and the condensed chromatin becomes more vesicular. Intermediate cells are normally found in clusters or solid sheets and are often amalgamated with the other cell types.

Mucous cells are the neoplastic cells in mucoepidermoid carcinoma that contain epithelial mucin, regardless of morphology. Inflammatory cells that have phagocytized mucin, of course, are excluded. Often mucin is evident only with the use of special stains such as Mayer's mucicarmine or Alcian blue. Morphologically, mucous cells resemble intermediate, epidermoid, clear, and columnar cells (fig. 5-5). They occur in small clusters or are

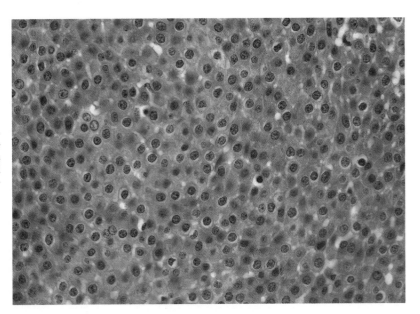

Figure 5-4
INTERMEDIATE CELLS
The cells are smaller than epidermoid cells, and some have perinuclear clearing of their cytoplasm. These cells are still predominantly round or ovoid and lack the polygonal shape of epidermoid cells.

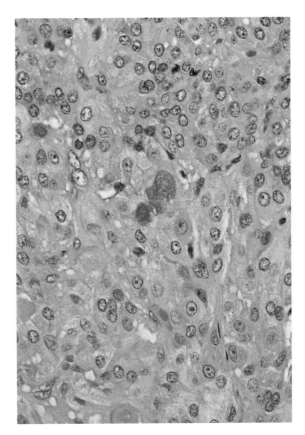
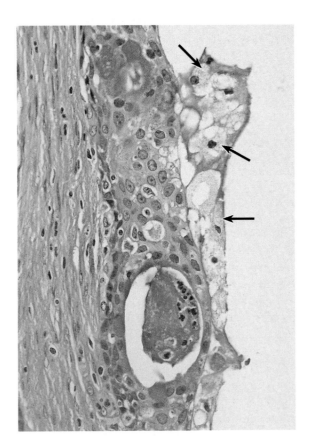

Figure 5-5
MUCOUS CELLS

Left: Mayer's mucicarmine stain highlights mucous cells that were outnumbered by epidermoid and intermediate cells and not appreciated with hematoxylin and eosin staining.

Right: Some of the large cells with foamy cytoplasm (arrows) that line a cystic space appear to be mucous cells but were mucin negative, foamy histiocytes.

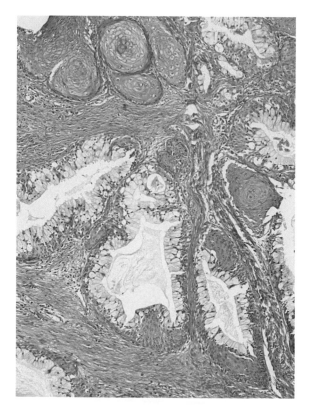

Figure 5-6
EPIDERMOID CELLS

In this example the epidermoid cells are distinct. They are in both the solid and cystic neoplastic structures. In the latter, they are outnumbered by mucous cells. A few smaller intermediate cells are evident in this area of the tumor.

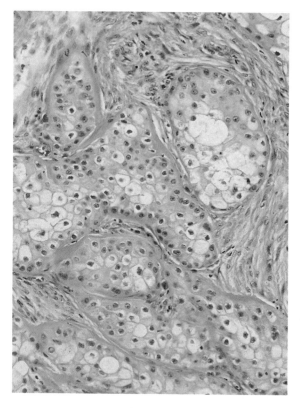

Figure 5-7
CLEAR CELLS

Clear cells in mucoepidermoid carcinoma are usually large, round or polygonal and have centrally placed nuclei. Their shape, size, and arrangement in this field suggest they are altered epidermoid cells.

randomly interspersed among other types of much more numerous cells. Occasionally, they are large, ovoid or goblet shaped; have abundant, foamy cytoplasm; and resemble mucous acinar cells (fig. 5-2). This form of mucous cell usually lines cystic or duct-like structures. Mucous cells comprise less than 10 percent of most tumors (7).

Epidermoid cells form small solid nests or partially lined cystic spaces (fig. 5-6). Epidermoid differentiation is relatively more subtle: in some cases it is only focal or limited to scattered polygonal cells among large intermediate cells. When islands and strands of epidermoid cells are present, they are usually surrounded by smaller, basaloid intermediate cells. Keratin pearl formation and individual cell keratinization are only rarely seen in mucoepidermoid carcinoma and usually occur in inflamed tumors.

Clear cells account for about 10 percent of most mucoepidermoid carcinomas (fig. 5-7) but,

on occasion, can comprise a large portion of the tumor (fig. 5-8). In some cases it appears that focally there is a transition between epidermoid and clear cells. Special stains reveal that the clear cells often contain glycogen and occasionally mucin (fig. 5-9). Columnar cells are less numerous than mucous cells but, when present, often line cystic and ductal structures.

The characteristic features of many mucoepidermoid carcinomas are a prominent cystic or, occasionally, papillary-cystic component (fig. 5-10) and small duct-like structures. The cysts are usually lined by mucous, intermediate, or epidermoid cells which also have focal extramural proliferations. The lumens are typically filled with mucus, which occasionally spills into surrounding connective tissue and forms pools (fig. 5-11) that dissect some distance from the neoplastic epithelium. Occasionally, origin from ductal epithelium is evident (fig. 5-12). In many

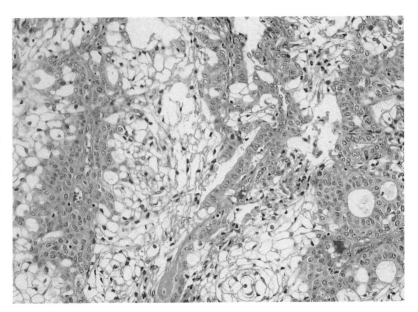

Figure 5-8
CLEAR CELLS

A large proportion of this tumor was composed of clear cells admixed with intermediate and columnar cells. Unlike the tumor in figure 5-7 most of the nuclei in these clear cells are peripherally rather than centrally located.

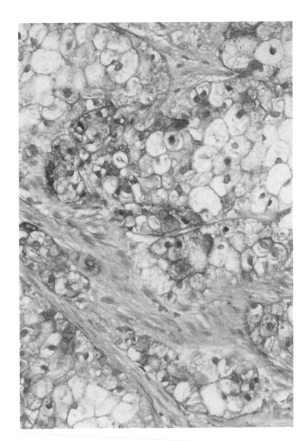 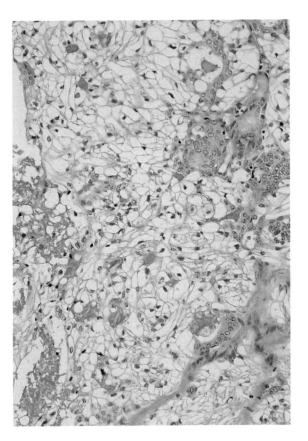

Figure 5-9
CLEAR CELLS

Left: Periodic acid–Schiff stain demonstrates that many of the clear cells contain glycogen since the material was diastase labile.
Right: Mayer's mucicarmine highlights the extracellular and intracytoplasmic mucin.

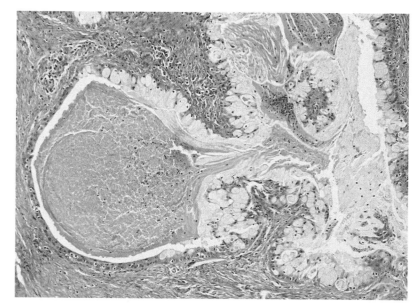

Figure 5-10
PAPILLARY-CYSTIC GROWTH IN
MUCOEPIDERMOID CARCINOMA
Prominent papillary growth extends into large, mucin-filled cystic spaces. Numerous goblet-type mucous cells normally comprise a large portion of the papillary structures.

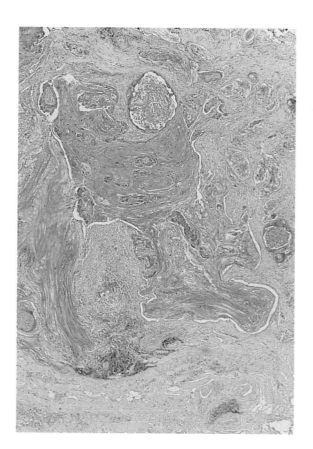

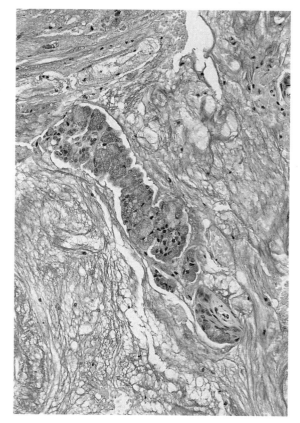

Figure 5-11
MUCUS POOLING
Left: Mayer's mucicarmine stain highlights mucus that has spilled into connective tissue and incited an inflammatory response. In tissue sections that have a limited amount of tumor, this feature might be misinterpreted as a mucus escape reaction rather than mucoepidermoid carcinoma.
Right: Higher magnification reveals an island of neoplastic cells within the large pool of mucus.

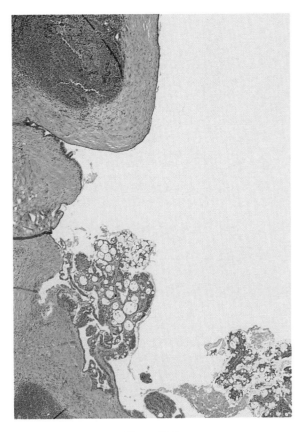

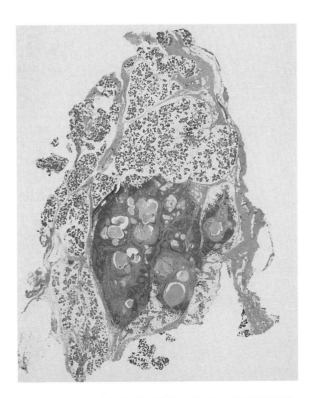

Figure 5-12
ORIGIN FROM DUCTAL EPITHELIUM

Neoplastic transformation (bottom) of the normal duct-lining epithelium (top) is seen. Infiltrative growth into parenchyma and connective tissue was evident elsewhere.

tumors solid cords, islands, and sheets of tumor cells are formed that are supported by fibrous stroma. The solid, cellular structures are composed primarily of intermediate cells with intermingled mucous, epidermoid, and clear cells; occasionally, even oncocytic cells are prominent (37). The fibrous stroma is usually abundant, and in some cases is hyalinized. Sometimes prominent lymphoid proliferation with well-formed follicles is associated with the tumor, which suggests metastatic carcinoma in a lymph node (fig. 5-13). Rarely, these tumors arise from ectopic salivary gland tissue located within a parotid or cervical lymph node (2,5,68,79), but without detailed clinical and surgical information these cases may be difficult to distinguish from tumor-associated lymphoid proliferation (TALP) (4). Unlike TALP, nodal tissue should have a capsule that has a lining of endothelium on its inner aspect and a subcapsular sinus.

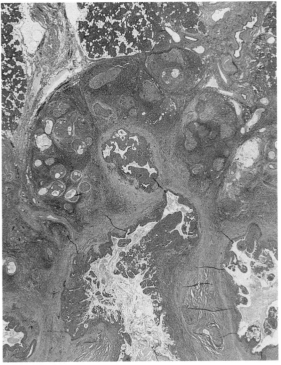

Figure 5-13
TUMOR-ASSOCIATED LYMPHOID PROLIFERATION

Top: In this superficial parotidectomy specimen, mucoepidermoid carcinoma incites a secondary lymphoid proliferation.

Bottom: Higher magnification of a different case shows the response extends along the periphery of the tumor.

Microscopic Grading. The original report of these tumors suggested dividing them into "relatively favorable" and "highly unfavorable" groups (76). Since then there has been a lack of universal agreement regarding which histologic grading criteria are most useful and whether two or three grades should be applied. This has led to doubts regarding the reproducibility of grading and, probably, indirectly to differences in expected treatment outcomes. Suggested grading criteria have included, either singly or in combination, the relative proportion of cell types, degree of "invasiveness," pattern of invasion, mitotic rate, degree of maturation of cellular components, necrosis, neural or vascular invasion, and proportion of tumor composed of cystic spaces relative to solid growth (1,7,16,24–26,42,48,57,58,73,82). Whereas some investigators concluded that most of these criteria are useful (58), one group recommended using only the ratio of solid to cystic growth (26). By this latter method, high-grade tumors have 90 percent or more of their area composed of tumor cells and 10 percent or less of cystic space; all others are low grade.

These grading criteria were analyzed in a retrospective study of mucoepidermoid carcinomas from 143 minor glands (7) and an ongoing investigation of 234 major glands. The histologic features found to be most useful in predicting high-grade, aggressive behavior were an intracystic component (space occupied by cysts) of less than 20 percent, 4 or more mitotic figures per 10 high-power fields, neural invasion, necrosis, and cellular anaplasia. The simultaneous assessment of these features improved prognostic correlation over individual parameters. Of these features, the most subjective evaluation and most difficult to standardize was anaplasia, which included nuclear pleomorphism, increased nuclear/cytoplasmic ratio, large nucleoli, anisochromia, and hyperchromasia. A quantitative grading system was devised to facilitate a more objective application of the criteria (Table 5-1) (7). The 5- to 6-point range was considered intermediate grade because the extremes of good and poor behavior were found below or above these points. This intermediate zone allows for interobserver variation and does not compel the pathologist to decide between low and high grades for a borderline tumor on the basis of interpretation of any one feature. The prognostic implications of the microscopic grade

Table 5-1

PARAMETERS FOR GRADING MUCOEPIDERMOID CARCINOMA AND POINT VALUES FOR EACH GRADE

Parameter	Parameter Point Value
Intracystic component <20%	+2
Neural invasion present	+2
Necrosis present	+3
Four or more mitoses per 10 HPF*	+3
Anaplasia	+4

Grade	Total Point Score
Low grade	0-4
Intermediate grade	5-6
High grade	7 or more

*HPF=high-power field. Example: A tumor whose entire area is estimated to be 40 percent cystic (0 points) but shows anaplasia (4 points) and 6 mitoses per 10 HPF (3 points) receives a total score of 7 points and is, therefore, considered a high-grade tumor.

using these criteria and this point system can be seen in Table 5-2.

The proportion of cell types does not correlate with behavior. Most low-grade tumors have numerous cystic spaces (fig. 5-14) formed by a variety of cell types (fig. 5-15), but some are solid and predominated by intermediate cells. Mitoses are rare and nuclei usually very bland. Intermediate-grade tumors often have cellular anaplasia and either cystic space comprising less than 20 percent of the entire tumor (figs. 5-16, 5-17) or neural invasion. Necrosis and solid growth are more often seen in the major than minor glands. By the suggested grading system (Table 5-1), the presence of anaplasia and either necrosis or 4 or more mitoses per 10 high-power fields (total of 7 points) signify high grade. Most high-grade mucoepidermoid carcinomas are relatively solid, anaplastic, and have 4 or more mitoses per 10 high-power fields (fig. 5-18). Necrosis and neural invasion are more frequent features (fig. 5-19). Some high-grade tumors have focal areas of limited cellular differentiation that resemble nonkeratinizing squamous cell carcinoma. Rarely, high-grade tumors contain distinct foci of lower-grade tumor (fig. 5-20).

Table 5-2

INFLUENCE OF MICROSCOPIC GRADE AND SITE ON PROGNOSIS*

Site	Number of Patients	Dead of Disease (number/% of same grade)
Minor glands	143	
Low grade	120	0 (0)
Intermediate grade	13	1 (8)
High grade	10	6 (60)
Parotid and sublingual glands	203	
Low grade	162	7 (4)
Intermediate grade	12	1 (8)
High grade	29	13 (45)
Submandibular gland	31	
Low grade	23	3 (13)
Intermediate grade	3	1 (17)
High grade	2	0 (0)
Total, all sites	377	
Low grade	305	10 (3.3)
Intermediate grade	31	3 (9.7)
High grade	41	19 (46.3)

*From reference 177 and ongoing study.

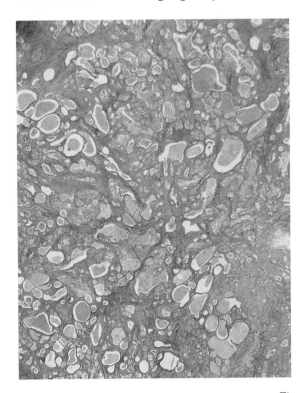
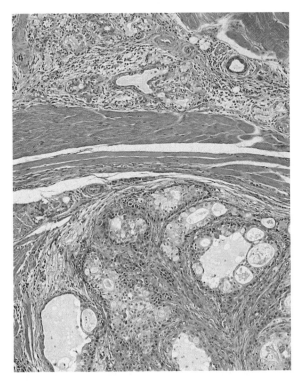

Figure 5-14

LOW-GRADE MUCOEPIDERMOID CARCINOMAS

Left: Low-power magnification shows a tumor of the parotid in which intracystic space comprises about half the tumor.

Right: This low-grade tumor arose from a minor salivary gland located within the muscle of the tongue. Tumor is at the bottom whereas normal acini and ducts are at the top. Normal glandular tissue within muscle, fat, and other tissues complicates evaluation of the degree of infiltration, a feature that, in the past, has been suggested as a grading criterion.

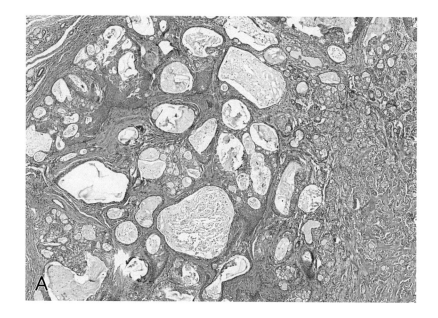

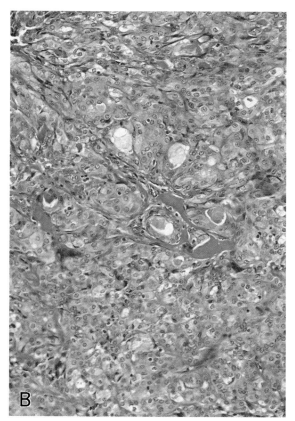
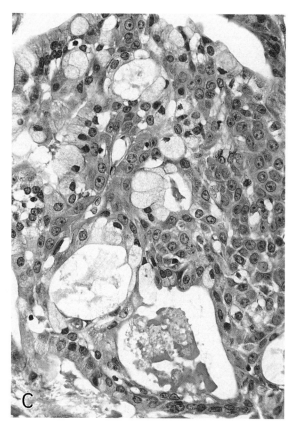

Figure 5-15
LOW-GRADE MUCOEPIDERMOID CARCINOMA

A: Although more than 20 percent of the total area of this tumor was composed of cystic space, a large portion (right) demonstrates solid growth. The tumor lacked neural invasion, necrosis, and anaplasia, and had very few mitoses.

B: A predominantly solid tumor has the characteristically bland cytomorphology of low-grade tumors.

C: This example shows mild nuclear enlargement and the presence of nucleoli. The size and shape of the nuclei are relatively uniform.

Figure 5-16
INTERMEDIATE-GRADE
MUCOEPIDERMOID CARCINOMA
This tumor has hyperchromatic nuclei that vary in size and shape. Several microcystic spaces are present in this field, but the tumor was predominantly solid. Although unimportant for grading this tumor, epidermoid differentiation is prominent at the left and individual cell keratinization is evident.

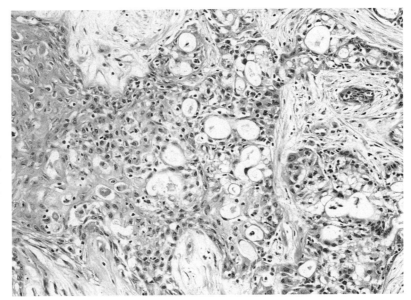

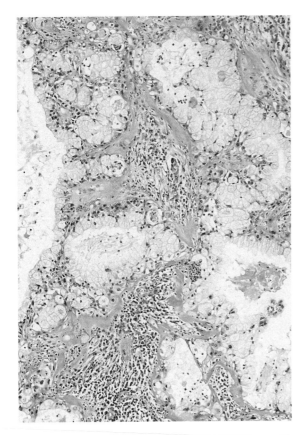

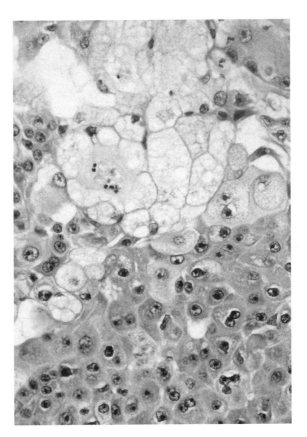

Figure 5-17
INTERMEDIATE-GRADE MUCOEPIDERMOID CARCINOMA
This example had predominance of mucous cells and more than 20 percent intracystic space, but neural invasion was found in addition to the cellular anaplasia shown. Inflammation is evident.

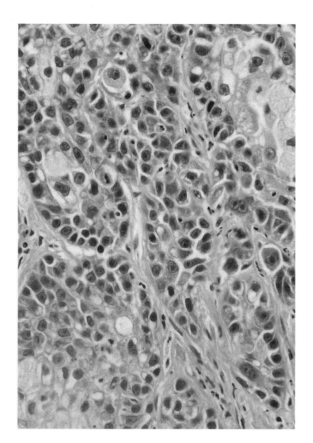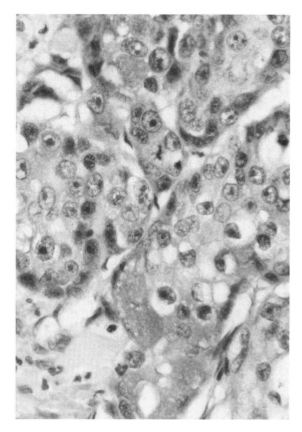

Figure 5-18
HIGH-GRADE MUCOEPIDERMOID CARCINOMA
Cellular anaplasia and solid growth are evident in these two examples. Neural invasion was seen in the example on the left, and both had more than 4 mitoses per 10 high-power fields. Intracytoplasmic mucin is confirmed with Mayer's mucicarmine stain.

The grade of mucoepidermoid carcinoma in the submandibular gland does not predict biologic behavior as reliably as for other sites. Of 23 low-grade tumors in that site, 6 either metastasized or caused the death of the patient. Spiro and colleagues (73) and others (40,72) have also found that submandibular gland tumors were the least predictable with respect to grade and stage.

Immunohistochemical Findings. Immunohistochemical studies of mucoepidermoid carcinomas with anti-cytokeratin have shown that intermediate, columnar, and epidermoid cells are consistently reactive; clear cells are variably reactive; and well-developed mucous cells generally unreactive. Most tumor cells are usually positive for epithelial membrane antigen and variably reactive with muscle-specific actin, vimentin, S-100 protein (more often with monoclonal than polyclonal anti-S-100-alpha), carcinoembryonic antigen, alpha-fetoprotein, and glial fibrillary acidic protein (39,41,44,53,62). The heterogeneity of the immunohistochemical staining does not correlate with tumor grade (53,62) although at least one report suggests that alpha-fetoprotein is more strongly expressed in high-grade than low-grade tumors (41). Another study using the monoclonal antibody B72.3 showed that immunoreactivity was strongest in mucoepidermoid carcinomas with prominent glandular differentiation (63).

Ultrastructural Findings. Earlier ultrastructural studies described six basic cell types: differentiated stem cells (cuboidal or basaloid on light microscopy), serous and mucoid secretory cells, mucus-producing goblet cells, epidermoid cells, and modified myoepithelial cells (17). Dardick and colleagues (21) have recently shown that there are essentially two basic types of cells,

167

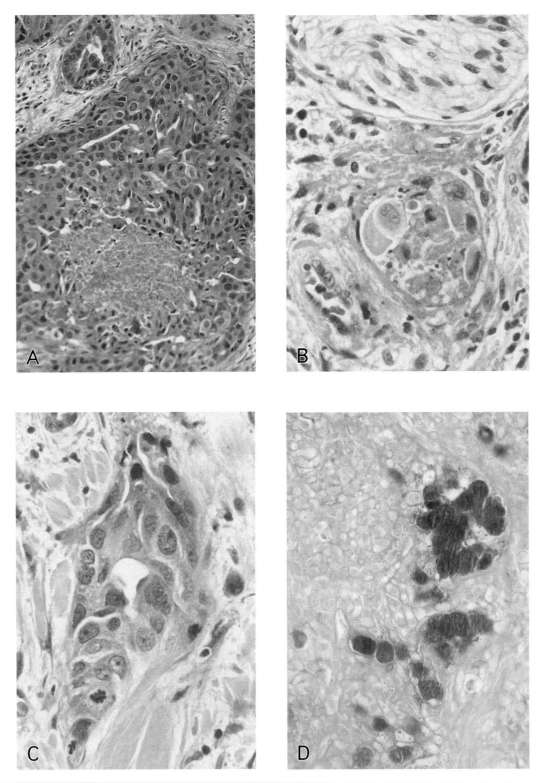

Figure 5-19
HIGH-GRADE MUCOEPIDERMOID CARCINOMAS
These tumors had focal necrosis, neural invasion, and increased and abnormal mitoses. Mucus was confirmed with the Alcian blue stain at pH 2.5 with hyaluronidase digestion.

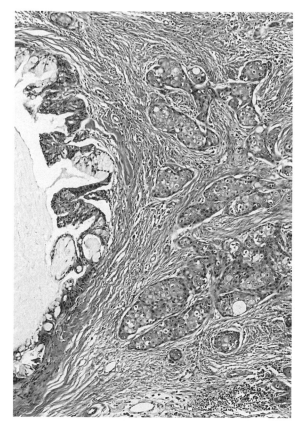

Figure 5-20
HIGH-GRADE MUCOEPIDERMOID CARCINOMA
This example of high-grade tumor (right) growing as solid cords was closely associated with prominently cystic tumor that by itself would be considered low grade (left). Both elements contained numerous mucous cells.

luminal and intermediate, that have specific organizational relationships. Luminal cells often have goblet cell formation and secrete mucus. Both types may contain tonofilaments and show epidermoid features, and both may accumulate excess glycogen that results in a light microscopic clear cell appearance. The luminal cells have microvilli on their apical surface and are surrounded by nonluminal (intermediate) cells that have basal lamina partially lining their surface (fig. 5-21). Unlike the impression with light microscopy, ultrastructurally the intermediate cell does not show bidirectional differentiation toward either mucous cells or epidermoid cells but, rather, is relatively distinctive in its morphology and relationship to the luminal cells. It has been suggested that these cells are the counterpart of the modified myoepithelial cell seen in mixed tumors (21).

Other Special Techniques. Several special methods have been used to study mucoepidermoid carcinomas in an attempt to identify those most likely to behave in an aggressive manner. Histochemical analysis has shown that both low- and high-grade tumors secrete a heterogeneous variety of mucosubstances (27). It has been suggested that the cells in most mucoepidermoid carcinomas demonstrate altered glycosylation and incomplete synthesis of their mucins, which is reflected by the presence of precursor substances (81). Cytophotometric analysis has shown that most tumors with atypical DNA are clinically aggressive but about one third of cytophotometrically normal tumors also behave aggressively (38). Mutation of the p53 gene is apparently infrequent in salivary gland neoplasms compared to lung carcinomas. Expression of p53 protein was seen in only 3 of 12 mucoepidermoid carcinomas (69). The proliferative capacity of the tumor cells has been evaluated by quantitation of the argyrophilic nucleolar organizer regions (AgNORs): the mucous cells show less activity than the intermediate and epidermoid cells (34). Studies have shown that the number of AgNORs is higher in mucoepidermoid carcinomas than in benign salivary tumors (55,90), and in one study a higher count correlated with an aggressive clinical course (19). Overlapping AgNOR counts among various tumors appears to preclude the routine use of this technique for definitive diagnosis (85).

Differential Diagnosis. Features of mucoepidermoid carcinoma that occasionally lead to consideration of other lesions include epidermoid and mucous cells; cystic or papillary-cystic growth with bland cytomorphology; and, conversely, solid, sheet-like areas with a predominance of intermediate, epidermoid, or clear cells.

Sialometaplasia, either secondary to nonspecific inflammation or as a component of necrotizing sialometaplasia (see Non-Neoplastic Tumor-Like Conditions), typically appears as a proliferation of nests of epidermoid or squamous cells that may contain occasional mucous cells. Squamous metaplasia is occasionally florid following fine-needle aspiration and in oncocytic neoplasms such as oncocytoma and Warthin's tumor, and may be accompanied by focal necrosis (80). The metaplastic nests vary in size but have smooth, regular edges; are often arranged in a lobular

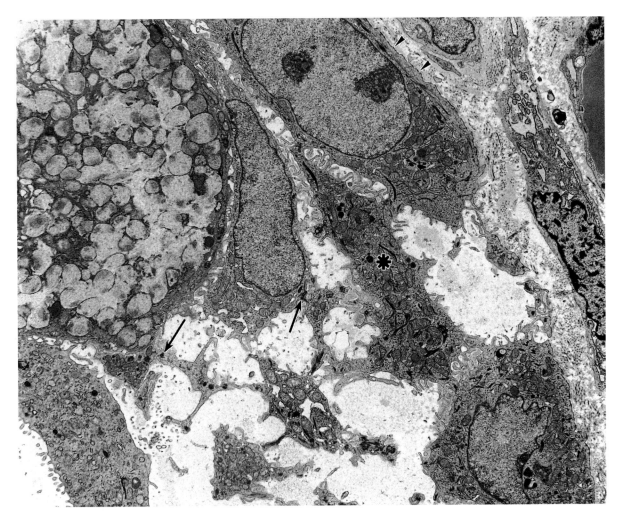

Figure 5-21
MUCOEPIDERMOID CARCINOMA

A portion of a lumen is in the lower left corner. A goblet-type lining cell (upper left) contains numerous mucous granules. Several nonluminal intermediate cells have widened intercellular spaces. The intermediate cells are attached to each other and to the luminal cell by desmosomes (arrows). The intermediate cells contain bundles of tonofilaments (asterisk) and are partially lined on their stromal surface by basal lamina (arrowheads). (Courtesy of Dr. Irving Dardick, Toronto, Canada.)

pattern outlined by the former salivary gland lobule; and are admixed with ductal remnants. Neither cystic growth nor the presence of other cell types, notably intermediate cells, are seen.

Inverted papillomas (see Papillomas) are composed of basaloid, epidermoid, and interspersed mucous cells and, like mucoepidermoid carcinoma, develop within an excretory duct. Compared to mucoepidermoid carcinoma, more of an inverted papilloma is composed of epidermoid cells. Furthermore, papillomas do not infiltrate surrounding tissues as small islands and cords of tumor cells.

Cystadenomas and cystadenocarcinomas are salivary gland tumors that demonstrate cystic or papillary-cystic growth and sometimes resemble mucoepidermoid carcinoma. Distinction from cystadenoma is discussed in more detail elsewhere (see Cystadenoma), but the most important distinguishing criteria are the more variable cell population and infiltrative, noncystic epithelial proliferation in mucoepidermoid carcinoma. Distinction from cystadenocarcinoma may also be difficult (see Cystadenocarcinoma); however, cystadenocarcinomas usually lack epidermoid differentiation, do not have the variety of cell types typically present in mucoepidermoid carcinoma, and usually lack solid islands and nests of tumor cells.

A predominance of epidermoid cells is unusual in mucoepidermoid carcinoma but does occur. In these instances, distinction from primary or metastatic squamous cell carcinoma relies on the histochemical demonstration of mucus within neoplastic cells. Interpretation may be complicated by the presence of residual ducts that contain small amounts of mucus within their lumens or within the cytoplasm of luminal cells. Squamous cell carcinomas are much more likely to show individual cell keratinization, a feature usually limited to small focal areas when present in mucoepidermoid carcinoma (see fig. 5-16).

Solid proliferations of intermediate cells in mucoepidermoid carcinoma are sometimes similar to cellular zones of modified myoepithelial cells in mixed tumors. Mucoepidermoid carcinomas, however, do not have myxoid or chondroid zones or small well-delineated ducts with round lumens characteristic of mixed tumors.

Tumors other than mucoepidermoid carcinomas that have a predominance of clear cells include clear cell carcinoma and epithelial-myoepithelial carcinoma. The clear cells in all three tumors often contain glycogen, but only the cells in mucoepidermoid carcinoma are associated with epidermoid and mucous differentiation. Epithelial-myoepithelial carcinoma demonstrates a characteristic biphasic pattern of cuboidal luminal cells surrounded by larger clear cells.

Prognosis and Treatment. The prognosis of mucoepidermoid carcinoma is largely dependent on clinical stage, tumor grade, and adequacy of treatment. Staging criteria for carcinoma of major salivary glands are well established (see General Considerations). Spiro and colleagues (8,74) have demonstrated that staging criteria currently used for head and neck squamous cell carcinoma are applicable to carcinoma of the minor salivary glands.

Despite disagreement on grading criteria, nearly all studies with follow-up data show that except for tumors of the submandibular gland low-grade tumors rarely recur or metastasize (82). In AFIP's data on mucoepidermoid carcinomas of the major and minor salivary glands, 5 and 2.5 percent, respectively, of low-grade tumors either metastasized to regional lymph nodes or resulted in the death of the patient whereas 55 and 80 percent, respectively, of the high-grade tumors did so (7). Furthermore, many low-grade tumors that later recurred or metastasized were advanced stage tumors. In comparison, 13 percent of patients with low-grade submandibular tumors died of disease.

Recurrences are much more likely if the margins of surgical resection contain tumor. Healey and colleagues (42) reported that of 33 low- and intermediate-grade neoplasms none recurred when the margins were free of tumor, but 6 of 12 tumors recurred when margins were involved. Thirteen of 16 high-grade tumors recurred when the margins were positive. Recurrences in the minor glands occur on average about 8 years after initial diagnosis (range, 3 months to 22 years) (7). In addition to the submandibular gland, the floor of the mouth and the tongue are sites of tumor with more aggressive and less predictable behavior. Maxillary sinus tumors are not included in this discussion but also have a relatively poor prognosis (73).

Regional metastasis of low-grade minor gland tumors is extremely rare and does not necessarily imply a poor prognosis, even if multiple nodes are involved (7). Metastases have been discovered synchronously with the primary or as long as 11 years later.

Distant metastasis of mucoepidermoid carcinoma does imply poor prognosis. The distant sites commonly involved are the lung, skeleton, and brain, but many other sites have been involved. Wide dissemination has occurred in some cases. Patients who died of disease often had recurrence, and both regional and distant metastases. Patients survive on average 2.3 and 2.6 years with minor and major gland tumors, respectively (7); however, the long-term survival rate of patients with high-grade tumors continues to decline for at least 8 years (1,25,26,43,49,58,75).

It is recommended that stage I and II mucoepidermoid carcinomas of the parotid gland be treated by conservative excision, with preservation of the facial nerve (73). Apparently, patients who have partial parotidectomies with clear margins of resection do as well as those who have total parotidectomies (84). The affected submandibular gland should be entirely extirpated. Combined surgery and radiotherapy as the first planned treatment may be indicated for tumors in this site because of its worse prognosis. Radical neck dissection is suggested for patients with T3 disease and indicated for patients with clinical evidence of cervical node metastases. Spiro and colleagues (73) performed elective neck dissection for selected patients with high-grade tumors of both major and minor glands and found that two thirds had occult metastases.

Treatment of minor gland tumors is usually wide surgical excision that ensures tumor-free margins. The wound is often left open to heal secondarily. When the tumor erodes or infiltrates underlying bone, removal of a portion of the maxilla or mandible is required to ensure complete removal. Some investigators advocate that mucoepidermoid carcinomas of the palate be routinely treated with partial maxillectomy regardless of grade or size (60), or if there are questionable margins (83). However, Melrose et al. (57) suggest local excision, with block excision of underlying bone only if there is evidence of bone destruction. Others agree with this approach for small low-grade tumors (28,32,64,70) and suggest that wide excision down to periosteum with at least 1-cm tumor-free lateral margins is appropriate therapy. High-grade and advanced-stage tumors must be treated aggressively at this and other sites. Indications for neck dissection are similar to those for major gland tumors. Tumors of the tongue, floor of mouth, and tonsillar area larger than 2 cm are particularly aggressive and consideration of elective neck dissection for these tumors may be justified (5,7,60).

In a study of tumors in the major glands, including 49 mucoepidermoid carcinomas, Tran et al. (84) concluded that adjuvant radiotherapy offered no increase in local control or survival among patients who had surgical excision with margins free of tumor. These investigators and others have noted that radiation might improve local control if residual disease was found at the surgical margins in a patient who was no longer amenable to surgery, but radiotherapy could not substitute for establishing tumor-free margins (20,52,56,84). In a study of major salivary gland carcinomas, Armstrong et al. (3) concluded that adjuvant radiotherapy improved survival only in patients with stage III or IV disease. In a similar study of minor gland carcinomas, no survival benefit was seen in patients who received combination therapy, although there was a trend towards better control of the primary tumor (74).

These investigators suggested that postoperative radiotherapy be used in patients who have high-stage disease, especially if high grade or when margins remain involved by tumor.

Several studies have evaluated the role of chemotherapy for salivary gland carcinomas (9, 50,61,77,87). Some investigators have suggested that high-grade mucoepidermoid carcinoma may show a sensitivity to chemotherapy that is similar to squamous cell carcinoma (50,77).

Central Mucoepidermoid Carcinoma

About 4 percent of all mucoepidermoid carcinomas in the AFIP files originate within the jaws, and the mandible is involved about four times more often than the maxilla. The mandibular predilection of previously published cases is 3 to 1 (12). These tumors arise in tissue that does not normally contain salivary glands. In most cases they are first discovered as asymptomatic radiolucencies. In the mandible, the third molar region is the most common area involved, and only rarely is the anterior segment affected. In the maxilla, the molar region is usually the preferred site. Mucoepidermoid carcinoma outnumbers all other types of salivary gland tumors that have been reported to arise in the jaws (11–13,23,33,47,67).

Theories explaining possible pathogenetic mechanisms have been discussed (14,15). The possible sources for the intrabony epithelium that gives rise to these tumors include: 1) ectopic salivary gland tissue resulting from a) developmentally entrapped minor salivary glands; b) inclusions of embryonic rests of submandibular or sublingual glands; or c) seromucous glands displaced from the maxillary sinus into the maxilla and 2) neoplastic transformation of the epithelial lining of odontogenic cysts. Because ectopic salivary gland tissue is rarely, if ever, observed in biopsies of the mandible or maxilla, it is suspected that origin from entrapped minor salivary glands in either jaw rarely, if ever, occurs. Far more mucoepidermoid carcinomas are seen in the jaws than biopsies that contain islands of ectopic salivary gland tissue.

There is ample evidence that mucoepidermoid carcinomas arise from the lining of odontogenic cysts. Transition of cyst lining to carcinoma is evident in some cases. The pluripotential capacity of odontogenic epithelium is further supported by the frequent occurrence of mucous cell prosoplasia, particularly in dentigerous cysts (fig. 5-22), and the development of cysts whose lining has small gland-like structures that have been referred to as sialo-odontogenic or glandular cysts (86,88). The lining of odontogenic cysts also gives rise to other neoplasms, including ameloblastoma and squamous cell carcinoma. Eversole and colleagues (29) reported that nearly 50 percent of central mucoepidermoid carcinomas are associated with a cyst or unerupted tooth, and Brookstone and Huvos (12) found that 8 of 11 central salivary gland tumors were associated with an odontogenic cyst or impacted tooth. It has been suggested that mucoepidermoid carcinoma be included as a type of primary intra-alveolar (odontogenic) carcinoma (89).

Clinically, some patients note a painless swelling or facial asymmetry. Occasionally, the tumor destroys a large portion of the jaw and may occupy the entire mandibular ramus. In the cases reviewed by Gingell et al. (35) about half the patients noted pain and a few experienced paresthesia or dysphagia.

Radiographically, diagnostic considerations might include dentigerous or other odontogenic cysts and ameloblastoma. Many of the cases in the AFIP files were associated with impacted third molars (fig. 5-23), and a few were in periapical locations. The radiolucencies often were surprisingly well circumscribed. Synchronous maxillary and mandibular mucoepidermoid carcinomas occurred in

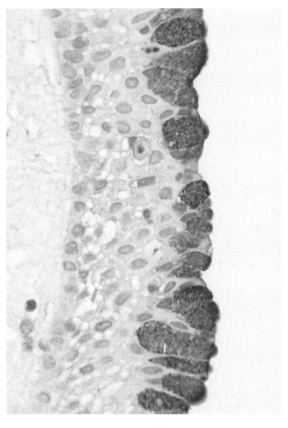

Figure 5-22
MUCOUS CELL PROSOPLASIA
IN DENTIGEROUS CYST
Mayer's mucicarmine stain highlights numerous mucous cells in the lining epithelium of an otherwise unremarkable dentigerous cyst.

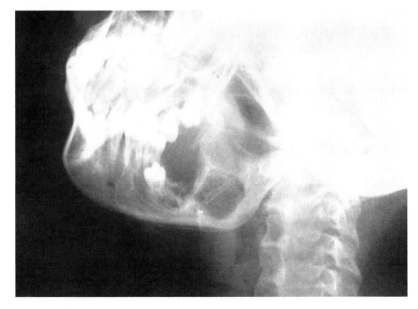

Figure 5-23
CENTRAL MUCOEPIDERMOID
CARCINOMA
The neoplasm is a large, destructive, radiolucent lesion that is associated with the impacted third molar and has extended into the ramus of the mandible.

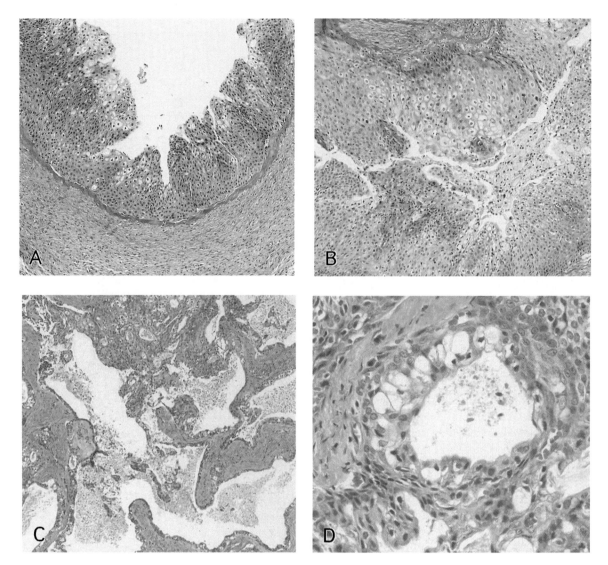

Figure 5-24
CENTRAL MUCOEPIDERMOID CARCINOMA
Uniformly thickened cyst lining is composed of intermediate, clear, epidermoid, and mucous cells (A) that are solid and infiltrative (B) in other areas. In a different example from the maxilla (C) there are many solid and cystic neoplastic areas. Higher magnification (D) reveals the characteristic variety of cell types.

a patient with adenomatous hyperplasia of the palatal salivary glands. In another patient an ameloblastoma was found in close association with a mucoepidermoid carcinoma, illustrating the proliferative and pluripotent capacity of odontogenic epithelium. Microscopically, similar diagnostic criteria apply to these tumors as to those in the major and minor glands (fig. 5-24) whereas grading criteria do not. Unlike glandular odontogenic cysts (fig. 5-25), mucoepidermoid carcinomas demonstrate infiltrative growth by noncystic elements.

Eversole et al. (29) found a recurrence rate for central mucoepidermoid carcinomas of 30 percent and a survival rate at both 2 and 5 years of 100 percent (29). One patient died of disease at 14 years, and at least one other was alive with disease at 10 years. Of 66 reported cases, only 9 percent metastasized (12).

Brookstone and Huvos (12) proposed a new staging system for central salivary gland tumors: lesions surrounded by intact cortical bone and no clinical expansion are designated stage I;

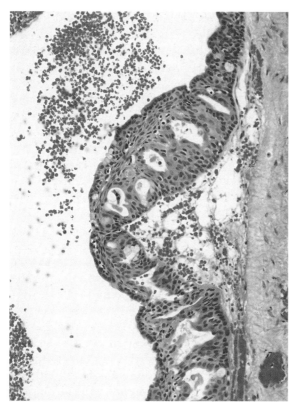

Figure 5-25
GLANDULAR ODONTOGENIC CYST
Slightly thickened cyst lining is composed of cuboidal, epidermoid, columnar, and mucous epithelial cells that form numerous gland-like structures. These cysts are often multilocular but solid growth is limited and infiltration of adjacent tissues does not occur.

lesions with intact cortical bone and expansion are stage II; and lesions with evidence of cortical perforation are stage III. They found that salivary gland tumors arising within bone behaved very differently than those arising in conventional sites. They noted no correlation between tumor grade and prognosis.

Of the 64 reported cases of mucoepidermoid carcinoma with treatment information, half were treated conservatively with either enucleation, curettage, or marsupialization, and the other half were treated more aggressively, with segmental resection with or without neck dissection or adjuvant therapy (12). The recurrence rate among patients treated conservatively was 40 percent while 13 percent of the radically treated cases recurred. These investigators suggest that the clinical stage of the tumor plays an important role in choice of treatment.

ADENOCARCINOMA, NOT OTHERWISE SPECIFIED

Definition. This is a salivary gland carcinoma that shows glandular or ductal differentiation but lacks prominence of any of the histomorphologic features that characterize the other, more specific carcinoma types. Because most epithelial salivary gland malignancies are also adenocarcinomas, the modifying term "not otherwise specified" (NOS) is used to distinguish these tumors.

General Features. Because of reporting variability, it is difficult to establish the frequency of occurrence and expected biologic behavior for this group of tumors. They have most often been designated as miscellaneous or unclassified adenocarcinomas or, simply, as adenocarcinomas (95,98,100,103–105,107,111). The authors of some of these reports, however, further subclassified the tumors into anaplastic, trabecular, solid, papillary, tubular, mucous cell, pseudoadamantine, cystic, mucinous, oncocytic, and typical subtypes (94,95,97,100,102,104). Based on the illustrations and descriptions within many of these reports, some cases would be better classified as polymorphous low-grade adenocarcinoma, papillary cystadenocarcinoma, basal cell adenocarcinoma, oncocytic adenocarcinoma, clear cell carcinoma, epithelial-myoepithelial carcinoma, and sebaceous carcinoma in the current classification system (92,99,104,106,110).

A study by Spiro et al. (104) of 204 patients with "adenocarcinoma" included 143 patients with tumors that arose in the major or minor salivary glands (the remainder arose from the seromucous glands of the nasal cavity, paranasal sinuses, and larynx, sites not included in this discussion). Of these 143, 108 were histologically designated as "typical," and most closely resemble the adenocarcinoma, NOS cases in the AFIP files. The major and minor salivary glands were affected nearly equally in their series. Importantly, their study included follow-up information that was correlated with the histologic grade (see Prognosis and Treatment).

Adenocarcinoma, NOS, is second only to mucoepidermoid carcinoma in frequency among malignant salivary gland neoplasms in AFIP files reviewed since 1985. They account for 9 percent of all salivary gland tumors and 16.8 percent of all malignancies. Women outnumber men 54 to 46 percent. The average age of the 279 AFIP patients on file is 58 years, with a range of 10 to 93 years; only 3 percent are under the age of 10 years. These tumors also account for a significant proportion of the tumors in most published series, but because of the reporting inconsistencies previously noted, their frequency ranges widely from 1.9 to 11.8 percent for both benign and malignant tumors and from 8.8 to 44.7 percent for malignant tumors (93).

At the AFIP, about 40 and 60 percent occur in the minor and major glands, respectively. Of the major gland tumors, only 10 percent occur in the submandibular gland, and the remainder involve the parotid gland. A few published cases arose in the sublingual gland (93,101). Of the minor gland tumors, the most common locations, in descending order, are palate (primarily hard palate), buccal mucosa, and upper and lower lips (each affected equally).

Clinical Features. Patients with tumors in the major glands usually present with solitary, asymptomatic masses (104). About 20 percent of patients with parotid tumors have pain or facial nerve weakness associated with tumors 2 to 8 cm in diameter. Nearly half of the tumors are fixed to the skin or deep tissues. In the submandibular gland, pain is more frequent (104). In the minor glands of the palate the lesion is usually asymptomatic but is ulcerated in one third of the cases and involves underlying bone in one quarter of the cases. Tumor duration ranges from less than 1 year to as long as 10 years for parotid tumors, 2 years or less when in the submandibular gland, and from 1 to 5 years in the minor glands (104).

Gross and Microscopic Findings. As with other malignant salivary gland tumors, adenocarcinoma, NOS, is often focally circumscribed, but otherwise the borders are irregular and in many areas not discernible from surrounding tissues. The cut surface is white or yellow-white and sometimes has hemorrhagic or necrotic zones.

Microscopically, despite being composed of relatively few cell types, adenocarcinoma, NOS, demonstrates a seemingly unlimited number of growth patterns (fig. 5-26) which often vary within individual tumors (fig. 5-27). The neoplastic epithelium forms small nests, islands, ramifying cords, tubules, or densely cellular, solid sheets. The only features common to all tumors in this group are the formation of glandular or duct-like structures and the presence of infiltrative growth. The diagnosis, therefore, largely depends on exclusion of the more characteristic types of salivary gland carcinoma and metastatic adenocarcinoma. Also, unlike most other salivary gland carcinomas this group displays great variability in degree of cytologic atypia that facilitates histologic grading into low-, intermediate-, and high-grade categories.

The tumors are composed of relatively distinct individual nodules separated by stromal connective tissue that is rich in collagen (fig. 5-28). The stroma in some cases is mucinous (fig. 5-29). However, in solid areas the cells are often so closely packed they appear to completely lack supporting stroma. Although some are focally circumscribed, unequivocal infiltration into salivary parenchyma or surrounding tissues is evident (fig. 5-30). Perineural and perivascular growth are common (fig. 5-31).

Ductal or glandular differentiation is evident in all cases. While it is obvious in low- to intermediate-grade tumors, it often is more subtle in high-grade tumors. In addition to the formation of ducts and tubules, small to medium-sized cysts are occasionally evident, and their lining is sometimes papillary. The cystic and papillary areas are limited and are considerably fewer than in cystadenocarcinoma.

Cuboidal, round, or ovoid cells have distinct borders and a tendency to aggregate in small cohesive clusters. Cytoplasm is abundant in some cells, and the cell borders in these are usually distinct. Clear cells and oncocytic features are occasionally evident (fig. 5-32). Globular or linear deposits of hyalinized acellular material are focally abundant in some tumors (fig. 5-33). In low-grade tumors the cells have nuclei that demonstrate minimal variation in size, shape, and staining characteristics, and few mitoses are evident (fig. 5-34). Small nucleoli are usually seen. Well-formed ductal and tubular structures are often prominent. Intermediate-grade tumors show some nuclear morphologic variability and more frequent mitoses (fig. 5-35). High-grade tumors have cells with enlarged, pleomorphic and hyperchromatic nuclei and many mitoses, including some that are atypical. Ductal and glandular differentiation is frequently limited but distinguishes adenocarcinoma, NOS, from undifferentiated carcinoma (fig. 5-36). Necrosis

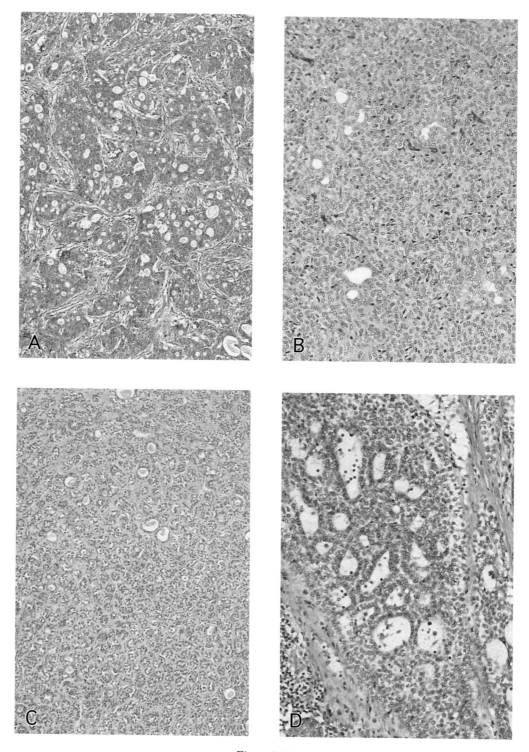

Figure 5-26
ADENOCARCINOMAS, NOT OTHERWISE SPECIFIED
Four different examples illustrate the architectural diversity of these tumors.
A: Numerous irregular trabeculae are separated by fibrous connective tissue stroma; ductal differentiation is prominent.
B: In many areas sheet-like, solid growth has focal glandular differentiation.
C: Most of the tumor is composed of individual ductal structures.
D: There are focal, larger, well-formed tubular structures.

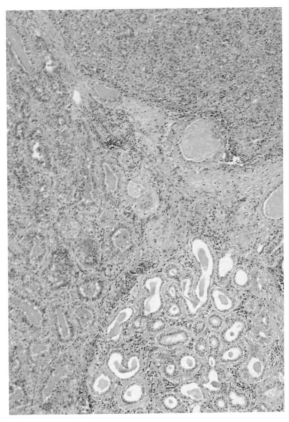

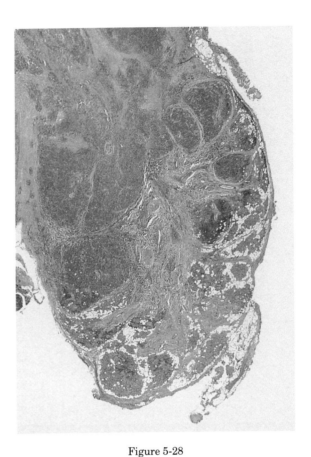

Figure 5-27

ADENOCARCINOMA, NOT OTHERWISE SPECIFIED

The solid growth on the top predominated in this tumor but as seen at the bottom of the illustration some areas demonstrate a tubular pattern.

Figure 5-28

ADENOCARCINOMA, NOT OTHERWISE SPECIFIED

Many small to medium-sized lobules have replaced the parotid parenchyma. A fair amount of fibrous stroma accompanies the neoplastic lobules.

Figure 5-29
ADENOCARCINOMA,
NOT OTHERWISE SPECIFIED

Anastomosing cords of tumor are separated by abundant mucinous rather than collagenous stroma.

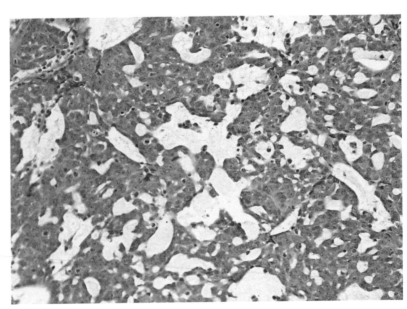

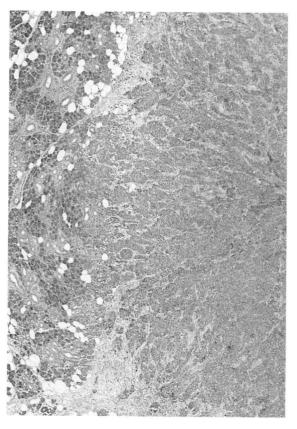

Figure 5-30
ADENOCARCINOMA, NOT OTHERWISE SPECIFIED
A thin band of connective tissue separates the tumor from the parotid tissue on either side, but in the center finger-like projections infiltrate into parenchyma.

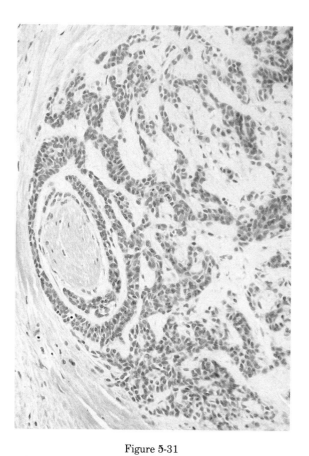

Figure 5-31
PERINEURAL GROWTH IN ADENOCARCINOMA, NOT OTHERWISE SPECIFIED
As with other salivary gland carcinomas, perineural growth is common.

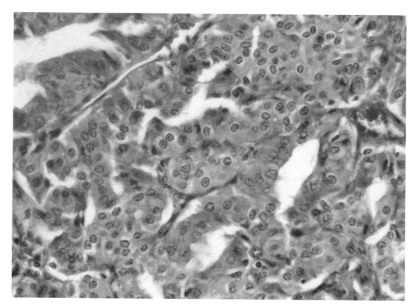

Figure 5-32
FOCAL ONCOCYTIC CHANGE IN ADENOCARCINOMA, NOT OTHERWISE SPECIFIED
Several small foci of cells having abundant granular, brightly eosinophilic cytoplasm were found in this tumor that was otherwise composed of much smaller cuboidal cells.

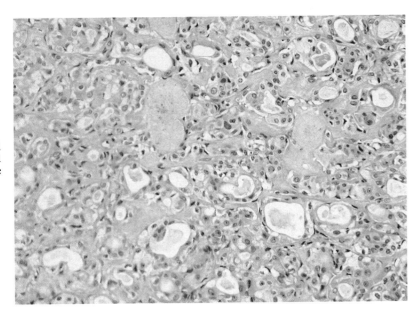

Figure 5-33
ADENOCARCINOMA,
NOT OTHERWISE SPECIFIED
This tumor has numerous ductal structures between which are scattered deposits of amorphous, eosinophilic material.

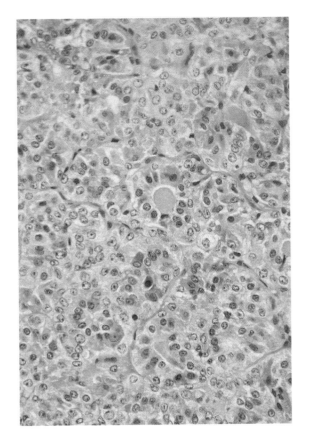

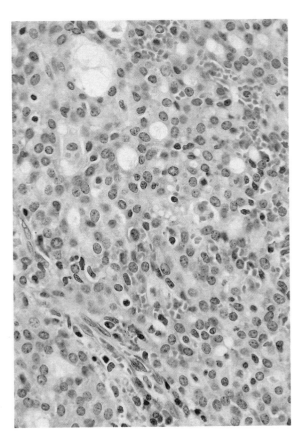

Figure 5-34
LOW-GRADE ADENOCARCINOMAS, NOT OTHERWISE SPECIFIED
The cells of these two low-grade tumors are cytomorphologically bland. The shape, size, and staining characteristics of the nuclei are relatively uniform and they have small, single nucleoli. Mitoses were rare in both. Some cells have abundant cytoplasm with distinct borders.

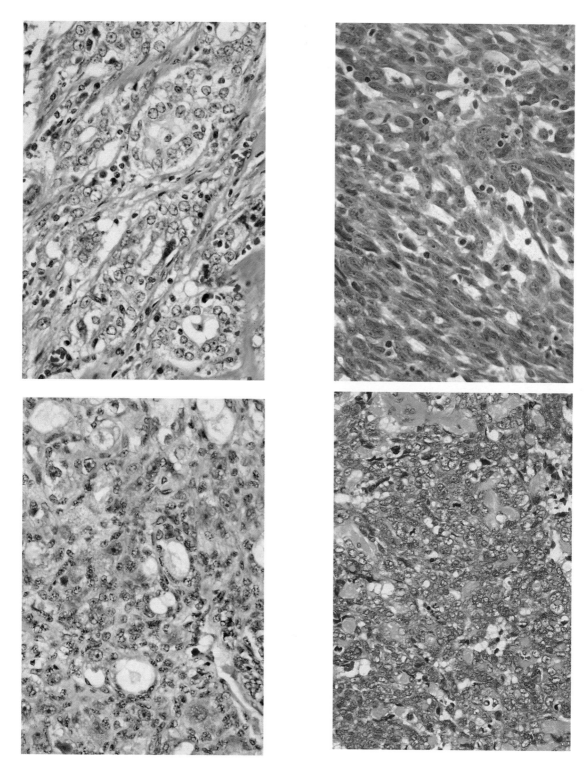

Figure 5-35
INTERMEDIATE-GRADE ADENOCARCINOMAS,
NOT OTHERWISE SPECIFIED

In these tumors the nuclei are larger and slightly more irregular, and scattered mitotic figures are evident. Ductal differentiation is obvious in most areas.

Figure 5-36
HIGH-GRADE ADENOCARCINOMAS,
NOT OTHERWISE SPECIFIED

Hyperchromatic, enlarged and pleomorphic nuclei characterize these two high-grade tumors. The cells are closely packed and there is focal ductal differentiation. Notice the spindling of cells in the case on the top.

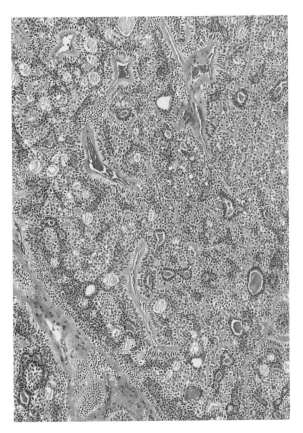

Figure 5-37
ADENOCARCINOMA,
NOT OTHERWISE SPECIFIED

Some areas of this tumor showed distinct ducts composed of darkly stained cells that were surrounded by clear cells, resembling the biphasic pattern of epithelial-myoepithelial carcinoma. This pattern also occurs focally in other salivary gland carcinomas, notably adenoid cystic carcinoma.

and hemorrhage are frequent. In all three grades special stains sometimes reveal luminal and, occasionally, intracytoplasmic mucin. Limited glycogen is occasionally present.

In some examples, small zones within the tumor exhibit features that mimic one or more other types of salivary gland carcinoma such as adenoid cystic carcinoma, acinic cell adenocarcinoma, and epithelial-myoepithelial carcinoma (fig. 5-37). Unlike these specific tumors, such features are limited to small areas in adenocarcinoma, NOS.

Differential Diagnosis. The diagnosis of adenocarcinoma, NOS, is essentially one of exclusion. Because low-grade adenocarcinoma, NOS, has relatively bland cytomorphologic features and well-formed ductal structures, the most difficult distinction is from adenomas. Infiltration

of parenchyma, nerves, blood vessels, or surrounding connective tissue distinguishes adenocarcinoma from adenoma. Although lack of encapsulation and even extracapsular extension occurs in some adenomas, tumor islands and strands that have permeated and replaced adjacent tissues are not acceptable in adenomas. Step sections may help resolve borderline cases.

Like low-grade adenocarcinoma, NOS, polymorphous low-grade adenocarcinoma (PLGA) has bland nuclear morphology and numerous ductal and tubular structures. However, PLGA often has a characteristic concentric whorl-like appearance, a mucohyaline background stroma, greater variability of cell types and morphologic patterns in any one tumor, a greater tendency to infiltrate tissues as small islands and tubules rather than finger-like projections extending from a central mass, and a characteristic pattern of uniformly sized and stained nuclei. Nearly all PLGAs have occurred in minor glands.

When adenocarcinoma is not readily classifiable as one of the better known types, consideration should be given to metastatic disease. A thorough review of the medical history and clinical examination are indicated. Immunohistochemical studies for antigens specific to other sites, such as the thyroid or prostate glands, can be useful. Metastasis of prostate cancer to the parotid gland is extremely unusual (96), however, and at least one case of salivary gland adenocarcinoma, NOS, has shown focal immunoreactivity with prostate-specific antigen and prostate-specific acid phosphatase (109).

Treatment and Prognosis. There are only two studies that include follow-up information for a relatively large number of adenocarcinomas, NOS (98,104). Some tumors in these studies involved the nasal cavity and paranasal sinuses, and others were probably specific forms of salivary adenocarcinoma. Nonetheless, these studies contain the most directly applicable data currently available. Matsuba et al. (98) concluded that survival was influenced by primary site: tumors of the oral cavity had a more favorable prognosis than those of the parotid or submandibular glands. Patients with low-grade disease had longer disease-free intervals and less frequent cervical node and distant metastases, but these investigators concluded that overall survival was not influenced significantly by grade. Distant metastases developed in some patients despite regional control of disease. Spiro et al. (104) found that recurrence was most frequent in patients with high-grade tumors. Distant metastases occurred in 26 percent of their patients and occurred more often in patients previously treated and in those with high-grade tumor. The lungs were involved in about half of those patients who had distant spread. Survival was better for tumors of the oral cavity than the parotid, and worse for patients with submandibular gland involvement. Prognosis also depended on clinical stage. There was a tendency for stage III tumors to be high histologic grade and stage I disease to be low grade. Unlike the findings of Matsuba et al., they found that survival was influenced by grade, and the 15-year survival for low-, intermediate-, and high-grade tumors was 54, 31, and 3 percent, respectively. Interestingly, the cure rate for low-grade adenocarcinoma, NOS, was similar to acinic cell adenocarcinoma, indicating the importance of separating this group from high-grade adenocarcinoma, NOS, a group that may be the most aggressive of all salivary gland carcinomas. As with most other forms of salivary gland carcinoma, even patients with the low-grade variant need long-term follow-up.

Spiro and colleagues concluded that surgery remains the primary treatment modality. They found that treatment decisions should include stage of disease: patients with stage I disease had a 10-year cure rate of 75 percent regardless of tumor grade. Adjuvant postoperative radiotherapy is indicated in intermediate- and high-grade tumors that have an advanced clinical stage. Matsuba et al. (98) found that local control of disease was better with combined therapy than with surgery or radiation alone.

ACINIC CELL ADENOCARCINOMA

Definition. Acinic cell adenocarcinoma is a malignant epithelial neoplasm in which the neoplastic cells demonstrate acinar differentiation. Although there are both serous and mucous type acinar cells in the various normal salivary glands, by conventional use the term acinic cell adenocarcinoma is defined by cytologic differentiation toward serous acinar cells, whose characteristic feature is cytoplasmic zymogen type secretory granules. As detailed below, this does not

mean that the cellular composition of these tumors is exclusively or even predominantly serous type cells, but a portion of the cell populations of these tumors demonstrates serous differentiation by light or electron microscopy.

The World Health Organization (WHO) monograph on the histologic typing of salivary gland tumors in 1972 (190) used the term acinic cell tumor for these neoplasms. In reference to both mucoepidermoid tumor and acinic cell tumor, the WHO monograph rationalized the preference for the word "tumor" rather than "carcinoma" by stating that many of these tumors are readily curable, that only a small minority metastasize, and that on histologic features alone it is not possible to readily identify which tumors are likely to metastasize. Therefore, the term tumor seemed to occupy an ambiguous middle ground between adenoma and carcinoma. Although the malignant potential of these tumors had been reported in the early 1950s (119,143,148), many other investigators also favored classifying acinic cell neoplasms as tumors rather than carcinomas (113,139,178, 181,189). However, undoubtedly influenced by studies and arguments subsequently presented by many other investigators (115–117,137,158,174), the WHO's revised classification of salivary gland tumors of 1991 (180) uses the term acinic cell carcinoma, and this Fascicle agrees with the carcinomatous designation for these neoplasms.

General Features. In AFIP data of salivary gland neoplasms, acinic cell adenocarcinoma is the third most common epithelial malignancy after mucoepidermoid carcinoma and adenocarcinoma, NOS; it comprises about 17 percent of primary malignant salivary gland tumors or about 6 percent of all salivary gland neoplasms. Other studies have reported a relative frequency of acinic cell adenocarcinoma from none to 19 percent of malignant salivary gland neoplasms (140,142,159,177,181,183,185,191,192,196). On average the incidence is about 10 percent. Both British and German registries of salivary gland lesions have reported an incidence of about 10 percent among epithelial malignancies (140,177). One series from South Africa reported an incidence of 11 percent while another series from Malawi had no acinic cell adenocarcinomas (191, 192). In a series of over 400 carcinomas from China, Yu and Ma (196) reported an incidence of

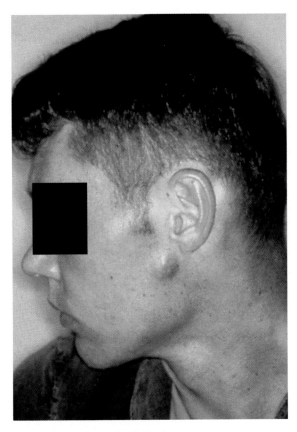

Figure 5-38
ACINIC CELL ADENOCARCINOMA:
CLINICAL PRESENTATION

A 2.0-cm raised subcutaneous nodule just anterior to the lower portion of the ear is a common clinical presentation for acinic cell adenocarcinoma. The tumor is in the superficial lobe of the left parotid gland of this 24-year-old man.

4.4 percent. On the other hand, they reported a remarkably high incidence of 11.6 percent for cystadenocarcinoma, which is much higher than the AFIP's experience. In fact, cystadenocarcinoma is a diagnostic category not even included in many other reported series, and the difference in classification among various investigators probably explains some of the variation in incidence reported for all types of salivary gland tumors. Papillary-cystic growth is one of the recognized architectural patterns that acinic cell adenocarcinomas manifest (112,117,130, 136,137,164,174,180,184), and perhaps some cystadenocarcinomas in the series of Yu and Ma might be classifiable as acinic cell adenocarcinoma by the histologic criteria given below.

Since the parotid gland is the largest salivary gland and is composed nearly exclusively of serous type acini, it is not surprising that 83 percent of acinic cell adenocarcinomas occur in this gland (fig. 5-38). About 4 percent arise in the submandibular gland, and most of the remainder develop in the intraoral minor salivary glands, most frequently in the buccal mucosa, upper lip, and palate (fig. 5-39). Origin in the sublingual gland is rare. Several small series of intraoral acinic cell adenocarcinomas have been reported (113,122,125,141,146,197). In the AFIP files acinic cell adenocarcinoma accounts for about 6.5 percent of all intraoral salivary gland tumors; other investigators have reported an incidence of

Figure 5-39
ACINIC CELL ADENOCARCINOMA:
CLINICAL PRESENTATION

The upper lip, or any other intraoral site, is an uncommon location for acinic cell adenocarcinoma.

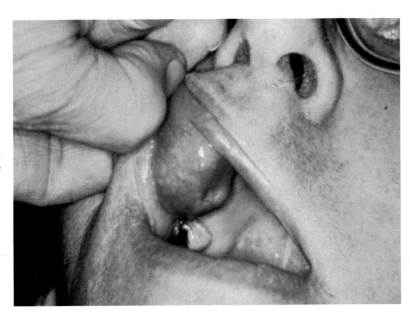

none to 4.2 percent (123,140,161,183, 191,192,194, 195). Although both serous and mucous acini are found in the intraoral salivary glands, Inoue et al. (160) have documented an acinic cell adenocarcinoma with serous cell differentiation in the glossopalatine glands, which typically have only mucous type acini. Rare intraosseous tumors of the jaws have been reported (113,124,130).

Although synchronous or metachronous neoplasia in multiple salivary glands is rare, up to 3 percent of acinic cell adenocarcinomas are bilateral (147). Acinic cell adenocarcinoma is the type of malignant salivary gland tumor that most often occurs bilaterally, usually in the parotid glands, but also in the submandibular and parotid glands (147). However, the number of cases is greatly exceeded by that of bilateral Warthin tumors and bilateral mixed tumors. It should be noted that some reported cases of bilateral clear cell type acinic cell adenocarcinoma appear to represent the clear cell variant of oncocytoma (see Oncocytoma) (147,170,171).

Women are affected more frequently than men in a ratio of 3 to 2. There is no predilection for any race evident in AFIP's data. Patients range from young children to centenarians. The mean age of patients is 44 years, but the age distribution is fairly even from the second to the seventh decades of life, with a slight peak in incidence in the fourth decade. Twelve percent of the patients in the AFIP case files were under 20 years old at the time of excision of their primary tumor. Thus, acinic cell adenocarcinoma trails only mixed tumor and mucoepidermoid carcinoma as the most common epithelial salivary gland tumor in children; however, most of these young patients were in the second decade of life. This incidence in children is analogous to that reported by others (120,163,166,179).

Clinical Features. The typical clinical history describes a slowly enlarging mass in the parotid region. Durations of symptoms prior to diagnosis have ranged from weeks to 40 years, but many patients report a duration of less than a year (112,128,130,150,174,184). A solitary, unfixed mass is typical, but in a few patients multiple nodules or fixation to skin or muscle has been reported (130,184). Pain or tenderness is a symptom for over a third of patients (112,128,130,137, 150,174), and the pain is often described as vague and intermittent. Facial muscle weakness occurs in 5 to 10 percent of patients (128,130,137).

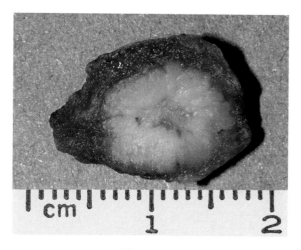

Figure 5-40
ACINIC CELL ADENOCARCINOMA: GROSS SPECIMEN
This tan, circumscribed but unencapsulated nodule in a small segment of lung tissue was a metastatic focus from an acinic cell adenocarcinoma of the parotid gland.

Gross Findings. Gross specimen examination may belie the malignant nature of acinic cell adenocarcinoma since most tumors are single, well-circumscribed nodules. Some even appear encapsulated. On the other hand, some tumors are irregular shaped, ill-defined, or multinodular. Tumors have ranged in size from 0.5 to 13.0 cm in largest dimension, but the majority are 1 to 3 cm. The cut surface is lobular and tan to reddish, and the consistency varies from firm to soft and solid to cystic (fig. 5-40).

Microscopic Findings. The archetypal acinic cell adenocarcinoma consists of sheets of large polygonal cells with granular, lightly basophilic cytoplasm and uniform, round, eccentric nuclei that are readily recognized as serous type acinar cells (fig. 5-41). However, the spectrum of architectural and cytologic features in acinic cell adenocarcinomas is much broader. Many investigators of large numbers of salivary gland tumors have consistently described several histologic architectural patterns and cellular types within the diagnostic spectrum of acinic cell adenocarcinoma (112,117,130,131,150,164,174, 175,180,184,189). While serous acinar cell differentiation characterizes this group of tumors, appreciation of the histopathologic variability should make recognition of this tumor easier.

Although the terms that various investigators have used to label the several histomorphologic

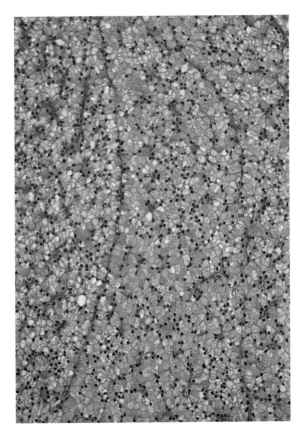

Figure 5-41
ACINIC CELL ADENOCARCINOMA
A sheet of acinar type cells with neither striated ducts nor the lobular arrangement of normal parotid acini readily identifies this tumor as acinic cell adenocarcinoma.

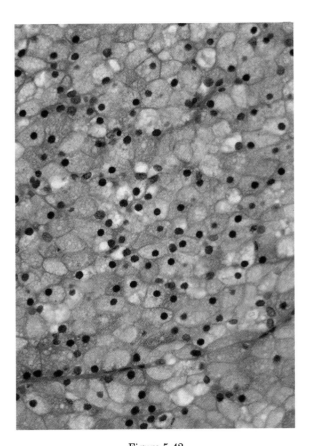

Figure 5-42
ACINIC CELL ADENOCARCINOMA: ACINAR CELLS
Typically, neoplastic acinar cells are large, round to polygonal cells with granular, slightly basophilic cytoplasm and dark, round, eccentrically located nuclei.

patterns and cellular features of these tumors have varied, the tumor descriptions have been similar. The descriptive categories presented by Abrams et al. in 1965 (112) have been useful to pathologists over the last 30 years and are still applicable today. Architectural growth patterns are categorized as solid, microcystic, papillary-cystic, and follicular. Cellular features are identified as acinar, intercalated ductal, vacuolated, clear, and nonspecific glandular. These descriptive categories do not define specific subtypes of acinic cell adenocarcinomas; the patterns are not exclusive of one another but rather help to define the spectrum of histologic features of these tumors. Although an individual tumor usually has a predominance of one pattern or cell type, many tumors have a mixture of features.

Serous acinar cell differentiation, of course, defines acinic cell adenocarcinomas, and the pro-duction of cytoplasmic zymogen-like secretory granules is the cytologic feature that most readily identifies acinar differentiation. Like their normal salivary gland counterpart, these tumor cells typically have abundant, pale basophilic cytoplasm with purplish cytoplasmic granules and eccentrically located, round, dark, basophilic nuclei (fig. 5-42). In some tumors small groups of acinar type tumor cells are clustered together in an organoid arrangement and are surrounded by a very thin fibrovascular stroma (fig. 5-43). These closely packed acinar cells resemble normal salivary gland, but the absence of striated ducts and a normal lobular configuration readily distinguishes this neoplastic proliferation. In other tumors the arrangement of the acinar cells varies from sheets to randomly scattered foci. Unlike normal acinar cells, neoplastic acinar cells are usually polygonal rather than

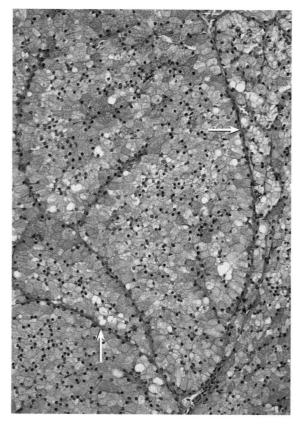

Figure 5-43
ACINIC CELL ADENOCARCINOMA: ACINAR CELLS
In this solid sheet of acinar type cells very thin fibrovascular septa (arrows) surround or partially surround and separate groups of cells.

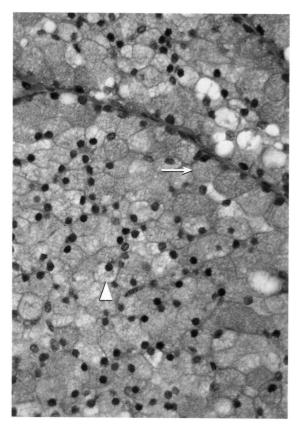

Figure 5-44
ACINIC CELL ADENOCARCINOMA: ACINAR CELLS
While some of the acinar type cells have distinctly granular cytoplasm (arrow), others have a finely reticular cytoplasm (arrowhead).

triangular or trapezoidal, exhibit greater variability in cellular and nuclear size, and have nuclei that vary from darkly basophilic to slightly vesicular. In many cells the cytoplasmic granules are inconspicuous and the cytoplasm has a finely reticular or foamy appearance (fig. 5-44). Periodic acid–Schiff (PAS) stain highlights the cytoplasmic secretory granules, which are resistant to diastase digestion (fig. 5-45). Mucicarmine stain helps distinguish zymogen-like granules from the mucinous granules of mucous cells. In over 40 percent of acinic cell adenocarcinomas acinar cells are the predominant cell type. However, in some tumors they comprise only a small percentage of the tumor cell population, and PAS stain in conjunction with mucicarmine stain can help confirm their identity.

Like the acinar type cells, the intercalated duct-like cells also resemble their normal gland counterpart. These cells are smaller than the acinar type cells, but their nuclear size is about the same. Therefore, the nuclear/cytoplasmic ratio of the intercalated duct type cells is greater than that of the acinar type cells. The cytoplasm is eosinophilic to amphophilic, and the cytoplasmic compartment is cuboidal (fig. 5-46). The nuclei are usually central within the cytoplasmic compartment and range from deeply basophilic to vesicular. There is greater variability in size of these cells than in normal glandular tissue. They surround luminal spaces that vary in size from small, duct-lumen size to large, cystic spaces. There is little resemblance to normal glandular architecture, and typically the ductal structures formed by these cells are arranged in a back-to-back fashion (fig. 5-47). Some intercalated duct type cells can be found in most acinic cell adenocarcinomas; they are the predominant cell type in about a third of tumors.

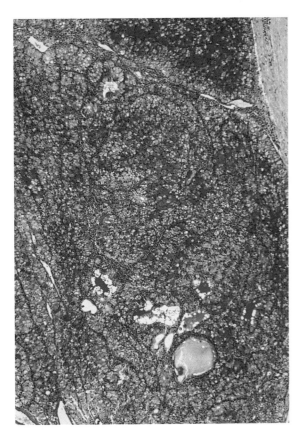

Figure 5-45

ACINIC CELL ADENOCARCINOMA: ACINAR CELLS

Like normal acinar cells, the secretory granules in neoplastic acinar cells react with PAS stain and are resistant to digestion with diastase. (PAS staining after diastase digestion)

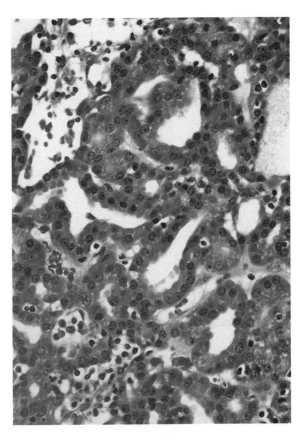

Figure 5-46

ACINIC CELL ADENOCARCINOMA:
INTERCALATED DUCTAL CELLS

Similar to normal intercalated duct cells, the cells in this field are cuboidal with round, centrally located, dark to pale nuclei. They surround variably sized luminal spaces. Many nuclei contain a small nucleolus.

Although not pathognomonic, vacuolated cells are characteristic of acinic cell adenocarcinomas; at least they are more conspicuous in acinic cell adenocarcinoma than any other salivary gland tumor. They are the predominant cell type in less than 10 percent of acinic cell adenocarcinomas, but when present they are an important diagnostic feature. These cells are characterized by vacuoles that fill most of the cytoplasmic compartment (fig. 5-48). The vacuoles are clear with hematoxylin and eosin stain and unreactive with PAS and mucicarmine; however, some vacuolated cells contain PAS-positive, diastase-resistant zymogen-like granules. The cells vary in size, and the cytoplasmic membranes of some appear expanded by the vacuoles. The number of vacuoles per cell varies from one to several, but the more vacuoles there are in a cell the smaller is each vacuole. The cytoplasm

that is unoccupied by vacuoles is eosinophilic to amphophilic. The nuclear features are similar to those of intercalated duct-like cells.

Clear cells might logically seem to be the extreme manifestation of vacuolated cells, but that does not always appear to be true. Some clear cells are associated with vacuolated cells, and these appear to be cells extended by a single large vacuole. Focal aggregates or sheets of clear cells are uncommon and occur unassociated with vacuolated cells. They have the cytologic configuration of acinar or nonspecific glandular cells but have nonstaining cytoplasm (fig. 5-49). In the experience of the AFIP and others, aggregates of clear cells are found in about 6 percent of acinic cell adenocarcinomas and form a significant portion of the neoplastic cell population in only 1 percent (137,174). Overemphasis of the importance of clear

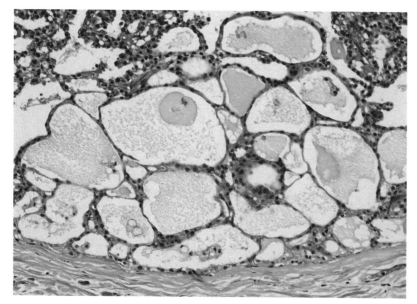

Figure 5-47
ACINIC CELL ADENOCARCINOMA:
INTERCALATED DUCTAL CELLS
Several of the luminal spaces are
cystically enlarged, and the lining duct-
type epithelial cells appear thinned and
flattened. The small cystic structures
abut one another and contain pale-
staining flocculent material.

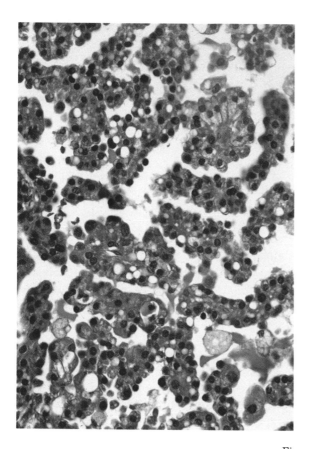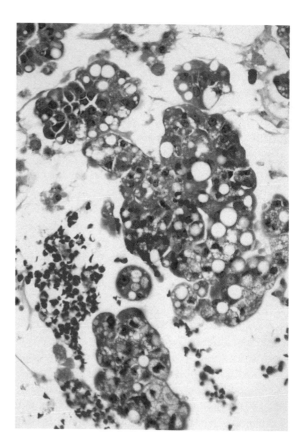

Figure 5-48
ACINIC CELL ADENOCARCINOMA: VACUOLATED CELLS
Left: Variably sized, small, clear cytoplasmic vacuoles are evident in many of the epithelial cells that form papillary
formations in a cystic area of this parotid gland tumor.
Right: A higher magnification of similar-appearing cells from another tumor shows some cells with several cytoplasmic
vacuoles. Some of the cells appear distended or even ruptured.

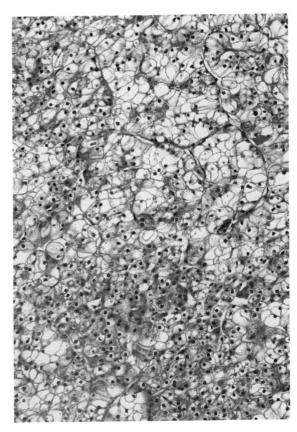

Figure 5-49
ACINIC CELL ADENOCARCINOMA: CLEAR CELLS
Most of the cells with pale or nonstaining cytoplasm are very similar in size and shape to the acinar type cells, which can be seen as the dark stained cells among the clear cells.

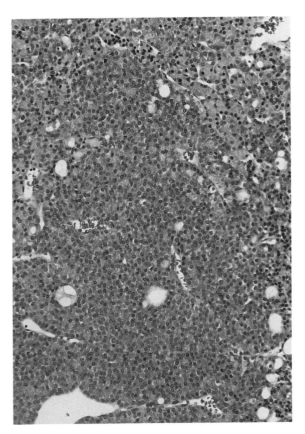

Figure 5-50
ACINIC CELL ADENOCARCINOMA:
NONSPECIFIC GLANDULAR CELLS
Cells that are generally smaller than acinar type cells, have eosinophilic to amphophilic cytoplasm, and typically proliferate as sheets of cells with indistinct cell boundaries are identified as nonspecific glandular cells because they lack unique characteristics of other cell types.

cells has lead to erroneous diagnoses of acinic cell adenocarcinoma (139,141,144,149,170,171). One report of "bilateral acinous cell tumors of the parotid gland" in a 59-year-old woman with multiple nodules of clear cells described and illustrated intracellular glycogen, oncocytes, and multifocal tumors in both parotid glands but no evidence of acinar cell differentiation (170). These features are most consistent with clear cell oncocytosis (see Oncocytoma). A purely clear cell variant of acinic cell adenocarcinoma probably does not exist (117, 133,137). Clear cells are a much more frequent component of mucoepidermoid carcinomas than acinic cell adenocarcinomas and are the principal diagnostic feature of epithelial-myoepithelial carcinomas and clear cell adenocarcinomas (see corresponding sections). The clear cells in acinic cell adenocarcinoma do not contain glycogen and probably represent fixation or tissue processing

artifactual changes and alterations of cytoplasmic organelles such as dilatation of endoplasmic reticulum (124). On the basis of immunohistochemical similarities, Takahashi et al. (187) speculated that the clear cells transform from neoplastic acinar cells.

Nonspecific glandular cells of acinic cell adenocarcinoma are round to polygonal, with amphophilic to eosinophilic cytoplasm and round, basophilic to vesicular nuclei (fig. 5-50). They are smaller but similar in shape to many acinar cells, but they lack cytoplasmic granules and are unreactive with PAS stain. They typically occur in syncytial sheets with poorly demarcated cell borders. Nuclear pleomorphism is more prominent in this cell population than the other cell types, and mitotic activity, when evident in acinic cell

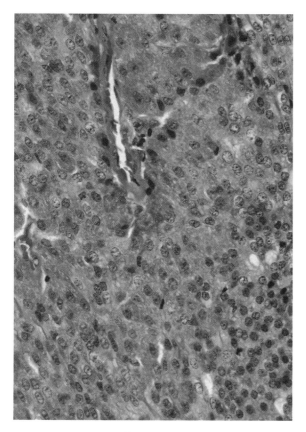

Figure 5-51
ACINIC CELL ADENOCARCINOMA:
NONSPECIFIC GLANDULAR CELLS

The nonspecific glandular cells, which have been characterized by some investigators as "undifferentiated," can demonstrate greater nuclear variability in size, staining, and mitoses than other cell types observed in acinic cell adenocarcinomas.

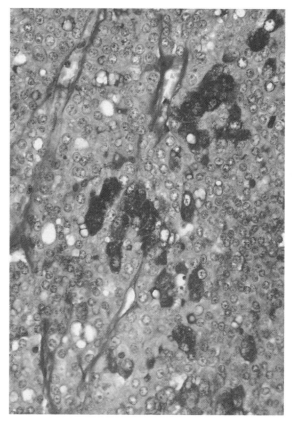

Figure 5-52
ACINIC CELL ADENOCARCINOMA: ACINAR AND
NONSPECIFIC GLANDULAR CELLS

The PAS-positive granular cytoplasm of the acinar differentiated cells distinguishes them from the sheet of unreactive, slightly smaller, nonspecific glandular cells. (PAS stain after diastase digestion)

adenocarcinomas, is mostly associated with the nonspecific glandular cells (fig. 5-51). Acinar cells with their cytoplasmic granules are often found scattered among the nonspecific glandular cells, and PAS stain helps identify them (fig. 5-52). Nonspecific glandular cells are present in most acinic cell adenocarcinomas, but they are the majority of the cell population in only about 15 percent of tumors.

In the solid growth pattern the tumor cells are closely apposed to one another to form sheets, nodules, or aggregates. The acinar type cell is usually the predominant cell type in the solid pattern, but in some tumors nonspecific glandular cells or, less often, clear cells form a significant portion of the cell population (fig. 5-53). Nodules of acinar cells with their basophilic cytoplasm,

cytoplasmic granules, and round dark basophilic nuclei have given rise to the description of these tumors as "blue dot tumors" (117); this form is the one most easily recognized as acinic cell adenocarcinoma. Some tumors, especially those less than 2 cm, have an apparent capsule of fibrous tissue. Apparent encapsulation and uniform, bland cytologic features transmit an impression of benignancy, but even these seemingly harmless tumors have a potential for malignant behavior if inadequately treated. A solid histomorphologic growth pattern predominates in over one third of acinic cell adenocarcinomas.

A microcystic pattern is a slightly more frequent component of acinic cell adenocarcinomas than the solid pattern. It is the principal pattern in about one third of tumors and a minor pattern

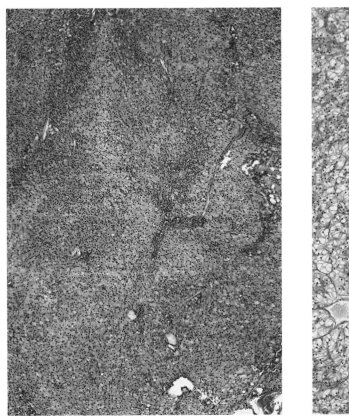 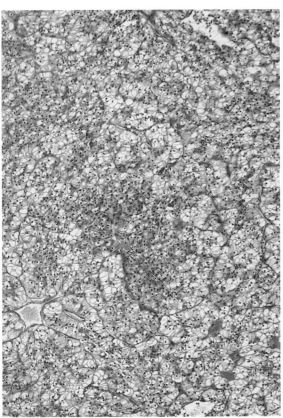

Figure 5-53
ACINIC CELL ADENOCARCINOMA: SOLID GROWTH PATTERN
The so-called solid growth pattern is characterized by large sheets of tumor cells.
Left: In many tumors the cells are mostly acinar type.
Right: Here the cells are mostly clear type with a cluster of darker staining acinar type cells in the center of the field.

in another third. The solid and microcystic patterns frequently occur in association with one another. The microcystic pattern is characterized by numerous small spaces within sheets or nodules of tumor cells (fig. 5-54). The microcystic spaces vary from several microns to a millimeter or more in size. Acinar type cells are usually easily identifiable in microcystic type tumors, but vacuolated and intercalated duct type cells are also often plentiful. The presence of vacuolated cells suggests that the microcystic spaces are coalesced ruptured vacuolated cells (fig. 5-55). These spaces are usually empty but sometimes contain amorphous, eosinophilic or pale basophilic material that stains with PAS and sometimes with mucicarmine. The microcysts are small and lack intraluminal epithelial proliferation.

The papillary-cystic pattern is characterized by prominent cystic spaces that are larger than those of the microcystic pattern and are sometimes even visible during gross examination. Tumor cells partially fill the cystic lumens in the form of papillary growths (fig. 5-56). The luminal epithelial proliferations vary from sparse, with only a few small projections or folds into mostly empty lumens, to extensive, with papillary epithelial proliferations nearly filling the lumens. Some of the luminal epithelial proliferations have a microcystic pattern, so these two patterns often overlap. Thin fibrovascular cores are visible within many of the papillary epithelial projections. Due to the two-dimensional nature of tissue sections, some of the epithelial proliferations appear to be "floating" within the cystic cavities. Acinar differentiated cells are usually less numerous in this pattern than in the solid or microcystic pattern and in some tumors are quite sparse. Intercalated duct type and vacuolated cells frequently

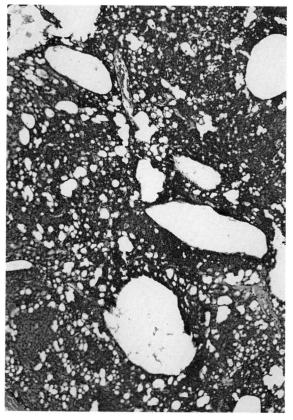

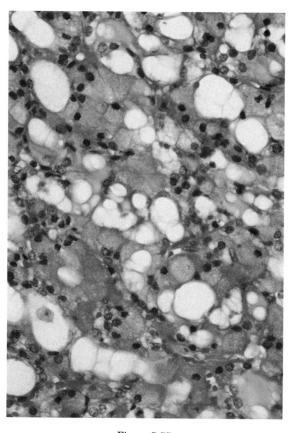

Figure 5-54
ACINIC CELL ADENOCARCINOMA:
MICROCYSTIC GROWTH PATTERN
Numerous small but variably sized spaces are inter-
spersed among the epithelial tumor cells.

Figure 5-55
ACINIC CELL ADENOCARCINOMA:
MICROCYSTIC PATTERN
Several granular acinar cells and vacuolated cells are
present in this microcystic area of acinic cell adenocarcinoma. Some of the microcystic spaces that are closely associated with cytoplasmic vacuoles give an impression that the
microcysts could result from rupture of the vacuoles.

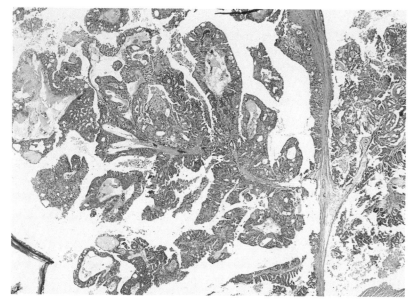

Figure 5-56
ACINIC CELL ADENOCARCINOMA:
PAPILLARY-CYSTIC GROWTH
PATTERN
Two large cystic spaces (right and
left) are lined by epithelium of variable
thickness, and branching projections of
epithelium occupy a large portion of the
cysts' lumens.

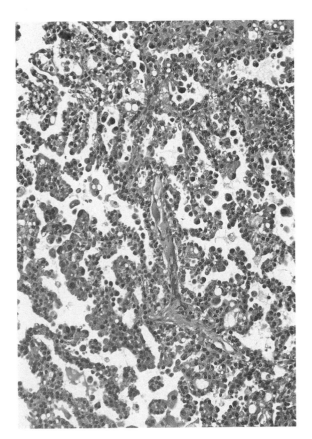

Figure 5-57
ACINIC CELL ADENOCARCINOMA:
PAPILLARY-CYSTIC GROWTH PATTERN

Thin, branching fibrovascular stalks are covered with a one to several cell–thick layer of epithelium. Some of the papillary fronds appear unattached to any adjacent papillary fronds due to the plane of section. The luminal surface of many of the epithelial cells bulges into the cystic cavity.

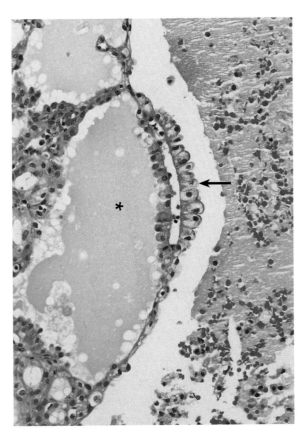

Figure 5-58
ACINIC CELL ADENOCARCINOMA:
PAPILLARY-CYSTIC PATTERN

High magnification of epithelial cells with their protruding luminal surface along a small cystic structure imparts a "tombstone row" appearance (arrow). The homogeneous, pale amphophilic material in the cyst lumen (asterisk) is usually PAS positive and may be weakly reactive with mucicarmine.

dominate. The epithelium covering the cyst walls and papillary projections varies from one to several cells in thickness (fig. 5-57). The surface of some of the epithelial cells bulges into the lumen and produces an undulating, "tombstone row" appearance (fig. 5-58). Many tumors contain extracellular, intraluminal mucinous material that is weakly to strongly reactive with PAS and sometimes with mucicarmine. Rarely, cytoplasmic mucicarminophilia of a few cells is observed. As long as convincing serous acinar cell differentiation is identified, some mucicarmine reactivity is compatible with a diagnosis of acinic cell adenocarcinoma. A few tumors are dominated by large cysts with only a small amount of luminal epithelial proliferation (fig. 5-59). This appearance suggests that these acinic cell adenocarcinomas either develop

within parotid cysts or experience marked cystic enlargement with minimal epithelial proliferation.

The follicular pattern is characterized by multiple cystic lumens filled with eosinophilic proteinaceous material (fig. 5-60). This pattern has a thyroid follicle–like appearance, which is heightened by the observation that most of the cystic spaces are lined by intercalated duct-like epithelial cells. Among the various architectural patterns of acinic cell adenocarcinoma, the follicular pattern is the least frequent and is prominent in only about 5 percent of the tumors. The cystic spaces are round to oval, variable in size, larger than those of the microcystic pattern, and generally lack luminal papillary epithelial proliferation (fig. 5-61). The luminal material stains well

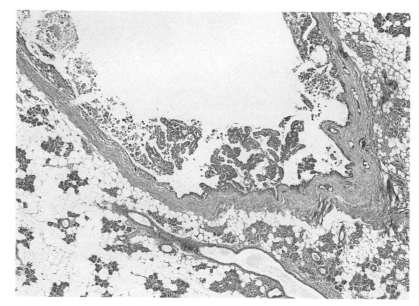

Figure 5-59
ACINIC CELL ADENOCARCINOMA:
PAPILLARY-CYSTIC PATTERN
Low magnification of a parotid
gland shows a large cystic structure
with a small amount of papillary epithelial growth into the lumen.

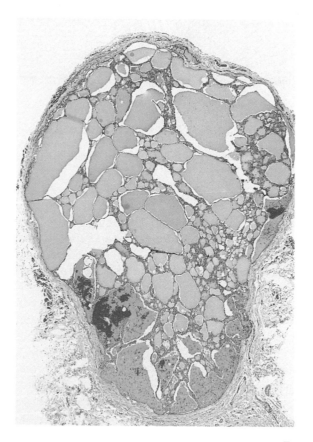 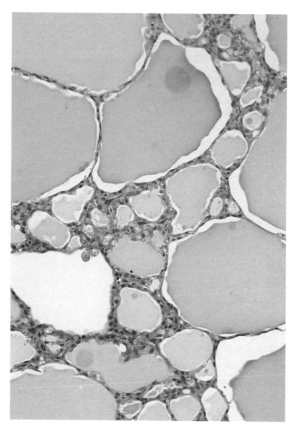

Figure 5-60
ACINIC CELL ADENOCARCINOMA: FOLLICULAR PATTERN
Left: This circumscribed tumor nodule has numerous, variably sized cystic structures that contain a homogeneous, eosinophilic proteinaceous material. The nodule resembles a thyroid follicle.
Right: At higher magnification the cystic spaces are mostly lined by intercalated duct-like cells.

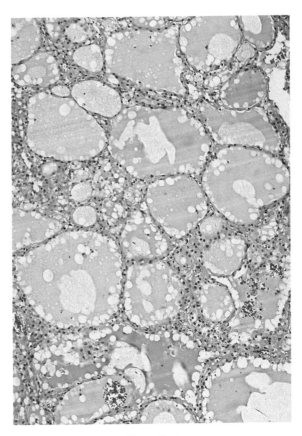

Figure 5-61
ACINIC CELL ADENOCARCINOMA:
FOLLICULAR PATTERN
Papillary configurations are absent or inconspicuous in the follicular pattern. The "interfollicular" regions contain vacuolated, nonspecific glandular, and acinar type cells.

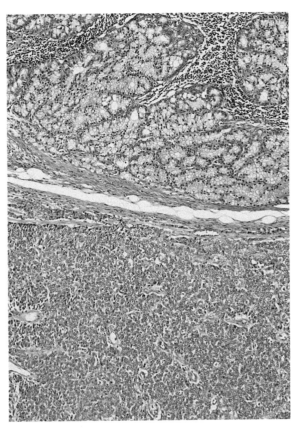

Figure 5-62
ACINIC CELL ADENOCARCINOMA
WITH UNDIFFERENTIATED CARCINOMA
Nodules of neoplastic acinar cells in a stroma with a prominent lymphoid infiltrate (top) are adjacent to a sheet of undifferentiated epithelial cells (bottom).

with PAS and sometimes weakly with mucicarmine. The epithelial cells in the interfollicular regions are mostly of nonspecific glandular type, with some vacuolated and acinar type cells.

Areas of "dedifferentiated" or undifferentiated carcinoma have been described as a component of a few acinic cell adenocarcinomas (117,135,186). The AFIP has identified four such tumors. These tumors are somewhat of an enigma since there is such a distinct contrast between the acinic cell adenocarcinoma and the adjacent undifferentiated carcinoma with its sheets and aggregates of epithelial cells with large nuclear/cytoplasmic ratios, many mitotic figures, cellular and nuclear pleomorphism, and no evidence of glandular or epidermoid differentiation (fig. 5-62). There is usually limited intermixing of the two patterns. Whether these tumors actually represent dedif-

ferentiation is difficult to determine. There is no evidence that the differentiated acinar portion of these tumors preceded that of the undifferentiated carcinoma portion, and they may represent the proliferation of two clones of neoplastic epithelial cells that have developed in proximity to one another. Deguchi et al. (132) has reported transformation of an acinic cell adenocarcinoma to adenocarcinoma with oncocytic features in a patient who experienced multiple recurrences over a 30-year period. Regardless of the histogenesis, we believe that the biologic potential and treatment of these tumors is dictated by the undifferentiated carcinoma component.

Acinic cell adenocarcinomas arising in intraparotid lymph nodes have been described (112, 165,167). However, some acinic cell adenocarcinomas are associated with prominent lymphoid

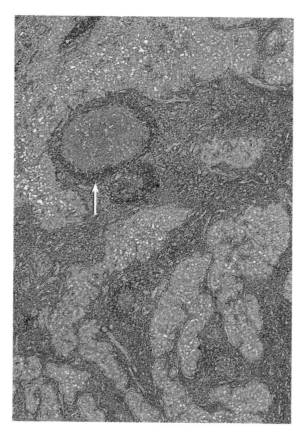

Figure 5-63
ACINIC CELL ADENOCARCINOMA
WITH LYMPHOID STROMA
The deeply basophilic tissue represents a lymphoid proliferation within the stroma of this acinic cell adenocarcinoma of the parotid gland. A lymphoid follicle is evident (arrow), but the lymphoid tissue does not have the configuration of a lymph node, such as a capsule and subcapsular sinus, medullary cords, and hilus.

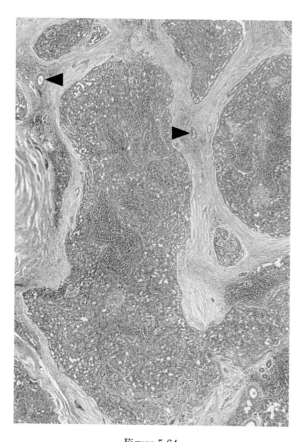

Figure 5-64
ACINIC CELL ADENOCARCINOMA: INFILTRATION
Several variably sized and shaped nodules of acinic cell adenocarcinoma in a densely collagenous stroma extend into parotid parenchyma (lower right). A few residual normal salivary gland ducts are entrapped within the tumor (arrowheads).

infiltrates of their stroma, even including lymphoid follicle formation, that appear to have proliferated along with the neoplastic epithelium as it infiltrates adjacent tissues (fig. 5-63). The intense lymphoid infiltrate appears to be an integral component of the stroma and unrelated to nodal tissue. Stromal lymphoid proliferation is not unique to acinic cell adenocarcinoma and occurs in other salivary gland tumors, especially mucoepidermoid carcinoma (114).

Most acinic cell adenocarcinomas infiltrate adjacent normal tissues (fig. 5-64), but some tumors, especially smaller ones, are well circumscribed even at the microscopic level (figs. 5-59, 5-60). The stroma varies from delicate fibrovascular tissue to extensively collagenous tissue.

Hemorrhage is most often noted in association with the papillary-cystic tumor growth pattern. Hemosiderin is deposited in the connective tissue, and, interestingly, many of the epithelial tumor cells often contain cytoplasmic hemosiderin granules (fig. 5-65). The intraepithelial hemosiderin pigment is finely granular and gives the epithelial cells a faint brownish cast. A positive PAS reaction is associated with this pigmented material and must be distinguished from zymogen granules in acinar differentiated cells (fig. 5-66). Iron stains, such as Perl's, can help correctly identify this granular pigmented material. Spherical calcifications, or psammomatous bodies similar to those that occur in papillary thyroid carcinoma, are present in a few tumors.

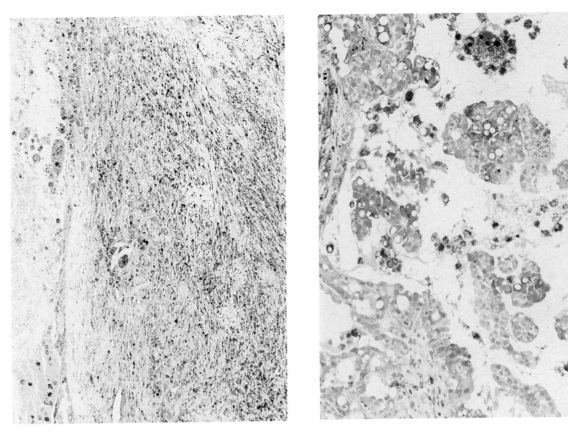

Figure 5-65
ACINIC CELL ADENOCARCINOMA: HEMOSIDERIN PIGMENT
Left: Iron stain shows that hemorrhage in a papillary cystic acinic cell adenocarcinoma has produced a focally dense deposition of hemosiderin pigment in the collagenous stroma.
Right: Blue iron pigment is evident in many of the epithelial tumor cells of a papillary cystic acinic cell adenocarcinoma that was associated with the hemorrhage. (Perl's iron stain)

Figure 5-66
ACINIC CELL ADENOCARCINOMA:
IRON PIGMENT
Much of the intraepithelial pigment that reacts with iron stain is also reactive with PAS stain, which may obscure staining of zymogen granules. (PAS stain after diastase digestion)

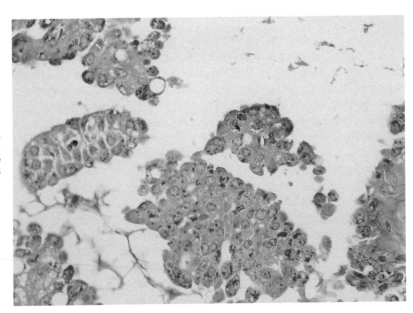

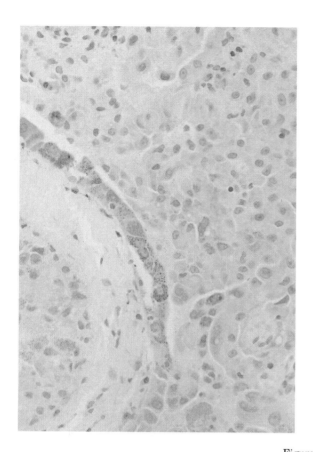 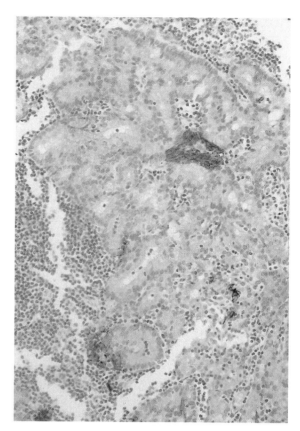

Figure 5-67
ACINIC CELL ADENOCARCINOMA: IMMUNOHISTOCHEMISTRY
Left: A few tumor cells are reactive with anti-amylase in this routinely formalin-fixed, paraffin-embedded and processed tissue section.
Right: Reactivity with a monoclonal antibody cocktail for cytokeratins is quite variable among acinic cell adenocarcinomas. In this section only a few tumor cells are reactive. (Avidin-biotin peroxidase stain)

Immunohistochemical Findings. Immunohistochemical studies have shown acinic cell adenocarcinomas to be reactive for cytokeratin, transferrin, lactoferrin, alpha-1-antitrypsin, alpha-1-antichymotrypsin, IgA, carcinoembryonic antigen, Leu-M1 antigen, and amylase (156,187). Reactivity for S-100 protein and glial fibrillary acidic protein has been described in some tumors (156,186). Many normal serous acinar cells are immunoreactive for amylase, and some investigators have advocated the use of anti-amylase for acinic cell adenocarcinomas (fig. 5-67) (121,176). At the AFIP and elsewhere, anti-amylase has been reactive in only a few acinic cell adenocarcinomas when formalin fixed and paraffin embedded, including tumors with numerous acinar type cells, and has not been very useful (134,168). Vasoactive intestinal polypeptide has been reported to be specifically reactive in acinic cell adenocarcinoma among various types of salivary gland tumors (157,187). Gustafsson et al. (153), who found a high content of cytokeratin 18 in two of four acinic cell adenocarcinomas, believed that they could distinguish among different salivary gland neoplasms on the basis of reactivity for various types of cytokeratins and vimentin (fig. 5-67).

Ultrastructural Findings. Mirroring the light microscopic findings, ultrastructural studies of acinic cell adenocarcinomas have revealed neoplastic epithelial cell populations of both acinar type and ductal type cells (118,124,131,138, 160,162). The characteristic feature of the acinar type cell is the presence of multiple, round, electron-dense cytoplasmic secretory granules (fig. 5-68). The number, size, and electron density of the secretory granules varies (151). Some of the acinar cells form small lumens with apical junctional

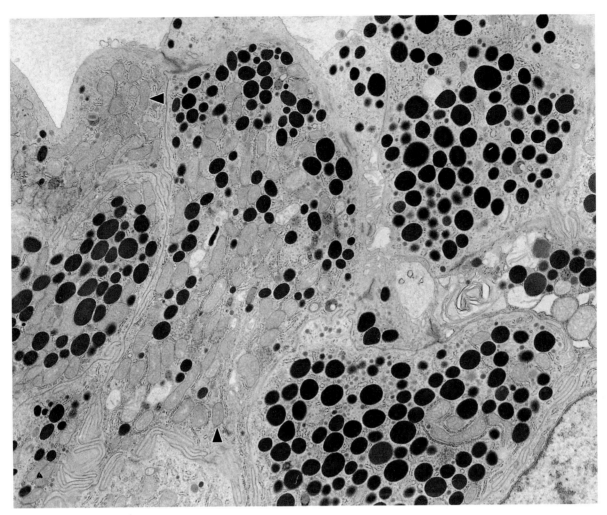

Figure 5-68
ACINIC CELL ADENOCARCINOMA: ULTRASTRUCTURE
Acinar differentiation is characterized in this cluster of neoplastic epithelial cells by numerous, variably sized, round, electron-dense cytoplasmic granules that are similar to the zymogen secretory granules of normal serous acinar cells. Many mitochondria are evident in some of the cells (arrowheads) (X4,600). (Courtesy of Dr. Irving Dardick, Toronto, Canada.)

complexes (zonulae occludentes) and sparse microvilli. Rough endoplasmic reticulum and numerous mitochondria are typically evident. The ductal and nonspecific glandular type cells lack secretory granules, have lesser amounts of endoplasmic reticulum, are joined by intercellular junctions, and are smaller than the acinar type cells. The ductal cells often border lumens and have apical junctional complexes and microvilli. Some cells contain vacuoles of varying size and shape, which are empty or appear to be autophagic vacuoles containing flocculent material (124). Dardick et al. (131) related the "microcysts" in tumors with a microcystic architecture to the

development of lumens that form in relation to groups of ductal type cells. These investigators and Chaudhry et al. (124) have described a few tumors with myoepithelial type cells; these cells had elongated, angular cell bodies and numerous longitudinally aligned microfilaments with focal linear densities. Basal lamina separates groups of acinar and ductal tumor cells from the stromal tissues. While Echevarria (133) indicated that the light microscopically clear cells are the result of artifactual changes, Chaudhry et al. found dilatations of rough endoplasmic reticulum, lipid inclusions, enzymatic degradation of secretory granules, and intracytoplasmic pseudolumens.

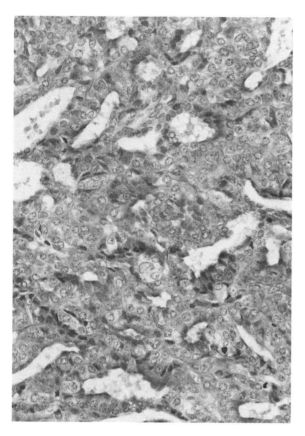

Figure 5-69
ACINIC CELL ADENOCARCINOMA

This papillary-cystic acinic cell adenocarcinoma can be distinguished from cystadenocarcinoma with PAS stain that highlights the secretory granules in acinar differentiated cells. (PAS stain after diastase digestion)

Differential Diagnosis. Tumors composed of numerous acinar differentiated cells pose little diagnostic challenge except in the recognition of neoplastic proliferations as different from normal salivary gland. Due to the absence of striated and interlobular ducts, alteration of the lobular architecture of normal salivary gland, and stromal fibrosis, this is usually not difficult. In tumors where acinar type cells are less obvious more attention must be given to a differential diagnosis, but in all cases recognition of acinar differentiated cells, sometimes with the help of special stains, is a key to diagnosis (fig. 5-69). The differential diagnosis for the papillary-cystic and follicular patterns includes cystadenocarcinoma, mucoepidermoid carcinoma, and metastatic thyroid carcinoma. In minor salivary glands, polymorphous low-grade adenocarcinoma is also considered. Although abun-dant clear cells are infrequent, acinic cell adeno-carcinoma is included in the differential diagnosis of clear cell neoplasms, which also includes muco-epidermoid carcinoma, epithelial-myoepithelial carcinoma, clear cell adenocarcinoma, clear cell oncocytoma, and metastatic renal cell carcinoma.

In AFIP files, cystadenocarcinomas, including papillary variants, are uncommon salivary gland tumors, but they share many features with papillary-cystic and follicular forms of acinic cell adenocarcinoma. A microcystic pattern and vac-uolated cells favor acinic cell adenocarcinoma while mucocytes, identified with mucicarmine stain, favor cystadenocarcinoma. Principally, identification of serous acinar differentiated cells distinguishes acinic cell adenocarcinoma. Therapy for these two neoplasms is similar, so distinction is not critical.

A papillary architecture is not very common in mucoepidermoid carcinoma, but epidermoid cells, mucocytes that are strongly mucicarminophilic, and absence of serous acinar cells distinguishes this tumor. Immunohistochemical staining for thy-roglobulin and the absence of serous acinar cells should readily distinguish metastatic thyroid car-cinoma from acinic cell adenocarcinoma.

In the minor salivary glands, acinic cell adenoc-arcinoma is an uncommon neoplasm while poly-morphous low-grade adenocarcinoma (PLGA) is common. A papillary-cystic pattern is not usually dominant in the latter, and there is a greater affinity for perineural growth, a more homoge-neous cell population, and a greater tendency for single-file cell infiltration at the tumor's periph-ery than in acinic cell adenocarcinoma (see Poly-morphous Low-Grade Adenocarcinoma). Similar to many acinic cell adenocarcinomas, PLGA has bland cytologic features and a tendency to form multiple growth patterns, such as solid, tubular, cystic, cribriform, and papillary.

In contrast to the clear cells in such tumors as epithelial-myoepithelial carcinoma, metastatic renal cell carcinoma, clear cell oncocytoma, and many clear cell adenocarcinomas, the clear cells in acinic cell adenocarcinoma are negative for glycogen. Features that distinguish acinic cell adenocarcinoma from clear cell mucoepidermoid carcinoma are the same as those already stated above. Clear cell adenocarcinoma lacks evidence of serous acinar cell differentiation.

Prognosis and Treatment. Many investigators have found that the biologic behavior of acinic cell adenocarcinoma cannot be reliably predicted on the basis of histomorphologic features (112,129,137,154,155,164,173,181). Other investigators have attempted to correlate a grading system with the biologic behavior of these neoplasms (116,117,126,130,150,152,172,184). Unfortunately, there has been little uniformity among investigators about the criteria for a grading system, and at least one of the grading schemes uses clinical staging criteria, such as size and site, as part of the grading criteria (117). Some who segregated these tumors by grade provided inadequate criteria for grading other than using terms such as well differentiated, poorly differentiated, and dedifferentiated (130, 152). In some reports the term poorly differentiated seems to refer to an absence of acinar cell or intercalated duct cell features, i.e., nonspecific glandular cells (126,152,172), while in others it seems to refer to undifferentiated carcinoma comparable to some nasopharyngeal carcinomas or large cell undifferentiated carcinoma of the lung (117,130). In this latter group, Colmenero et al. (130) remarkably included 9 of 20 tumors, an extremely high incidence in the AFIP experience. In these unusual cases the prognosis is dictated by the undifferentiated carcinoma and is poor. Overall, no correlation of prognosis with any of the four architectural patterns described above has been consistently established. Spiro et al. (184) found that patients with the papillary-cystic pattern had 100 percent mortality, but Perzin and LiVolsi (174) and Colmenero et al. (130) found that patients with a solid growth pattern had a worse prognosis. In general, features that are associated with tumors that recur or metastasize include frequent mitoses, focal necrosis, neural invasion, pleomorphism, infiltration (not circumscribed), stromal hyalinization, incomplete resection, large size, and involvement of the deep lobe of the parotid gland (116,117,135,137, 150,174,184). For acinic cell adenocarcinoma staging is probably a better predictor of outcome than histologic grading.

Cytometric studies of acinic cell adenocarcinoma have produced disparate results. Some investigators have found a positive correlation between DNA aneuploidy and an increased incidence of metastases and reduced patient survival (135), while other investigators have found no such correlation (152,154,155,193).

Argyrophilic nucleolar organizer regions (AgNORs), which have been correlated with proliferative activity and biologic behavior of many tumors, have been reported to have a greater mean count and smaller mean area in acinic cell adenocarcinoma than in normal parotid tissue or benign mixed tumor (127,145). By comparing the AgNOR count of acinic cell adenocarcinoma and several types of salivary gland carcinomas, Fujita et al. (145) classified the former as a low-grade malignancy. Chomette et al. (127) found a correlation between AgNOR count and biologic behavior in a study of 17 acinic cell adenocarcinomas whereas Timon et al. (193) found no significant correlation in 45 cases.

Ki-67 is a monoclonal antibody that is believed to be specifically reactive with proliferating cells. Using Ki-67 antibody in a study of salivary gland tumors that only included one acinic cell adenocarcinoma, Murakami et al. (169) reported the proliferating capacity of this single acinic cell adenocarcinoma to be 21.5 percent compared to a frequency of 18.3 percent as an average for several types of carcinomas, 4.7 percent for normal salivary gland, and 1.0 percent for mixed tumor.

Reported incidences of recurrence, metastasis, and patient deaths for acinic cell adenocarcinomas vary widely; these are probably influenced by the type of institution, the criteria used for diagnosis, treatment modalities employed, and length of follow-up. On average among several studies, these tumors have a recurrence rate of about 35 percent and a metastatic rate and death incidence of about 16 percent (126,130, 137,150,155,164,173,174). In a literature review that included nearly 2,300 cases, Hickman et al. (158) found that acinic cell adenocarcinoma had the best 5- and 10-year survival rates when compared to mucoepidermoid carcinoma, adenoid cystic carcinoma, and malignant mixed tumor. Multiple recurrences or metastases to cervical lymph nodes are associated with a poor prognosis: rarely do patients survive with distant metastases. Patients with short duration of symptoms have a worse prognosis than patients with pretreatment symptoms of long duration (137, 150). A couple of studies have found that recurrences are most likely within the first 5 years after resection of the primary tumor (137,150).

Since several studies have noted tumor metastasis and patient death many years after initial treatment, 5-year survival is not a reliable indicator of cure (164,174).

A number of studies of acinic cell adenocarcinomas arising in minor salivary glands indicate that these tumors are much less aggressive than those that occur in the parotid and submandibular glands (113,122,125,146,197). Tumors in the minor salivary glands rarely metastasize and rarely lead to death.

Complete surgical excision of the primary tumor in the form of parotidectomy or submandibular glandectomy offers the best opportunity for cure (116,150,159,173,184). Incomplete excision of the primary tumor portends a poor prognosis (116,150,174). Radiation therapy is not indicated as the primary form of treatment, but may contribute to improved survival of patients for whom complete excision cannot be accomplished (130,150,174,182).

ADENOID CYSTIC CARCINOMA

Definition. Adenoid cystic carcinoma is a malignant epithelial tumor that is often slow to metastasize but persistent and relentless in growth. Myoepithelial (abluminal) differentiated cells predominate, but there are some ductal differentiated cells. Growth patterns are characterized as cribriform, tubular, and solid.

Because the cribriform pattern of this tumor forms cylindrical accumulations of basal lamina, glycosaminoglycans, and stroma, the term *cylindroma* has been applied. Although it is probably the oldest term used in reference to this tumor, cylindroma is an undesirable synonym because of possible confusion with the benign dermal eccrine tumor of the same name. *Adenocystic carcinoma* is another synonymous term that can be confused with the mucinous (adenocystic) carcinoma of eccrine origin, which is histologically very similar to the mucinous adenocarcinoma of salivary glands. The term adenoid cystic carcinoma has been in use for 40 years and is preferred.

General Features. With the recognition of several new types of salivary gland carcinoma, concepts about long-established entities are modified. The perceived incidence of adenoid cystic carcinoma has been affected since the delineation of polymorphous low-grade adenocarcinoma (terminal duct carcinoma), a tumor that frequently has been misinterpreted as adenoid cystic carcinoma. Polymorphous low-grade adenocarcinoma (PLGA) was first described in 1983 (203,220), and since 1985 the AFIP has identified twice as many PLGAs as adenoid cystic carcinomas in the minor salivary glands. PLGA has become the second most common malignant tumor of minor salivary glands during this period. In their large series, Waldron et al. (282) also found PLGA to be more common in the minor salivary glands than adenoid cystic carcinoma. In this period the AFIP has found adenoid cystic carcinoma to be the fifth most common malignant epithelial tumor of the salivary glands behind mucoepidermoid carcinoma; adenocarcinoma, not otherwise specified (NOS); acinic cell adenocarcinoma; and PLGA. It constitutes about 7.5 percent of all epithelial malignancies and 4 percent of all benign and malignant epithelial salivary gland tumors. In the older literature, adenoid cystic carcinoma was reported as the most common malignant tumor of intraoral salivary glands, and several recent studies are in agreement (264,275) including reports from Britain (217), South Africa (232), Japan (269), and Germany (257). This contrasts with AFIP data and other studies (250), including reports from Australia (207), Nigeria (198), and China (236) and the large series of minor salivary gland tumors reported by Waldron et al. (282) which shows that mucoepidermoid carcinoma is considerably more common in both the intraoral and the parotid salivary glands than adenoid cystic carcinoma.

The ratio of female to male patients has been just slightly higher than 3 to 2, which is about the same ratio as that for all salivary gland tumors as a group. All ages of patients, from children to elderly, have been affected, but adenoid cystic carcinoma is predominantly a tumor of adults with a definite peak incidence in the fourth through sixth decades of life.

The parotid gland, submandibular gland, and palate, in descending order, are the sites of most frequent occurrence: 55 percent of adenoid cystic carcinomas have occurred in the parotid or submandibular glands. While all intraoral sites of salivary gland tissue have been involved, nearly half of the intraoral tumors occur in the palate. The lower lip, retromolar-tonsillar pillar region, and sublingual gland are less common sites for

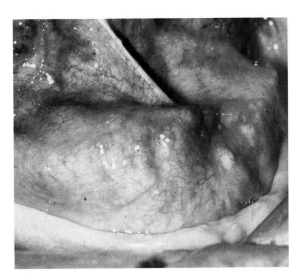
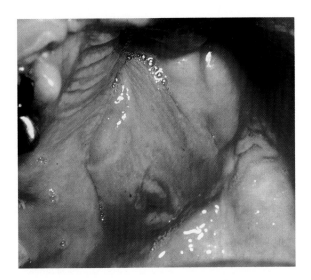

Figure 5-70
ADENOID CYSTIC CARCINOMA

Left: This sublingual gland tumor slowly enlarged to produce a large, lobulated mass in the anterior floor of the mouth. The oral mucosa is intact.

Right: On the other hand, the oral mucosa overlying this palatal adenoid cystic carcinoma has ulcerated.

adenoid cystic carcinoma, just as they are for salivary gland neoplasms in general.

Relatively little information on cytogenetic abnormalities in salivary gland neoplasms is available, but anomalies of the terminal part of 6q and 9p have been reported for adenoid cystic carcinomas by Stenman et al. (267) and others (228).

Clinical Features. In the major salivary glands adenoid cystic carcinoma characteristically develops as a slowly growing swelling in the para-auricular or submandibular region. In exceptional cases, the swelling may develop rapidly. Small tumors are often movable by palpation, but larger tumors usually become fixed to the skin or deeper surrounding tissues. Tenderness, pain, and even facial nerve paralysis frequently develop during the course of the disease and are probably related to the high incidence of nerve invasion associated with this tumor.

Intraoral tumors also generally present as slowly growing submucosal nodules (fig. 5-70). Assessment of fixation to adjacent structures is difficult for palatal tumors because these tissues are normally bound tightly to the palatal and alveolar bone. Ulceration of the mucosa overlying intraoral tumors is common, especially for palatal tumors (fig. 5-70). Pain is a variable finding, but the incidence increases with increasing tumor duration and size.

Gross Findings. Adenoid cystic carcinomas are usually firm and white to gray-white (fig. 5-71). Small tumors occasionally appear well circumscribed and, rarely, even encapsulated, although this is not typical. Circumscription is deceptive because tumor tissue has often infiltrated beyond the tumor margin that is evident by unaided visual examination. Because of the propensity for adenoid cystic carcinoma to insidiously extend along nerve tracts, surgeons often request multiple frozen section examinations of peripheral nerve segments removed from regions beyond the visual extent of the tumor.

Microscopic Findings. The morphologic growth patterns observed in adenoid cystic carcinoma can be categorized into three types: cribriform, tubular, and solid. The cribriform pattern is the most common whereas the solid pattern is the least common. However, a mixture of patterns within a single neoplasm is typical. Cribriform and tubular areas frequently occur together, and even when the solid pattern is predominant, foci of either the cribriform or tubular type, or both, can usually be found somewhere within the neoplasm (fig. 7-72).

The cribriform pattern imparts a sieve-like or Swiss cheese–like appearance to the tumor, i.e., islands of neoplastic epithelial cells contain several small, round, pseudocystic structures. The cystic structures vary slightly in diameter but are rarely very large. These cyst-like spaces are not true ductal or glandular lumens but are actually contiguous with the supporting connective tissue stroma of the tumor. Although in two-dimensional tissue sections these pseudocystic spaces usually appear completely encompassed by neoplastic epithelial cells, in some foci the pseudocystic spaces are in continuity with the collagenous stroma (fig. 5-73). These cylindrical structures usually contain either basophilic material, eosinophilic hyalinized material, or both (fig. 5-73). Ultrastructurally, the basophilic substance represents accumulation of glycosaminoglycans, and the eosinophilic material is due to excessive production of basal lamina (fig. 5-74).

The majority of the neoplastic cells are abluminal type cells of myoepithelial differentiation. The

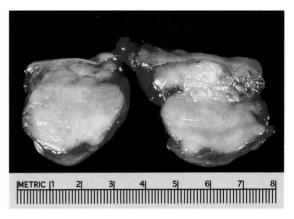

Figure 5-71
ADENOID CYSTIC CARCINOMA
This carcinoma of the submandibular gland appears deceptively well circumscribed with unaided visual examination.

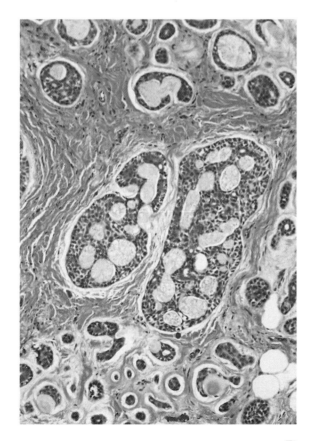 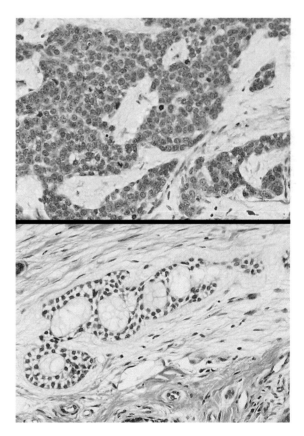

Figure 5-72
ADENOID CYSTIC CARCINOMA
Various morphologic patterns commonly exist within a single neoplasm.
Left: A tubular pattern is evident at the top and bottom portion of the figure while a cribriform pattern with variable amounts of mucohyaline material is present in the center.
Right: Within this palatal neoplasm are areas of solid growth (top) and tubular-cribriform growth (bottom).

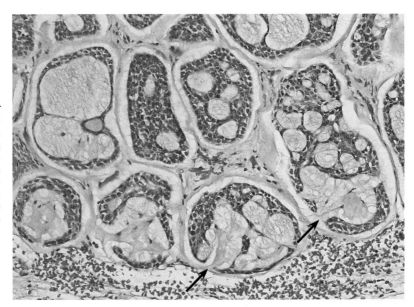

Figure 5-73
ADENOID CYSTIC CARCINOMA:
CRIBRIFORM PATTERN

Interconnecting cords and nests of tumor cells surround multiple, variably sized, small cyst-like structures. Although the cyst-like spaces resemble duct lumens, they are actually pseudolumens and are in continuity with the stroma of the tumor (arrows). The basophilic and hyalinized eosinophilic materials within the pseudocysts are glycosaminoglycans and basal lamina produced by the epithelial cells.

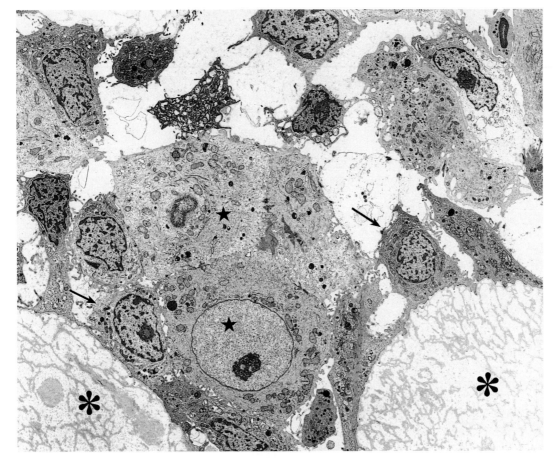

Figure 5-74
ADENOID CYSTIC CARCINOMA

Electron micrograph illustrates abluminal, myoepithelial type cells (arrows) peripheral to ductal cells (stars). The luminal surface of the ductal cells has microvilli (not seen in this section). The pseudolumens (asterisks) adjacent to the myoepithelial differentiated cells contain basal lamina and glycosaminoglycans (X4700). (Courtesy of Dr. Irving Dardick, Toronto, Canada.)

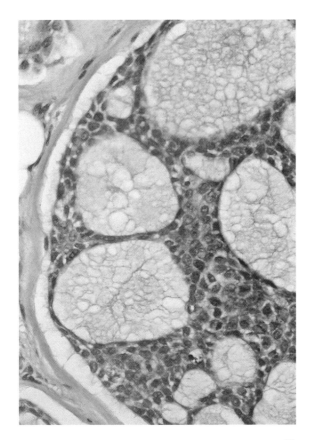 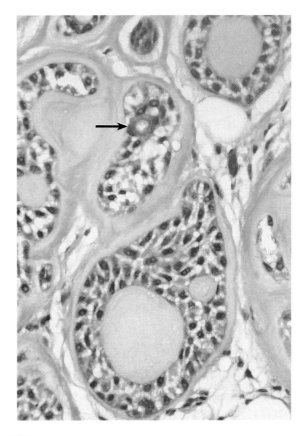

Figure 5-75
ADENOID CYSTIC CARCINOMA
Left: In this field the majority of epithelial tumor cells are uniform in size and shape, with pale eosinophilic to amphophilic cytoplasm and poorly defined boundaries. They surround extra-epithelial cyst-like spaces that contain basophilic material.
Right: Most of these epithelial cells have clear cytoplasm with poorly defined borders and irregular-shaped nuclei. Within these groups of myoepithelial type cells foci of ductal type cells with true lumens can be found. A focus of duct type cells with round nuclei and eosinophilic cytoplasm (arrow) is within a cord of more irregular myoepithelial type cells with clear cytoplasm.

cell borders are indistinct, and the cytoplasm varies from amphophilic to clear. The nuclei are rather uniform in size and vary from darkly basophilic to lightly basophilic with a homogeneous chromatin pattern. Small nucleoli are sometimes evident. The nuclear/cytoplasmic ratio is about 1 to 1. The nuclei are frequently smoothly round to oval, but many are angular and irregular. This angular nuclear pattern is characteristic of adenoid cystic carcinoma; the angular nuclei typically are seen in cells with pale to clear cytoplasm (fig. 5-75).

Among the prominent basaloid myoepithelial cells are scattered foci of ductal cells. These cells surround tiny lumens, which are much smaller than the pseudolumens of the stromal cyst-like spaces (fig. 5-75). The cells are about the same size as the more numerous basaloid myoepithel-

ial cells, but they have eosinophilic cytoplasm; a larger nuclear/cytoplasmic ratio; and uniform, round nuclei, sometimes with small nucleoli.

The tubular pattern is composed of the same two cell types as described for the cribriform pattern. In this pattern, however, the tumor cells are arranged in small nests that are separated from one another (fig. 5-76). The tumor cells may surround individual cyst-like spaces, but continuity of the pseudolumens with the connective tissue stroma is usually more evident than in the cribriform pattern. True duct-type lumens surrounded by differentiated ductal cells are more conspicuous in the tubular pattern (fig. 5-77). Individual tumor nests may contain an inner lumen lined by ductal cells that in turn are surrounded by myoepithelial type cells. The angular nuclei and clear cytoplasm characteristic

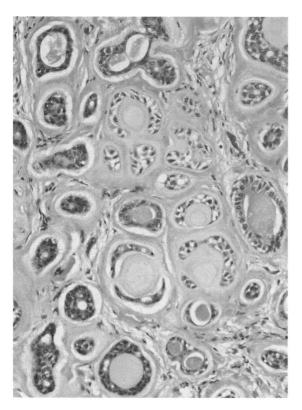

Figure 5-76
ADENOID CYSTIC CARCINOMA:
TUBULAR PATTERN

Tumor cells form small tumor islands in a circular (tubular) pattern around eosinophilic hyalinized or basophilic material. Some of the tubular epithelial structures are embedded within a hyalinized stroma.

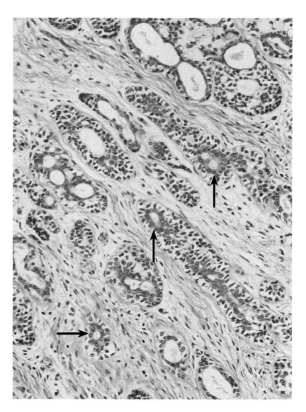

Figure 5-77
ADENOID CYSTIC CARCINOMA:
TUBULAR PATTERN

The myoepithelial type cells with clear cytoplasm and irregular nuclei are very distinct from the more uniform, eosinophilic duct type cells that surround lumens (arrows).

of adenoid cystic carcinoma can usually be identified. The islands of tumor cells are frequently in a hyalinized stroma and may be closely aggregated or more widely separated. Sometimes, the eosinophilic hyaline stroma is so prominent that the tumor cells appear to be squeezed into thin strands, which has been called a trabecular pattern by some (fig. 5-78) (205).

The solid pattern of adenoid cystic carcinoma is characterized by variably sized, rounded or lobulated aggregates of tumor cells in which cyst-like spaces are absent or few (fig. 5-79). The individual tumor cell morphology is similar to that seen in the cribriform and tubular patterns, but many cells are larger, less angular, and have larger nuclei. The cell population is dominated by basaloid myoepithelial type cells, but foci of duct cell differentiation can be found in the tumor lobules (fig. 5-80). Whereas mitotic figures are usually sparse

in the cribriform and tubular patterns, they are more numerous in the solid pattern, in which counts of 5 or more per 10 high-power fields may occur. Also, more cellular and nuclear pleomorphism can be seen in the solid pattern. Tumor cell necrosis is distinctly uncommon in the cribriform and tubular patterns, but it is often a feature of the solid pattern, with individual cell necrosis and comedonecrosis (fig. 5-81). Cribriform and tubular patterns are usually found in association with the solid pattern (see fig. 5-72).

Peripheral nerve invasion is one of the hallmarks of adenoid cystic carcinoma. In fact, the reputation of this tumor to invade nerves has led to the misdiagnosis of other salivary gland carcinomas with neural invasion as adenoid cystic carcinoma. While peripheral nerve invasion is characteristic, it is not pathognomonic of adenoid cystic carcinoma (fig. 5-79). Nerve invasion is

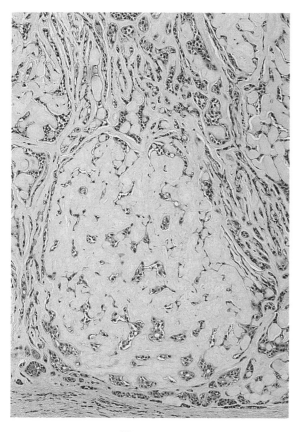

Figure 5-78
ADENOID CYSTIC CARCINOMA
Eosinophilic hyalinized stroma, due to excessive production of basal lamina, contains thin strands of tumor cells.

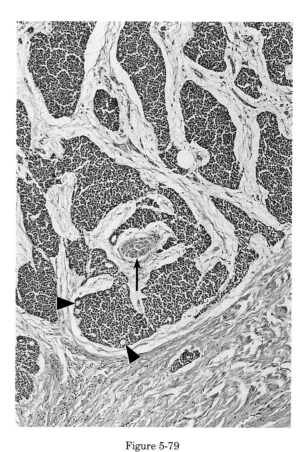

Figure 5-79
ADENOID CYSTIC CARCINOMA: SOLID PATTERN
Densely cellular, irregular-shaped islands of tumor contain only a few small pseudocysts (arrowheads). A peripheral nerve is located in the center of the photograph (arrow).

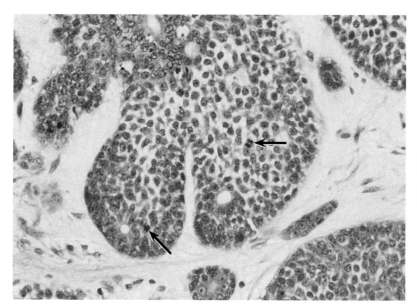

Figure 5-80
ADENOID CYSTIC CARCINOMA:
SOLID PATTERN
At high magnification characteristic cells of adenoid cystic carcinoma have indistinct borders, clear cytoplasm, and irregular nuclei. Mitotic figures are also evident (arrows). A few small lumens form a minor component.

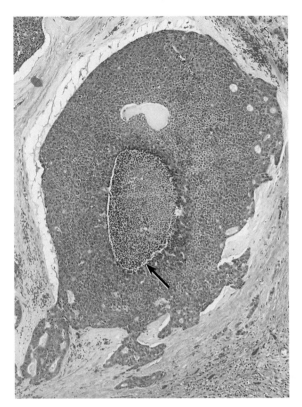

Figure 5-81
ADENOID CYSTIC CARCINOMA: SOLID PATTERN

A central area of comedo-type necrosis (arrow) is evident in this large island of tumor.

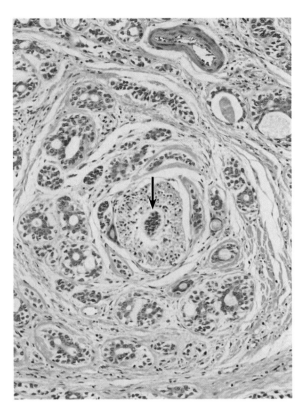

Figure 5-82
NEURAL INVASION BY
ADENOID CYSTIC CARCINOMA

In addition to the tumor nests along the periphery of the nerve, there is a tumor nest within the central portion of the nerve bundle (arrow).

usually perineural within the nerve sheath, but tumor can sometimes be found within the nerve itself (fig. 5-82).

Infiltration of adjacent tissues is characteristic of most malignant tumors and adenoid cystic carcinoma is certainly no exception (fig. 5-83). However, occasionally, small adenoid cystic carcinomas appear remarkably well circumscribed, with minimal evidence of infiltrative growth (fig. 5-84). For these uncommon tumors, diagnosis relies on the characteristic architecture and cytologic features of the tumor.

Ultrastructural Findings. Ultrastructural studies have agreed with the light microscopic findings of bidirectional differentiation of adenoid cystic carcinoma with luminal (ductal) and abluminal (myoepithelial and basal) cells (fig. 5-74) (208,248). The duct-type luminal cells have microvilli on their luminal surface and are joined by desmosomes, interdigitating processes, and terminal bars. They often contain tonofilaments and

rough endoplasmic reticulum. The more abundant abluminal cells that surround the ductal cells and are adjacent to the pseudocysts vary in their ultrastructural features. Many have irregular nuclei and narrow cytoplasmic processes similar to normal myoepithelial cells, and some have prominent amounts of fine filaments with focal dense bodies in their cytoplasm. Other cells lack dense bodies but still have abundant fine filaments. Still others have few fine filaments. Tonofilaments are present in some cells, and desmosomes and hemidesmosomal attachments to the basal lamina in the pseudocysts can be found. The pseudocysts contain reduplicated basal lamina and granulofibrillar proteoglycans. Basal lamina also surrounds the epithelial cell islands. In addition to the pseudocysts, smaller intercellular spaces between the abluminal cells contain granulofibrillar proteoglycans.

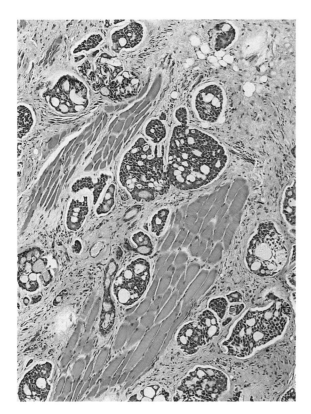

Figure 5-83
INFILTRATION BY ADENOID CYSTIC CARCINOMA
Intermuscular and intramuscular infiltration is evident in this carcinoma of the tongue.

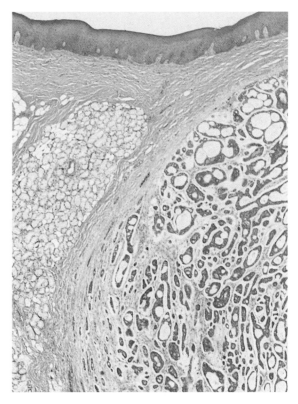

Figure 5-84
ADENOID CYSTIC CARCINOMA OF THE PALATE
This adenoid cystic carcinoma appears remarkably well circumscribed and demarcated from the adjacent mucous salivary gland lobules (left).

Histochemical and Immunohistochemical Findings. The pseudocysts in the cribriform and tubular types of adenoid cystic carcinoma are typically Alcian blue positive. Chondroitin sulfate and heparin sulfate have been identified immunohistochemically (244,246), and Alcian blue positivity is abolished with heparinase and chondroitinase but not hyaluronidase (273). The epithelial-stromal interface and pseudocysts are also reactive to laminin, fibronectin, and type IV collagen (209,214,260,273). These results indicate that the pseudocysts contain components of basement membrane. Differing results have been reported for anti-S-100 protein staining, but most investigators have identified S-100 protein in tumor cells of adenoid cystic carcinoma (fig. 5-85) (213,242,245,250,274). Likewise, disparate results have been reported for anti-glial fibrillary acidic protein (GFAP) (226,245). In studies at the AFIP, limited GFAP reactivity has been observed in some adenoid cystic carcinomas. Coexpression of keratin and vimentin (200,204,211,225,243,260, 274), as well as reactivity for muscle actin and myosin (200,229,253), are indicative of myoepithelial differentiation (fig. 5-85). The ductal differentiated cells that line true lumens are reactive for carcinoembryonic antigen (CEA) (fig. 5-85), epithelial membrane antigen (EMA), and lactoferrin and unreactive for muscle-specific actin, vimentin, and alpha-1-antichymotrypsin; the nonluminal and pseudocyst lining cells react conversely (209,210,224, 270,271). Interestingly, estrogen, progesterone, and progesterone receptor have been immunohistochemically localized in adenoid cystic carcinoma (249); other investigators were unable to demonstrate estrogen receptors in formalin-fixed adenoid cystic carcinoma tissue (240).

The argyrophil staining technique for nucleolar organizer regions (AgNORs) has shown a

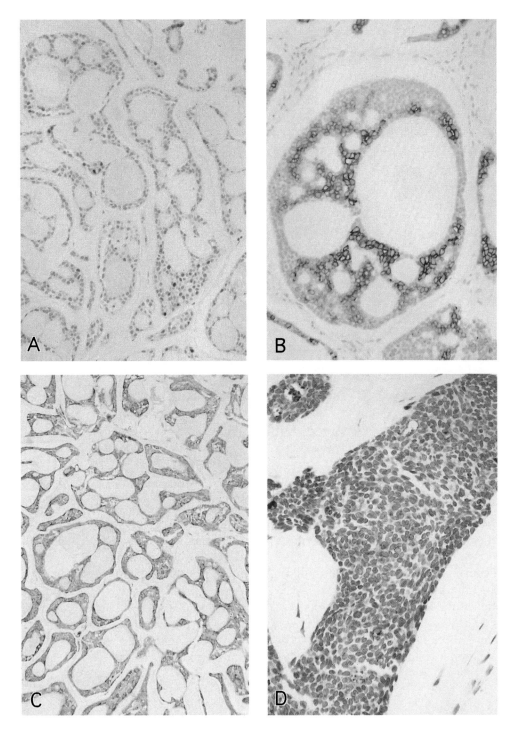

Figure 5-85
ADENOID CYSTIC CARCINOMA: IMMUNOHISTOCHEMISTRY

A: There is mostly nuclear and some cytoplasmic immunoreactivity for S-100 protein in a few of the tumor cells, but reactivity can vary markedly from tumor to tumor and area to area.

B: The immunoreactivity of the tumor cells for cytokeratin is variable in this photograph. In other areas or other adenoid cystic carcinomas the number of reactive cells and the intensity may be more or less.

C: Immunoreactivity for alpha–smooth muscle actin is prominent in this tumor but may be less in other tumors.

D: Luminal surfaces of ductal differentiated cells are most immunoreactive for CEA in this solid type adenoid cystic carcinoma. (Avidin-biotin peroxidase stain)

significantly increased number of AgNORs in adenoid cystic carcinoma compared to normal salivary gland tissue and benign salivary gland tumors (218,221,239,241,278).

Differential Diagnosis. Following its elucidation as a distinct type of salivary gland carcinoma in 1983, PLGA has become one of the principal considerations in the differential diagnosis of adenoid cystic carcinoma; distinguishing between these two tumors is important because of their significantly different biologic behaviors (see Polymorphous Low-Grade Adenocarcinoma). Since PLGA is primarily a tumor of intraoral minor salivary glands, this diagnostic differential is not usually a problem in the major salivary glands. Both tumors are composed of ductal and abluminal myoepithelial differentiated cells, so some histologic similarity is to be expected. Furthering their similarity is the marked propensity of both tumors to infiltrate around peripheral nerves. However, both morphologic and cytologic features allow distinction between these two tumors. PLGA is characterized by a very uniform population of epithelial cells with round, vesicular to euchromatic nuclei and eosinophilic cytoplasm. Mitotic figures and cellular pleomorphism are uncommon in cribriform and tubular types of adenoid cystic carcinoma but are distinctly rare in PLGA. In adenoid cystic carcinoma the characteristic cells are pale to clear staining and angular with angular nuclei, which are usually more hyperchromatic than the nuclei of PLGA. As described above, these cells surround scattered foci of ductal type cells. In PLGA the cells are arranged in variable patterns, which is one of the hallmarks of PLGA. These patterns include cribriform, hyalinized, cystic, sheet-like, glandular, tubular, canalicular, and single-file cords. At low magnification, PLGA often has a swirled appearance that can be described as eye-of-a-storm–like. The pseudocystic, cribriform, and tubular patterns that characterize most adenoid cystic carcinomas are limited when present in PLGA. The solid type adenoid cystic carcinomas nearly always have foci of cribriform or tubular patterns and the characteristic cytologic features described above.

It has been suggested that immunohistochemical staining may help distinguish PLGA from adenoid cystic carcinoma. CEA and EMA reactivity have been reported to be more diffuse in PLGA,

whereas they are confined to the ductal type cells in adenoid cystic carcinoma (222). S-100 protein reactivity also has been described as more prominent and diffuse in PLGA than adenoid cystic carcinoma (222,251), and actin reactivity is greater in adenoid cystic carcinoma (251). On the other hand, Simpson et al. (262) found that the immunohistochemical reactions of the two tumors were not dissimilar enough to be of practical value.

Epithelial-myoepithelial carcinoma (EMC) can be a difficult diagnostic challenge because, like adenoid cystic carcinoma, it has a biphasic cell pattern of ductal cells surrounded by abluminal cells that demonstrate myoepithelial differentiation. This biphasic pattern is usually more conspicuous in EMC than adenoid cystic carcinoma (see Epithelial-Myoepithelial Carcinoma). The periductal cells in EMC are large, polygonal clear cells with rounded nuclei rather than the smaller, angular cells of adenoid cystic carcinoma. These large clear cells often dominate EMC, may grow in sheets, and contain notable amounts of glycogen. EMC does not grow in a cribriform pattern, but it may have a tubular appearance and marked basal lamina production that forms hyalinized areas in the stroma. Since the same two cell types are proliferating in both neoplasms, immunohistochemistry is not much help although the clear cells in EMC react weakly or not at all for cytokeratin.

Mixed tumor is not often confused with adenoid cystic carcinoma, but since both are composed of neoplastic myoepithelial and ductal type cells, foci within mixed tumors may resemble adenoid cystic carcinoma (see Mixed Tumor). The characteristic myxochondroid areas and the plasmacytoid and spindled myoepithelial cells that are common in mixed tumor are not evident in adenoid cystic carcinoma. In mixed tumors dense aggregates of myoepithelial type cells are arranged around ductal type cells but become less dense with increasing distance from the ductal structure as they blend into the myxochondroid areas. In adenoid cystic carcinoma the tumor cells are usually well demarcated from the surrounding stroma.

Basaloid squamous cell carcinoma is a recently described variant of squamous cell carcinoma of the upper aerodigestive tract and has features that resemble adenoid cystic carcinoma (fig. 5-86) (201,235,281). Basaloid squamous cell carcinoma has a predilection for the hypopharynx, base of

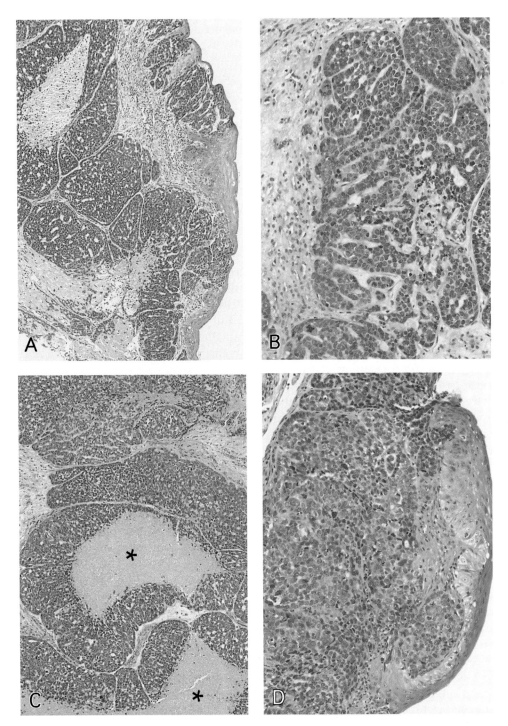

Figure 5-86
BASALOID SQUAMOUS CELL CARCINOMA

A: Variably shaped aggregates of small, basaloid cells involve the mucosal stratified squamous epithelium as well as the lamina propria of the posterior tongue.

B: Relatively uniform, small, round cells with scant cytoplasm compose tumor islands with focal, small lumen-like spaces that impart a glandular appearance. Some of these pseudoluminal areas contain eosinophilic hyaline material.

C: Areas of comedonecrosis (asterisks) are common.

D: The basaloid epithelial cells are in intimate association with dysplastic stratified squamous epithelium of the mucosal surface.

tongue, and supraglottic larynx, regions where adenoid cystic carcinoma occurs infrequently. This tumor is composed of small, hyperchromatic cells that form solid lobules, adenomatoid arrangements, and cords. The tumor aggregates are frequently associated with eosinophilic hyaline material and comedonecrosis. However, basaloid squamous cell carcinoma has a squamous component that distinguishes it from the solid type of adenoid cystic carcinoma. This component usually involves the mucosal epithelium in the form of epithelial dysplasia, carcinoma in situ, or invasive squamous cell carcinoma, but foci of squamoid cells also occur in the basaloid lobules. Immunohistochemically, basaloid squamous cell carcinoma is reported to be unreactive for muscle-specific actin, and CEA reactivity occurs in the squamoid cells rather than the ductal cells, in contrast to adenoid cystic carcinoma (201).

Prognosis and Treatment. Adenoid cystic carcinoma has an undesirable but deserved reputation for indolent but persistent and recurrent growth, late onset of metastases, and eventual death of patients. In contrast to other carcinomas with poor survival statistics, adenoid cystic carcinoma, in general, has a good 5-year survival rate. However, the 10- to 20-year survival rates are low. Therefore, categorizing adenoid cystic carcinomas into high- and low-grade types is somewhat deceptive since the long-term survival is often poor even with so-called low-grade tumors. Nevertheless, different biologic courses can be predicted for adenoid cystic carcinoma by histologic criteria. These prognoses are based upon morphologic growth patterns.

The general consensus is that adenoid cystic carcinomas with tubular or cribriform growth patterns have a better prognosis than those with solid growth patterns (202,223,227,237,247,254,265, 268). Although there is some disagreement about whether there is any difference in survival rates between the tubular and the cribriform patterns, all investigators agree that carcinomas with a solid growth pattern have the most fulminant course, which is characterized by early metastasis and a poor 5-year survival. The cribriform pattern has been reported to have a higher rate of local recurrence and local failure than the tubular pattern (237). Since many adenoid cystic carcinomas display multiple patterns, grading is not always straightforward. Szanto et al. (268) found that any

solid areas worsened the prognosis (their grade II) and that tumors with more than 30 percent solid areas had the worst prognosis (their grade III). They reported 15-year cumulative survival rates for patients with tumors that had none, less than 30 percent, and more than 30 percent solid areas to be 39 percent, 26 percent, and 5 percent, respectively. Greiner et al. (223) also found that survival was very poor for patients with tumors with more than 30 percent solid pattern. In the cribriform pattern, however, Santucci and Bondi (255) found a positive correlation between the number of gland-like spaces per square millimeter of tumor and the survival interval of the patient.

Contradictory results have been reported on the relationship between perineural tumor invasion and development of metastases: van der Wal et al. (277) found no significant correlation; Vrielinck et al. (280) found that 40 percent of tumors with perineural invasion subsequently metastasized but none without perineural growth metastasized. Luna et al. (234) correlated invasion of nerves larger than 0.25 mm with aggressive clinical behavior for submandibular adenoid cystic carcinoma.

Of course, in addition to histologic pattern, clinical stage has a major influence on prognosis and may be a better predictor than grade. Spiro and Huvos (265) reported cumulative 10-year survivals of 75 percent, 43 percent, and 15 percent for patients with stages I, II, and III and IV, respectively. Hamper et al. (227) found that tumor size greater than 4 cm was correlated with an unfavorable clinical course in all cases. Primary site may also be a factor. Parotid gland tumors have a better prognosis than submandibular gland tumors. Nascimento et al. (247) reported that minor salivary gland tumors had an overall worse prognosis than major gland tumors, but others have found no such difference (212,238).

Cytophotometry to evaluate nuclear DNA content has had mixed results as a predictor of clinical outcome. Several investigators have found that patients with diploid tumors had longer survival times and less morbidity than those with aneuploid histograms (219,227,234). Greiner et al. (223) reported that 35 of 37 adenoid cystic carcinomas were diploid, and thus DNA content was not very useful for prognosis. However, they did find that there was a higher incidence of tumors with high S-phase fractions among patients who did poorly. Eibling et al. (216) found that DNA ploidy had only limited value. Aneuploidy and high S-phase fraction seem to correlate with the solid histologic pattern (219,234,252). Yamamoto et al. (283) found that as the disease progresses tumors may actually transform from a tubular pattern in the early stages to a cribriform pattern and finally to a solid pattern in the later stages.

Unlike most other types of salivary gland carcinoma, distant metastases are far more frequent than regional lymph node metastases with adenoid cystic carcinoma. About 40 to 60 percent of patients develop distant metastases (199,212, 238,259), most commonly to the lung, bone, and soft tissues (261), and distant metastases often develop despite local control of the tumor (237).

Wide to radical surgical excision and postoperative radiation therapy offer the best chance for long-term survival (206,215,266). While radiation therapy alone seems to be inadequate for adenoid cystic carcinoma, as an adjunct to surgery it has been shown to improve local control of tumor, especially when there is microscopic residual tumor (199,230,231,233,238,247,259, 272,276,279). However, gross residual tumor portends a poor outcome. Chemotherapeutic treatment of adenoid cystic carcinoma has received limited attention, but in the past cisplatin and recently, high-dose melphalan has shown some favorable results (256,258,263).

POLYMORPHOUS LOW-GRADE ADENOCARCINOMA

Definition. Polymorphous low-grade adenocarcinoma (PLGA) is a malignant epithelial tumor that is essentially limited to occurrence in minor salivary gland sites and is characterized by bland, uniform nuclear features; diverse but characteristic architecture; infiltrative growth; and prominent neurotropism.

General Features. PLGA was first identified as a specific salivary gland adenocarcinoma in 1983 by two independent groups of investigators. Freedman and Lumerman (292) first reported 12 cases as lobular carcinoma and the following month Batsakis et al. (286) reported 12 as terminal duct carcinoma. The term lobular carcinoma was suggested because of the resemblance of the neoplasm to infiltrating lobular carcinoma of the

breast whereas terminal duct implied the histogenetic origin. The following year the term polymorphous low-grade adenocarcinoma was suggested as a clinically and morphologically descriptive term (290) and is currently preferred (308). Since some cases demonstrated prominent papillary-cystic growth, papillary and nonpapillary variants were distinguished in subsequent reports (291,294,302,311). It was observed that the so-called papillary variant was more likely to recur, metastasize to regional and distant sites, and result in the death of the patient (316). While PLGA may have a focal papillary component, tumors that have an exclusive papillary pattern and lack other characteristic features of PLGA are best classified as cystadenocarcinomas or other carcinomas, depending on the features present (310).

Since the original recognition and description of PLGA, it has been recognized that its frequency among all minor salivary gland tumors is substantial. In a series of 426 minor salivary gland tumors, Waldron and colleagues (315) found that PLGA represented 11 percent of all tumors and 26 percent of those that were malignant. A similar frequency was observed in a study of a predominantly black population (excluding the two papillary cases for the reasons cited above); PLGA was the most common salivary malignancy in that series (313). In AFIP data since 1985, PLGA comprises 7.4 percent of minor salivary gland tumors and 19.6 percent of those that are malignant. These data indicate that in minor gland sites PLGA is twice as frequent as adenoid cystic carcinoma, and among all benign and malignant salivary gland tumors only mixed tumor and mucoepidermoid carcinoma are more common.

PLGA occurs almost exclusively in minor salivary gland sites. Over 60 percent of tumors in the AFIP files occurred in the mucosa of either the soft or hard palates, about 16 percent occurred in the buccal mucosa, and 12 percent in the upper lip. Only one tumor occurred in the lower lip. The remaining tumors were found at scattered sites such as the retromolar region, floor of mouth, and tongue. Although the AFIP has not seen any tumors in the major glands, single examples in American (307) and Australian (301) patients and two instances each in patients from Japan (297,299) and the Netherlands (310) have been reported. PLGA has also been reported in the major glands as the carcinomatous component of carcinoma ex mixed tumor (286,312). One tumor involved both the submandibular and parotid glands but occurred 8 years after the diagnosis of mixed tumor and may also represent carcinoma ex mixed tumor (295). Origin from the seromucous glands of the nasopharynx (317) and nose (289,293) has also been reported.

The initial report of PLGA noted that all 12 patients were female (292) but subsequent reports included a substantial number of male patients (284,286,290). Nevertheless, over 70 percent of civilian patients in AFIP data are female, a proportion greater than for malignant salivary gland tumors in general. The female to male ratio is about 2 to 1 among published cases (314). The average age of patients is 59 years, with a range of 21 to 94 years; over 70 percent of patients are between the ages of 50 and 79 years. It appears that there may be a predilection for this tumor to occur in blacks. Whereas less than 11 percent of all malignant salivary gland tumors in AFIP files occur in blacks, 27 percent of these tumors do. At least one other study of Americans has reported a similar observation (290), and a preponderance of PLGA in an African population has been noted (313).

Clinical Features. PLGA characteristically presents as a firm, nontender swelling of otherwise normal mucosa of the hard and soft palates, often at their junction; the cheek; or upper lip (fig. 5-87). Discomfort is sometimes experienced. As with other tumors in these sites, bleeding, telangiectasia, or ulceration of the overlying mucosa may occasionally occur. The duration of lesion has varied from weeks to as many as 30 years (284,286,290,292,314). Most tumors are less than 2 cm in diameter, but examples with dimensions as large as 6 cm have been observed (284). Large tumors of the floor of the mouth infrequently secondarily involve the sublingual gland and result in a clinically observable neck mass. Lesions overlying bone occasionally erode or infiltrate bone, and this warrants routine radiographic evaluation of tumors at these sites.

Gross Findings. PLGA usually appears as an ovoid, circumscribed but unencapsulated mass that approximates the surface epithelium, which is rarely ulcerated. Although some tumors focally appear distinctly separate from adjacent salivary gland lobules, in other areas they usually are poorly demarcated. The cut surface is

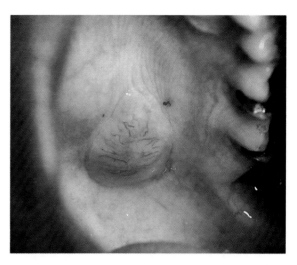

Figure 5-87
POLYMORPHOUS LOW-GRADE ADENOCARCINOMA
This tumor presented as a well-circumscribed, slow growing mass at the junction of the hard and soft palates. Pronounced telangiectasia of the overlying mucosa is evident. (Courtesy of Dr. Richard Canaan, Ocean Springs, MS.)

homogeneously tan and has a glistening surface and uniformly firm texture.

Microscopic Findings. As its name implies, PLGA demonstrates a wide variety of morphologic growth patterns from one tumor to the next and within the same tumor. However, its recognition is facilitated by the unique combination of certain architectural features and the bland cytomorphologic features that are present in all cases.

With low-power examination, PLGA often appears well circumscribed but focally infiltrative (fig. 5-88). The central portion of the tumor is usually solid or lobulated, but in the peripheral areas small lobules, islands, and columns of cells extend into surrounding connective tissue or salivary parenchyma (fig. 5-89). These neoplastic structures in many tumors approximate the overlying surface epithelium (fig. 5-90). The solid areas frequently resemble one or more of several other benign and malignant salivary gland tumors, so it is important that microscopic examination is not limited to the central portion of the tumor.

Various growth patterns within individual tumors and among different tumors include solid, trabecular, ductular, and tubular formations, and these usually account for large portions of each lesion (fig. 5-91). Cribriform, cystic, and papillary-cystic architecture are often present in focal areas but they do not predominate (fig. 5-92). One

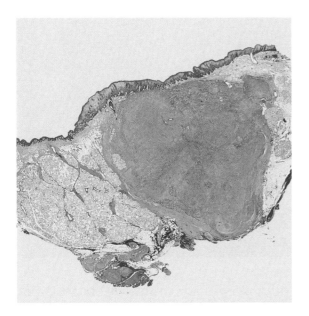

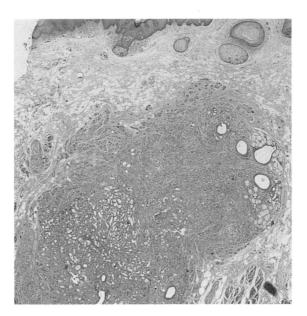

Figure 5-88
POLYMORPHOUS LOW-GRADE ADENOCARCINOMA
At low magnification these two examples appear at least partially circumscribed but lack encapsulation.

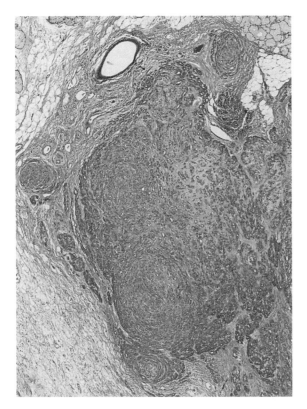

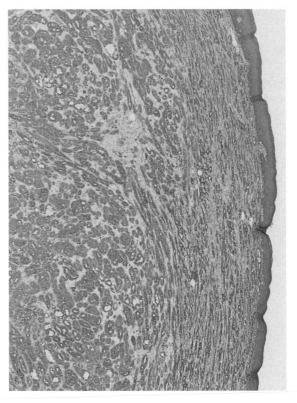

Figure 5-89
POLYMORPHOUS LOW-GRADE ADENOCARCINOMA
Characteristically, small islands of tumor cells are found distant from the central portion of the tumor and infiltrate salivary gland parenchyma, fat, and fibrous connective tissue.

Figure 5-90
POLYMORPHOUS LOW-GRADE ADENOCARCINOMA
Parallel cords of tumor cells extend from the more tubular, main part of the tumor to the surface epithelium.

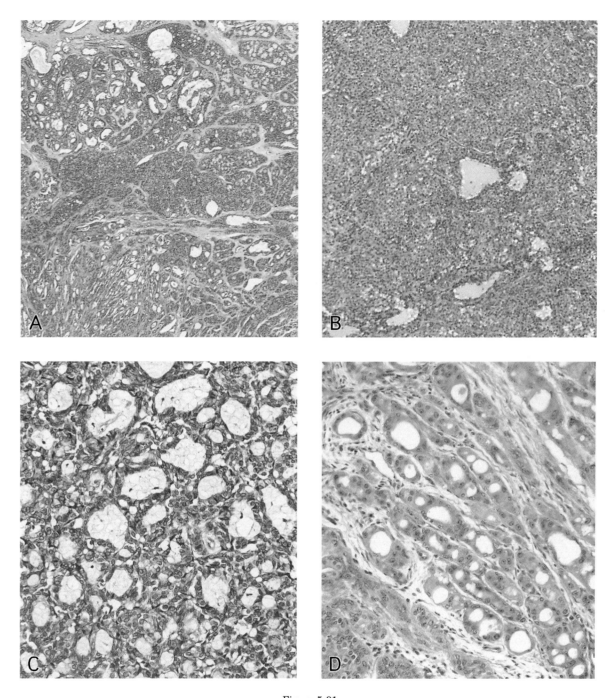

Figure 5-91
MORPHOLOGIC VARIABILITY
Architecturally, polymorphous low-grade adenocarcinoma shows various combinations of solid, ductal, trabecular, and tubular growth.

of the characteristic features is formation of small tubular structures that have distinct central lumens lined by a single layer of cuboidal cells. These occur as isolated structures or in clusters. In either case they are often more numerous peripheral to the central area of the tumor where they are seen infiltrating muscle, connective tissues, and salivary glands (fig. 5-93). They are often closely

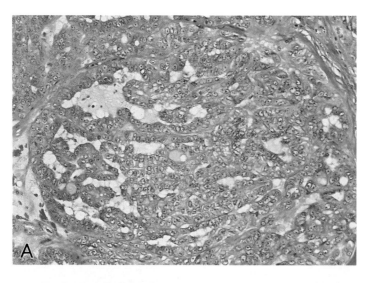

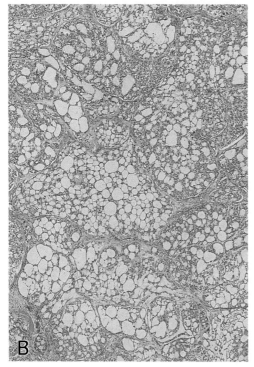

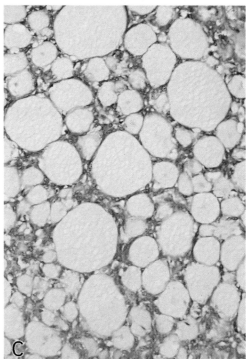

Figure 5-92
POLYMORPHOUS LOW-GRADE ADENOCARCINOMA

A: This tumor focally demonstrates minimal papillary growth into ductal or small cystic spaces.

B: Cribriform growth is focally predominant in this unusual case. The pseudocystic spaces contain pale-staining, amorphous, amphophilic mucoid material.

C: High-magnification examination reveals spaces partially encircled by uniform vesicular nuclei that are unlike the small, angular, hyperchromatic nuclei of adenoid cystic carcinoma.

associated and aligned with streaming columns and trabeculae of cells that display concentric whorling, creating a target-like appearance (fig. 5-94). This concentric arrangement is present in about one third of tumors (292). An orderly arrangement of individual and interconnecting cords of tumor cells are often parallel to the convex, more solid, central body of tumor or

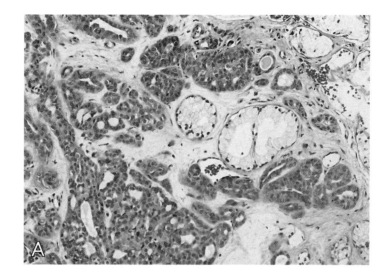

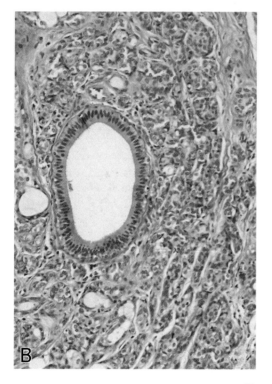

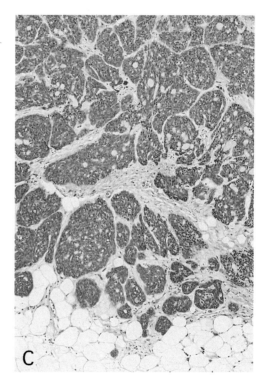

Figure 5-93
INFILTRATIVE GROWTH
A: Individual and groups of small, tubular structures that have morphologically bland nuclei have infiltrated and partially replaced minor salivary gland tissue. This is one of the most characteristic features of polymorphous low-grade adenocarcinoma.
B: Although all acini have been replaced in this field, a single persistent duct is completely surrounded by tumor.
C: Infiltration into peripheral fat and connective tissue is evident.

haphazardly infiltrate a considerable distance into surrounding tissues (fig. 5-95). Because PLGA can invade bone, histologic evaluation of maxillary or mandibular bone specimens is indicated (fig. 5-96).

The majority of tumor cells are isomorphic. They have round, ovoid, or fusiform nuclei that have finely stippled chromatin and either inconspicuous or slightly enlarged nucleoli (fig. 5-97).

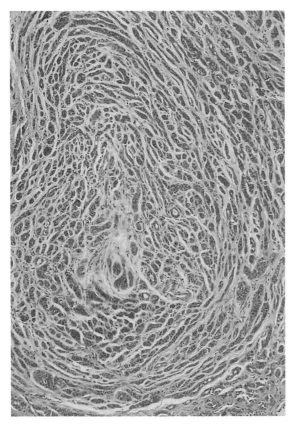

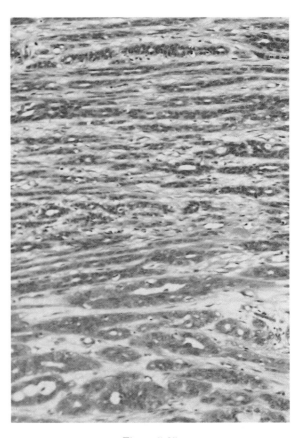

Figure 5-94
POLYMORPHOUS LOW-GRADE ADENOCARCINOMA
Tumor cells are often concentrically arranged around a central point, as in this example, creating a unique targetoid appearance.

Figure 5-95
POLYMORPHOUS LOW-GRADE ADENOCARCINOMA
Streaming rows and cords of tumor cells contain numerous tubular formations with distinct lumens.

Figure 5-96
INFILTRATION OF BONE
This decalcified section of maxilla reveals destruction of bone by tumor. Maxillary involvement was radiographically detected prior to surgery in this case.

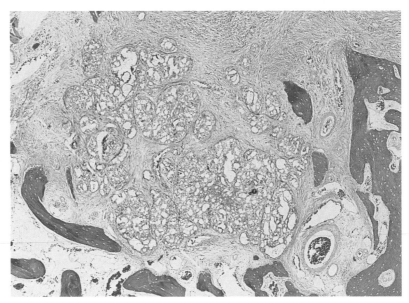

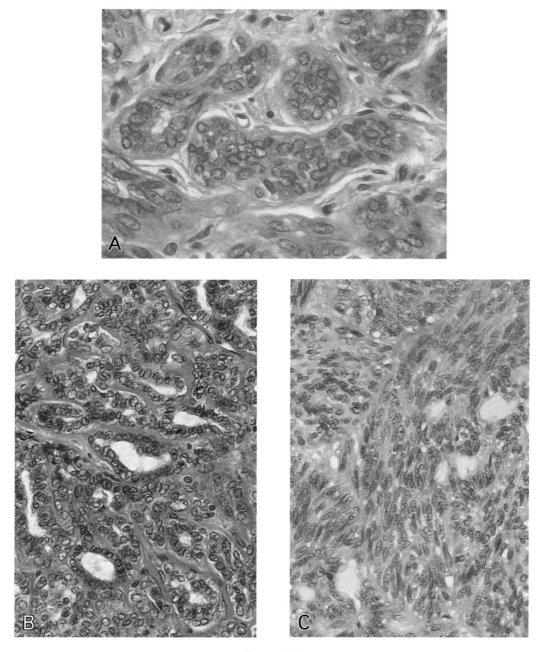

Figure 5-97
BLAND NUCLEAR MORPHOLOGY
The nuclei in these polymorphous low-grade adenocarcinomas are round, ovoid, or spindled; have only slightly irregular contours and finely dispersed chromatin; and have either inconspicuous or small, single nucleoli.

The tumor nuclei stain with the same intensity as the nuclei in normal salivary tissue. Mitoses are rare, and atypical mitoses are not seen. The eosinophilic cytoplasm is scant and the cell borders indistinct. Variably present are oncocytes (fig. 5-98), clear cells, and, rarely, mucous cells which are often difficult to distinguish from residual mucous acini or cells. The neoplastic epithelium is usually associated with limited collagenous stroma, but more abundant hyaline or muco-hyaline stroma often develops around more widely spaced epithelial structures (fig. 5-99).

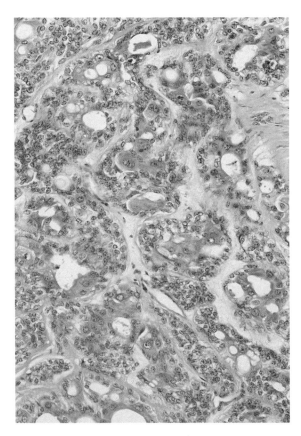

Figure 5-98
FOCAL ONCOCYTIC CHANGE
Discrete collections of cells with abundant, brightly eosinophilic cytoplasm comprise portions of many of the neoplastic structures.

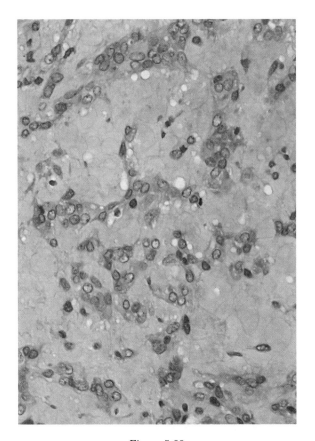

Figure 5-99
VARIABLE STROMA
Most tumors contain relatively limited stroma, but some have areas with abundant mucohyaline or mucoid stroma, adding to their polymorphous appearance.

Crystalloids that resemble the tyrosine-rich crystals in some mixed tumors have been reported in 3 to 5 percent of cases (288,305). They occur within either the neoplastic epithelial or stromal elements (fig. 5-100). Psammoma-like calcifications also are occasionally evident.

A frequent finding is perineural infiltration (fig. 5-101); this occurs more often than with any other salivary gland carcinoma, including adenoid cystic carcinoma. Perivascular involvement is also common but less frequent than perineural infiltration. The involved nerves and blood vessels are often wrapped in several layers of concentrically arranged tumor cells.

Immunohistochemical and Ultrastructural Findings. The neoplastic cells of PLGA are immunoreactive with antibodies to cytokeratin, vimentin, muscle-specific actin, epithelial membrane antigen, carcinoembryonic antigen, and glial fibrillary acidic protein (GFAP) (285,296, 298,300,304,306). It has been suggested that immunohistochemistry can help distinguish PLGA from mixed tumor and adenoid cystic carcinoma (285, 296). Although some subtle differences may be apparent when series of tumors are studied, the variability in cellular immunoreactivity among these tumors and the subjectivity inherent in some interpretations limit the usefulness of immunohistochemistry in individual cases.

Electron microscopy demonstrates the presence of sheets of randomly arranged cells with occasional areas that contain duct-like structures; these structures have peripheral basal lamina and short intraluminal microvilli (294,300,303, 304). Ovoid and fusiform cells with electron-lucent cytoplasm are intermingled with

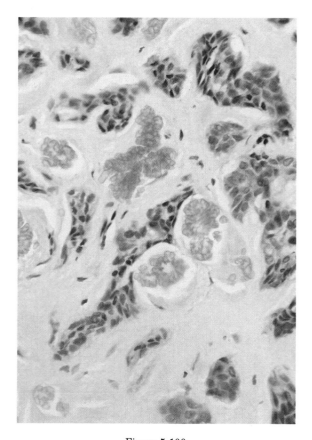

Figure 5-100
CRYSTALLOIDS
Radially arranged cylinders form petal-like structures in the stroma of this polymorphous low-grade adenocarcinoma.

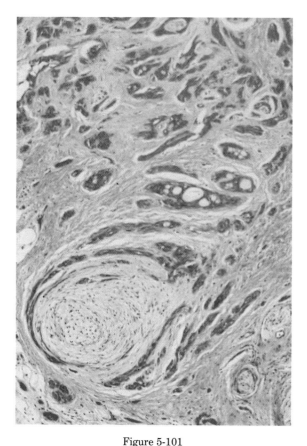

Figure 5-101
PERINEURAL INFILTRATION
Involvement of peripheral nerves is nearly always seen with this tumor. However, because neural invasion occurs in any malignant salivary gland tumor, this finding is not used as a feature for tumor classification.

those having denser cytoplasm. Some cells are widely separated by abundant, amorphous intercellular material (fig. 5-102). The cytoplasm of some cells contains intermediate filaments, and well-formed junctional complexes are evident.

Differential Diagnosis. Based on published reports and AFIP cases, the salivary gland tumors most apt to create problems in distinction from PLGA are mixed tumor, carcinoma ex mixed tumor, and adenoid cystic carcinoma (286,287,292).

Mixed tumor and PLGA have hyaline or mucohyaline stroma that contains sheets of neoplastic epithelial cells with morphologically bland nuclei and scattered, well-formed ductal or tubular structures (fig. 5-103). Although mixed tumors of the minor glands are typically not encapsulated, they do not infiltrate surrounding connective tissue, fat, parenchyma, nerves, or

blood vessels like PLGA. For this reason, it is critical that the biopsy tissue include the interface of tumor with surrounding tissue (fig. 5-104). Unlike mixed tumor, the tubular or ductal structures in PLGA often are entirely isolated from the more solid tumor areas and more often than mixed tumors are lined by a single row of similar cells. Although myxoid tissue is present in mixed tumor and PLGA, the myxochondroid and chondroid zones present in mixed tumor are not evident in PLGA (fig. 5-105).

The diagnosis of carcinoma ex mixed tumor is based upon identification of characteristic benign mixed tumor and focal transformation to carcinoma. The carcinomatous areas usually demonstrate atypical nuclear morphology (see section Carcinoma Ex Mixed Tumor). In rare instances, carcinomas arising in mixed tumors

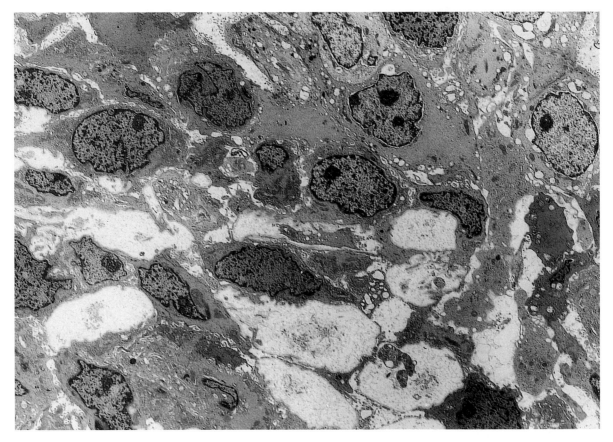

Figure 5-102
POLYMORPHOUS LOW-GRADE ADENOCARCINOMA
This stroma-rich area shows haphazardly arranged cells that vary in electron density. Abundant intercellular deposits are present and formation of microvilli is seen in several areas (X1,100).

Figure 5-103
POLYMORPHOUS LOW-GRADE
ADENOCARCINOMA
The ductal structures are surrounded by loosely arranged ovoid and spindled cells, resembling the myoepithelial-rich zones in mixed tumors.

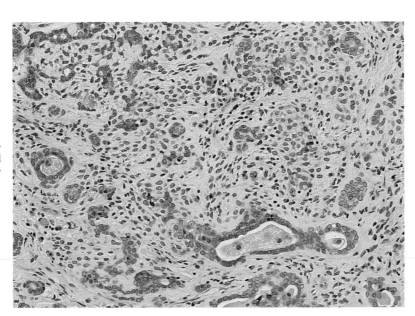

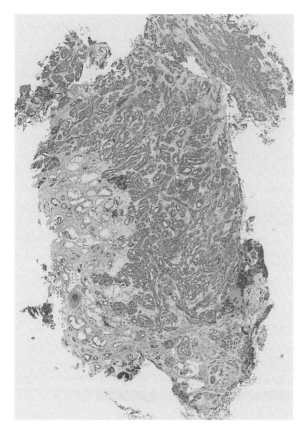

Figure 5-104
FRAGMENTED BIOPSY
Unlike fragmented biopsies of mixed tumor, fragments of PLGA may contain ductal structures that infiltrate and destroy minor salivary gland tissue.

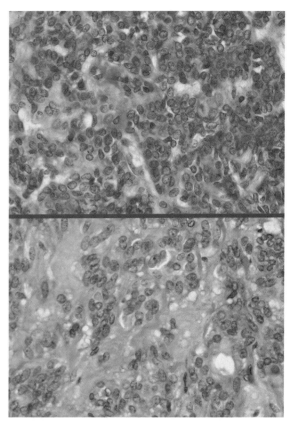

Figure 5-105
MIXED TUMOR VERSUS POLYMORPHOUS LOW-GRADE ADENOCARCINOMA
Distinguishing mixed tumor from PLGA is often not possible on a cytomorphologic basis, and necessitates evaluation of the tumor interface with adjacent tissues. The nuclear features of mixed tumor (top) are similar to those of PLGA (bottom). In this instance, mucoid stroma is more abundant in the PLGA.

resemble PLGA (286,312). Nevertheless, in typical PLGA the nuclei of the epithelium in all areas, including those that contain mucohyaline stroma, are uniformly bland.

Most adenoid cystic carcinomas, like PLGA, are characterized by isomorphic nuclei, little mitotic activity, focal mucohyaline stroma, extensive infiltration of adjacent tissues, prominent neurotropism, and cribriform tubular and solid growth. These similarities have led some investigators to consider that PLGA may represent a less aggressive variant of adenoid cystic carcinoma (284,286). There are features that help distinguish the two. The nuclei in PLGA are slightly larger, rounder, and more uniform than the angular hyperchromatic nuclei in adenoid cystic carcinoma (fig. 5-106). Cytoplasmic staining of the cells is usually eosinophilic in PLGA and clear in ade-

noid cystic carcinomas. PLGA does not have large cribriform pseudocystic spaces that contain pools of hematoxyphilic glycosaminoglycans. Solid cellular areas in PLGA, unlike those in the solid variant of adenoid cystic carcinoma, contain many tubular structures and do not show nuclear pleomorphism, focal necrosis, or increased mitotic activity (see Adenoid Cystic Carcinoma).

Prognosis and Treatment. Although the number of cases of PLGA with long-term follow-up is limited, mean follow-up of patients in one study was over 14 years (290), and other studies have followed individual cases as long as 11 to 37 years (284,311). Excluding those cases reported as PLGA in which there was prominent papillary-cystic growth, only one patient has died of disease,

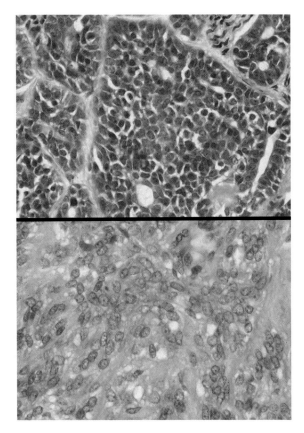

Figure 5-106
ADENOID CYSTIC CARCINOMA
The smaller, more angular and hyperchromatic nuclei of adenoid cystic carcinoma (top) contrast with those of PLGA (bottom).

apparently as a result of direct tumor extension into vital structures of the head (284). The reported recurrence rate in these studies ranged from 0 to nearly 30 percent and included patients whose tumors were incompletely excised (284, 285,290,300,309,314). A recent review of 204 published cases revealed a 17 percent recurrence rate and a regional metastasis rate of 9 percent (314). Some patients have multiple recurrences, and recurrences develop from months to many years after initial treatment, which indicates a need for long-term follow-up. In large series with follow-up data, metastasis to regional lymph nodes occurred in just under 10 percent of patients and there was no metastasis to distant sites (284,290,300).

For most PLGAs wide but conservative surgical excision is appropriate. The size of the tumor and whether or not there is bone involvement determine the extent of the excisional procedure. In instances where tumor overlies bone, such as the palate and retromolar region, radiographic evaluation is recommended. Involvement of the maxilla may necessitate a partial maxillectomy; however, maxillectomy is unnecessary in the absence of invasion into bone. Likewise, invasion of mandibular bone requires en bloc resection. Soft tissue and bony surgical margins should be free of tumor. Neck dissection is not warranted unless there is clinical evidence of lymph node involvement (316). There is no evidence that indicates a benefit from postoperative radiation or adjuvant chemotherapy, although both modalities have been used (284,286,290,292).

MALIGNANT MIXED TUMORS

The broad, generic heading for this section, malignant mixed tumors, includes three distinct pathologic entities. Carcinoma ex mixed tumor comprises the vast majority while carcinosarcoma (true malignant mixed tumor) and metastasizing mixed tumor are extremely rare.

Carcinoma Ex Mixed Tumor (Carcinoma Ex Pleomorphic Adenoma)

Definition. This is a carcinoma that shows histologic evidence of arising in or from a benign mixed tumor. Diagnosis requires identification of benign tumor. Unlike carcinosarcomas, only the epithelial component is malignant. Although most of these tumors are obviously infiltrative, rarely the carcinoma may be confined by the capsule; these are further categorized as in situ or noninvasive. Most often the carcinomatous element represents undifferentiated carcinoma or adenocarcinoma, not otherwise specified, but occasionally other types, such as mucoepidermoid carcinoma or adenoid cystic carcinoma, occur (328).

In the past, some investigators suggested that some of these tumors develop as de novo malignancies in which the carcinomatous element has morphologic and cytologic characteristics of benign mixed tumor (319,325,334). This concept was disputed by Livolsi and Perzin (332) who reported that these tumors all contained residual benign mixed tumor. They were able to identify zones of transition between benign and malignant tumor in many cases. Among AFIP cases, malignant transformation of benign mixed tumor can often be histologically substantiated. To satisfy the definition of carcinoma ex mixed tumor: 1) at least a focus of benign mixed tumor must be identified or 2) a previously benign mixed tumor must have been excised from a site in which recurrent tumor is carcinomatous. In some cases carcinoma probably completely replaces a preexisting benign mixed tumor; however, history of a longstanding mass, by itself, is not acceptable evidence of the preexistence of mixed tumor.

General Features. Gnepp (326) reviewed 60 recently published series of carcinoma ex mixed tumors: the average incidence was 3.6 percent of all salivary gland tumors, 6.2 percent of all mixed tumors, and 11.6 percent of all malignant tumors. There was considerable variation in the incidence of carcinoma ex mixed tumor among these series. For instance, the proportion of carcinoma ex mixed tumor among all malignant salivary gland tumors ranged from 2.8 to 42.4 percent. At the AFIP, material reviewed since the beginning of 1985 showed carcinoma ex mixed tumors to be 8.8 percent of all mixed tumors and 4.6 percent of all malignant salivary gland tumors. This ranks it as the sixth most common salivary gland malignancy following mucoepidermoid carcinoma; adenocarcinoma, not otherwise specified; acinic cell adenocarcinoma; polymorphous low-grade adenocarcinoma; and adenoid cystic carcinoma.

In the Grepp review, the approximate frequencies for occurrence of carcinoma ex mixed tumors in the parotid, submandibular, sublingual, and minor glands are 67, 15, less than 1, and 18 percent, respectively (326). The frequency of occurrence in major glands is higher than would be predicted solely on the basis of the distribution of benign mixed tumors. At the AFIP 86 percent of all carcinoma ex mixed tumors occur in the major glands compared to only 71 percent of all mixed tumors. This difference probably relates to the much higher recurrence rate of benign mixed tumors in the major than in the minor glands. Longevity and recurrence are risks for malignant transformation. Eneroth and Zetterberg (321,323, 324) have shown that the incidence of malignant transformation in mixed tumors increases with the duration of the tumor: the incidence was 1.6 percent for tumors with durations of 5 years or less

but 9.6 percent in those present for more than 15 years. Microspectrophotometric analysis of a small number of their cases showed that tumor cells in mixed tumor of longer duration developed a tetraploid fraction similar to that found in the carcinomas.

A comparison of patient age between carcinoma ex mixed tumors and benign mixed tumors in the AFIP's cases showed that the carcinomas occur, on average, about 13 years later than the adenomas (46.9 verses 60.1 years). Carcinoma ex mixed tumor is extremely unusual in patients under 30 years of age (2.9 percent in AFIP cases) and was not encountered in two large series of salivary gland tumors in children (329,330). Like others (340,342), the AFIP has seen a slight female predilection (53 percent), but in one series female patients comprised 75 percent (332).

Clinical Features. Livolsi and Perzin (332) found that about 20 percent of patients had one or more operations for mixed tumor before the diagnosis of carcinoma ex mixed tumor was established. Most patients with carcinoma ex mixed tumor, however, had been aware of a previously untreated salivary gland mass for many years. In slightly more than half of their patients, the mass was present for a period of 3 to 41 years, and one third of these were aware of recent, rapid growth or ulceration. Spiro and colleagues (340) noted that about 20 percent of their patients had known of their tumors for more than 20 years. As previously noted, the risk of malignant transformation correlates with the duration of the mixed tumor.

The most common clinical presentation of carcinoma ex mixed tumor, regardless of the history, is a painless mass (332,340), although sometimes the mass is associated with pain or facial nerve palsy. Seifert and colleagues (336) found that 36 percent of their patients had facial paralysis. The neoplasm is sometimes freely movable but often fixed to underlying soft tissue or bone, especially in patients with recurrent tumors (340).

Gross and Microscopic Findings. Grossly, carcinoma ex mixed tumor is usually poorly circumscribed and often extensively infiltrative (326); occasionally it is circumscribed or even completely encapsulated (332,335). The average sizes recorded by LiVolsi and Perzin (332) were 4.4, 5.0, and 2.2 cm, respectively, for tumors in the parotid, submandibular, and minor salivary glands, with a

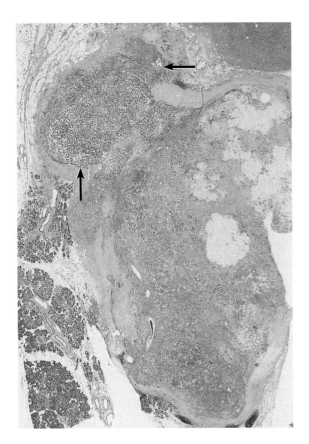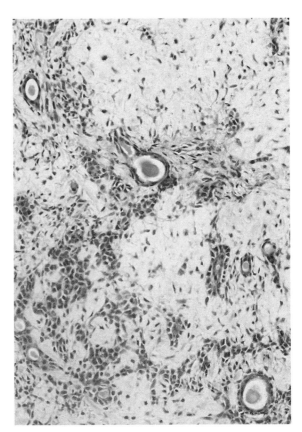

Figure 5-107
CARCINOMA EX MIXED TUMOR

Left: There is a prominent myxochondroid element characteristic of benign mixed tumor in the right center and top of this illustration. A hypercellular carcinomatous component extends into periparotid fat (arrow).

Right: Higher magnification of the benign element shows complete lack of cytologic abnormalities and a typical chondromyxomatous elements.

range of 0.5 to 12 cm for all sites. The tumors are white or tan-gray, and hemorrhage, necrosis, and central cystic degeneration are common.

Microscopically, benign mixed tumor comprises a variable proportion of the entire mass. Myxoid, chondroid, and hyalinized stroma contain strands and tubules of proliferating epithelium that lack cytomorphologic abnormalities (fig. 5-107). In some sections the benign element appears clearly demarcated from the carcinoma (fig. 5-108), but scattered foci of malignant transformation within the benign element are more frequent (figs. 5-109, 5-110). If there is a sudden change in growth rate of a longstanding tumor, and the initial microscopic sections show only malignant tumor, serial sections are indicated to search for a benign component.

The carcinomatous element displays both cytomorphologic abnormalities and infiltration of surrounding tissues. Rarely, however, the carcinoma is at an early stage of development and confined by capsular tissue (fig. 5-111). Because such tumors have a markedly better prognosis than the more common invasive type, they are designated by several synonymous terms that include *encapsulated, in situ, preinvasive*, and *noninvasive carcinomas ex mixed tumor* (332,337).

The carcinomatous element typically is composed of cells with enlarged, pleomorphic, and hyperchromatic nuclei; prominent nucleoli (fig. 5-112); and a high mitotic rate (fig. 5-113). All in situ carcinomas need to be extensively sampled to ensure that extracapsular involvement has not occurred (fig. 5-114). Carcinoma ex mixed

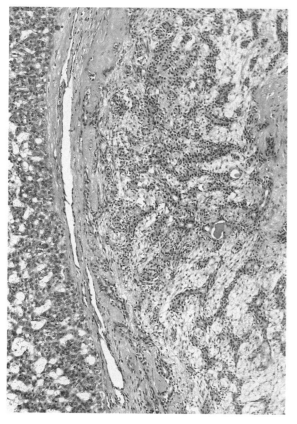

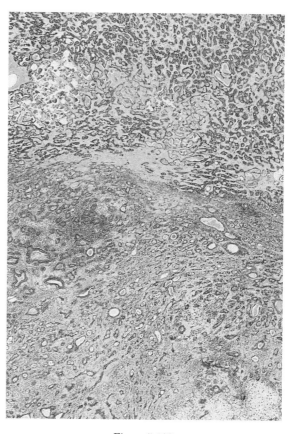

Figure 5-108
CARCINOMA EX MIXED TUMOR

The carcinomatous element (left) appears separated from the benign element (right) by a band of hyalinized connective tissue. More direct evidence of malignant transformation was found in other sections where the two elements were contiguous.

Figure 5-109
MALIGNANT TRANSFORMATION
OF MIXED TUMOR

Benign tumor is on the bottom and the more darkly staining carcinoma on the top.

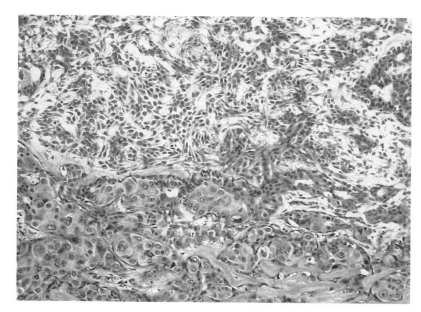

Figure 5-110
MALIGNANT TRANSFORMATION
OF MIXED TUMOR

Apparent malignant transformation of benign mixed tumor (top) to carcinoma is evident. Cellular atypia is present in some of the duct-like structures in the benign mixed tumor.

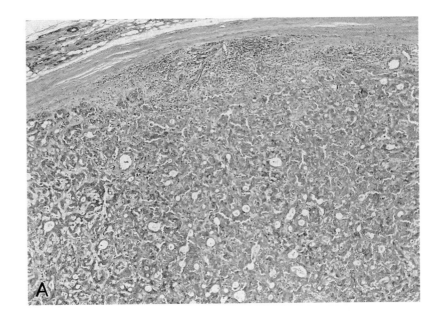

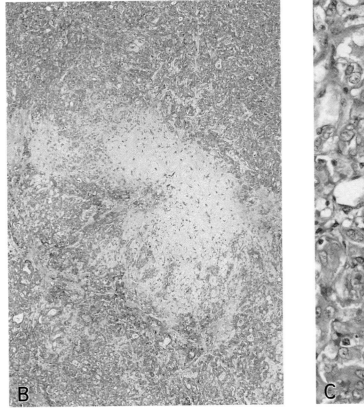
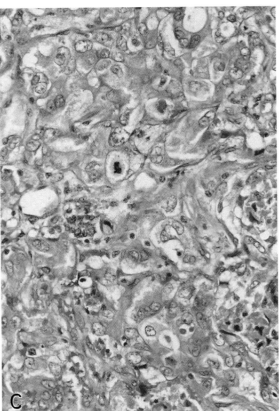

Figure 5-111
CARCINOMA IN SITU EX MIXED TUMOR
This carcinoma was entirely confined by capsular tissue, a portion of which is seen in A. In B residual benign mixed tumor is evident whereas high magnification (C) reveals the malignant cytomorphologic features.

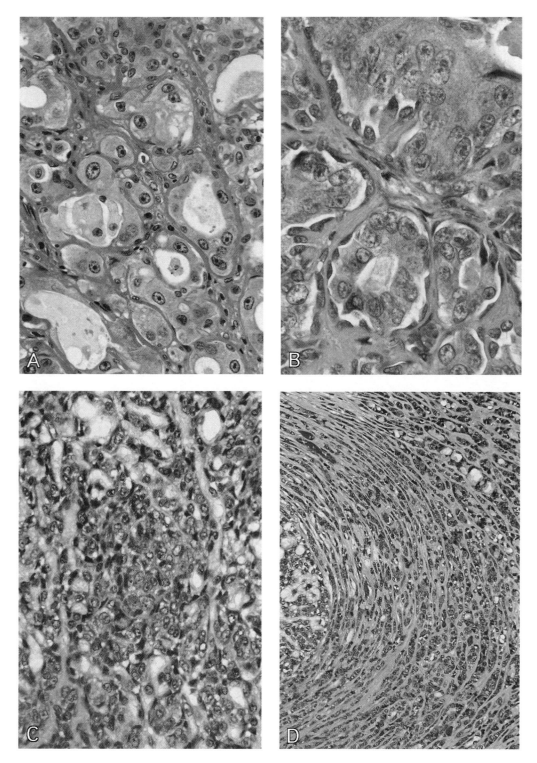

Figure 5-112
CARCINOMA EX MIXED TUMOR
The carcinomatous component of these three different examples demonstrates variations in cellularity and degree of adenocarcinomatous differentiation, but all demonstrate nuclear abnormalities, including large nucleoli. The bottom two illustrations are from the same case and show the variation in growth pattern within a single tumor. The degree of cellular pleomorphism in all examples is unacceptable in benign mixed tumors.

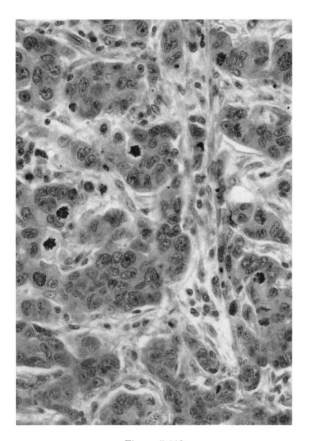

Figure 5-113
INCREASED MITOSES IN
CARCINOMA EX MIXED TUMOR
Mitotic activity varies considerably but is not usually as
prominent as in this field.

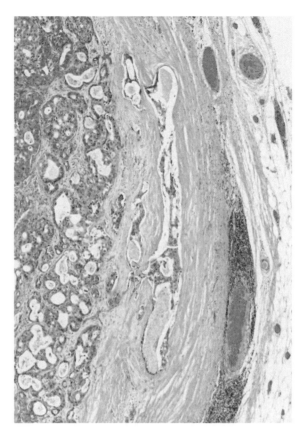

Figure 5-114
FOCAL CAPSULAR INVASION
Although this tumor has a thick capsule that is infiltrated by tumor, the tumor appears contained. However, serial sections showed infiltration of adjacent parenchyma and periparotid connective tissue.

tumor often shows neural and vascular invasion (fig. 5-115). In one study perineural invasion was found in 55 percent of cases (332). Prominent hyalinization (fig. 5-116) and hemorrhage are common. Necrosis is frequently evident in high-grade tumors (fig. 5-117).

In most tumors, the carcinomatous component is adenocarcinoma that can not be further classified (not otherwise specified or NOS). As with other adenocarcinomas, NOS, grading based on the degree of cytologic anaplasia has prognostic importance. In the series of Tortoledo and colleagues (342), which included 37 carcinomas ex mixed tumor, the carcinomatous component was designated as ductal in 13, undifferentiated in 10, terminal duct (polymorphous low-grade) in 9, myoepithelial in 3, and unclassified in 2 because of limited tissue (342). Other

types observed at the AFIP or reported in the literature include mucoepidermoid carcinoma (fig. 5-118), epidermoid carcinoma, adenoid cystic carcinoma, clear cell adenocarcinoma, acinic cell adenocarcinoma, and myoepithelial carcinoma (fig. 5-119) (326,331,332,336,338,340). Subclassification requires that features of a specific carcinoma predominate within the malignant component (332).

Differential Diagnosis. Mixed tumors with focally atypical features occasionally cause concern about malignant transformation. Fine-needle aspiration or other surgical procedures sometimes result in infarction, hemorrhage, and inflammation that is associated with reactive cytologic atypia, metaplasia, and focal proliferation of adjacent epithelial elements. Knowledge of previous surgical manipulation is helpful for

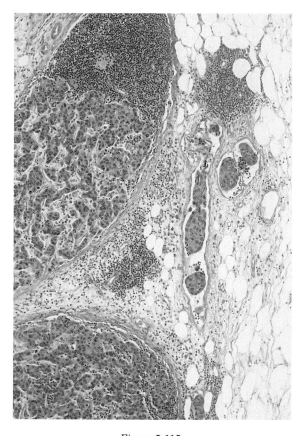

Figure 5-115
VASCULAR INVASION
Intravascular tumor is evident in this field (right center).
The lymphoid tissue at the top was a hyperplastic response
to the tumor rather than residual lymph node.

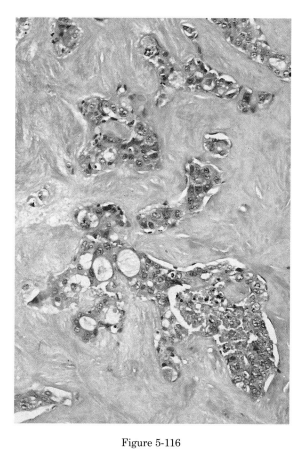

Figure 5-116
PROMINENT HYALINIZATION
The carcinomatous islands are surrounded by abundant,
hyalinized connective tissue. This is a nonspecific finding
that may be present in other types of salivary gland carcinoma. Necrotic tumor is evident (bottom right).

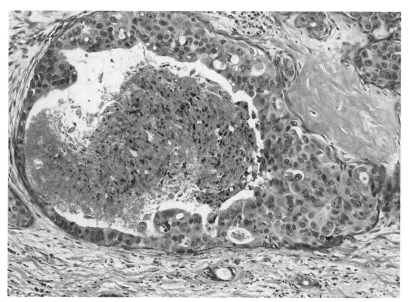

Figure 5-117
FOCAL NECROSIS
A large focus of necrotic tumor is pres-
ent in this island of high-grade carcinoma.

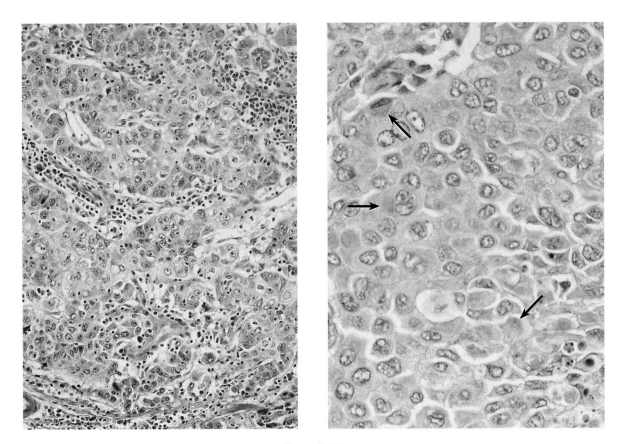

Figure 5-118
MUCOEPIDERMOID CARCINOMA EX MIXED TUMOR
The carcinomatous component of this tumor had solid and cystic growth and was composed of several cell types including epidermoid and mucous cells. The mucicarmine stain helps highlight the intracytoplasmic mucin (arrows).

Figure 5-119
MYOEPITHELIAL CARCINOMA
EX MIXED TUMOR
The carcinoma in this case was composed entirely of spindle and ovoid cells that were strongly and diffusely immunoreactive for cytokeratin and smooth muscle actin.

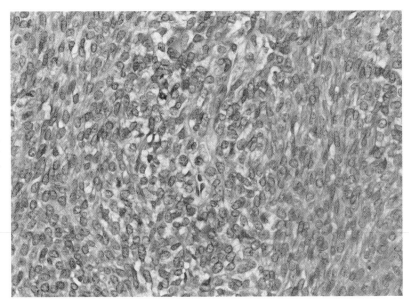

the evaluation of atypical features. In these situations cellular anaplasia is usually minimal. Epithelial islands are sometimes isolated by fibrosis and inflammation but invasion into surrounding tissues is not evident.

Some salivary gland adenocarcinomas have foci of tubular structures embedded within myxoid zones that resemble carcinoma ex mixed tumor; abnormal cytologic features throughout the tumor distinguish these zones from benign mixed tumor. On the other hand, chondromyxoid differentiation, if present, would be extremely unusual in the absence of mixed tumor.

Carcinosarcoma ex mixed tumor and pure carcinosarcoma may be confused with carcinoma ex mixed tumor because hyalinized or myxoid stroma in the latter occasionally simulates sarcoma (326). Distinguishing features in carcinoma ex mixed tumor include the lack of nuclear atypia of the stromal cells and absence of osteosarcoma, chondrosarcoma, or undifferentiated sarcoma.

Treatment and Prognosis. Data from two studies has shown that 38 to 53 percent of patients develop one or more recurrences (332,340). Livolsi and Perzin (332) observed that 75 percent of recurrences develop within 5 years from initial treatment, but they and others have noted recurrences as long as 25 years later (320,326,340). Spiro et al. (340) found the likelihood of recurrence higher in the submandibular and minor glands than in the parotid. Livolsi and Perzin noted that the recurrence rate in the parotid and submandibular glands was similar but was lower for minor gland tumors, especially those that occurred in the palate. It has also been demonstrated that recurrence indicates a poorer prognosis (322,332): of 16 patients with local recurrence, 14 died of disease compared to only 1 of 5 patients without recurrence.

Although few cases of in situ carcinoma ex mixed tumor have been followed long-term, it appears that with complete surgical excision prognosis is similar to that of benign mixed tumor. A review by Gnepp (326) of published series found that the survival of conventional, invasive carcinoma ex mixed tumor ranged from 25 to 65 percent at 5 years, 24 to 50 percent at 10 years, 10 to 35 percent at 15 years (318,322,325,327,340,341), and 0 to 38 percent at 20 years (322,339). These same studies reported that lymph node involvement occurred in 15 to 24 percent of patients with previously unresected tumors and in 40 percent of those with recurrent tumors. Distant metastasis to the lung, bone, brain, liver, or subcutaneous tissue occurs most often in patients whose treatment failed at the primary site (332,340).

Unlike some other salivary gland carcinomas, the gross dimensions of the tumor do not correlate with the prognosis, presumably because the proportion of the benign to malignant component varies considerably (340,342).

Tortoledo et al. (342) evaluated the prognostic importance of both the measured distance of invasion and the histologic subclassification of the carcinoma. As measurement landmarks they used: 1) persistent capsule or stromal condensation around the mixed tumor and 2) identifiable residual benign mixed tumor, such as chondroid matrix. Measurements were made at right angles from the residual benign component nearest the capsule to the most distant infiltrative edge of the carcinoma. They found that patients whose carcinoma extended for more than 8 mm beyond the residual capsule or benign residual tumor died of their disease whereas none of those with less invasive tumor died. They also found that the extent of invasion correlated with the presence of perineural invasion and metastasis to lymph nodes. Of the patients with low-grade carcinomas (polymorphous low-grade adenocarcinoma), only 1 of 9 died of disease compared to 7 of 10 patients with undifferentiated carcinomas. Patients whose surgical specimens had tumor-positive margins had a higher recurrence rate and higher death rate from disease (332, 333,342). However, some patients with surgical margins negative for tumor still had recurrences and metastases, and died of tumor (342).

In the series by Spiro and colleagues (340), the treatment for two thirds of the patients with parotid tumors consisted of subtotal parotidectomy with preservation of the facial nerve in most cases. Total parotidectomy with sacrifice of at least part of the nerve was required for the remaining patients, most of whom had large or recurrent tumors. Neck dissection in conjunction with the initial surgical treatment was performed in about 20 percent of the cases. Patients with tumors of the submandibular gland had the involved gland removed and about half had a neck dissection. Tumors of the minor glands often required removal of at least portions of the mandible or maxilla, and neck dissection in some cases. Livolsi and Perzin (332) recommend radical neck dissection for major gland disease whether or not there is clinical evidence of lymph node enlargement and for minor gland tumors only when lymphadenopathy is present. However, based on the data presented by Tortoledo et al. (342) modification of this approach should be considered for tumors with a low-grade carcinomatous element or those that show limited invasion. Radiotherapy alone has proven ineffective although it may have a beneficial role when used in conjunction with surgery (332,340,342).

Carcinosarcoma

Definition. Carcinosarcoma is a rare malignant neoplasm of salivary glands that manifests both carcinomatous and sarcomatous components, and either or both components are expressed in metastatic foci.

Within the generic category malignant mixed tumor, carcinosarcoma has been referred to as *true malignant mixed tumor* (347,350,351,359, 363) to distinguish it from carcinoma ex mixed tumor in which there is only a carcinomatous malignant component. The World Health Organization (WHO) classification of 1991 (358) does not list carcinosarcoma as a specific type of salivary gland neoplasm but describes it as a variant of carcinoma in pleomorphic adenoma. By the WHO definition, this tumor should develop within the context of a benign mixed tumor; however, some carcinosarcomas develop de novo while others develop in association with benign mixed tumors (345–347,357,361). Two groups of investigators have described carcinosarcomas that developed in preexisting carcinoma ex mixed tumors (350,360).

Dual carcinomatous and sarcomatous neoplasia raises questions about histogenesis. Does this neoplasm result from synchronous malignant transformation of parenchymal and stromal elements of the salivary gland; does the sarcomatous component represent modulation of malignant myoepithelial cells similar to the chondromyxoid modulation in benign mixed tumors; or are two independent cell lines derived from a primitive, pluripotential cell? Some investigators have reported no evidence of myoepithelial differentiation in carcinosarcoma by light microscopic or immunohistochemical techniques (345), but others have cited evidence from similar investigations and ultrastructural studies that support myoepithelial modulation for the sarcomatous component of carcinosarcomas (347,353,359–361).

General Features. The rarity of carcinosarcoma is denoted by the fact that there are only eight documented cases in the AFIP files, only three of which have been reviewed in the last decade. These represent less than 0.1 percent of salivary gland neoplasms. Because of its rarity, little other data on incidence has been published. Kirklin et al. (356) found 4 carcinosarcomas among 909 parotid tumors in a study performed in the early 1950s (346). Stephen et al. (359) reported the largest series, 12 cases, of which 11 were accessioned at M. D. Anderson Hospital in Houston over a 32-year period. Garner et al. (350) reported only 2 cases at the University of Iowa over a 60-year period. About 33 adequately documented cases have been reported in the English language literature (345–347,350–355,357, 359–361,363,364).

About 65 percent of carcinosarcomas occurred in the parotid gland and 22 percent in the submandibular gland. Four tumors were described in the palate, and one each was reported in the tongue and upper lip. Patient age ranges from 14 to 87 years, with a mean of 57 years; most patients are over 50 years old at the time of diagnosis. Men and women are affected equally.

Hellquist and Michaels (353) reported two carcinosarcomas in the palate that developed 30 and 36 years following radiation therapy for benign mixed tumors; they speculated that radiation may have been an etiologic factor. Other reports have not noted an association with previous radiation therapy.

Clinical Features. Similar to many patients with carcinoma ex mixed tumors, some patients with carcinosarcomas report slow growth of their tumors over several years followed by sudden rapid growth; these carcinosarcomas are most often associated with benign mixed tumors. Other patients, however, describe development of their tumors over only a few months to a year; these tumors are unlikely to be associated with benign mixed tumor. Swelling, pain, nerve palsy, and ulceration have been frequent manifestations. Cervical lymphadenopathy is infrequent.

Gross Findings. Primary neoplasms have ranged from 2 to 13 cm in largest dimension. Most tumors have been over 3 cm, and the mean size has been about 4 cm. Recurrent tumors as large as 8 cm have been described. Small tumors sometimes appear well circumscribed, but larger tumors are unencapsulated and infiltrative. The cut surface is usually grayish but often contains areas of necrosis, hemorrhage, or calcification.

Microscopic Findings. Analogous to benign mixed tumor, carcinosarcomas are composed of both epithelial- and mesenchymal-appearing neoplastic tissues. Cytologic atypia, including cellular and nuclear pleomorphism, hyperchromatism, and mitotic figures, and invasive growth distinguish carcinosarcoma from benign mixed tumor. Both carcinomatous and sarcomatous tissues are evident and differentiate these neoplasms from carcinoma ex mixed tumors in which only carcinomatous features are present. In most tumors the two components are intermixed with one another (fig. 5-120), but occasionally the carcinoma and sarcoma elements occur adjacent to one another (fig. 5-121). Comparable to the chondroid differentiation that is common in benign mixed tumors, the sarcomatous constituent is most often characterized as chondrosarcoma (fig. 5-122); however, osteosarcoma (fig. 5-123), fibrosarcoma (fig. 5-124), myxosarcoma (fig. 5-125), malignant fibrous histiocytoma (fig. 5-126), and even liposarcoma also have been identified. In two tumors in the AFIP files the sarcomatous component contained numerous multinucleated giant cells in a fibrohistiocytic proliferation consistent with malignant giant cell tumor (giant cell malignant fibrous histiocytoma) (fig. 5-127). Osteoclast-like giant cells in malignant mixed tumors have been noted by other investigators as well (345,349,352).

In most cases, the sarcomatous component dominates the carcinomatous component. Most frequently the carcinomatous elements are ductal carcinoma (fig. 5-128), but squamous cell carcinoma and undifferentiated carcinoma have also been identified (fig. 5-129). Most of the carcinomatous elements are high grade on the basis of cytomorphologic features and mitoses, but at the AFIP adenoid cystic carcinoma (fig. 5-130) and papillary cystadenocarcinoma (see fig. 5-121) also have been identified in carcinosarcomas.

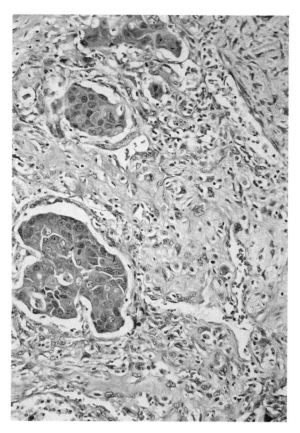

Figure 5-120
CARCINOSARCOMA
Islands of malignant epithelial cells are surrounded by very pleomorphic, sarcomatous fibromyxoid tissue. The clear spaces around the carcinomatous islands are retraction artifact produced by tissue processing.

Metastatic and recurrent tumors also usually manifest both carcinomatous and sarcomatous elements, but in some recurrent tumors only sarcoma has been recognized. Occasionally, in areas where carcinomatous and sarcomatous elements are closely associated or intermingled, there is a transitional zone that resembles the zone of modified myoepithelial cells of mixed tumors around ductal cells adjacent to chondroid tissue.

In some tumors foci of benign mixed tumor have been identified (fig. 5-131). Sometimes, sites of excised mixed tumors later develop carcinosarcomas.

Ultrastructural studies show chondrocytic and epithelial differentiation (347,360,361). The chondrocytic tissue has a considerable stromal matrix of glycosaminoglycans and collagen surrounding cells with an irregular configuration,

239

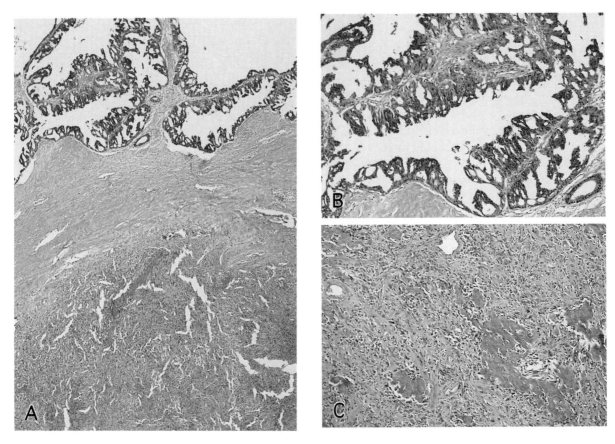

Figure 5-121
CARCINOSARCOMA

A: A fibrous band separates carcinoma (top) from sarcoma in a carcinosarcoma of the parotid gland.

B: The carcinoma is a papillary cystadenocarcinoma.

C: Higher magnification shows that the sarcoma is of osteogenic type.

Figure 5-122
CHONDROSARCOMA
IN CARCINOSARCOMA

A pale, basophilic extracellular chondroid matrix separates neoplastic chondrocytes. At the top right of the field atypical spindle cells are adjacent to the chondroid area.

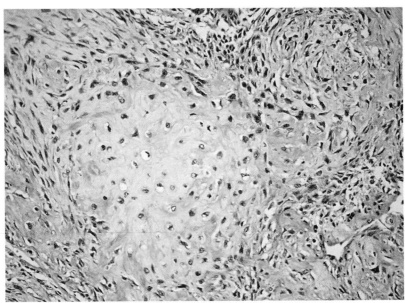

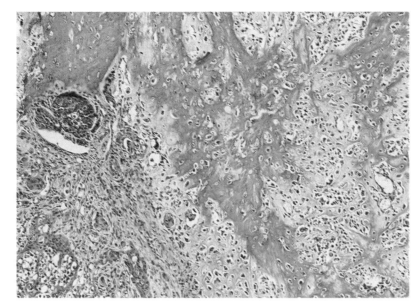

Figure 5-123
OSTEOSARCOMA
IN CARCINOSARCOMA

An osteoid-appearing matrix contains atypical lacunar cells and is bordered by malignant osteoblast-type cells in a carcinosarcoma from the parotid gland. Islands of carcinomatous tissue are evident in the lower left portion of the field.

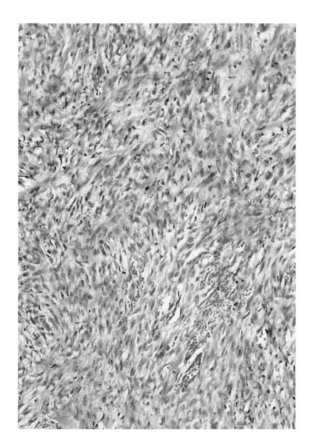

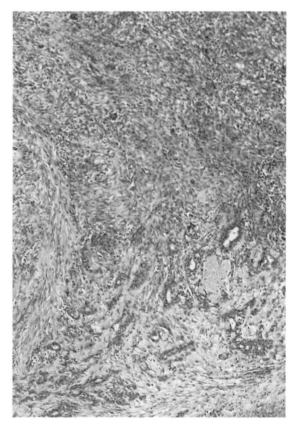

Figure 5-124
FIBROSARCOMA IN CARCINOSARCOMA

Left: Ill-defined fascicles of plump spindle cells with mitoses and a scant fibrillar matrix produce a fibrosarcomatous appearance in a carcinosarcoma from the submandibular gland.

Right: Low magnification shows adenocarcinoma (bottom) associated with the sarcomatous spindle cells.

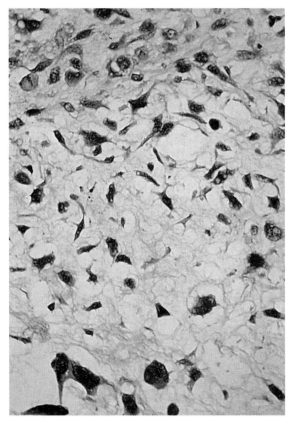

Figure 5-125
MYXOSARCOMA IN CARCINOSARCOMA
Markedly pleomorphic, stellate, spindle, and round cells in an abundant, loose, finely fibrillary matrix produce a myxosarcomatous appearance.

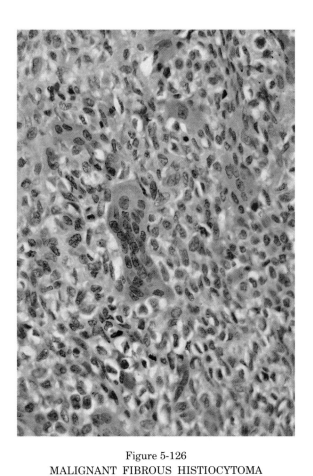

Figure 5-126
MALIGNANT FIBROUS HISTIOCYTOMA
IN CARCINOSARCOMA
Multinucleated giant cells among a dense population of atypical, ovoid and round, mononuclear cells give this area of a carcinosarcoma of the parotid gland a malignant fibrous histiocytoma-like appearance.

Figure 5-127
MALIGNANT GIANT CELL
TUMOR IN CARCINOSARCOMA
Numerous pleomorphic, multinucle-ated giant cells lie adjacent to an island of ductal carcinoma (upper left) in this parotid tumor. The clear spaces are due to processing artifact.

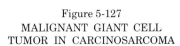
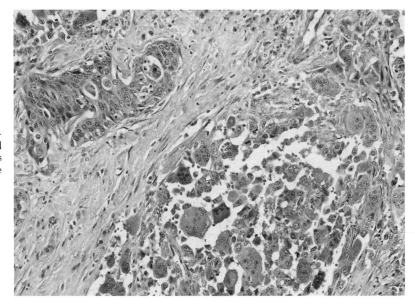

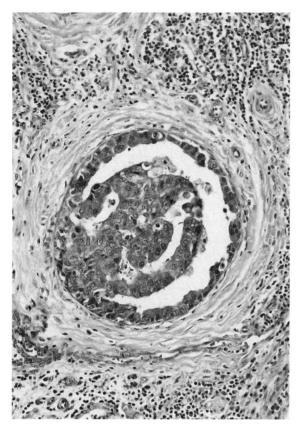

Figure 5-128
DUCTAL CARCINOMA IN CARCINOSARCOMA
This island of malignant ductal epithelium is representative of the carcinomatous component that was associated with the giant cell tumor illustrated in figure 5-127.

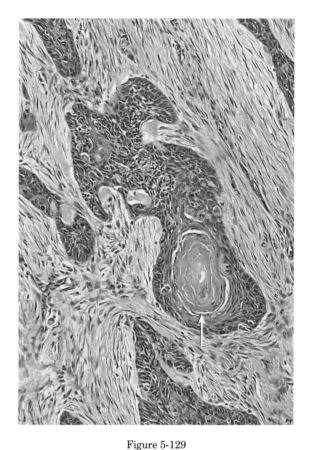

Figure 5-129
SQUAMOUS CELL CARCINOMA
IN CARCINOSARCOMA
Keratinization (arrow) is evident in irregular-shaped islands of epidermoid carcinoma from carcinosarcoma of the parotid gland.

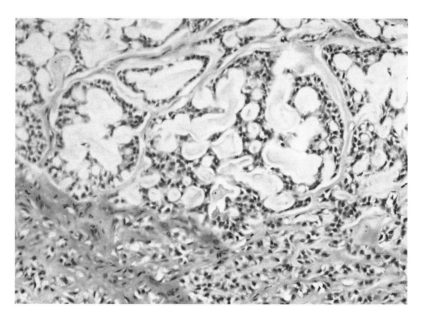

Figure 5-130
ADENOID CYSTIC CARCINOMA
IN CARCINOSARCOMA
The cribriform pattern and pseudocystic spaces with eosinophilic hyalinized material give the carcinomatous portion (top) of this carcinosarcoma an adenoid cystic appearance. The carcinosarcoma was associated with the spindle cell proliferation seen in figure 5-124.

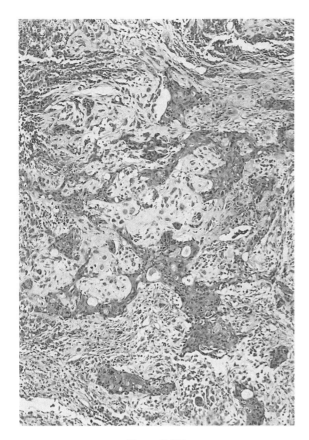

Figure 5-131
CARCINOSARCOMA WITH ARCHITECTURAL
PATTERN OF MIXED TUMOR
The relationship of the myxochondroid and epithelial tissues suggests that this carcinosarcoma developed in a mixed tumor.

extension of cytoplasmic processes from the cell surface, prominent rough endoplasmic reticulum, and cytoplasmic glycogen and lipid. Epithelial cells typically have desmosomal attachments; some have microvilli, tonofilaments, and basal lamina. In addition, myoepithelial features, such as bundles of fine cytoplasmic filaments, desmosomal attachments, and subplasmalemmal pinocytotic vesicles, have been identified in the chondrocytic areas. These latter features suggest that the sarcomatous component is derived from modulation of myoepithelial cells in at least some tumors.

Immunohistochemical studies have generally demonstrated reactivity for cytokeratin, epithelial membrane antigen, and S-100 protein in the carcinomatous cells and reactivity for vimentin in the sarcomatous tissue. Anti-S-100 protein is frequently reactive in the sarcomatous type cells (345,361,363,364). Toynton et al. (363) reported reactivity for glial fibrillary acidic protein in both sarcomatous and carcinomatous elements of a carcinosarcoma from the upper lip.

Differential Diagnosis. In the major salivary glands the differential diagnosis includes benign mixed tumor and primary and metastatic sarcomas. In the intraoral minor salivary glands, spindle cell carcinoma is also a consideration.

A mild to moderate degree of cytologic atypia within benign mixed tumors is not rare and is compatible with benignancy (see Mixed Tumor). However, marked cytologic atypia of epithelial and mesenchymal-type tissues and invasive growth discern carcinosarcoma from mixed tumor. In some cases, both benign mixed tumor and carcinosarcoma are evident. Early malignant transformation in an encapsulated mixed tumor is problematic, but, fortunately, has little impact on therapy because absent or minimal invasion by malignant mixed tumors is still associated with an excellent prognosis (362).

Sarcomas of the major salivary glands are uncommon but not as rare as carcinosarcomas (343,344); however, extraskeletal chondrosarcoma in the major salivary glands is extremely rare. There is only one case in the AFIP files. Since chondrosarcoma is the most common mesenchymal component of carcinosarcomas, a salivary gland tumor that manifests chondrosarcomatous features is most likely a carcinosarcoma and should be thoroughly sampled for a carcinomatous component. Fibrosarcoma, osteosarcoma, and malignant fibrous histiocytoma are other sarcomas frequently identified in carcinosarcomas. Although immunoreactivity for cytokeratin is rarely observed in these mesenchymal neoplasms, anti-cytokeratin immunohistochemistry can be helpful in identifying carcinomatous elements in sarcomatoid salivary gland tumors. Synovial sarcoma is an exception since both immunohistochemistry and histochemical staining for salivary mucins are similar to carcinosarcoma. Tightly interlacing fascicles of uniform spindle cells with embedded epithelioid cells and gland-like structures are more characteristic of synovial sarcoma than carcinosarcoma, which has more pleomorphic, less integrated carcinomatous and sarcomatous tissues.

Spindle cell carcinomas of the oral mucosa often histologically resemble malignant fibrous histiocytomas and, occasionally, contain osteosarcoma- or chondrosarcoma-like features (348). Since they occur in tissues that contain minor salivary glands, they need to be differentiated from carcinosarcoma. Diagnostic features include malignant dysplasia or overt epidermoid carcinoma of the mucosal epithelium, continuity with atypical basaloid cells of the surface epithelium, and absence of adenocarcinomatous features, both cytological and architectural.

Prognosis and Treatment. Among 24 cases of carcinosarcoma in the literature with follow-up data, 14 patients (58 percent) died of disease; 4 patients (17 percent) were living with persistent, recurrent, or metastatic disease; 2 patients (8 percent) died of unrelated causes; and 4 patients (17 percent) were alive and well (345347, 350,352,355,356,359,360,363). In the largest series studied (359), the average survival period was 3.6 years. Recurrent disease, often multiple episodes, developed in approximately two thirds of patients, and metastases in about half. Although unusual for salivary gland carcinomas, most metastases were hematogenous rather than lymphatic. Lung has been the most common site of metastasis.

Carcinosarcoma is an aggressive, high-grade malignancy, and aggressive therapy employing radical surgery, with and without adjunctive radiation therapy and chemotherapy, is used. Since hematogenous metastases are more common than lymphatic metastases, radical neck dissection is appropriately reserved for patients with lymphadenopathy.

Metastasizing Mixed Tumor

Definition. Metastasizing mixed tumor is a very rare salivary gland neoplasm that histologically is a benign mixed tumor that inexplicably metastasizes. The metastatic foci closely resemble the primary neoplasm and contain a mixture of cytologically benign epithelial and mesenchymal-like chondromyxoid tissue. The term *benign metastasizing mixed tumor* has been applied to these tumors (374,375), but the occurrence of metastases and death of some patients indicate that the adjective "benign" is inappropriate and misleading. Unfortunately, diagnosis of these tumors is only established in retrospect after the metastases have been identified.

General Features. After an extensive search, Wenig et al. (378) located 32 case reports in the literature; they also added 8 new cases to their series for a total of 11 cases. One case reported by Hellquist and Michaels (371) was described as a mixed tumor of the palate that metastasized to a lymph node, but the palatal tumor subsequently developed into a carcinosarcoma. At least three additional cases have been reported (372,375), but the case reported by Minic (372) is most unusual because the primary parotid tumor was described as both benign mixed tumor and carcinosarcoma, and the metastases in the lymph nodes were described as having both benign- and malignant-appearing histologic patterns.

There is often a long interval between diagnosis of the primary mixed tumor and metastasis. Intervals as long as 52 years have occurred; in the series of 11 cases studied by Wenig et al. (378) the intervals averaged 20 years and ranged from 6 to 52 years. A long interval between occurrence of the primary tumor and the metastasis creates problems for both clinicians and pathologists correlating a metastasis with a primary tumor that was excised in the distant past. The metastatic foci can be interpreted as primary neoplasms (375), and some cases of metastasizing mixed tumor probably go unrecognized. An accurate medical history is essential.

Recurrence of tumor, often multiple episodes, in the primary site prior to development of metastases has characterized most metastasizing mixed tumors. Metastases have developed synchronous with recurrence and up to 29 years after the most recent recurrence (369,375,378, 379). Wenig et al. (378) postulated that the increased frequency of surgical intervention may result in vascular permeation by the neoplasm and ultimately lead to metastasis. However, they noted no evidence of vascular infiltration in the primary or recurrent tumors they studied. At the AFIP vascular permeation has been observed in the capsule of some benign-appearing mixed tumors, but none of these tumors have been known to metastasize; however, the long interval before metastasis can make this difficult to assess.

Radiation therapy for primary or recurrent disease in some patients with metastasizing

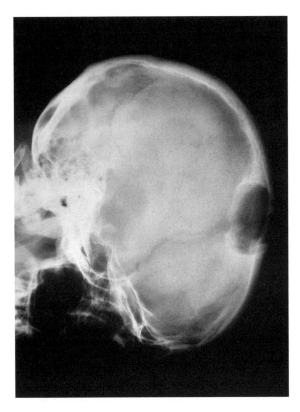
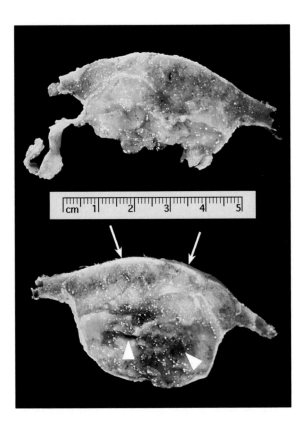

Figure 5-132
METASTASIZING MIXED TUMOR

Left: This well-demarcated radiolucency of the skull has sclerotic borders and represents metastatic tumor from a mixed tumor of the parotid gland that had been initially resected 16 years previously. The patient had complained of headaches.

Right: The resection specimen is bounded by a rim of bone (arrows), is pale tan with focal hemorrhage, and is focally cystic (arrowheads).

mixed tumors has led to speculation that radiation may have contributed to the subsequent malignant manifestations in these cases (371, 373,375,377). To the contrary, Wenig et al. (378 pointed to the fact that none of the 11 patients they studied had received radiation therapy prior to the development of metastases.

Of primary mixed tumors that subsequently metastasize, 80 percent are found in the parotid gland, 12 percent in the submandibular gland, and 8 percent in the minor salivary glands. Hematogenous metastases are more prevalent than lymphatic metastases to regional lymph nodes. Bone, lung, and lymph nodes have been the most common sites of metastatic disease, but kidney, liver, central nervous system, retroperitoneum, and skin have also been involved (370,378).

On the basis of the relatively few cases, there appears to be no significant sex predilection. Pa-

tients have ranged in age from 8 to 72 years, with a mean age of about 28 years at the time of presentation of their primary salivary gland tumors. The median age for diagnosis of metastatic disease has been about 60 years (378). These data are similar to those for carcinoma ex mixed tumor.

Clinical Features. The clinical manifestations of the primary mixed tumors are notable for the absence of features that are often associated with malignant neoplasms. Like most other benign mixed tumors, the primary neoplasm is usually a single, well-defined mass. Pain, facial paralysis, or rapid growth are absent. The duration of the primary tumor before diagnosis has ranged from months to years (366,375). Signs and symptoms of metastatic disease are related to the sites involved and have included bone pain, pathologic fracture, abdominal pain, headaches, swellings, and abnormal chest radiographs (fig. 5-132) (378).

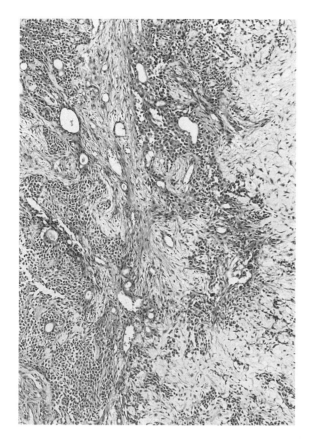 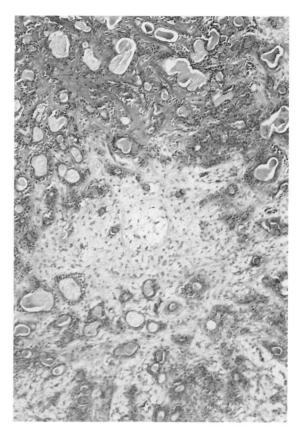

Figure 5-133
METASTASIZING MIXED TUMOR

Left: Mixed tumor of the submandibular gland has an equal mixture of typical epithelial and myxochondroid tissue.

Right: The metastatic tumor that was discovered in the humerus 20 years after excision of the primary tumor and 9 years after excision of a third recurrence has an appearance similar to the primary tumor.

Gross Findings. The primary neoplasms are indistinguishable from other mixed tumors of salivary gland. They are circumscribed and usually encapsulated. They have ranged from 0.5 to 15 cm in largest dimension, and a relative increased size over conventional mixed tumors has not been noted. Recurrent neoplasms are often multinodular and have been as large as 15 cm (378). Metastases are single or multiple, well-circumscribed and even encapsulated, gray to tan, sometimes glistening nodules that have varied from 1 to 15 cm (fig. 5-132).

Microscopic Findings. The histologic features of the primary neoplasm are within the spectrum of features that characterize benign mixed tumors (figs. 5-133, 5-134) (see Mixed Tumor). Populations of cells with ductal and myoepithelial differentiation are present, and the myoepithelial cells may have both plasmacytoid and spindled forms. Mesenchymal-like myxoid and myxochondroid tissue are intermixed with epithelial areas in varying proportions. The cellular density of the tumors is variable, just as it is in conventional mixed tumors. Mixed tumors with a predominantly myxoid architecture have been reported to be associated with increased risk for recurrence (376), and El-Naggar et al. (368) stated that metastasizing mixed tumors manifest a preponderance of stromal, often myxoid, tissue (fig. 5-135). Contrary to that, Wenig et al. (378) found that only 1 of their 11 tumors had a predominantly mesenchymal appearance. Features associated with malignant transformation such as anaplasia; numerous mitoses; marked cellular pleomorphism; invasion of adjacent tissues, vessels, or nerves; necrosis; and hemorrhage are not present. Several investigators have noted some cytologic atypia, such as cellular and nuclear

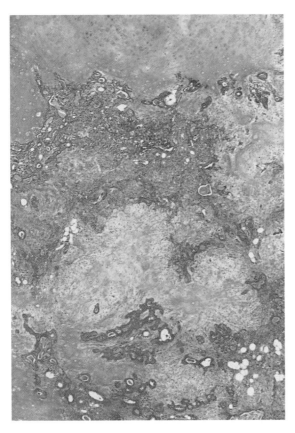
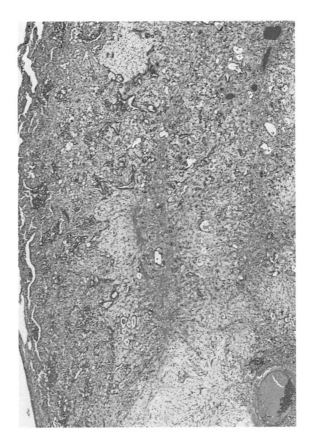

Figure 5-134
METASTASIZING MIXED TUMOR
The variegated appearance of this mixed tumor of the parotid gland (left) with hyalinized, myxoid, and densely cellular areas is similar but not exactly duplicated in the pulmonary metastasis (right) that occurred after 19 years and three recurrences of the primary tumor.

pleomorphism and mitotic figures, within the primary or recurrent mixed tumors, but these features have been within parameters acceptable for benign mixed tumors and insufficient to identify malignancy (fig. 5-136) (365,368, 378, 380). On average the number of mitoses has been about 1 per 10 high-power fields (378).

The histopathologic appearance of the metastatic foci is similar to the primary salivary gland neoplasm (figs. 5-133, 5-134). Some have a slight variation in cell density and proportion of epithelial and mesenchymal-like tissues from the primary tumor, but the features are characteristic of benign mixed tumor. Immunohistochemical reactions are identical to those of mixed tumors and include reactivity for cytokeratin, S-100 protein, smooth muscle actin, vimentin, and glial fibrillary acidic protein (fig. 5-137).

Differential Diagnosis. Metastatic tumor foci need to be differentiated from skeletal and extraskeletal chondrosarcoma, chordoma, and chondroid hamartoma of the lung. Chondrosarcomas are generally more atypical with more pleomorphism and mitotic figures than metastatic mixed tumors. The presence of an epithelial component with ductal differentiation and immunoreactivity for cytokeratin distinguishes metastatic mixed tumors from chondrosarcoma. Distinction from chordoma and chondroid hamartoma of the lung is more problematic. Physaliferous cells are not present in mixed tumors. Chondroid chordomas nearly always occur in the spheno-occipital region, a site where metastatic mixed tumors have not been found. The cartilage nests in hamartomas of the lung are usually surrounded by cellular fibrous tissue, and the

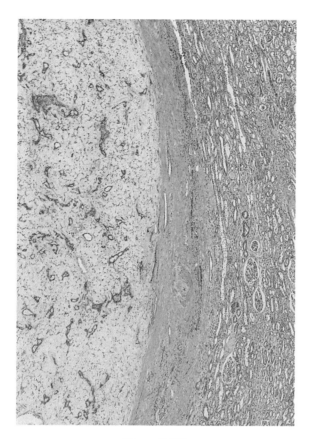

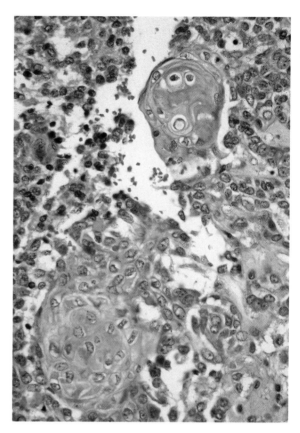

Figure 5-135
METASTASIZING MIXED TUMOR
This metastatic tumor in the kidney is well demarcated from the adjacent renal tissue and has a predominantly myxoid appearance, with widely separated islands and cords of ductal structures.

Figure 5-136
METASTASIZING MIXED TUMOR
High-magnification field from a mixed tumor that metastasized to the ischium shows focal squamous differentiation and some cytologic variability; however, the tumor is not overtly malignant.

epithelial elements merge with adjacent alveoli or bronchioles (370). A complete and accurate medical history is one of the most helpful elements in the differential diagnosis.

Prognosis and Treatment. Up to 90 percent of patients experience recurrence at the primary site of their mixed tumor prior to or concurrent with the appearance of metastases. Recurrences develop up to 26 years after excision of the primary neoplasm (378). Seven of the 11 patients in the Wenig et al. (378) study had multiple recurrences. Among reports with adequate follow-up, 7 of 32 patients died as a result of their tumors, a mortality rate of 22 percent (378). The interval to death ranged from 2 to 8 years after a diagnosis of metastasis (370).

Flow cytometric analysis has not proven reliably useful for identifying potentially metasta-

sizing mixed tumors. Wenig et al. (378) found that 9 of the 11 metastasizing mixed tumors they examined were DNA diploid. In one case the primary tumor had a DNA aneuploid population, and in another case aneuploidy was identified in the metastatic tumor. Cresson et al. (367) found that both the primary and metastatic mixed tumor were aneuploid in the one tumor they studied while El-Naggar et al. (368) reported that both primary and metastatic tumor were diploid in their case.

One of the most significant clinicopathologic correlations for metastasizing mixed tumors has been the high incidence of recurrence in the primary tumor site before metastasis. Therefore, avoidance of recurrence of primary mixed tumor would seem to be the best preventive method for metastasizing mixed tumors, and prevention of

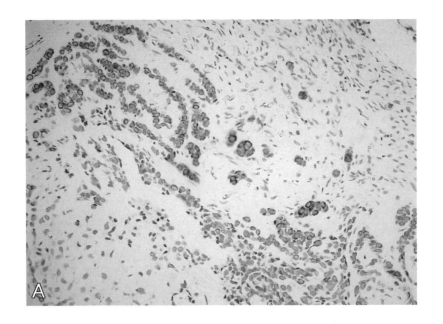

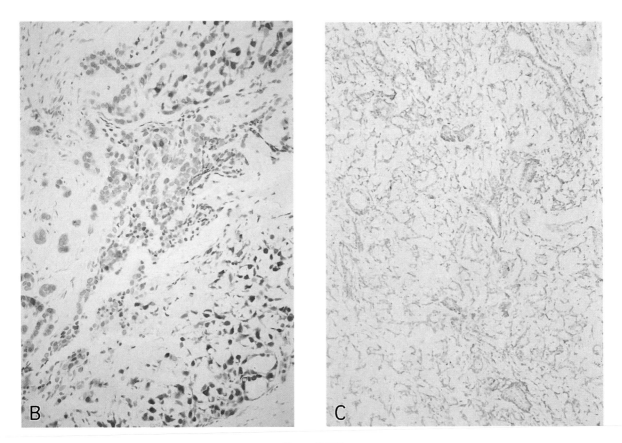

Figure 5-137
METASTASIZING MIXED TUMOR: IMMUNOHISTOCHEMISTRY
A metastatic mixed tumor in the ischium is immunoreactive for cytokeratin (A) and S-100 protein (B), and a metastatic mixed tumor in the lung demonstrates immunoreactivity for glial fibrillary acidic protein (C). (Avidin-biotin peroxidase stain)

recurrence of salivary gland mixed tumors correlates best with the completeness of surgical removal. Wide surgical excision results in very low recurrence rates of mixed tumors.

Surgery has been the principal treatment for metastatic foci. The extent and technique are dependent on the site and size of the metastatic tumor, but complete removal is the objective. Although adjuvant radiotherapy has been utilized (378), it is not expected that these metastatic foci are any more responsive to radiation or chemotherapy than the primary mixed tumor.

PRIMARY SQUAMOUS CELL CARCINOMA

Definition. This is a malignant epithelial tumor of the major salivary glands composed of epidermoid cells. There is no history or current evidence of a similar primary tumor elsewhere in the head and neck region. Diagnosis, therefore, requires the clinical exclusion of primary disease located in some other site. This diagnosis is not made in minor salivary glands because distinction from the much more common mucosal squamous cell carcinoma is not feasible. The terms *primary squamous* and *primary epidermoid cell carcinoma* are used synonymously.

General Features. Past exposure to radiation therapy appears to increase the risk of developing this tumor (387,392,396,400,402,405). Affected patients often have been previously irradiated for acne; benign or malignant neoplasms; or an enlarged thymus, thyroid gland, or tonsils (396,402,405). The median time between irradiation and diagnosis of salivary carcinoma is about 15.5 years (405), with a range of 7 to 32 years (400). However, radiation seemed less important in one series of 18 patients with primary squamous cell carcinoma in which only one patient had been previously irradiated (390).

The reported frequency of primary squamous cell carcinoma among all major gland tumors in large series has varied from 0.9 (388) to 4.7 percent (389). In a review of 2,807 benign and malignant salivary gland tumors, Spiro (403) found that they represented 1.9 percent of all tumors and 7.1 percent of 748 malignant major gland tumors. They have been reported to represent between 1.9 and 9 percent of malignant parotid tumors (390,413), and between 2.1 and 5.5 per-

cent of malignant submandibular tumors (383, 387,404). Of AFIP's major gland accessions since 1985, they comprise 2.7 percent of all tumors; 5.4 percent of malignant tumors; and 2.8 and 2.5 percent, respectively, of all parotid and submandibular tumors.

The average age of patients with primary squamous cell carcinoma is between 61 and 68 years, with an age range of 20 to 89 years (390, 402,406). The average age of patients in the AFIP registry is 64 years, with a range of 13 to 93 years; the 13-year-old is the only patient below 20 years of age, but other examples in children have been reported (381,397). At the AFIP, patients with parotid disease are about 9 years older than those with submandibular tumors, similar to statistics reported by Shemen et al. (402).

Although examples of primary squamous cell carcinoma originating in the minor glands have been reported (385,391), the diagnosis can be made confidently only in the major glands. It occurs in the parotid gland nearly nine times more often than in the submandibular gland. In both the series by Shemen et al. and the AFIP cases, nearly 90 percent affected the parotid, and in this gland they occurred almost exclusively in the superficial lobe (402). There is no report of a case in the sublingual gland. There is a strong male predilection: in four published series, 75 of 104 patients (72 percent) were male (390,402, 405,406) and in AFIP cases, 77 percent of civilian patients were men.

Clinical Features. In the series of Shemen et al. (402), just over half the patients with parotid gland disease presented with an asymptomatic mass. Another 19 percent complained of a painful mass, 11 percent had facial nerve palsy, and 7 percent had a lump in the neck. Seifert et al. (401) reported that primary squamous cell carcinoma is one of the salivary carcinomas that most often causes preoperative facial nerve paralysis. Submandibular tumors are usually painful. The duration of symptoms at either site is usually less than 1 year and rarely exceeds 2 years (402). Fixation to skin or deep structures, or ulceration occurs in some cases. Rare patients with the tumor in Stensen's duct have presented with painful swellings in the cheek (412).

Gross and Microscopic Findings. The tumors are typically unencapsulated and difficult to distinguish from surrounding tissues. They are firm and the cut surface is light gray or white.

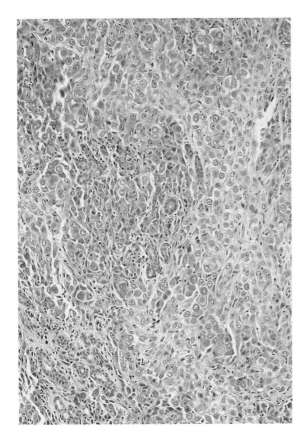 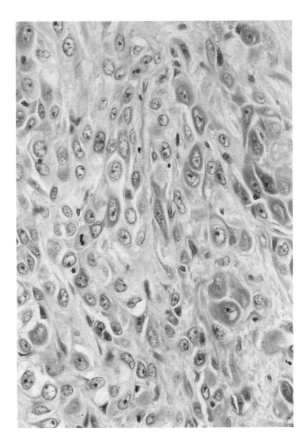

Figure 5-138
PRIMARY SQUAMOUS CELL CARCINOMA

Left: This example from the parotid gland demonstrates prominent intracellular keratinization and loosely cohesive tumor cells. Several residual ducts are in the center and bottom left portion of the illustration.

Right: Higher magnification of a different tumor shows variation in cellular keratinization.

Microscopically, these tumors are typical keratinizing squamous cell carcinomas that are usually well to moderately differentiated (fig. 5-138). Intracellular keratin and intercellular bridges are normally evident, but keratin pearl formation is less frequent. About 7 percent of tumors in the AFIP files are poorly differentiated, mostly nonkeratinizing tumors, but unlike undifferentiated carcinoma they have at least focal epidermoid differentiation (407,409). In all cases, special stains fail to reveal intracytoplasmic mucin.

Typically, anastomosing strands and islands of tumor infiltrate and replace glandular parenchyma (fig. 5-139). Remnants of normal or metaplastic ducts and degenerating acini often are surrounded by the advancing tumor, which may superficially resemble adenocarcinomatous differentiation, especially when tumors lack prominent keratinization (fig. 5-140). Gland lobules are often completely destroyed and replaced by tumor, but ductal epithelium is sometimes surprisingly resistant to advancing tumor (fig. 5-141). Mitoses are typically frequent (fig. 5-142), and perineural involvement (fig. 5-143) as well as vascular invasion are common. Although most tumors contain a fibrous stromal component (fig. 5-139), a minority incite a prominent desmoplastic response that surrounds and exceeds the amount of scattered tumor islands (fig. 5-144). Radiation-induced fibrosis occurs in patients that were previously irradiated for some other disease. Occasionally, fortuitous sections reveal origin from dysplastic ductal epithelium (fig. 5-145) (394). Rare tumors appear to originate from the epithelium that lines large cystic ducts (fig. 5-146). Transition of the epithelium from normal to dysplastic to neoplastic is evident.

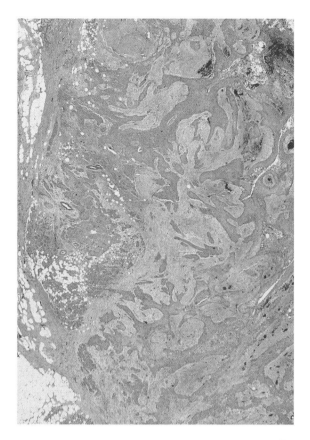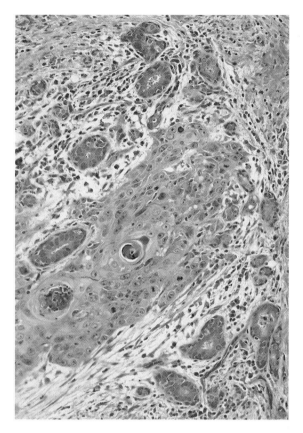

Figure 5-139
PRIMARY SQUAMOUS CELL CARCINOMA
Left: Low magnification shows interconnected strands of tumor separated by fibrous stroma. A remaining salivary gland lobule is at left center of illustration.
Right: Higher magnification demonstrates obvious squamous differentiation and residual ducts.

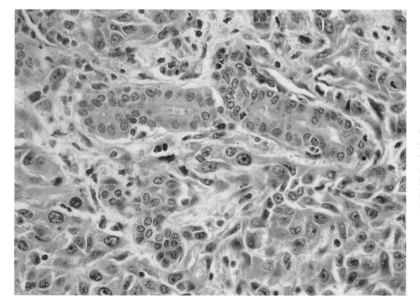

Figure 5-140
PRIMARY SQUAMOUS CELL CARCINOMA
Residual ducts are surrounded by tumor cells. The tumor cells have large, irregular nuclei and large nucleoli whereas the duct cell nuclei are bland and have indistinguishable or small nucleoli. The difference between ductal and neoplastic epithelium is occasionally much more subtle.

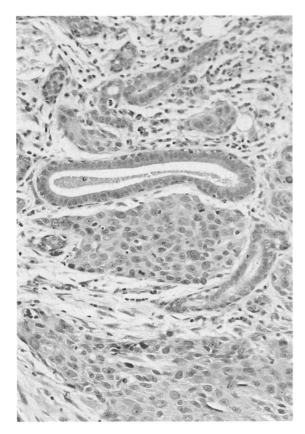

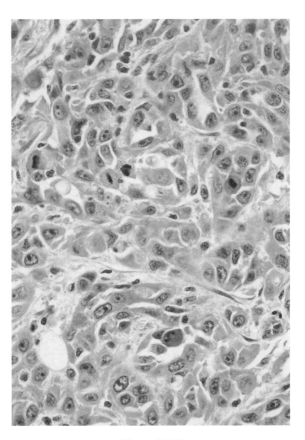

Figure 5-141
PRIMARY SQUAMOUS CELL CARCINOMA

Despite widespread replacement of most glandular elements in this tumor, isolated ducts persist. In some tumors the identification of such ducts is the only evidence that the tumor involves the salivary gland. The lumen of the largest duct appears partly compressed by tumor.

Figure 5-142
PRIMARY SQUAMOUS CELL CARCINOMA

Sheet-like growth of polygonal cells with several mitoses is seen in addition to individual cell keratinization, pleomorphic nuclei, and prominent nucleoli.

Figure 5-143
PERINEURAL GROWTH
OF PRIMARY SQUAMOUS
CELL CARCINOMA

As with many other types of salivary gland carcinoma, perineural growth is often present.

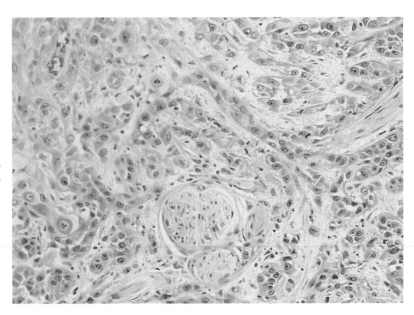

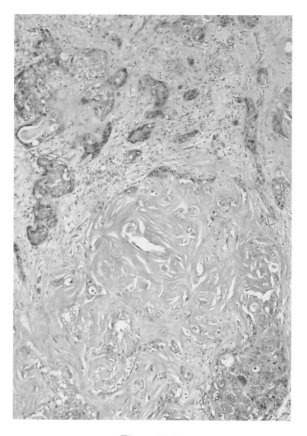

Figure 5-144
PRIMARY SQUAMOUS CELL CARCINOMA
This is one of several areas in this tumor that demonstrated prominent desmoplasia with hyalinization.

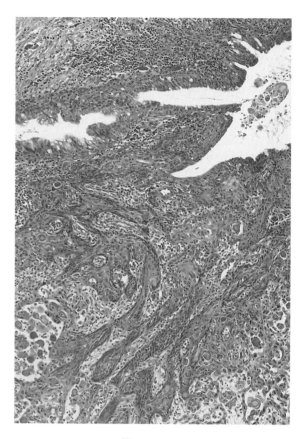

Figure 5-145
PRIMARY SQUAMOUS CELL CARCINOMA
ARISING FROM DUCT
Origin from ductal epithelium is evident. Transformation of the ductal epithelium from normal (top) to neoplastic (bottom) is seen.

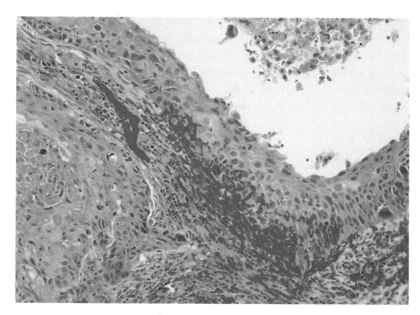

Figure 5-146
PRIMARY SQUAMOUS CELL
CARCINOMA
Epithelium lining a cyst or ectatic duct is shown that demonstrates dysplastic changes. Invasive carcinoma that appeared to originate from this lining is at the left.

Differential Diagnosis. Ductal squamous metaplasia may simulate squamous cell carcinoma. Ductal metaplasia occurs secondary to inflammation and surgical manipulation, such as fine-needle aspiration and as a component of necrotizing sialometaplasia (NSM). NSM is rare in the major salivary glands and characteristically shows lobular necrosis of the affected salivary gland in addition to the squamous changes. Squamous metaplasia lacks the cytomorphologic atypia and frank infiltrative growth of squamous cell carcinoma.

In contrast to primary squamous cell carcinoma, high-grade mucoepidermoid carcinoma has at least scattered cells that contain intracytoplasmic mucin. In addition to mucous and epidermoid cells, smaller basaloid and intermediate cells often focally predominate within even some of the high-grade mucoepidermoid carcinomas. Squamous cell carcinomas are composed of a much more homogeneous cell population and are more likely to have intracellular keratinization than mucoepidermoid carcinomas. However, in high-grade mucoepidermoid carcinomas the number of mucocytes is often limited, and their identification requires careful examination with special stains because ultimately it is the presence or absence of mucous cells on which distinction rests.

The most difficult distinction is between primary versus metastatic squamous cell carcinoma. In all studies of squamous cell carcinomas that involve the parotid gland, metastatic tumors outnumber primary tumors (382,384,390, 396,408). Only rarely do primary tumors originate from ductal epithelium, so interpretation in most cases depends on clinical evaluation of the patient. However, if tumor is only found within parotid or submandibular lymph nodes with no parenchymal involvement, an extrasalivary gland primary is highly probable. Unlike most primary salivary gland squamous cell carcinomas, metastatic nasopharyngeal squamous carcinomas are usually only moderately or poorly differentiated and often are composed of individual, large cystic islands with comedonecrosis. In a study of 2,802 patients with squamous cell carcinoma of the skin of the head and neck, 1.5 percent had parotid gland metastases (389). As with primary salivary gland squamous cell carcinoma, patients were usually in their sixth or seventh decade of life and there was a strong male predilection. The skin of the preauricular area, ear (including the external auditory canal), and cheek were the most common primary sites. Primaries may also be located in skin of the neck, nose, temple, and forehead (396,399). More than 72 percent of the patients with metastatic carcinoma had primary skin lesions greater than 2 cm in diameter and a duration of symptoms of 24.7 months (399). This implies that in most instances, small or occult skin cancers rarely manifest in the parotid gland. Uncommon sites that may harbor primary squamous cell carcinoma that metastasizes to the parotid include larynx, tongue, and lung. Lee et al. (395) found that skin of the ear was the primary site of squamous cell carcinoma in 19 of 28 patients with metastasis to parotid lymph nodes.

Prognosis and Treatment. Ulceration or fixation, advanced patient age, and advanced tumor stage are associated with a poor prognosis (402). Other investigators have noted low rates of survival in patients with facial paralysis (386, 390). Shemen et al. (402) found that the cure rates at 5, 10, 15, and 20 years were 24, 18, 17, and 17 percent, respectively, excluding patients who died of other causes with no evidence of disease or who were lost to follow-up. They noted that these 5-year follow-up periods were in contradistinction to the continually declining rates of most other malignant salivary gland tumors. Similar findings were observed by others (390).

Follow-up information on 41 patients showed treatment failure in 61 percent, all within the first year (402). With parotid tumors, distant metastasis occurred in 9 percent and regional failure in 51 percent of patients. Regional failure occurred in 66 percent of patients with submandibular tumors. Metastasis to cervical lymph nodes, discovered at the time of initial diagnosis, were found in 46 percent of patients.

Parotidectomy is performed for parotid tumors, and the facial nerve is spared if possible (402). However, in 45 percent of patients the facial nerve is excised because of involvement by tumor. Involved submandibular glands are resected. Concurrent neck dissection is performed for tumors in either gland if cervical metastases are detected or suspected. Because regional failure is the most significant concern, it is suggested that a composite resection might be appropriate for most tumors that involve the capsule of the submandibular gland. Gaughan et al. (390) recommended neck dissection on all patients; 30 percent of their patients with no palpable cervical disease who had neck dissection had microscopic disease. Stylohamular dissection with neck dissection has been used with some success for advanced cases that invade the infratemporal fossa or parapharyngeal space (393). There appears to be some evidence that postoperative radiotherapy may help control regional recurrence (398,402,406,408,410,411).

BASAL CELL ADENOCARCINOMA

Definition. Basal cell adenocarcinoma is an epithelial neoplasm that is cytologically and histomorphologically similar to basal cell adenoma, but is infiltrative and has a slight potential for metastasis.

Basal cell adenocarcinoma is a recently defined entity in the classification of salivary gland tumors and is included in the recent WHO monograph on the classification of salivary gland tumors (435). Although pathologists at the AFIP have identified this type of tumor for several years, only a few descriptions of this neoplasm have appeared in the literature (415,418,421,423,426,427,432,440). The largest series reported at the time of preparation of this Fascicle is that of Ellis and Wiscovitch (423). Terms used to refer to this or similar types of neoplasms include *basaloid salivary carcinoma, carcinoma ex monomorphic adenoma, malignant basal cell adenoma, malignant basal cell tumor,* and *basal cell carcinoma* (418,421,424, 426,427,429). As early as 1970, Evans and Cruickshank (424) mentioned the existence of malignant basal cell tumors in their monograph, but they provided no details other than that these tumors infiltrate and metastasize.

A few investigators have described adenoid cystic carcinomas arising from or developing in association with basal cell adenomas and speculated that basal cell adenoma is the benign counterpart of adenoid cystic carcinoma (419,425). Batsakis et al. (417) later repudiated one of these reports. These cases are questionable and appear to represent multifocal membranous basal cell adenomas or basal cell adenocarcinomas. Similar reports of hybrid basal cell adenoma-adenoid cystic carcinoma occurring in infants are probably best reclas-

sified as sialoblastoma, another newly described entity (414,436) (see Sialoblastoma).

Chomette et al. (422) described 24 tumors in a paper titled, "Basaloid carcinoma of salivary glands, a variety of undifferentiated adenocarcinoma"; however, the authors clearly indicated that the tumors they reported were solid variants of adenoid cystic carcinoma. Likewise, Seifert et al. (434) considered malignant basal cell adenoma to be synonymous with the basaloid (solid) type of adenoid cystic carcinoma. Histomorphologic features and biologic behavior demonstrate that the tumors now classified as basal cell adenocarcinomas are not solid variants of adenoid cystic carcinoma.

Pingitore and Campani (433) described a man with multiple dermal cylindromas and basal cell adenomas who developed pulmonary metastases, but the authors believed that the lung metastases were from a dermal cylindroma of the scalp rather than a very large membranous basal cell adenoma of the parotid gland. Lo et al. (428) reported a basal cell adenocarcinoma of the palate, but their limited photomicrographs are more suggestive of polymorphous low-grade adenocarcinoma, a diagnosis they did not consider in their discussion.

It is difficult to determine whether a particular basal cell adenocarcinoma develops within a pre-existing basal cell adenoma. Most basal cell adenocarcinomas probably arise de novo. Luna et al. (429), however, reported a series of eight carcinomas that they believe arose in basal cell adenomas.

General Features. Since this is a recently defined salivary gland neoplasm, it has not been included in large published series of salivary gland tumors. In the files at the AFIP since 1985, it has comprised 1.6 percent of all salivary neoplasms and 2.9 percent of malignant salivary neoplasms. Nearly 90 percent of these tumors occurred in the parotid gland, and only three tumors were identified in the minor salivary glands of the oral cavity. One of eight tumors reported by Luna et al. (429) was in the palate. The tumor of the palate reported by Lo et al. (428) was questionably a basal cell adenocarcinoma. The incidence among carcinomas of the parotid gland is about 5 percent.

Luna et al. (429) and the AFIP have found that patients are equally divided in gender. Thus far, this tumor has not occurred in a child, and the average age of the patients is 60 years.

Clinical Features. Pain or tenderness has been a complaint of a few patients, but, similar to most salivary gland neoplasms, swelling has usually been the only sign or symptom experienced. Sudden increase in size was noted by a few patients (423,429), but apparently this had no influence on the outcome. Duration of tumor before excision has been weeks to 10 years. In one case reported by Luna et al. (429), the one reported by Hyma et al. (426), and at least four of the AFIP cases there was a diathesis of multiple dermal adenomas and parotid basal cell adenocarcinomas.

Gross Findings. The gross features are quite similar to those of basal cell adenoma. Like most parotid gland tumors, basal cell adenocarcinomas most frequently occur in the superficial (lateral) lobe of the gland. The color of the cut surface is variable and may be gray, tan-white, or brown. Some tumors have visible cystic formations, but the texture is usually homogeneous. They may be well circumscribed but not encapsulated or may infiltrate the adjacent parotid parenchyma or surrounding tissues.

Microscopic Findings. As indicated by the nomenclature, both the cytologic and histomorphologic characteristics of basal cell adenocarcinoma are similar to those of basal cell adenoma. In fact, examination of only limited foci may not distinguish the two. Yet, basal cell adenocarcinoma manifests the parameters of a malignant neoplasm that segregates it from basal cell adenoma, the most important of which is infiltrative growth.

Infiltrative growth is more than just the absence of a fibrous capsule, and it must be differentiated from the multinodular pattern that is common in the membranous type of basal cell adenoma (see Basal Cell Adenoma). Infiltration is manifested by extension of nodules, nests, or cords of tumor cells from the main tumor mass into adjacent lobules of parotid parenchyma, dermis, skeletal muscle, or periglandular fat (figs. 5-147–5-149). The tumor penetrates between parotid acini, causing degeneration of some acini and entrapping other acini in the tumor (fig. 5-150). A fibrous tissue stroma usually accompanies the infiltrating adenocarcinoma and frequently contains lymphocytic and plasmacytic inflammatory cells (fig. 5-151). Vessel or peripheral nerve invasion is evident in about a fourth of the tumors (figs. 5-152, 5-153).

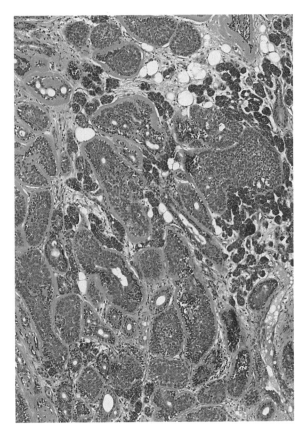

Figure 5-147
BASAL CELL ADENOCARCINOMA
In this low-magnification micrograph, numerous small nests of basaloid epithelial cells in a fibrous stroma infiltrate the parotid parenchyma without any evidence of a capsule or circumscription.

Encroachment or entrapment of peripheral nerves is common, but nerve encroachment by itself is not necessarily indicative of malignancy.

Prior to the establishment of basal cell adenocarcinoma as a diagnostic entity, Strauss et al. (437) described an infiltrating basaloid neoplasm of the parotid gland that bound to the facial nerve; a portion of the nerve had to be excised for resection of the tumor. Due to an absence of cytologic atypia, such as nuclear and cytoplasmic pleomorphism and high mitotic figure count, the tumor was interpreted as an unusual basal cell adenoma. Today, this tumor would be classified as basal cell adenocarcinoma. The degree of cytologic atypia is variable among these tumors (figs. 5-154, 5-155) but is usually mild to moderate with a notable resemblance to basal cell adenoma (fig. 5-156). Counts of mitotic

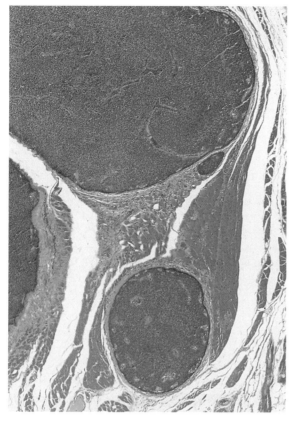

Figure 5-148
BASAL CELL ADENOCARCINOMA
Large and medium-sized nodules of a basaloid cell neoplasm of the parotid gland have infiltrated the masseter muscle.

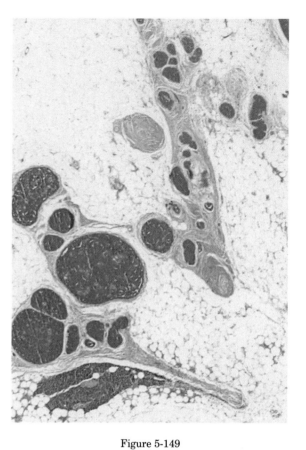

Figure 5-149
BASAL CELL ADENOCARCINOMA
Varying sized nodules of basaloid cells have infiltrated the buccal adipose tissue adjacent to the parotid gland.

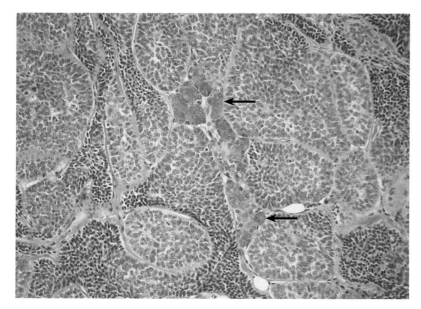

Figure 5-150
BASAL CELL ADENOCARCINOMA
Foci of serous acinar cells (arrows) remain in this lobule of parotid gland tissue that has been infiltrated by large nests or islands of basaloid cells.

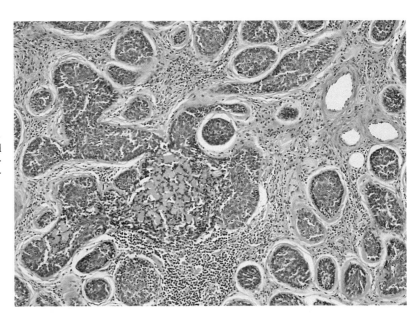

Figure 5-151
BASAL CELL ADENOCARCINOMA
Proliferation of variably sized and shaped nests of basaloid tumor cells occurs in a dense fibrous stroma with scattered and focally dense lymphocytes.

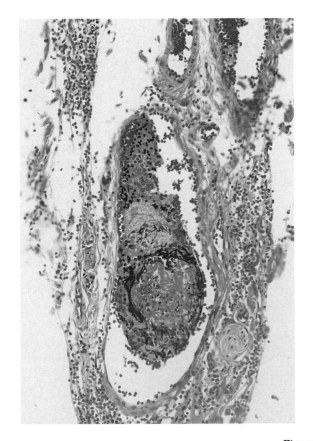
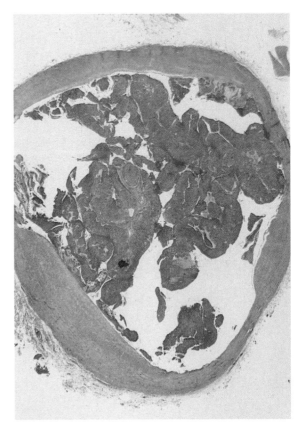

Figure 5-152
VASCULAR INVASION BY BASAL CELL ADENOCARCINOMA

Left: Basaloid epithelial cells from a basal cell adenocarcinoma of the parotid gland are associated with fibrin clot and blood cells in the intravascular compartment of a thin-walled blood vessel.

Right: An irregular mass of tumor cells is in the intravascular compartment of a dilated vein excised as part of a parotidectomy specimen that contained a basal cell adenocarcinoma.

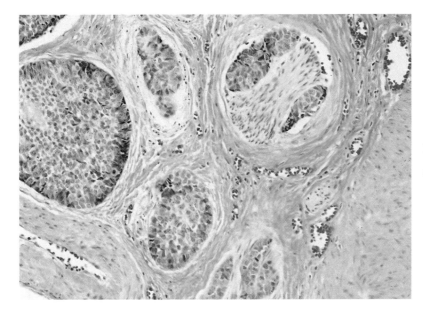

Figure 5-153
PERINEURAL INVASION BY
BASAL CELL ADENOCARCINOMA
The perineural space of a branch of
the facial nerve has been invaded by
basaloid epithelial cells of a parotid
gland neoplasm.

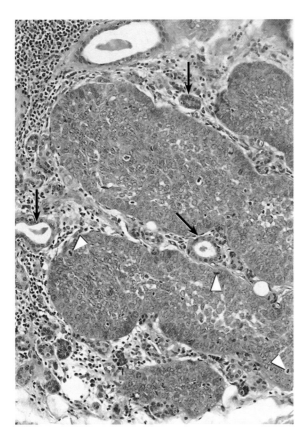

Figure 5-154
BASAL CELL ADENOCARCINOMA

Foci of normal ducts (arrows) remain after infiltration of
a parotid gland lobule by basal cell adenocarcinoma. The
tumor cells are relatively uniform, but some pleomorphism
and mitotic figures (arrowheads) are present. Palisading of
cell nuclei along the stromal interface is not distinct.

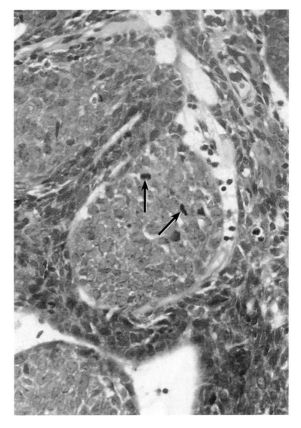

Figure 5-155
BASAL CELL ADENOCARCINOMA

High-magnification micrograph of basaloid tumor cells
shows two mitotic figures (arrows), but cytologic atypia is not
prominent. Cells are fairly uniform except that cells with slightly
darker, smaller nuclei seem to partially surround cells with paler,
larger nuclei. Unlike most solid-type basal cell adenomas, peripheral palisading of nuclei is inconspicuous.

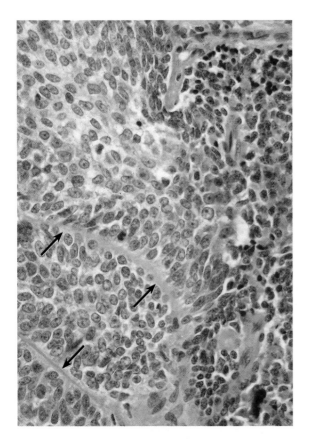

Figure 5-156
BASAL CELL ADENOCARCINOMA
Nests of uniform basaloid cells without cytologic atypia (but a mitotic figure) are segregated by thin hyaline septa (arrows). There are both small, dark (right) and larger, pale (left) basaloid cells, but palisading of nuclei of peripheral cells is minimal.

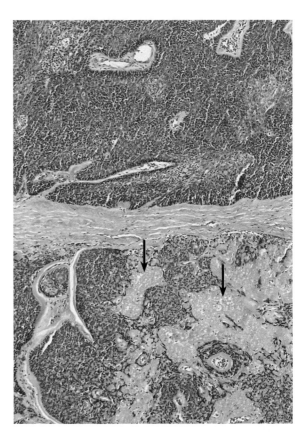

Figure 5-157
NECROSIS IN BASAL CELL ADENOCARCINOMA
Areas of tumor cell necrosis (arrows) are an uncommon feature of basal cell adenocarcinoma.

figures vary from less than 1 to up to 10 per 10 high-power fields (at X400 magnification) but are most often in a range of 2 to 3 per 10 high-power fields. A few tumors have foci of necrosis (fig. 5-157), but this feature is not typical.

Basal cell adenocarcinomas manifest histomorphologic patterns similar to those associated with basal cell adenomas: solid, membranous, trabecular, and tubular. Most have a solid pattern. Basaloid epithelial cells are aggregated in variably sized and shaped nests that are separated from one another by thin septa or thick bands of collagenous stroma (figs. 5-147, 5-148, 5-150, 5-151, 5-154–5-157). Many of these tumors produce an excessive amount of basal lamina material in the form of intercellular droplets and peripheral membranes of eosinophilic hyalinized material, hence the term membranous type (fig.

5-158). This hyaline material stains with periodic acid–Schiff stain. Luna et al. (429) reported that the membranous (or dermal analogue) type of basal cell adenoma was the type that most frequently underwent malignant transformation in their series of carcinomas ex monomorphic adenomas. Circular foci of squamous differentiation, with or without keratin production, are present among the basaloid cells in some tumors (figs. 5-159, 5-160). In contrast to the solid pattern, a latticework of interconnecting bands of basaloid cells characterizes the trabecular growth pattern. In some tumors small pseudocysts or lumens and duct cell differentiation are evident among the trabeculae of basaloid cells and produce a tubulotrabecular appearance (fig. 5-161). Lumens are prominent in the tubular type, but this is an uncommon pattern among basal cell adenocarcinomas (fig. 5-162).

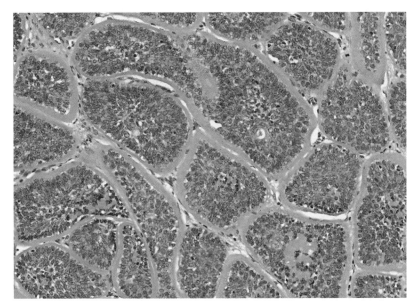

Figure 5-158
MEMBRANOUS BASAL CELL
ADENOCARCINOMA

Eosinophilic, membrane-like bands of basal lamina around islands of basaloid cells as well as intranodular globules of eosinophilic hyalinized material characterize the membranous or dermal analogue type of basal cell adenocarcinoma. On the basis of this field alone distinction from basal cell adenoma is not possible.

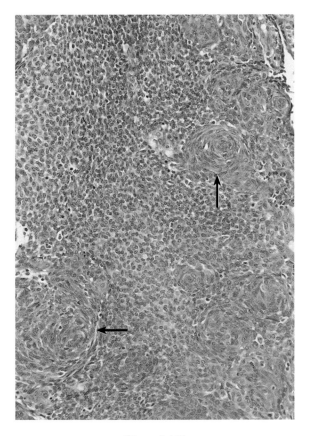

Figure 5-159
SQUAMOID SWIRLS IN
BASAL CELL ADENOCARCINOMA

Focal, roughly circular areas of cells with a squamoid epithelial appearance (arrows) blend into a sheet of basaloid cells.

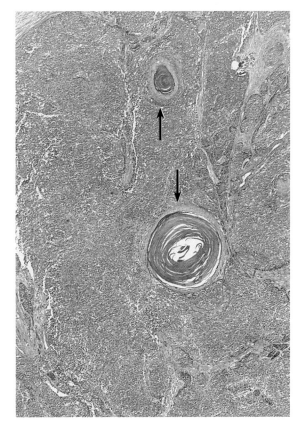

Figure 5-160
FOCAL SQUAMOUS DIFFERENTIATION
IN BASAL CELL ADENOCARCINOMA

Two foci (arrows) of squamous differentiation with keratin production are within a large mass of basaloid cells of a tumor from the parotid gland.

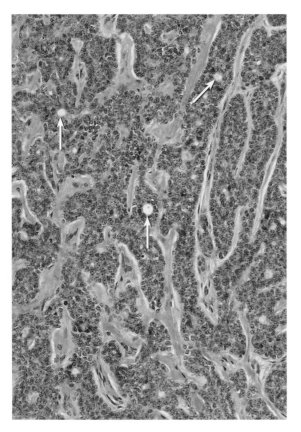

Figure 5-161
TRABECULAR BASAL CELL
ADENOCARCINOMA
Bands of basaloid cells interconnect in an irregular pattern. Within the bands small lumens or pseudolumens are evident (arrows) and produce what may be called a tubulotrabecular pattern.

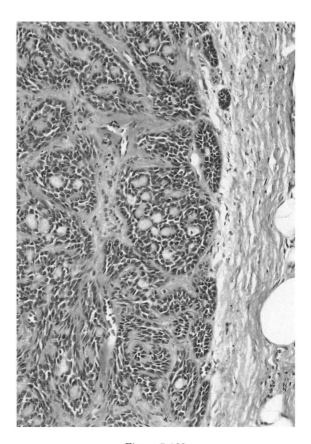

Figure 5-162
TUBULAR BASAL CELL ADENOCARCINOMA
Numerous small lumens or pseudolumens characterize the tubular form of basal cell adenocarcinoma.

Akin to basal cell adenoma, palisading of nuclei along the stromal interface of the basaloid cells is observed in basal cell adenocarcinomas, but this peripheral palisading appears less frequently and less prominently than in the adenomas (figs. 5-155, 5-156, 5-163). It is also more evident in the solid and membranous patterns than the trabecular or tubular patterns.

Similar to basal cell adenomas, the basaloid cell population has two cellular forms (fig. 5-164). The most conspicuous cells are relatively uniform with pale eosinophilic to amphophilic cytoplasm, indistinct cell borders, and round to oval, pale basophilic nuclei. The other cells are smaller and have less cytoplasm and more basophilic nuclei that give the tissue a more basophilic appearance. When they are evident, the

smaller, darker cells tend to be clustered at the periphery of the epithelial islands or bands, and these cells often have palisaded nuclei along the stromal interface. In addition to basaloid cells, some cuboidal, ductal cells are present within most basal cell adenocarcinomas (fig. 5-165). These cells are least evident in the solid and membranous patterns and most prominent in the tubular pattern.

Immunohistochemical staining is variable from tumor to tumor but in many tumors supports myoepithelial differentiation of some of the basaloid cells (fig. 5-166). Williams et al. (440) found smooth muscle actin and vimentin reactivity in 83 and 78 percent, respectively, of 23 basal cell adenocarcinomas they studied. This reactivity tended to be concentrated in the more peripheral

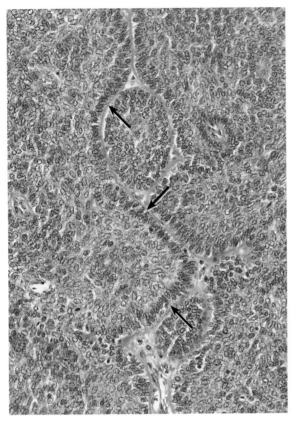

Figure 5-163
PALISADING OF NUCLEI IN
BASAL CELL ADENOCARCINOMA
Focally, palisading of the nuclei of the basaloid cells is
evident along the periphery of the tumor nodules (arrows).
In general, this feature is less evident in basal cell adeno-
carcinomas than in basal cell adenomas.

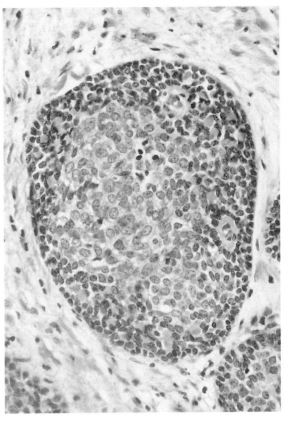

Figure 5-164
CYTOLOGIC FEATURES OF
BASAL CELL ADENOCARCINOMA
High magnification of a small nodule in basal cell adeno-
carcinoma shows cells with small, dark nuclei clustered
around the periphery of cells with larger, paler nuclei.

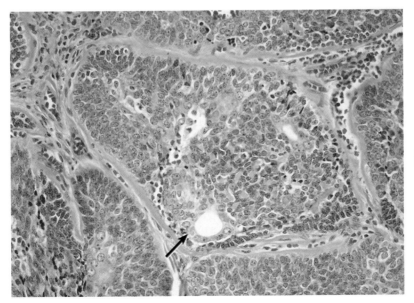

Figure 5-165
DUCT CELL DIFFERENTIATION
IN BASAL CELL
ADENOCARCINOMA
Cuboidal ductal cells surround a
small lumen (arrow) within a nodule of
basaloid cells.

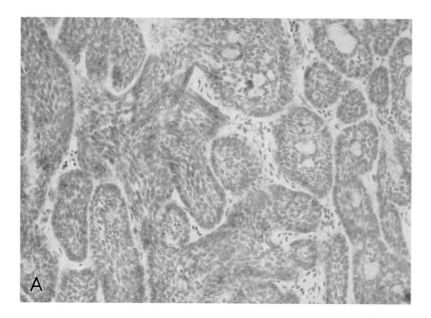

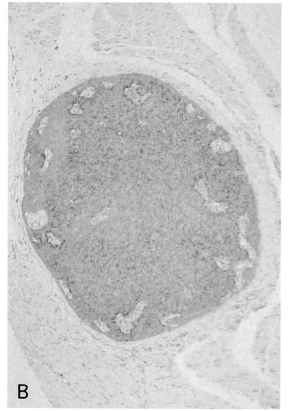

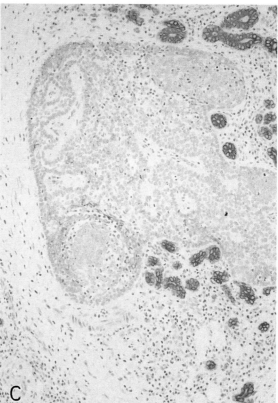

Figure 5-166
BASAL CELL ADENOCARCINOMA: IMMUNOHISTOCHEMISTRY

A: Immunohistochemical staining for smooth muscle actin is mostly evident in the basaloid cells located along the stromal interface. Like most immunohistochemical reactions in basal cell adenocarcinomas, the number of reactive cells varies from tumor to tumor.

B: In this focus of basal cell adenocarcinoma that has infiltrated skeletal muscle, many of the tumor cells are immunoreactive for vimentin. Along with smooth muscle actin, vimentin is thought to be a marker for myoepithelial differentiation.

C: All basal cell adenocarcinomas demonstrate some reactivity for cytokeratin although it may be focal, as in this tumor. (Avidin-biotin peroxidase stain)

cells of the basaloid cell proliferations. All of the tumors were reactive for cytokeratins, and focal reactivity for S-100 protein, epithelial membrane antigen, and carcinoembryonic antigen was detected.

Differential Diagnosis. The principal entity in the differential diagnosis of basal cell adenocarcinoma is basal cell adenoma. Cytologic features alone are frequently insufficient for distinction. While cellular atypia and number of mitotic figures, in general, are greater in basal cell adenocarcinoma than basal cell adenoma, in any specific neoplasm they are of equivocal help by themselves. Infiltrative, destructive growth, as distinct from expansile or multifocal growth, and neural and vascular invasion are the most important factors in differentiating these two tumors.

Adenoid cystic carcinoma is also considered in the differential diagnosis. Distinction from adenoid cystic carcinoma is more critical than distinction from basal cell adenoma since the difference in prognosis in the former is more profound. Both adenoid cystic carcinoma and basal cell adenocarcinoma are composed of relatively uniform, basaloid-appearing cells; however, basal cell adenocarcinoma lacks the cribriform pattern and pseudocysts of amorphous, basophilic glycosaminoglycans characteristic of adenoid cystic carcinoma. Even the solid type of adenoid cystic carcinoma usually contains some cribriform foci. Cytologic features also help: the pale to clear cells with irregular, angular nuclei characteristic of adenoid cystic carcinoma contrast with the oval to round, eosinophilic cells and round nuclei of basal cell adenocarcinoma (see Adenoid Cystic Carcinoma). The mixture of large pale and small dark cells common to basal cell adenocarcinoma is not a feature of adenoid cystic carcinoma. Although focal necrosis and high mitotic figure counts are not infallible discriminators, they are more consistently a feature of solid adenoid cystic carcinoma than basal cell adenocarcinoma.

Basaloid squamous carcinoma is a recently defined type of squamous cell carcinoma of the upper aerodigestive tract that has basaloid features (416,430,438). It has a predilection for the hypopharynx, base of tongue, and supraglottic larynx, regions in which basal cell adenocarcinoma rarely or never occurs. A case of basaloid squamous carcinoma that involved the buccal mucosa has been reported (420). This tumor is composed of small, hyperchromatic cells that form solid lobules, adenomatoid arrangements, and cords. The tumor aggregates are commonly associated with eosinophilic hyaline material and comedonecrosis (see section on Adenoid Cystic Carcinoma for illustrations of basaloid squamous carcinoma). In contrast to basal cell adenocarcinoma, basaloid squamous carcinoma has a malignant squamous component that involves the mucosal epithelium in the form of epithelial dysplasia, carcinoma in situ, or invasive squamous cell carcinoma. Immunohistochemically, basaloid squamous cell carcinoma is reported to be unreactive for muscle actin, and anti-carcinoembryonic antigen reactivity occurs in the epidermoid cells rather than the ductal and basaloid cells as in basal cell adenocarcinoma (416).

Prognosis and Treatment. Basal cell adenocarcinomas are low-grade carcinomas. They are infiltrative, locally destructive, and tend to recur, but they only occasionally metastasize. None of the few individually reported cases metastasized, but follow-up was limited (421,425–427,432). None of the eight cases reported by Luna et al. (429) as carcinomas ex monomorphic adenoma metastasized; but six patients had local recurrences, and four of these still had recurrent disease from 7 to 10 years after primary treatment. Ellis and Wescovitch (423) reported recurrences in 7 and metastases in 3 of 25 patients. The metastases were to cervical lymph nodes and, in one case, to lung. Luna et al. (431) have reported basal cell adenomas that arose in heterotopic salivary gland tissue in periparotid and upper cervical lymph nodes, and these tumors must be distinguished from metastatic basal cell adenocarcinoma. In addition to basal cell adenoma, other types of salivary gland tumors also have been described in heterotopic salivary gland tissue (439). In general, a primary intraglandular neoplasm needs to be documented before a salivary-type tumor in periparotid lymph nodes is accepted as metastatic disease.

Considering the low-grade biologic potential of basal cell adenocarcinomas, surgical excision is appropriate treatment. At least partial parotidectomy or complete submandibular glandectomy are indicated. Rare intraoral basal cell adenocarcinomas should be excised with margins of normal tissue to ensure complete removal. Enucleation or curettage are to be avoided.

EPITHELIAL-MYOEPITHELIAL CARCINOMA

Definition. Epithelial-myoepithelial carcinoma is an uncommon, low-grade malignant epithelial neoplasm composed of variable proportions of ductal and large, clear-staining, myoepithelial differentiated cells. The clear cells are typically arranged peripherally around the ductal cells and usually predominate.

Since this tumor is composed of ductal and myoepithelial types of epithelial cells, ductal-myoepithelial carcinoma might be more appropriate terminology, but epithelial-myoepithelial carcinoma is now the established term. Tumors of this type have been reported under a variety of names, including *adenomyoepithelioma* (443), *clear cell adenoma* (448,466), *tubular solid adenoma* (452), *monomorphic clear cell tumor* (441), *glycogen-rich adenoma* (454), *glycogen-rich adenocarcinoma* (460), *clear cell carcinoma* (445), and *salivary duct carcinoma* (456,467). From this list of terms it is evident that these tumors were often considered benign before studies with sufficient follow-up identified their metastatic potential. In fact, the second series Fascicle on major salivary gland tumors (471) includes an illustration of epithelial-myoepithelial carcinoma under the heading of clear cell adenoma. Donath et al. (451) first introduced the term epithelial-myoepithelial carcinoma in the German language literature in 1972, and Corio et al. (447) helped establish this term in the English language literature with their report of 16 cases in 1982. The WHO classification of 1972 (472) did not specifically include this tumor, but in the discussion of "other types of monomorphic adenomas" the monograph refers to biphasic tumors with duct-like structures surrounded by clear cells and mentions the term clear cell adenoma. The WHO monograph of 1991 (468) includes epithelial-myoepithelial carcinoma in its classification. Also reporting in the German language literature, Kleinsasser et al. (456) appear to have been the first to use the term salivary duct carcinoma, which is also a new entity in the recent WHO classification (see Salivary Duct Carcinoma), but today two of their five cases would be better classified as epithelial-myoepithelial carcinomas.

Investigators have noted that some epithelial-myoepithelial carcinomas are composed predominantly of clear cells (442,446,459). On the other hand, some clear cell neoplasms, especially those that occur in the intraoral minor salivary glands, are almost exclusively a monomorphous population of clear cells that have morphologic features uncharacteristic of most epithelial-myoepithelial carcinomas. Little long-term follow-up information is available for these cases, and future investigations might clearly establish that some clear cell carcinomas are variants of epithelial-myoepithelial carcinoma. However, since the term epithelial-myoepithelial carcinoma implies a biphasic neoplasm, other investigators (444, 445,457,469,470) and the authors currently classify monomorphous clear cell carcinomas separately (see Clear Cell Adenocarcinoma).

Tumors with similar if not identical histologic features to epithelial-myoepithelial carcinomas of salivary gland have been identified in breast and skin (462,465).

General Features. Epithelial-myoepithelial carcinoma is an uncommon neoplasm of salivary glands. It is difficult to assess the reported incidence of this tumor among large surveys of salivary gland neoplasms since it has not often been included as a specific entity. Recent evaluations indicate an average incidence of about 1 percent of salivary gland neoplasms (441,442,449,458, 469). This corresponds to the AFIP experience of 1.1 percent of all epithelial salivary gland neoplasms reviewed over the last decade.

It is predominantly a tumor of the major salivary glands, specifically the parotid gland. The proportion of epithelial-myoepithelial carcinomas that have been reported in the intraoral minor salivary glands has ranged from none to 41 percent, but on average the range is 10 to 15 percent (442,453,463). The AFIP's data show a frequency of about 11 percent in the minor glands and about 10 percent in the submandibular gland, similar to other reports.

The youngest patient in the AFIP case files was 15 years old, and a tumor in an 8-year-old child has been reported (461); however, epithelial-myoepithelial carcinoma is primarily a tumor of adults. The peak incidence is in the seventh decade of life, and the mean age of patients is about 60 years. About 60 percent of patients are female.

Clinical Features. Localized swelling is frequently the only sign, but occasionally patients experience pain or facial weakness (446,449).

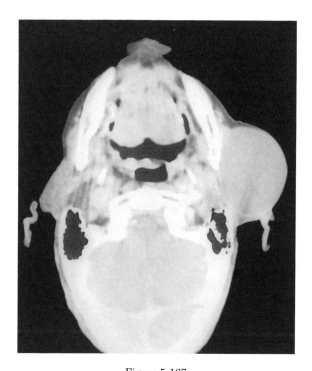

Figure 5-167
COMPUTERIZED TOMOGRAPHIC IMAGE OF
EPITHELIAL-MYOEPITHELIAL CARCINOMA
A large, well-circumscribed mass with uniform radio-density is clearly evident in the left parotid gland region.

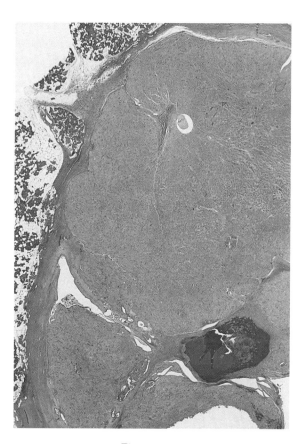

Figure 5-168
EPITHELIAL-MYOEPITHELIAL CARCINOMA
A dense fibrous connective tissue capsule separates the tumor from the normal parotid gland parenchyma (left).

The duration of symptoms before diagnosis has ranged from a few months to years (458).

Gross Findings. Primary tumors range in size from 1 to 12 cm in largest dimension, but 2 to 3 cm is typical (453). They are frequently well circumscribed (fig. 5-167), but recurrent tumors and some primary tumors are multinodular and irregular and sometimes hemorrhagic or necrotic. The tumors are firm, and the cut surfaces are gray-white to tan-white.

Microscopic Findings. Confirming the gross examination impression, many epithelial-myoepithelial carcinomas are well circumscribed. Belying their malignant potential, some are partially encapsulated (fig. 5-168), and many are multilobular (fig. 5-169).

As the name for this group of tumors indicates, they are composed of a biphasic cell population: myoepithelial cells and ductal cells. The myoepithelial cells are characterized by their large size, polygonal shape, and clear-staining cytoplasm. Myoepithelial differentiation of the clear cells is indicated by their peripheral posi-

tion relative to the ductal cells and by immunohistochemical and ultrastructural evidence. In most tumors the clear myoepithelial cells are the dominant cellular component and are evident even at low magnification (fig. 5-170). High magnification shows ductal elements surrounded by clear cells (fig. 5-171). The ductal elements are composed of intercalated duct-like cells that usually border small lumens. The ductal cells are cuboidal, with eosinophilic cytoplasm and uniform, round nuclei that occupy most of the cytoplasmic compartments. The lumens frequently contain an eosinophilic proteinaceous material that ordinarily reacts with periodic acid–Schiff (PAS) stain but not mucicarmine stain. The clear cells are arranged peripheral to the ductal cells and are usually more numerous. They are distinctly larger and more variable in size than the duct cells and have larger, more

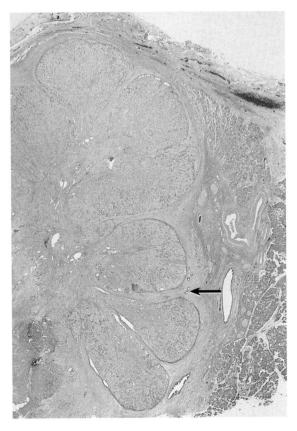

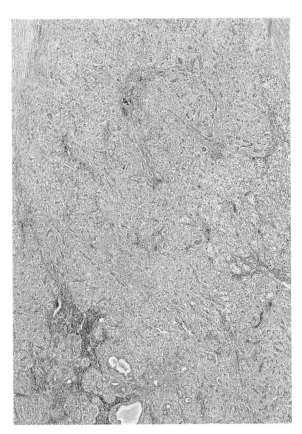

Figure 5-169
EPITHELIAL-MYOEPITHELIAL CARCINOMA
Fibrous connective tissue bands separate lobules of this multilobular tumor. The tumor seems well circumscribed, but residual ducts of parotid parenchyma (arrow) are present adjacent to and between tumor lobules.

Figure 5-170
EPITHELIAL-MYOEPITHELIAL CARCINOMA
With low-magnification microscopy the biphasic cellular composition is difficult to discern, but pale-staining and clear cells are evident.

irregularly shaped nuclei. The cytoplasm does not usually stain with hematoxylin and eosin, although variable amounts of pale eosinophilic or amphophilic cytoplasm are present in some cells. PAS staining before and after digestion of the tissue with diastase (amylase) usually demonstrates significant glycogen in the clear cells (fig. 5-172). These "myoepithelial" clear cells are mostly polygonal but sometimes are elongated or spindle shaped (fig. 5-173). They often have indistinct cytoplasmic borders.

The ratio of clear cells to ductal cells is variable from tumor to tumor and within the same tumor. The proportion of ductal cells ranges from about a third of the cell population to nearly absent (figs. 5-174–5-176). In most tumors the ductal structures are conspicuous among the clear cell population; however, in some tumors the ductal

cells are more difficult to distinguish from the myoepithelial clear cells, and a careful search is sometimes needed to identify them (fig. 5-177).

The epithelial tumor cells are arranged in sheets (figs. 5-173, 5-177), an organoid pattern (figs. 5-175, 5-178), or discrete tumor nests (figs. 5-174, 5-176, 5-179). Eosinophilic, hyalinized membranes that are highlighted with PAS often surround aggregates of tumor cells, whether in an organoid pattern or as separate nests (fig. 5-180), and are quite extensive in some tumors (figs. 5-171, 5-174). In still other tumors the stroma is a loose, collagenous, almost myxoid tissue (fig 5-176). The tumors are solid (fig. 5-170) or cystic (fig. 5-181). When cystic, papillary epithelial proliferations often occupy some or most of the cyst luminal spaces (fig. 5-182). The epithelium lining the cystic spaces usually retains the

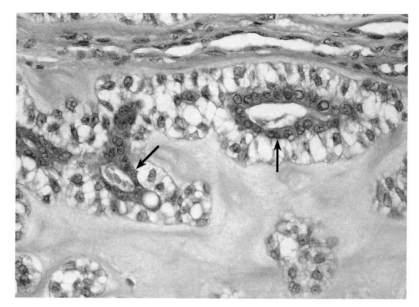

Figure 5-171
EPITHELIAL-MYOEPITHELIAL
CARCINOMA
Eosinophilic cuboidal, intercalated duct-like cells (arrows) surround lumens and are themselves surrounded by larger, polygonal cells with nonstaining cytoplasm.

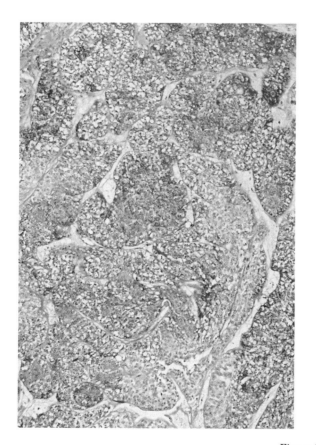
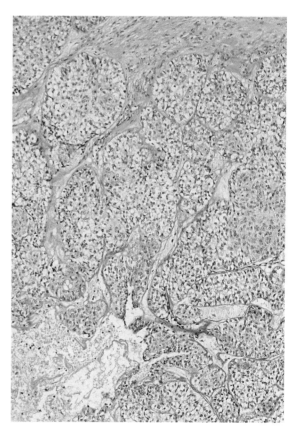

Figure 5-172
EPITHELIAL-MYOEPITHELIAL CARCINOMA CONTAINING GLYCOGEN
Cytoplasmic periodic acid–Schiff staining (left) that is abolished when the tissue section is digested with diastase before staining (right) indicates significant glycogen in the clear cells.

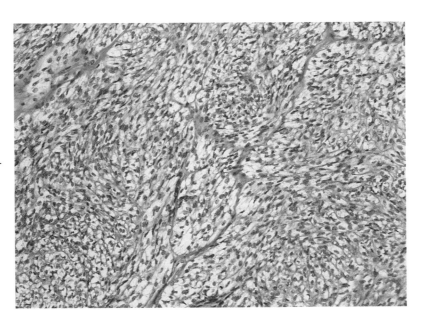

Figure 5-173
SPINDLED CELLS IN
EPITHELIAL-
MYOEPITHELIAL CARCINOMA
These myoepithelial clear cells are distinctly spindle shaped.

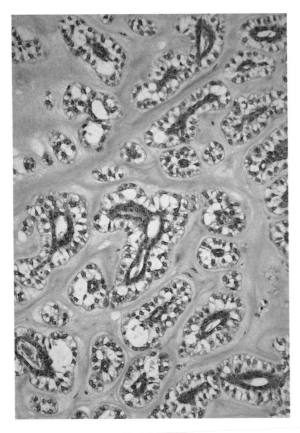

Figure 5-174
EPITHELIAL-MYOEPITHELIAL CARCINOMA
Smaller, eosinophilic ductal cells are relatively numerous and conspicuous within small groups of larger clear cells. The periepithelial stromal tissue is hyalinized.

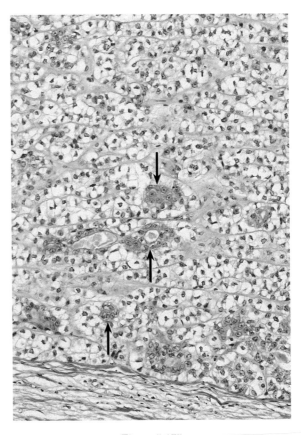

Figure 5-175
EPITHELIAL-MYOEPITHELIAL CARCINOMA
Within this sheet of clear cells the ductal elements (arrows) are not very prominent and comprise only about a tenth of the total cell population. Very thin fibrous bands surround groups of clear cells.

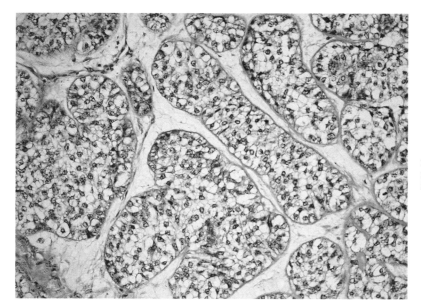

Figure 5-176
EPITHELIAL-MYOEPITHELIAL
CARCINOMA
Multiple irregular nests of polygonal clear cells lie within a very loose, myxoid stroma. No ductal cells are evident in this field.

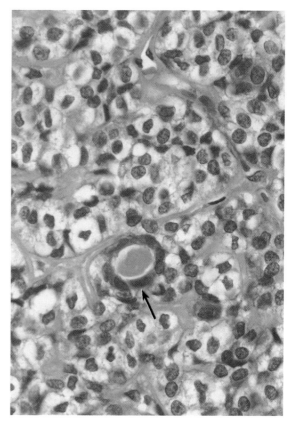

Figure 5-177
EPITHELIAL-MYOEPITHELIAL CARCINOMA
Left: Ductal elements are inconspicuous in this sheet of clear cells.
Right: At high magnification a focus of subtle but definite duct formation is evident (arrow).

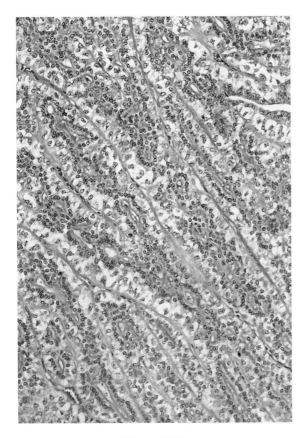

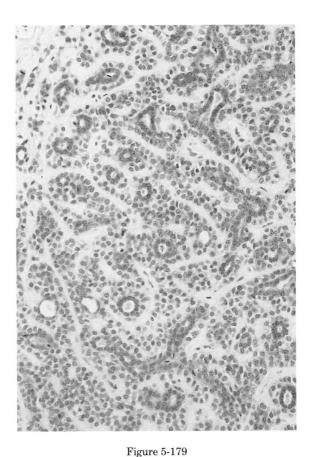

Figure 5-178
EPITHELIAL-MYOEPITHELIAL CARCINOMA

Thin fibrovascular septa encompass groups of ductal and clear myoepithelial cells in an organoid arrangement.

Figure 5-179
EPITHELIAL-MYOEPITHELIAL CARCINOMA

The clear myoepithelial cells that surround the ductal cells are smaller in this case than those in most epithelial-myoepithelial carcinomas, and their demarcation from the stroma is less distinct. These features are reminiscent of the ductal-myoepithelial configurations seen in mixed tumors.

Figure 5-180
HYALINE MEMBRANES
IN EPITHELIAL-
MYOEPITHELIAL CARCINOMA

Periodic acid–Schiff stain highlights the eosinophilic, hyalinized basal lamina material that surrounds nests of tumor cells.

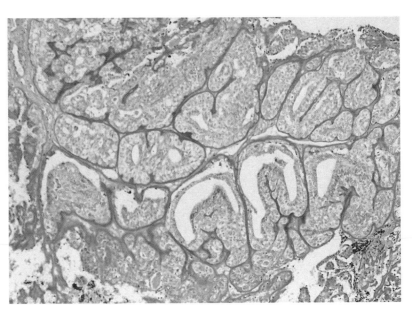

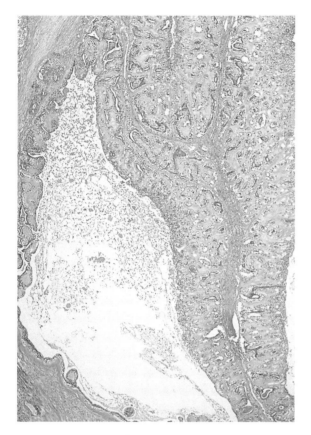

Figure 5-181
CYSTIC EPITHELIAL-
MYOEPITHELIAL CARCINOMA
Cystic spaces that are lined by tumor cells frequently occur in epithelial-myoepithelial carcinomas.

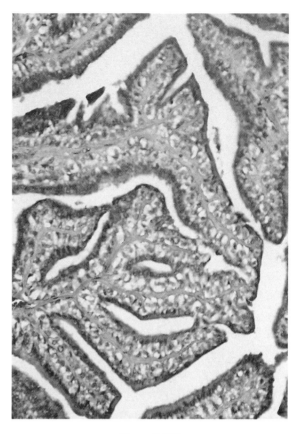

Figure 5-182
PAPILLARY EPITHELIAL-
MYOEPITHELIAL CARCINOMA
Branching papillae of tumor with thin fibrovascular cores extend into a cystic space. The epithelial lining of the cystic structure and papillae has maintained the basic biphasic cellular relationship of lumen-lining ductal cells and peripheral clear cells.

biphasic relationship of myoepithelial clear cells peripheral to ductal cells.

In most tumors cytologic atypia is mild or absent, but occasional tumors manifest cellular and nuclear pleomorphism and increased mitotic figures (figs. 5-183, 5-184). Mitotic figure counts of 2 or less per 10 high-power fields (at X400 magnification) are typical but range up to 8 to 10 per 10 high-power fields in rare tumors. Even though gross and low-magnification examination may show these tumors to be well circumscribed, nests of tumor cells frequently infiltrate adjacent parenchyma or tissues (fig. 5-185), including peripheral nerves (fig. 5-186). Central necrosis of tumor lobules occurs in some tumors. Rarely, foci of mucicarminophilic cells are present (fig. 5-187).

Immunohistochemical and Ultrastructural Findings. Immunohistochemical studies have characteristically described the ductal cells as immunoreactive for cytokeratin (fig. 5-188) and the clear cells as immunoreactive for S-100 protein (fig. 5-189) (446,453,459,469). This is relative, however, and immunoreactivity for S-100 protein is variable: in some tumors most of the clear cells are unreactive, and in other tumors the ductal cells are weakly reactive. While the ductal cells usually react intensely for cytokeratin, the clear cells are often reactive for cytokeratin as well. Immunoreactivity for smooth muscle actin is frequently intense in the clear cells (fig. 5-190). Occasionally, some reactivity for glial fibrillary acidic protein is found (fig. 5-191). Investigators

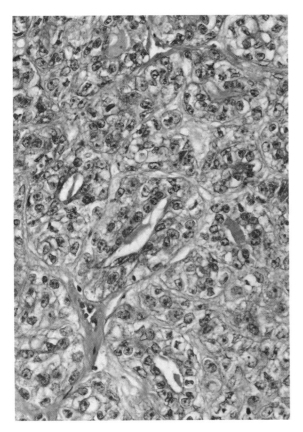

Figure 5-183
CYTOLOGIC ATYPIA IN EPITHELIAL-
MYOEPITHELIAL CARCINOMA

In this tumor both the ductal and clear cells have more irregular-shaped and -sized nuclei than typical epithelial-myoepithelial carcinoma, and nucleoli are distinct.

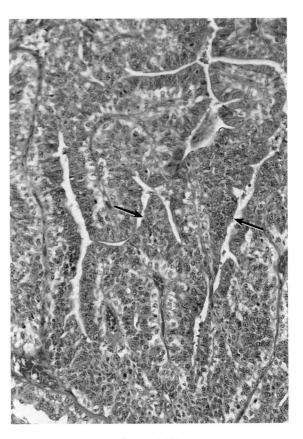

Figure 5-184
CYTOLOGIC ATYPIA IN EPITHELIAL-
MYOEPITHELIAL CARCINOMA

The ductal cells have more vesicular nuclei and scattered mitotic figures. They are multilayered in foci (arrows).

Figure 5-185
EPITHELIAL-MYOEPITHELIAL
CARCINOMA

Two small nests of tumor cells that are located adjacent to a blood vessel and away from the main tumor mass are associated with a chronically inflamed fibrous connective tissue stroma.

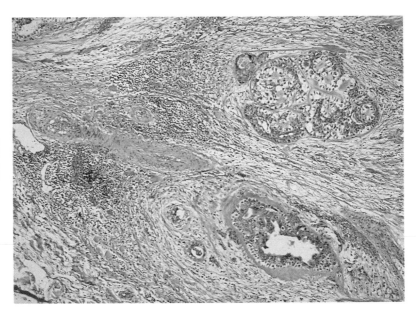

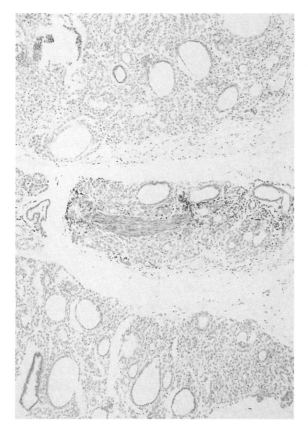

Figure 5-186
PERINEURAL GROWTH OF EPITHELIAL-
MYOEPITHELIAL CARCINOMA
Immunohistochemical staining for S-100 protein high-
lights a peripheral nerve that is enveloped by tumor cells.
(Avidin-biotin peroxidase stain)

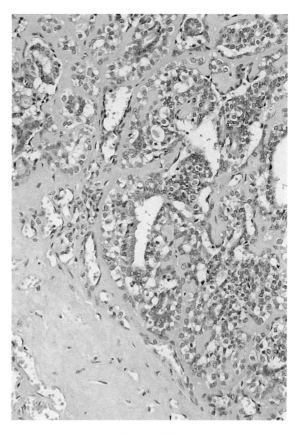

Figure 5-187
MUCOUS CELLS IN EPITHELIAL-
MYOEPITHELIAL CARCINOMA
Most epithelial-myoepithelial carcinomas are unreactive
with mucicarmine stain, but rare tumors such as this one
may have a few mucous cells.

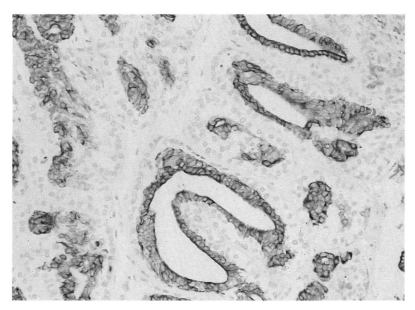

Figure 5-188
CYTOKERATIN IN EPITHELIAL-
MYOEPITHELIAL CARCINOMA
Immunoreactivity for cytokeratin
with a cocktail of monoclonal antibodies
is intense in ductal cells, but there is also
faint immunostaining of some clear
cells. (Avidin-biotin peroxidase stain)

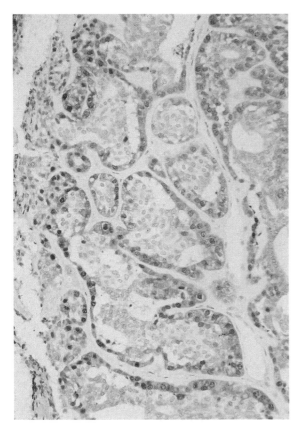

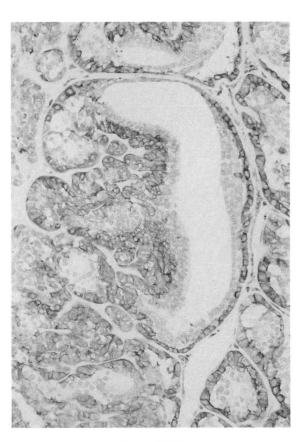

Figure 5-189
S-100 PROTEIN IN EPITHELIAL-
MYOEPITHELIAL CARCINOMA

Immunohistochemical staining for S-100 protein shows intense staining of the most peripheral clear cells and less intense staining of more central clear and ductal cells. (Avidin-biotin peroxidase stain)

Figure 5-190
SMOOTH MUSCLE ACTIN IN EPITHELIAL-
MYOEPITHELIAL CARCINOMA

The clear cells react intensely with anti-smooth muscle actin, but the ductal cells are unreactive. (Avidin-biotin peroxidase stain)

Figure 5-191
GLIAL FIBRILLARY ACIDIC
PROTEIN IN EPITHELIAL-
MYOEPITHELIAL CARCINOMA

Although less frequent than in mixed tumors, immunoreactivity for glial fibrillary acidic protein can occasionally be observed in the myoepithelial cells of epithelial-myoepithelial carcinoma. (Avidin-biotin peroxidase stain)

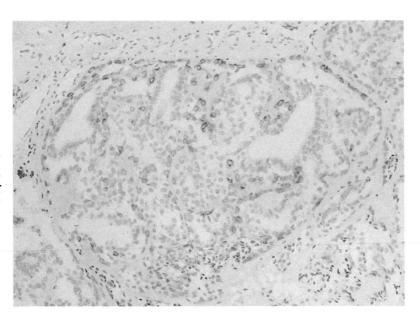

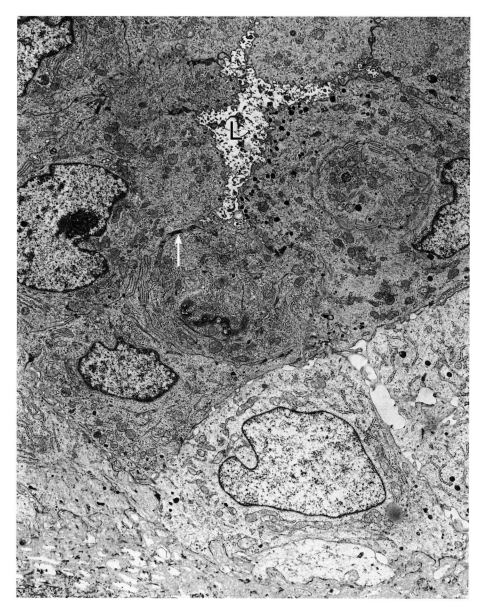

Figure 5-192
EPITHELIAL-MYOEPITHELIAL CARCINOMA: ULTRASTRUCTURE
Electron micrograph shows electron-lucent cells adjacent to more electron-dense cells. The electron-dense cells surround a small lumen (L), have microvilli on the luminal surface, and are joined by desmosomes (arrow). Along the basal surface of the more electron-lucent cells is a thickened basal lamina (BL) (X9,600). (Courtesy of Dr. Irving Dardick, Toronto, Canada.)

have reported reactivity for myosin and vimentin in the clear cells, amylase in the ductal cells, and type IV collagen in the periepithelial membranes (446,450,459,464).

The bicellular features observed with light microscopy are also evident with electron microscopy (fig. 5-192). Electron-dense cells are surrounded by electron-lucent cells. The electron-dense cells en-

compass small lumens, have microvilli on their luminal surface, and are attached to one another by well-formed junctional complexes and desmosomes. Some of these cells have dense core secretory granules, a dilated endoplasmic reticulum, tonofilaments, and a conspicuous Golgi complex. The electron-lucent cells contain fewer organelles and often have large aggregates of glycogen;

some have a conspicuous rough endoplasmic reticulum, arrays of microfilaments with focal densities, subplasmalemmal plaques, and multilayered basal lamina (447,449,459,460).

Differential Diagnosis. Several other types of salivary gland neoplasms also are composed of both luminal (ductal) and abluminal (myoepithelial) cells, including mixed tumors, adenoid cystic carcinomas, and polymorphous low-grade adenocarcinomas. Epithelial-myoepithelial carcinomas lack the mesenchymal-appearing myxochondroid tissue that characteristically occurs in mixed tumors. In the myoepithelial component of mixed tumors the cells are usually smaller than those of epithelial-myoepithelial carcinomas and generally are not optically clear.

Similar to some epithelial-myoepithelial carcinomas, adenoid cystic carcinomas often have inconspicuous ductal differentiated cells and many myoepithelial-type cells with lightly hematoxylin and eosin stained or unstained cytoplasm. However, the cells in adenoid cystic carcinoma are smaller and typically have more hyperchromatic nuclei; in addition, many nuclei are irregular and angular shaped. Both epithelial-myoepithelial carcinoma and adenoid cystic carcinoma have tubular and solid growth patterns, but the characteristic cribriform pattern of adenoid cystic carcinoma is not a feature of epithelial-myoepithelial carcinoma.

Some clear cells can be found in polymorphous low-grade adenocarcinoma, but they are not a predominant component and are not arranged in a bicellular pattern with ductal cells. Polymorphous low-grade adenocarcinoma is primarily a tumor of intraoral minor salivary glands while epithelial-myoepithelial carcinoma occurs most frequently in the parotid glands.

Clear cells can be a prominent component of mucoepidermoid carcinomas, acinic cell adenocarcinomas, sebaceous carcinomas, and oncocytomas. All of these tumors lack the characteristic biphasic cellular pattern of epithelial-myoepithelial carcinomas. In contrast to epithelial-myoepithelial carcinomas, mucoepidermoid carcinomas have epidermoid and mucous differentiated cells. Acinic cell adenocarcinomas have acinar differentiated cells, and the clear cells are negative for glycogen. Likewise, sebaceous carcinomas are negative for glycogen, but frozen sections stain for lipids. Clear cells in oncocytomas contain glycogen, have the cellular morphology

and organoid pattern of typical oncocytomas, and usually have typical eosinophilic oncocytes associated with the clear cells.

By definition, clear cell adenocarcinomas are composed of epithelial cells with cytoplasm that does not stain with hematoxylin and eosin and lack apparent intercalated duct cell differentiation (see Clear Cell Adenocarcinoma). There are arguments for and against inclusion of these monomorphous clear cell tumors within the epithelial-myoepithelial category. In favor of one inclusive category are the observations that: some biphasic epithelial-myoepithelial carcinomas have areas with few ductal differentiated cells; many monomorphous clear cell carcinomas contain glycogen; and some monomorphous clear cell carcinomas are immunoreactive for S-100 protein. Reasons for segregating monomorphous clear cell carcinomas from epithelial-myoepithelial carcinoma are: the unique biphasic appearance of epithelial-myoepithelial carcinomas; the occurrence of most epithelial-myoepithelial carcinomas in the major salivary glands while the majority of monomorphous clear cell carcinomas occur in the minor salivary glands; and the observation that the growth pattern of many monomorphous tumors is uncharacteristic of growth patterns of most epithelial-myoepithelial carcinomas. This Fascicle segregates monomorphous clear cell carcinomas because of their different clinical and histologic features.

Although rare in the salivary glands, metastatic renal cell carcinoma is usually considered in the differential diagnosis of clear cell neoplasms. The lipid content (if unprocessed tissue is available), prominent vascularity, and lack of biphasic cell pattern help distinguish renal cell carcinoma from epithelial-myoepithelial carcinoma, but in some cases clinical evaluation for a renal neoplasm may be necessary.

Prognosis and Treatment. As a whole, most reported follow-up information indicates that epithelial-myoepithelial carcinoma is a low-grade malignancy with frequent recurrences, has a tendency to metastasize to periparotid and cervical lymph nodes, and occasionally results in distant metastasis and death (442,446,447,455,458,463, 469). Recurrences are seen in slightly over 30 percent of patients, and lymph node metastases in about 18 percent. Most recurrences manifest within 5 years of resection of the primary tumor, but intervals as long as 9 years to first recurrence have been reported (463). Multiple recurrences up to 28 years after initial surgery have been described (447). About 8 percent of patients have distant metastases, such as to lung, kidney, and brain, and a similar number of patients die as a result of their tumors. In contrast, Fonseca and Soares (453) recently reported 20 patients with follow-up in which 35 percent had metastases and 40 percent died of disease. Distant metastases at intervals as long as 14 and 28 years after initial surgery have been reported (447,463). Most investigators have not been able to correlate an unfavorable clinical course with specific histologic features, but Fonseca and Soares (453) found that nuclear atypia of more than 20 percent of tumor cells was the only histologic variable that indicated a poorer prognosis.

No conclusions can yet be made on the basis of the limited cytometric analyses of the DNA content of epithelial-myoepithelial carcinomas. Hamper et al. (455) found no aneuploid tumors among the 12 they studied, and none of their patients died. Fonseca and Soares (453) reported that 3 of the 8 patients in their series who died had aneuploid tumors, and no survivor had an aneuploid tumor.

Little definitive data for treatment recommendations are available. Most patients have been treated by surgical excision of tumor, but several received radiation therapy in addition (459). Most low-grade malignancies of salivary glands are primarily treated by surgical excision: partial or complete parotidectomy, submandibular glandectomy, or wide local excision of minor salivary gland tumors. Adjunctive radiation therapy is sometimes used, especially when the completeness of excision is in doubt.

CLEAR CELL ADENOCARCINOMA

Definition. Clear cell adenocarcinoma is a malignant epithelial neoplasm composed of a monomorphous population of cells that have optically clear cytoplasm with standard hematoxylin and eosin stains and lack features of other specific neoplasms.

The WHO's most recent classification of salivary gland neoplasms (487) does not define a specific category for clear cell tumors. The monograph states that clear cells are a feature of a wide variety of salivary gland neoplasms, including pleomorphic adenoma, clear cell oncocytoma, sebaceous adenoma, mucoepidermoid carcinoma, acinic cell adenocarcinoma, epithelial-myoepithelial carcinoma, and sebaceous carcinoma. Most tumors with clear cells can be categorized into one of these types on the basis of other characteristic features. Epithelial-myoepithelial carcinoma is defined as a bicellular tumor of duct-like structures composed of an inner layer of duct lining cells and an outer layer of clear cells. Because clear cells are the predominant feature in some epithelial-myoepithelial carcinomas, it might be presumed that monomorphous clear cell tumors should be included in this category. On the other hand, some monomorphous clear cell neoplasms have features that are uncharacteristic of most epithelial-myoepithelial carcinomas (481,484,489). Ogawa et al. (484) found that monomorphous clear cell tumors were immunohistochemically and ultrastructurally variable. While future investigations might clearly establish which monomorphous clear cell carcinomas are variants of epithelial-myoepithelial carcinoma, for reasons previously stated (see previous section) this Fascicle and other literature (474,475,478,479,481,484,488,489) classify monomorphous clear cell carcinomas separately.

General Features. Since controversy and inconsistency have characterized the reporting of clear cell neoplasms and since these tumors are not often included in surveys of salivary gland neoplasms, it is difficult to derive meaningful incidence rates from the literature. Spiro et al. (492) included clear cell adenocarcinoma as a subtype in their study of 204 salivary gland adenocarcinomas, but no specific data were provided. Waldron et al. (495) found 2 clear cell carcinomas of the palate among 426 minor salivary gland tumors while Simpson et al. (489) had 2 clear cell carcinomas in a series of 40 minor salivary gland tumors. Among 190 salivary gland tumors, Thomas et al. (493) reported 1 clear cell carcinoma of the cheek. It is clear that these are uncommon salivary gland neoplasms. About 12 case reports have been described in the literature (484,489), and Milchgrub et al. (481) have reported a series of 11 cases that they called "hyalinizing clear cell carcinoma." Since 1985, monomorphous clear cell adenocarcinomas have comprised about 1 percent of the epithelial salivary gland neoplasms reviewed at the AFIP.

Unlike the bicellular epithelial-myoepithelial carcinomas that primarily occur in the major salivary glands, nearly 60 percent of clear cell adenocarcinomas in the AFIP files have involved the minor salivary glands; most reported cases have also involved the minor salivary glands (481,484,489). About 35 percent of the tumors in the intraoral salivary glands have occurred in the palate, but the buccal mucosa, tongue, floor of the mouth, lip, and retromolar and tonsillar areas also have been involved.

These are tumors of adults: most occur in the fifth to seventh decades of life. The mean age of patients is about 58 years. Patients' ages for the tumors reviewed at the AFIP have ranged from 18 to 90 years although a tumor in the tongue of a 17-month-old boy was reported (494). Women and men are affected nearly equally.

Clinical Features. Swelling has been the only manifestation in most cases, but ulceration of the overlying mucosa and pain have been associated with some intraoral tumors. Erosion of palatal bone and fixation to adjacent tissues have been described (489). Tumor duration before surgery has ranged from 1 month to as long as 15 years (489).

Gross Findings. The size of the tumor at first occurrence is usually 3 cm or less in largest dimension. The cut surface is grayish white, and the tumors are poorly circumscribed and frequently infiltrate adjacent tissues, including the mucosal surface and bone.

Microscopic Findings. Clear cell adenocarcinomas are composed of a monomorphous population of polygonal to round cells that have optically clear cytoplasm when stained with hematoxylin and eosin (fig. 5-193), although in some tumors a portion of the cells have pale eosinophilic cytoplasm (fig. 5-194). The cells are variably sized but most are as large or larger than normal acinar cells. The nuclei are round, often eccentric, lightly to moderately basophilic, and frequently contain small nucleoli (fig. 5-195). The nuclear/cytoplasmic ratio is generally small, but some tumors have a moderate degree of nuclear pleomorphism (fig. 5-196). Mitotic figures are scarce.

Many tumors demonstrate a significant glycogen content with PAS stain before and after tissue digestion with diastase (fig. 5-197), similar to epithelial-myoepithelial carcinoma, but other tumors exhibit little or no glycogen. In-

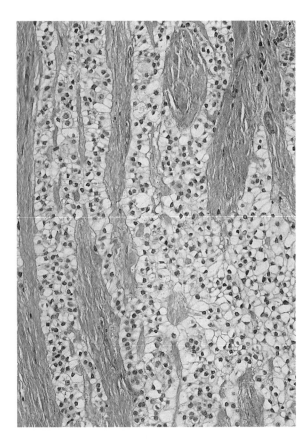

Figure 5-193
CLEAR CELL ADENOCARCINOMA
Sheets of polygonal cells with optically clear cytoplasm have well-defined cell boundaries and are separated by bands of fibrous connective tissue. While most of the tumor cells have clear cytoplasm, a few have pale amphophilic cytoplasm.

tracytoplasmic mucins are not evident with mucicarmine or Alcian blue stain.

The tumor cells are arranged in sheets, nests, and cords in a variable amount of fibrous stroma (figs. 5-198, 5-199). Microcysts infrequently occur, and ductal structures are rare or absent. The connective tissue stroma of these tumors is as variable as the configuration of the tumor cells. The islands, cords, and individual epithelial cells are separated by: 1) interconnecting, thin fibrous septa (figs. 5-198, 5-200); 2) thick, cellular collagenous bands (fig. 5-201); 3) sclerotic or hyalinized collagenous tissue (fig. 5-202); and 4) short, fine wisps of collagen (fig. 5-203).

Clear cell adenocarcinomas are unencapsulated, generally poorly circumscribed, and infiltrative (figs. 5-204, 5-205). Involvement of peripheral nerves is common (fig. 5-206).

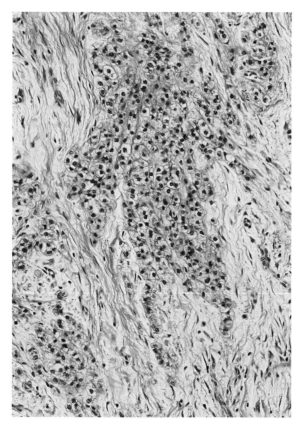

Figure 5-194
CLEAR CELL ADENOCARCINOMA
In this irregular-shaped focus of tumor from an intraoral clear cell adenocarcinoma, many of the cells have variable amounts of eosinophilic cytoplasm.

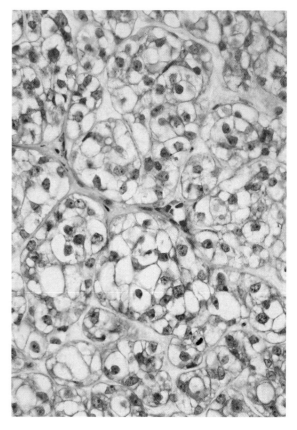

Figure 5-195
CLEAR CELL ADENOCARCINOMA
The polygonal clear cells have well-defined cell borders, and most have eccentrically located round nuclei. The cellular and nuclear morphology is uniform with little pleomorphism.

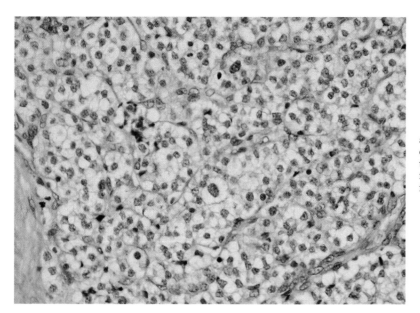

Figure 5-196
CLEAR CELL ADENOCARCINOMA
There are occasional larger nuclei and a mild degree of variability in nuclear size of the cells in this tumor, but the nuclear staining intensity is uniform. Mitotic figures are typically fewer than 2 per 10 high-power fields.

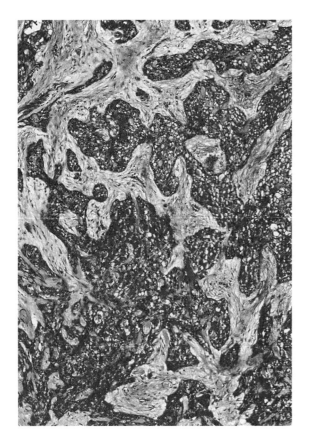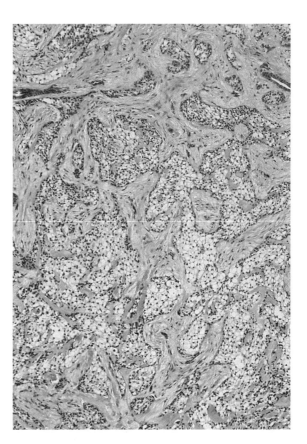

Figure 5-197
GLYCOGEN IN CLEAR CELL ADENOCARCINOMA
Intense PAS staining of the tumor cells before (left) and absence of PAS staining after (right) digestion of the tissue with diastase indicate significant cytoplasmic glycogen. The glycogen content varies among tumors but can be influenced by fixation and processing.

Figure 5-198
CLEAR CELL
ADENOCARCINOMA

In this carcinoma from the tongue, thin fibrous connective tissue septa separate sheets of closely apposed clear cells.

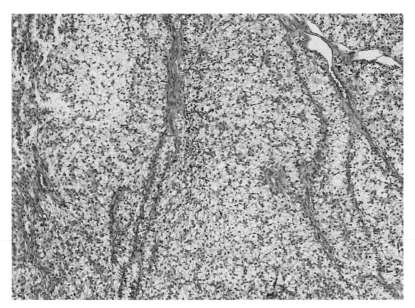

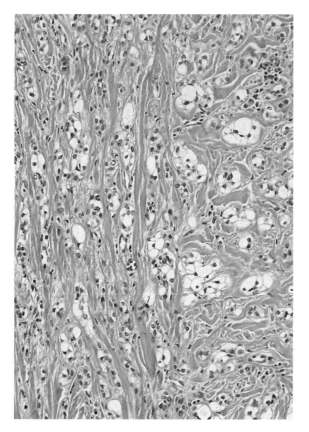

Figure 5-199
CLEAR CELL ADENOCARCINOMA
Small nests of clear cells are surrounded by dense collagenous tissue in a carcinoma from the lower lip.

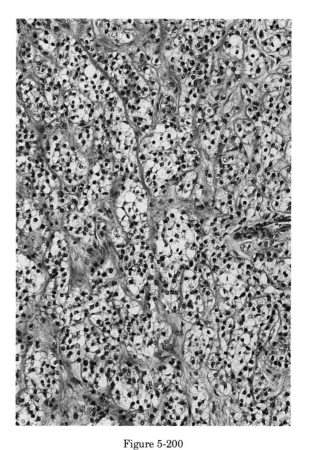

Figure 5-200
CLEAR CELL ADENOCARCINOMA
Thin fibrovascular septa surround groups of clear cells from a tumor of the buccal mucosa.

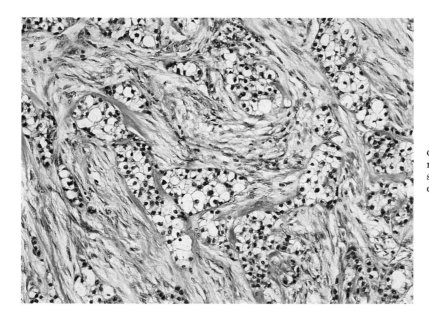

Figure 5-201
CLEAR CELL ADENOCARCINOMA
A tumor from the sublingual gland is composed of irregularly shaped and sized nests and cords of clear cells that are supported by a moderately cellular fibrous connective tissue stroma.

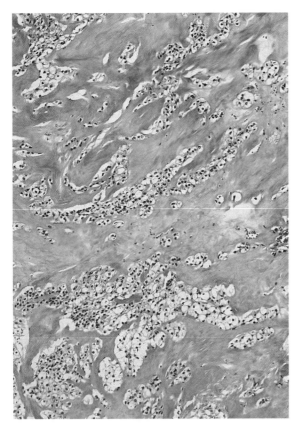

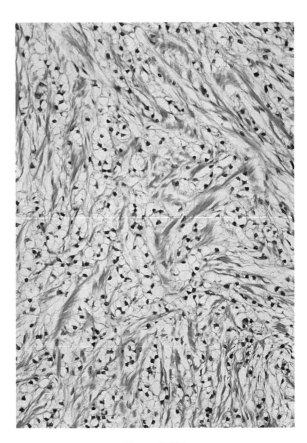

Figure 5-202
CLEAR CELL ADENOCARCINOMA

A dense, hyalinized collagenous stroma segregates cords and small groups of clear cells and produces a scirrhous appearance in this tumor from the floor of the mouth.

Figure 5-203
CLEAR CELL ADENOCARCINOMA

It is difficult to discern the boundaries of the nests of clear cells in this tumor from the palate because of the feathery stromal collagen.

Figure 5-204
CLEAR CELL ADENOCARCINOMA

Tumor cells have extended to the mucosal surface epithelium and infiltrated and destroyed the normal salivary gland lobules in this carcinoma of the hard palate. A few ducts of the residual salivary gland lobule are evident (arrows).

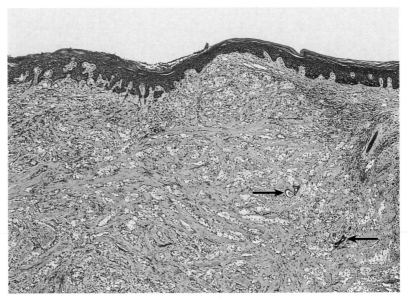

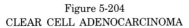

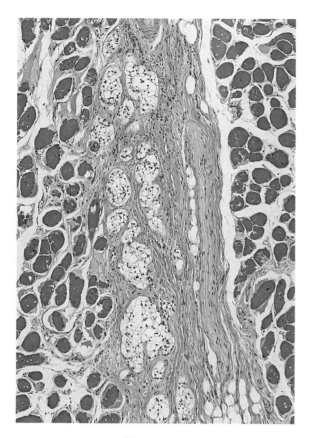

Figure 5-205
CLEAR CELL ADENOCARCINOMA
Aggregates of clear cells in a dense fibrous stroma have invaded skeletal muscle.

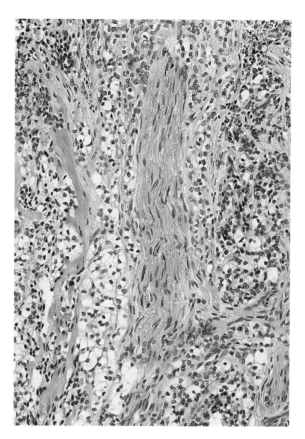

Figure 5-206
PERINEURAL INFILTRATION OF
CLEAR CELL ADENOCARCINOMA
Clear cells surround a peripheral nerve branch in palatal tumor.

Immunohistochemical studies have produced differing results (478,481,484,489,494). Most tumors have been focally to diffusely immunoreactive for cytokeratin (fig. 5-207), but both positive and negative immunoreactivity for S-100 protein, glial fibrillary acidic protein, actin, and vimentin have been reported (fig. 5-208). The few ultrastructural investigations have shown features of epithelial and duct cell differentiation, including tight junctions, desmosomal attachments, tonofilaments, microvilli, and basal lamina, but specific features of myoepithelial differentiation, including arrays of fine filaments with focal dense bodies and pinocytotic vesicles, are absent (474,478,481,483,484,489).

Differential Diagnosis. Clear cells may be a conspicuous component of a number of salivary gland neoplasms, most notably mucoepidermoid carcinoma, acinic cell adenocarcinoma, epithe-

lial-myoepithelial carcinoma, clear cell oncocytoma, sebaceous adenoma, and sebaceous carcinoma, as well as metastatic carcinomas, especially renal cell carcinoma. The diagnosis of clear cell adenocarcinoma requires exclusion of these other specific tumor types.

Mucoepidermoid carcinoma is the most common clear cell–containing salivary gland neoplasm, and the clear cells may or may not demonstrate glycogen. In addition to any clear cells that are present, mucocytes that stain with mucicarmine and Alcian blue as well as epidermoid cells identify mucoepidermoid carcinoma. The infrequent clear cell component of acinic cell adenocarcinoma is glycogen negative. Acinar cell differentiation is evinced by diastase-resistant, PAS-positive, intracytoplasmic granules. In addition, the microcystic, papillary-cystic, and follicular patterns that characterize many acinic cell

287

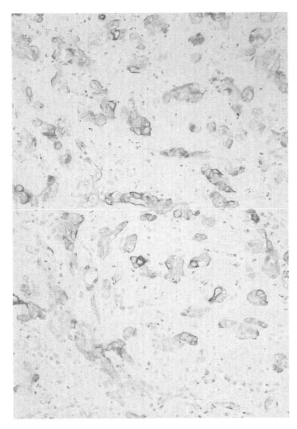

Figure 5-207
CLEAR CELL ADENOCARCINOMA:
IMMUNOHISTOCHEMISTRY
Tumor cells are immunoreactive with a cocktail of monoclonal anti-keratin antibodies. The tumor cells were unreactive for S-100 protein and glial fibrillary acidic protein. (Avidin-biotin peroxidase stain)

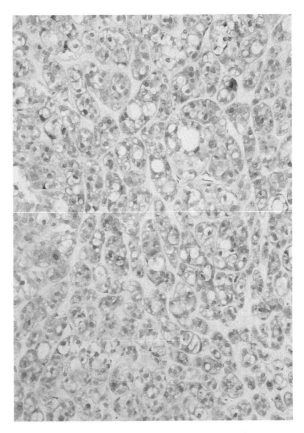

Figure 5-208
CLEAR CELL ADENOCARCINOMA:
IMMUNOHISTOCHEMISTRY
Unlike the tumor in figure 5-207, most of the clear cells in this clear cell adenocarcinoma are immunoreactive for S-100 protein. (Avidin-biotin peroxidase stain)

adenocarcinomas are not features of clear cell adenocarcinoma. Clear cells in oncocytomas contain glycogen; but, in contrast to clear cell adenocarcinomas, clear cell oncocytomas are circumscribed and not infiltrative, usually contain some intensely eosinophilic cells, are reactive with phosphotungstic acid–hematoxylin stain, and demonstrate excessive mitochondria when examined ultrastructurally. The rare sebaceous adenomas and adenocarcinomas are glycogen negative, generally have foamy rather than water-clear cytoplasm, and contain cytoplasmic lipids, which are best demonstrated with lipid stains on frozen sections of unprocessed tissue.

Epithelial-myoepithelial carcinoma is distinguished from monomorphous clear cell adenocarcinoma by its biphasic cell population: cuboidal, eosinophilic, luminal duct cells surrounded by larger, polygonal, clear cells, which ultrastructurally and immunohistochemically have features of myoepithelial differentiation (see Epithelial-Myoepithelial Carcinoma). The ratio of clear cells to duct cells is variable, and in clear cell–predominant epithelial-myoepithelial carcinomas careful microscopic examination is sometimes necessary to identify the biphasic pattern. In addition, a collagenous stroma that separates small nests and cords of clear cells or individual clear cells is more consistent with clear cell adenocarcinoma than epithelial-myoepithelial carcinoma.

Metastasis of infraclavicular primary neoplasms to salivary gland tissues is infrequent, but the AFIP and others have reviewed several metastatic renal cell carcinomas in the major salivary glands (see Secondary Tumors) (473,476, 480,485,486,490,491). Discovery of metastatic tumor may be the first indication of a primary renal carcinoma. Both primary clear cell adenocarcinoma and metastatic renal cell carcinoma are frequently glycogen positive, exhibit infiltration, have little cytologic atypia, have few mitoses, and are composed of nearly all clear cells. Mucicarmine positivity would rule out renal cell carcinoma, but primary clear cell adenocarcinoma of salivary gland is usually negative for intracytoplasmic mucin as well. Demonstration of intracytoplasmic lipid favors renal cell carcinoma, but lipids are usually eluted during tissue processing. A subtle difference is the vascularity of renal cell carcinoma. Small capillaries are present in clear cell adenocarcinoma, but the vascular channels in metastatic renal cell carcinoma are often conspicuous, dilated, and even sinusoidal, and hemorrhage and hemosiderin are generally more prominent. The greater pleomorphism and cytologic atypia evident the less likely the tumor is a primary clear cell carcinoma. It is not always possible to confidently differentiate between primary and metastatic carcinoma, and clinical evaluation for a renal primary tumor often is important.

Histologic distinction of clear cell adenocarcinoma in mucosa near the maxillary or mandibular alveolar ridges from clear cell odontogenic carcinoma is difficult and requires clinical, radiologic, and histopathologic correlation (5,10). Odontogenic clear cell carcinoma is a rare neoplasm. Radiographic evidence of a centralized, destructive osseous lesion indicates odontogenic rather than salivary gland origin.

Prognosis and Treatment. On the basis of the limited number of cases with follow-up information, clear cell adenocarcinomas are low-grade neoplasms. While infiltration of surrounding tissues, including peripheral nerves and vessels, is indicative of malignancy, only three reported cases and two cases reviewed at the AFIP have metastasized to cervical lymph nodes. No patient is known to have died as a result of tumor. Excision has been the primary therapy in all cases, and four patients received adjunctive radiotherapy.

CYSTADENOCARCINOMA

Definition. Cystadenocarcinoma is a rare malignant tumor histologically characterized by prominent cystic and, frequently, papillary growth, but lacking features that characterize cystic variants of several more common salivary gland carcinomas. Conceptually, cystadenocarcinoma is the malignant counterpart of benign cystadenoma.

General Features. Until only recently, cystadenocarcinoma was not included as a separate neoplasm in any of the well-known published salivary gland classification schemes, including those of Evans and Cruikshank (510), Thackray and Lucas (526), or the WHO in 1972 (527). Presumably most cases were included in the heterogeneous group of tumors labeled "adenocarcinoma." In 1991, papillary cystadenocarcinoma was included in the new WHO classification (519), and cystadenocarcinoma, with or without a papillary component, in the AFIP classification (507). Examples have been reported under other terminology including *malignant papillary cystadenoma* (507), *mucus-producing adenopapillary (nonepidermoid) carcinoma* (499,509), *low-grade papillary adenocarcinoma of the palate* (496,514, 515,528) and *papillary adenocarcinoma* (503, 518,523,524). Several investigators used the term cystadenocarcinoma descriptively prior to 1991 (497,500–504,506,511–513,520,529). The mucinous adenocarcinoma described and illustrated in the WHO monograph (519) represents cystadenocarcinoma with mucus-filled cysts described in this Fascicle.

The AFIP recently studied 57 cystadenocarcinomas and found that men and women were affected equally. The average age of patients was about 59 years. Although the age range was relatively broad (20 to 86 years) over 70 percent of patients were over 50 years of age. About 65 percent of tumors occurred in the major salivary glands, and most of these were in the parotid gland. Although occurrence in the sublingual gland of any salivary gland tumor is unusual, the collective experience with cystadenocarcinoma indicates its frequency in that gland is proportionately greater than other benign or malignant tumors (498,505,525). In descending order of frequency, the minor gland sites include the lips, buccal mucosa, palate, tongue, retromolar area, and floor of the mouth.

Clinical Features. Most patients present with a slowly growing, asymptomatic mass. The tumor is often compressible but only rarely is associated with pain or facial paralysis. Its innocuous clinical appearance is highlighted by an example of a sublingual tumor that was at first thought to be a mucous retention cyst (ranula) in the floor of the mouth (505). Palatal tumors have eroded bone and infiltrated into the nasal cavity and maxillary sinuses.

Gross and Microscopic Findings. Grossly, tumors seen at the AFIP are cystic or multicystic, partially circumscribed masses that range in size from 0.4 to 6.0 cm.

Microscopically, the predominant low-power feature is the presence of numerous cystic structures that typically form a circumscribed but unencapsulated mass (fig. 5-209). The cystic spaces are separated by connective tissue or closely appose one another. The spaces usually anastomose with one another, vary in size and shape within each tumor, and are haphazardly arranged. However, in some cases the majority of the tumor is composed of a limited number of more uniform and larger spaces (fig. 5-210). The lumens are often filled with mucus, and dystrophic calcifications occur in this material or in the intercystic stromal tissue. Small to medium-sized duct-like structures are often present. Occasionally, solid epithelial islands present between the larger cysts develop various sized duct-like structures (fig. 5-211). The solid elements typically account for a small portion of the entire tumor but are sometimes numerous along the advancing front of tumor.

The cystic tumor element, as well as the smaller duct-like structures and solid islands, demonstrate infiltrative growth through the salivary gland parenchyma and into the surrounding connective tissues (fig. 5-212). The smaller neoplastic structures often extend a considerable distance from the main portion of the tumor. Typically, however, infiltration is focal and some areas have a noninfiltrative border more characteristic of an adenoma than adenocarcinoma. Ruptured cysts with hemorrhage and granulation tissue are frequently evident.

The epithelium lining the neoplastic cysts and duct-like structures demonstrates a wide range of morphologic appearances and proliferative capacity. In the AFIP material about 75 percent of cases have a conspicuous papillary component.

The papillae range in number, appearance, and complexity from single, peninsular structures from which smaller fronds project, to multiple, more solid proliferations that nearly fill the entire lumen (figs. 5-209, 5-213). The epithelial lining of the cystic spaces and papillae vary from a single cell layer to many cells in thickness. When thickened, the lining sometimes focally forms numerous spaces that have a cribriform appearance (fig. 5-214). Occasionally, as in other salivary gland adenocarcinomas (517), a dense tumor-associated lymphoid response occurs, which on low-power examination resembles Warthin's tumor (fig. 5-215).

Many cell types are present (fig. 5-216). In AFIP cases, the predominant cell type is small cuboidal in over 60 percent of tumors; others are either large cuboidal (16 percent) or tall columnar (12 percent). Mixed cell types are found in other tumors: mucous, clear, oncocytic, and rarely even epidermoid cells are present focally. The columnar cells in some cases have a gastrointestinal appearance; however, the pale eosinophilic, mucin-rich–appearing cytoplasm in these cells usually fails to stain with mucicarmine. Either columnar or tall cuboidal cells typically predominate in papillary areas, and the cell population is often limited to a single cell type.

Regardless of the type of cells found, the size, shape, and staining qualities of their nuclei normally vary little. Nucleoli are usually evident but mitotic figures are rare. Several tumors have a moderate degree of nuclear pleomorphism, but thus far this has not been found to correlate with a more aggressive clinical course.

Differential Diagnosis. A cystic component is present in many different types of benign and malignant salivary gland tumors, but it predominates in only a few. Of these, some, such as Warthin's tumor, have such characteristic features that their distinction is relatively easy. Tumors that have some features that overlap with those of cystadenocarcinoma include cystadenoma, polymorphous low-grade adenocarcinoma (PLGA), mucoepidermoid carcinoma, the papillary cystic variant of acinic cell adenocarcinoma, and salivary duct carcinoma.

Both cystadenoma and cystadenocarcinoma are composed of epithelial cells that have bland cytomorphology and a tendency to form papillae. Cystadenomas are often not encapsulated, and

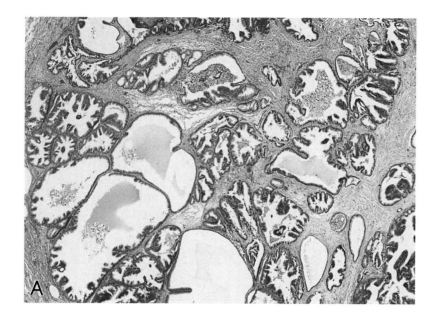

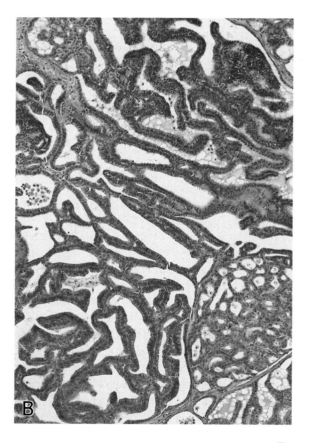

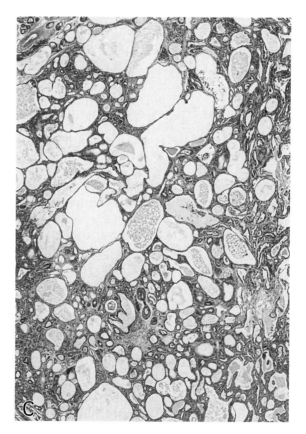

Figure 5-209
CYSTADENOCARCINOMA

Some of the variations commonly seen in cystadenocarcinomas are shown. In A, numerous neoplastic cystic spaces, some of which are slightly separated by connective tissue, form a mass that exhibits a relatively well-circumscribed interface with surrounding fibrous tissue (left). Note the prominent papillary growth in A compared to the growth in two different tumors (B and C) that lack a papillary component.

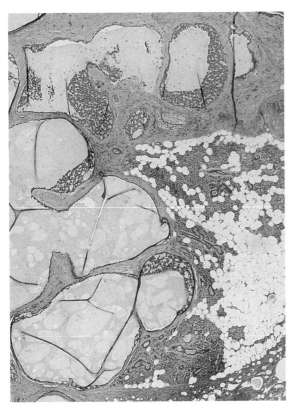

Figure 5-210
CYSTADENOCARCINOMA
This example is characterized by having fewer but larger cystic spaces than the previous tumors. Note the focal proliferation of the lining epithelium and extension into the gland.

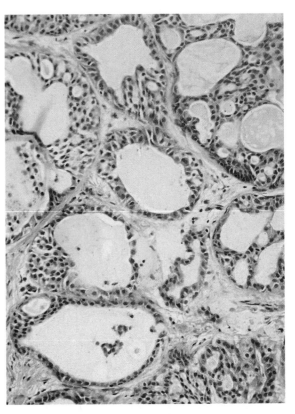

Figure 5-211
CYSTADENOCARCINOMA
The numerous small luminal spaces within the tumor islands appear to progressively enlarge or coalesce and eventually form duct-like structures and small cysts.

sometimes the smaller cystic structures are separated from the main portion of the tumor, which suggests infiltrative growth. Distinction between the two tumors may be difficult but ultimately depends on the presence or absence of frank infiltration into salivary gland parenchyma or surrounding connective tissue. Review of step sections of borderline tumors for evidence of invasion is recommended.

PLGA often has small cystic spaces that demonstrate papillary growth. Compared to cystadenocarcinoma, PLGA occurs almost exclusively in minor glands; infiltrates as islands, cords, tubules, and linearly arranged concentric whirling fascicles of tumor cells; has a mucinous or hyalinized stroma; and frequently shows perineural growth. The papillae in PLGA are usually part of a more extensive epithelial proliferation and are not as distinct as in cystadenocarcinoma. Furthermore, in cystadenocarcinoma the papil-

lae are usually composed of tall columnar or goblet cells, and variation in the type of cells is minimal compared to that in PLGA. As suggested by Slootweg (26), some of the tumors previously diagnosed as the papillary variant of PLGA are better designated as papillary cystadenocarcinoma.

Low-grade mucoepidermoid carcinoma often has papillary cystic areas; has a variety of cell types that include cuboidal, columnar, and clear cells; and invades salivary parenchyma in a subtle manner. Unlike cystadenocarcinoma, the cystic structures in mucoepidermoid carcinoma are composed of admixtures of both mucous and epidermoid cells, and a solid proliferative component usually represents a larger portion of the entire tumor. Epidermoid differentiation in cystadenocarcinoma is rare. Nonetheless, distinction from rare examples of cystadenocarcinoma that have focally prominent mucous cells may be problematic (fig. 5-217).

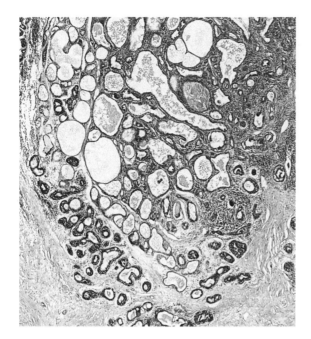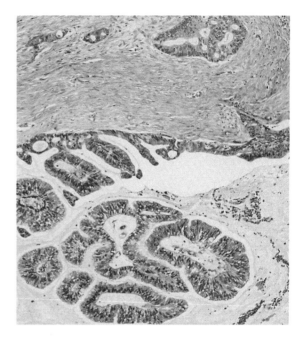

Figure 5-212
INFILTRATIVE GROWTH IN CYSTADENOCARCINOMA

Left: Although this tumor was relatively well circumscribed elsewhere, in this area many small cysts infiltrate paraglandular connective tissue.

Right: A portion of a large cyst is present at the bottom. On the top several smaller, more solid islands of neoplastic epithelium have infiltrated adjacent connective tissue. The islands have a tendency to form luminal spaces and many would probably have eventually developed into larger cysts.

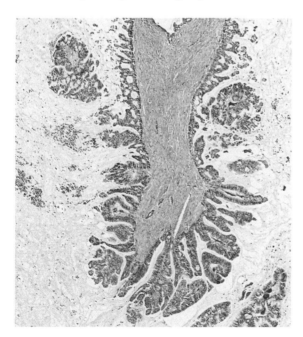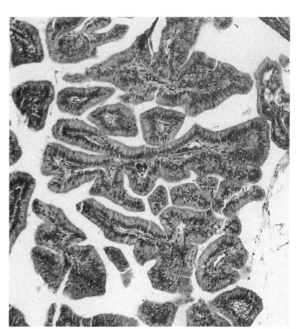

Figure 5-213
PAPILLARY GROWTH OF CYSTADENOCARCINOMA

Left: Numerous small papillae proliferate from a central luminal projection that has a core of fibrous connective tissue. The lumen also contains abundant mucus.

Right: The papillae are larger, more complex, and partially fill the luminal space.

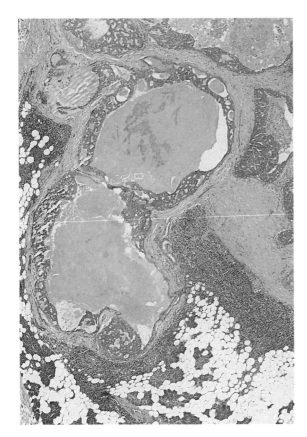
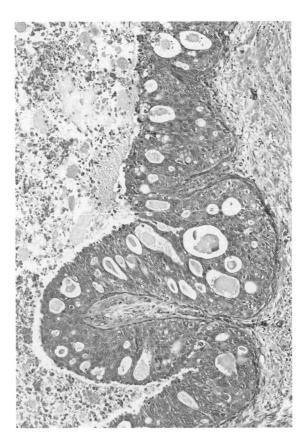

Figure 5-214
CYSTADENOCARCINOMA

The lining epithelium of this case showed both a moderate degree of proliferation and the tendency to form cribriform spaces, features that are reminiscent of salivary duct carcinoma. Higher magnification shows bland nuclear features and numerous small spaces that contain mucin.

Figure 5-215
CYSTADENOCARCINOMA

Many portions of this tumor were accompanied by a prominent lymphoid proliferation. One of the few germinal centers present is seen in the lower right corner. No evidence of lymph node architecture was found.

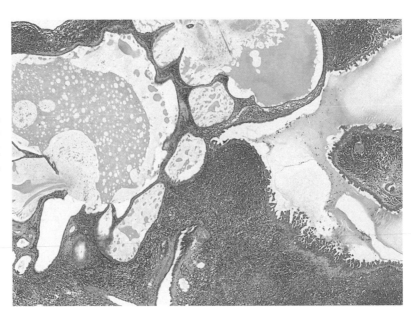

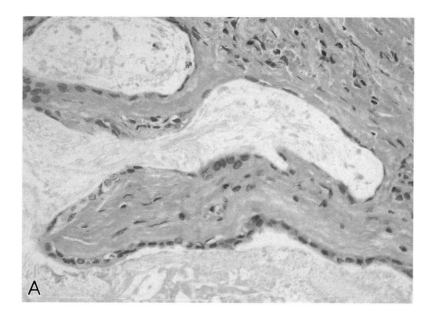

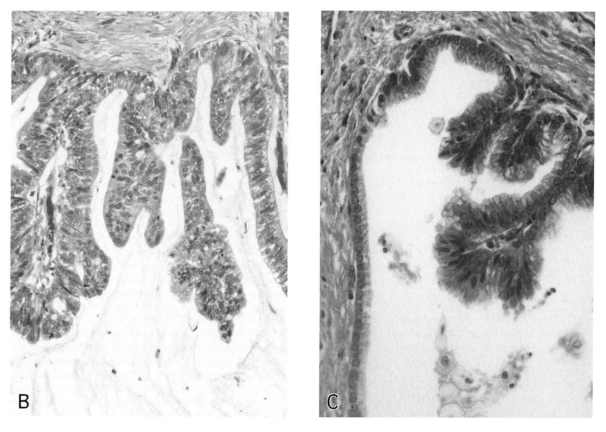

Figure 5-216
CELL TYPES IN CYSTADENOCARCINOMA
Lining epithelium varies from cuboidal (A) to columnar (B). In C a transition from tall cuboidal to columnar is present. The nuclear features in all types are uniformly bland.

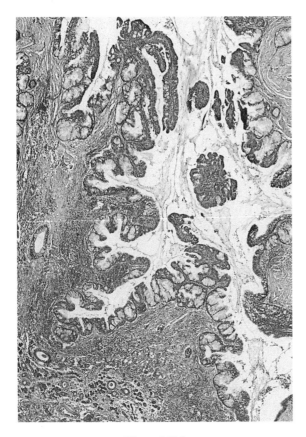

Figure 5-217
CYSTADENOCARCINOMA

On low-power examination distinction of this papillary cystadenocarcinoma from low-grade mucoepidermoid carcinoma is not possible. Cystadenocarcinoma was favored because neither epidermoid differentiation nor focally solid growth were found. Fortunately, the treatment and prognosis are similar for both.

The papillary cystic form of acinic cell adenocarcinoma often shows microcystic growth, a feature not expected in cystadenocarcinoma (508). Additionally, the presence of solid areas composed of large, basophilic cells that contain periodic acid–Schiff, diastase-resistant granules further supports acinic cell adenocarcinoma.

Compared with cystadenocarcinoma, the tumor cells in salivary duct carcinoma usually have large, pleomorphic nuclei with ample eosinophilic cytoplasm. Mitoses are often numerous and necrosis is normally evident. These morphologic differences help distinguish salivary duct carcinoma from examples of cystadenocarcinoma with cystic structures lined by epithelium that form cribriform spaces (fig. 5-214).

Prognosis and Treatment. Because of their rarity very limited follow-up data are available that pertain specifically to cystadenocarcinoma. Additionally, published series include cystadenocarcinoma among other types of tumors (515). In a series of AFIP cases, follow-up information was available for 39 of 57 patients studied. All 39 patients were either alive or had died of other causes and were free of tumor at a mean interval of 52 months after initial surgery. Three patients (7.7 percent) had recurrences at an average of 76 months from initial therapy. Four patients had metastases to regional lymph nodes (10 percent), three at the time of diagnosis and one 55 months later. The outcome of these and other cases supports the opinion that cystadenocarcinomas are low-grade neoplasms (504,505,520). It would, therefore, seem appropriate to use the same treatment principles as applied to other low-grade salivary adenocarcinomas (522). Therapy includes superficial parotidectomy, glandectomy for submandibular or sublingual disease, and wide excision of minor gland tumors, with bone resection only when involved by tumor. Facial nerve branches should be sacrificed only when involved by tumor, and neck dissection is only performed to resect obvious metastases (522).

UNDIFFERENTIATED CARCINOMAS

Undifferentiated carcinomas of salivary glands are a group of uncommon, malignant epithelial neoplasms that lack the specific light-microscopic morphologic features of other types of salivary gland carcinomas. In general, they have neither glandular or epidermoid features although occasional foci might suggest such differentiation. Electron microscopic examination demonstrates some features associated with ductal, epidermoid, or neuroendocrine differentiation in some tumors, but these ultrastructural features do not seem to have any specific prognostic significance.

These tumors are composed of either small cells (which are about 30 μm or less in diameter) with scant cytoplasm and uniform nuclei or larger, more pleomorphic cells that are three or more times the size of small cells. This difference in cell size and morphology permits segregation of undifferentiated carcinomas into a *small cell type* and a *large cell type*. Because these are rare neoplasms, published studies are few. A few investigations have focused on either the small or large cell type (531–534,536), but other investigators have combined small cell and large cell variants in their analyses (530,535,537). Although this makes analysis of published data on each type more difficult, the distinct morphologic difference between the small and large cell types makes it convenient to categorize them separately, as done by the WHO in their recent classification scheme for salivary gland tumors (538).

In addition, some large cell undifferentiated carcinomas are characterized by an extensive, dense lymphoid stroma, which is sometimes the dominant histopathologic feature, and are separately classified as *lymphoepithelial carcinoma*. The microscopic architecture of these undifferentiated carcinomas resembles both benign lymphoepithelial lesions (BLEL), within which some of these carcinomas develop, and some nasopharyngeal carcinomas. They also have a racial predilection that has not been identified in other salivary gland carcinomas (see Lymphoepithelial Carcinoma). And similar to nasopharyngeal carcinoma, an association with Epstein-Barr virus (EBV) infection has been established. Although they are rare, these carcinomas have received considerably more attention in the published literature than large cell undifferentiated carcinomas without lymphoid stroma. Because of the lymphoid stroma, racial predilection, viral association, and special identification by investigators, this group of carcinomas is separately categorized and discussed.

The undifferentiated carcinomas of salivary gland are histologically similar to undifferentiated carcinomas that arise in other organs and tissues. Therefore, metastatic carcinoma is a principal concern in the differential diagnosis of all types of primary undifferentiated carcinoma of the salivary glands.

Small Cell Carcinoma

Definition. Small cell carcinoma of the salivary glands is a rare, primary malignant tumor that with conventional light microscopy is composed of undifferentiated cells and with ultrastructural or immunohistochemical studies demonstrates neuroendocrine differentiation. This tumor has also been referred to as *extrapulmonary oat cell carcinoma* (557,559). Because of the morphologic similarity to the more common small cell carcinomas of the lung or other sites, metastatic disease must be clinically excluded.

General Features. Small cell carcinomas occur in many head and neck sites including the salivary glands, nasal cavity and paranasal sinuses, hypopharynx, cervical esophagus, proximal trachea, and, most commonly, larynx (540, 549,550,557,559,569). In the parotid gland the frequency of occurrence as a proportion of all parotid epithelial malignancies has been reported as high as 6.8 percent (565). Koss et al. (559) reported that they represented 3.5 percent of all malignant tumors of minor salivary glands in their series; however, this series included cases that arose from the seromucous glands of the nose and paranasal sinuses. Of the cases in the AFIP files since 1985, small cell carcinoma represents 1.7 percent of primary malignant epithelial parotid tumors, 2.2 percent of submandibular malignancies, and 1.8 percent of all major gland malignancies. Over 80 percent of the most recent cases occurred in the parotid gland, but in older AFIP cases reviewed by Gnepp et al. (549) the parotid and submandibular glands were equally involved. No tumors in minor glands are recorded in recent material at the AFIP.

Review of previously published cases and AFIP material shows that these tumors typically occur in the fifth through the seventh decades of life (mean age, 56 years; range, 5 to 86 years) (547, 555). Among AFIP's civilian patients, men have outnumbered women 6 to 1. A less striking male predilection of 1.6 to 1 has been previously reported (547).

It has been assumed that the argentaffin Kulschitzky-like cells of the bronchus serve as progenitors of small cell carcinoma of the lung (580). Whether or not this is the case, no such population of cells normally populates the salivary glands. However, several groups of investigators have provided some evidence for the presence of neuroendocrine differentiation in the major salivary glands of humans and other mammals (544,549,558,566,571). For instance, neuroendocrine granules have been demonstrated in serous acini and intercalated ducts of human parotid and submandibular glands and may be increased in noninsulin dependent diabetes (558). In this regard, it has been noted at the AFIP that normal parotid tissue may rarely demonstrate chromogranin immunoreactivity. Whatever the source of the tumor cells, there is a population of cells within salivary gland tissue that possesses the capacity to proliferate and to manifest neuroendocrine differentiation.

Clinical Features. In half the cases, patients present with a nonpainful parotid mass of 3 months or less duration (542,549,555,556,560, 563,570). Pain has been experienced but surprisingly is only occasionally associated with these tumors (555). Lymph nodes that are enlarged by tumor are often found clinically at the time of the initial examination (555).

Gross and Microscopic Findings. Grossly, tumors are usually poorly circumscribed, firm, occasionally multilobulated, and vary from grayish white to yellow (549,567,570).

The WHO and others (549,560,562,570,572) distinguish between two types of small cell carcinoma of salivary glands: small cell neuroendocrine carcinoma and small cell ductal carcinoma, depending on whether neurosecretory granules or ductal differentiation is present. It has been suggested by some of these investigators that most salivary gland small cell carcinomas are small cell ductal carcinomas rather than true neuroendocrine carcinomas largely because ultrastructurally they lack neurosecretory granules. A recent study by Gnepp and Wick (551) of some of the same tumors that in a previous study lacked dense core granules ultrastructurally, showed neuroendocrine characteristics when studied immunohistochemically. For this reason, they concluded that dividing small cell carcinomas of the salivary glands into two histologic subtypes is not justified. Furthermore, Hui and colleagues (555) have shown that the presence or absence of neuroendocrine differentiation has no prognostic significance, and that separation of small and large cell types of undifferentiated carcinoma may not be necessary. It should be noted that dense core granules are also difficult to find in small cell carcinomas of the lung (580); it has been suggested that formalin fixation results in the destruction of neurosecretory granules (553).

Microscopically, the tumors are composed of solid sheets, nests (fig. 5-218), and irregular cords of closely packed cells that extensively infiltrate the salivary parenchyma and paraglandular tissues (fig. 5-219). At low magnification, small, well-demarcated, darkly hematoxyphilic zones are often focally apparent; these represent artifactually crushed nuclei, a phenomenon to which this tumor seems particularly susceptible (fig. 5-220). The cellular structures are separated by fibrous stroma that is often hyalinized and vascular. Focal necrosis is frequently seen. In some cases necrosis is extensive (fig. 5-221).

The histomorphologic features of small cell carcinoma of the salivary glands closely parallels those of lung carcinomas. As with oat cell type of small cell carcinoma of the lung, most salivary cases are composed of uniform cells that are larger than lymphocytes (fig. 5-222) and have dense round to oval nuclei with diffuse chromatin; small, typically inconspicuous nucleoli; and sparse cytoplasm (fig. 5-223) (579). Nuclei may contain small single or multiple nucleoli, and nuclear molding is often observed. In some cases the cells are focally more polygonal or fusiform (fig. 5-224). Some tumor cells have more abundant cytoplasm, resembling the intermediate cell type of small cell carcinoma of the lung (545,579). Ductal differentiation occasionally is evident (551), but more often pseudoglandular spaces are formed by loosely cohesive cells (fig. 5-225). In the review of 12 cases by Gnepp et al. (549), 4 had foci that demonstrated ductal differentiation. Limited squamous changes are only rarely evident (554,562).

The cells are usually about 1 1/2 to 2 times the size of lymphocytes (fig. 5-222). In their study of undifferentiated carcinomas of major salivary glands Hui and colleagues (555) designated tumors composed of cells smaller than 30 μm as small cell carcinoma and those with larger cells as large cell carcinoma. The periphery of some of the cell nests may exhibit a vague palisading arrangement, suggesting rosette formation (fig. 5-226). Homer-Wright type rosettes have been described in these tumors (556). Mitoses are frequent, and there is occasional neural and vascular invasion (fig. 5-227).

Immunohistochemical Findings. Most cells are immunoreactive for keratin although focal areas are nonreactive (551,555,575). The paranuclear, globular staining pattern seen in many of these tumors is not evident in other types of salivary gland carcinoma (fig. 5-228). The globules are thought to represent filament whorls that may be seen ultrastructurally (539). In one study, 7 of 11 salivary small cell carcinomas

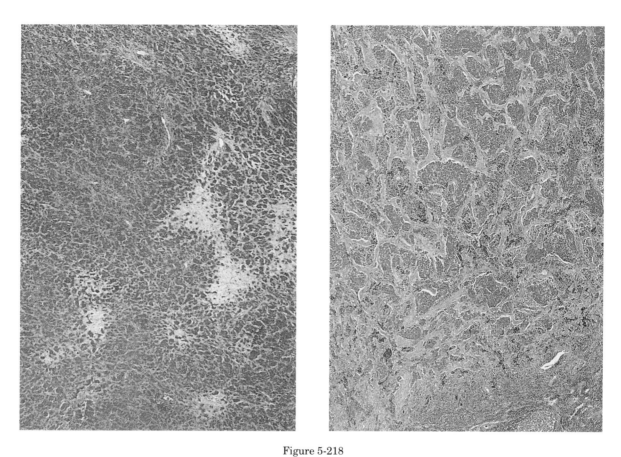

Figure 5-218
SMALL CELL CARCINOMA
Left: Sheets of tumor are formed by discrete, individual small nests and cell clusters.
Right: A different example is composed of irregular, interconnected tumor islands separated by hyalinized stroma.

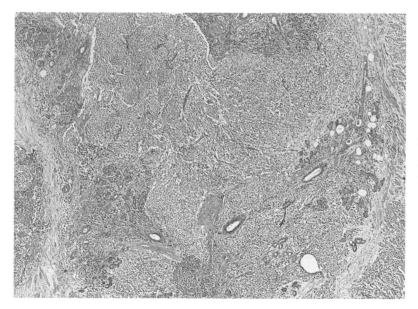

Figure 5-219
SMALL CELL CARCINOMA
A salivary gland lobule is largely replaced by irregular solid sheets of small, densely basophilic tumor cells. Several groups of residual acini and ducts are evident.

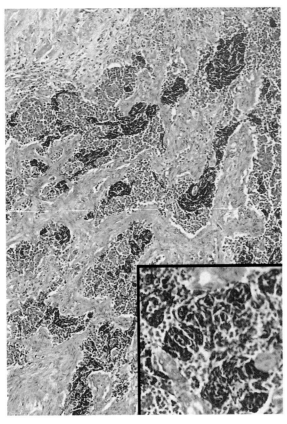

Figure 5-220
SMALL CELL CARCINOMA

Numerous anastomosing cords of tumor cells are separated by fibrous connective tissue. Darkly hematoxyphilic foci represent crush artifact that is better seen at higher magnification (inset).

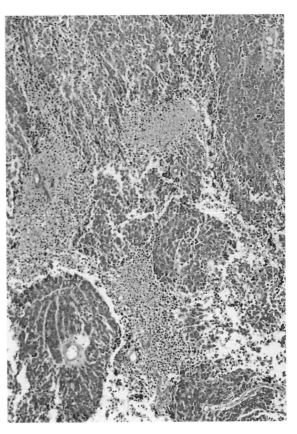

Figure 5-221
SMALL CELL CARCINOMA

Tumor with extensive necrosis is shown. A rim of viable tumor surrounds a small blood vessel in the lower left corner.

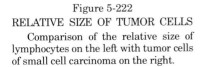

Figure 5-222
RELATIVE SIZE OF TUMOR CELLS

Comparison of the relative size of lymphocytes on the left with tumor cells of small cell carcinoma on the right.

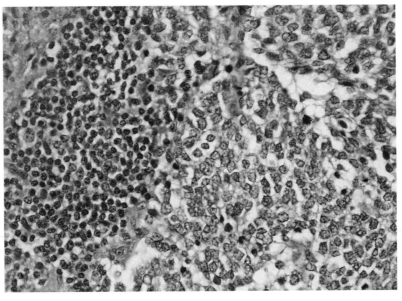

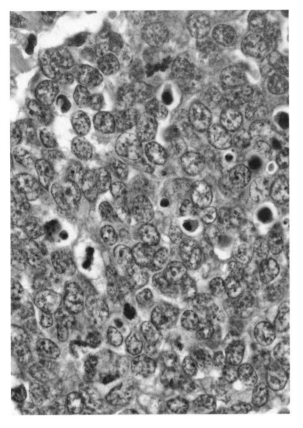

Figure 5-223
SMALL CELL CARCINOMA
High magnification of tumor cells shows ill-defined cytoplasmic borders, overlapping round nuclei with dispersed chromatin, and only rare, small nucleoli.

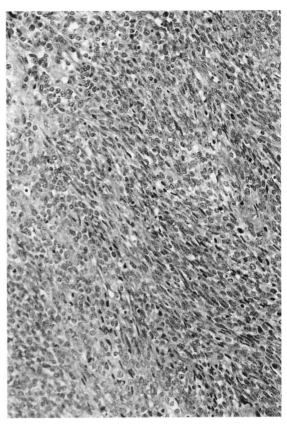

Figure 5-224
SMALL CELL CARCINOMA
The nuclei are focally elongated and arranged in vague fascicles.

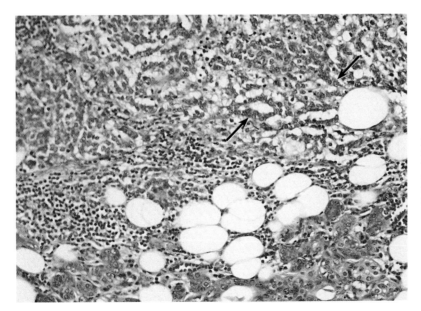

Figure 5-225
SMALL CELL CARCINOMA
The tumor infiltrates into and replaces salivary tissue that contains normal fat. Focally the arrangement of tumor cells around small empty spaces suggests an attempt at ductal differentiation (arrows). Many small cell carcinomas contain well-formed ductal structures.

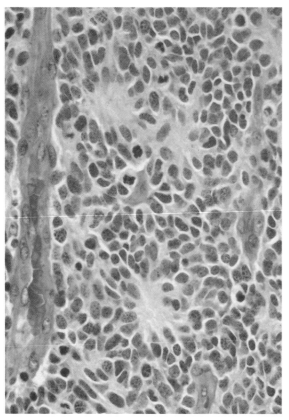

Figure 5-226
PSEUDOROSETTES
Two pseudorosettes in this field result from regimentation of tumor nuclei around fibrillary eosinophilic material.

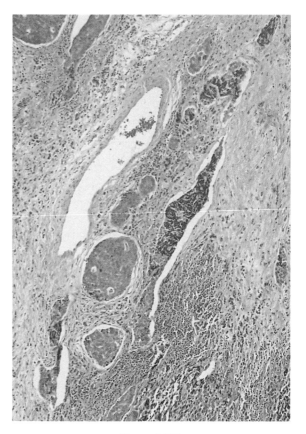

Figure 5-227
VASCULAR INVASION
Several blood vessels are filled by tumor cells, some of which are artifactually crushed and, therefore, more hematoxyphilic.

Figure 5-228
CYTOKERATIN
IMMUNOREACTIVITY OF
SMALL CELL CARCINOMA
The tumor cells are diffusely immunoreactive. The punctate perinuclear globular staining results in the characteristic "dotted" pattern.
Inset: Higher magnification of a different tumor shows that the chromogen is sharply localized at one pole of the nucleus.

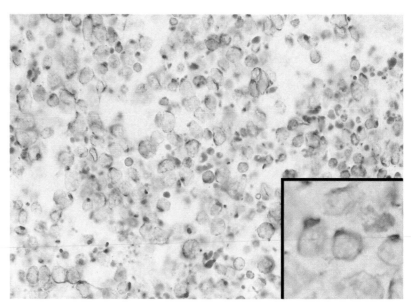

exhibited this finding (551). Although this peculiar staining pattern is not usually found in oat cell carcinomas of the lung, it is seen in neuroendocrine carcinomas of the skin (Merkel cell carcinoma) and in pulmonary and intestinal carcinoids (589,574).

In addition to the paranuclear staining with anti-cytokeratin, other determinants that indicate neuroendocrine differentiation include immunoreactivity of tumor cells with anti-Leu-7, synaptophysin, chromogranin, and neuron-specific enolase (fig. 5-229) (552,561,564,576,577). Gnepp and Wick (551) found that all 11 salivary gland small cell carcinomas in their study showed at least one of these five determinants despite the finding that only four of the tumors had secretory granules by electron microscopy. Similarly, chromogranin immunoreactivity has been seen in Merkel cell carcinomas even when electron microscopy failed to reveal neurosecretory granules (553). Immunoreactivity for epithelial membrane antigen (EMA) is also usually seen in small cell carcinomas of both salivary and pulmonary origin, but anti-EMA also nonspecifically stains various salivary and nonsalivary carcinomas (551,568). Immunoreactivity with antivimentin is seen in some cases but not with anti-S-100 protein or HMB-45 (551,555).

Ultrastructural Findings. Electron microscopy shows small, closely apposed, primitive but uniform cells that have scant cytoplasm and pyknotic nuclei (546,555,556,560,563,565,567, 578). The cells are joined by sparse, poorly or well-formed cell junctions. Tonofilaments are normally inconspicuous. Organelles include mitochondria, polyribosomes, microtubules, a rough endoplasmic reticulum, and a well-developed Golgi apparatus. Membrane-bound dense core neurosecretory granules that typically have diameters of 60 to 150 nm are present in only about 20 percent of small cell carcinomas of the salivary glands (fig. 5-230) (556), a frequency similar to that for small cell carcinomas of the lung (580).

Differential Diagnosis. The differential diagnosis for primary small cell carcinoma includes both epithelial and nonepithelial primary and metastatic tumors. Distinction from the much more common non-Hodgkin lymphomas is greatly facilitated by immunohistochemical analysis for cytokeratin and leukocyte common antigen (LCA). Only rarely are small cell carcinomas not immunoreactive with anti-cytokeratin, and they do not react with anti-LCA (551,539). Conventional light microscopy shows that compared to malignant lymphoma the cells of small cell carcinomas are larger, have nuclei with more uniform peripheral contours and more finely stippled chromatin, often form pseudoglandular spaces, have a greater number of mitoses, and have a propensity for necrosis. Compared to the extensive destruction of the glandular tissue usually associated with small cell carcinomas, most lymphomas permeate the gland in a manner that leaves many residual ducts and acini. Lymphomas do not usually form separate cords and nests.

The solid variant of adenoid cystic carcinoma is composed of solid nests and sheets of small, isomorphic cells that often show focal necrosis and numerous mitotic figures. For these reasons, distinction from small cell carcinoma may be difficult. Features that favor adenoid cystic carcinoma include focal cribriform or occasional well-formed tubular pseudoglandular structures, even in the solid variant. Immunohistochemically, adenoid cystic carcinoma expresses cytokeratin but the paranuclear globular pattern characteristic of small cell carcinoma is not present. Neuroendocrine differentiation is not evident immunohistochemically or ultrastructurally (565).

Distinguishing primary small cell carcinoma from metastatic disease of the lung, skin, sinonasal region, or other sites may be difficult. Hui and colleagues (555) found that their series of undifferentiated salivary gland carcinomas included two cases each of oat cell carcinoma of the lung and Merkel cell carcinoma of the scalp. In the AFIP material metastases of oat cell carcinoma from the lung outnumber metastases from Merkel cell carcinoma from the skin (548). While paranuclear cytokeratin reactivity is not seen in small cell carcinoma of the lung, it is expected in Merkel cell carcinoma (539). It has also been reported that most Merkel cell carcinomas express neurofilament, usually in a perinuclear globular pattern, and salivary small cell carcinomas do not, although further investigation in this area is needed (542). Occult primary disease is more likely in the lung than the skin of the head and neck, so in most cases evaluation of the patient for lung disease is indicated. Metastases to the parotid and submandibular glands from the lung have been reported as the first manifestation of disease (541,543,573).

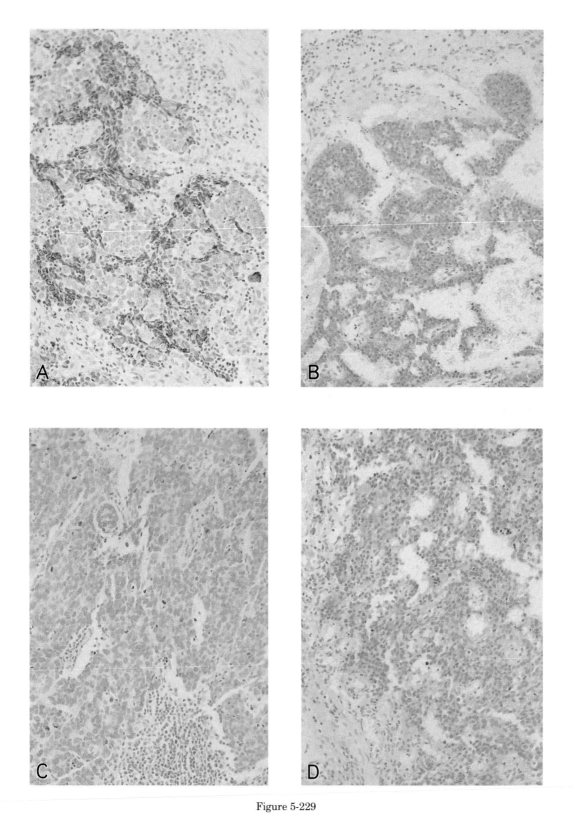

Figure 5-229
IMMUNOREACTIVITY OF SMALL CELL CARCINOMA
Neuroendocrine differentiation is supported by immunoreactivity of many of the tumor cells for chromogranin (A) or synaptophysin (B). Often seen but less specific is reactivity for Leu-7 (C) and neuron-specific enolase (D).

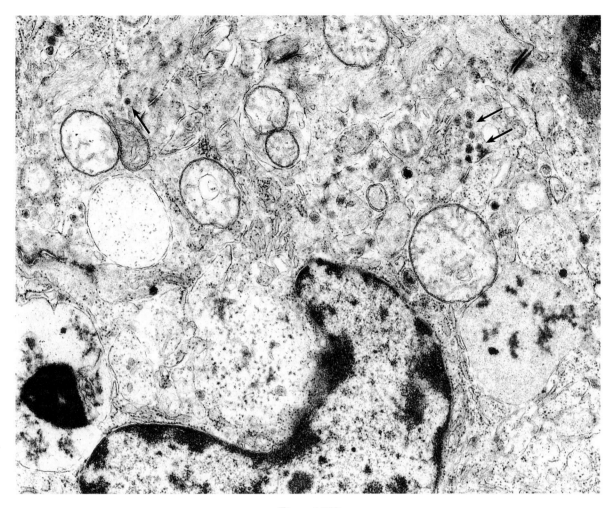

Figure 5-230
ELECTRON MICROSCOPY OF SMALL CELL CARCINOMA
Abundant electron-dense neurosecretory granules are scattered among other cellular organelles (arrows). A well-developed desmosome is seen in the upper right corner.

One other malignancy that metastasizes to the parotid region with some frequency is malignant melanoma (548) (see Metastatic Disease). Compared to small cell carcinoma, the nuclei of melanoma are usually larger, have clumped rather than finely dispersed chromatin, and have large and often multiple nucleoli. Unlike small cell carcinoma, melanoma cells are often immunoreactive for S-100 protein and HMB-45 antigen and nonreactive for cytokeratin.

Prognosis and Treatment. Although the prognosis for patients with small cell carcinoma of the salivary glands is better than for those with small cell carcinoma of the lung or larynx, it is a high-grade malignancy that is treated aggres-

sively. A review of 189 published cases observed that 121 patients had died of tumor (555). Gnepp and colleagues (549) found that the 2-year and 5-year survival for major gland tumors was 70 and 46 percent, respectively. Three of their six patients who died of disease did so in less than 1 year. Distant metastatic sites include the liver, brain, and mediastinum. Hui et al. (555) found that of 16 undifferentiated carcinomas of the major salivary glands, 12 of which were small cell carcinomas, the most important predictor of behavior was the tumor size (555). Ten of their 16 patients died of disease within 4 1/2 years. All patients with tumors measuring greater than 4 cm died and were about twice as likely to have perineural invasion, extrasalivary extension, and regional failure as those with smaller tumors. Three of the 4 patients with carcinomas measuring 2 cm or less were alive after 5 years. Unlike one previous report (562), they found that neither the presence or absence of neuroendocrine differentiation nor cell size (small versus large) influenced prognosis.

Most patients have been treated with surgical excision, with or without ipsilateral neck dissection, and postoperative radiation (547,555,560). Radical neck dissection has been successful for patients who develop cervical lymphadenopathy (556). Radiation doses have varied from 5,000 to 6,000 rads to the gland and slightly less to the neck. Chemotherapy has been given for regional recurrences or distant metastases (555,556,570,578).

Large Cell Undifferentiated Carcinoma

General Features. The reported incidence of undifferentiated carcinoma has varied from less than 1 to 20 percent of malignant epithelial neoplasms of salivary glands (581,583,584,586, 588–590,593–596,598,601,606). However, some examples of "undifferentiated" or "anaplastic" carcinoma are actually the lymphoepithelial type of undifferentiated carcinoma, which is discussed separately below as *lymphoepithelial carcinoma*. Batsakis and Luna (583) and Hui et al. (588) have suggested that the marked variance in the reported incidence of undifferentiated carcinoma may be because some investigators: 1) include carcinomas that are not recognized as metastatic tumors to the salivary glands; 2) include some high-grade carcinomas that are classifiable as other specific types of carcinoma, such as solid adenoid cystic carcinoma or carcinoma ex mixed tumor; or 3) use the qualifying adjective "undifferentiated" inappropriately for nonmalignant tumors, such as sialoblastoma or basal cell adenoma. In fact, in a study of 22 undifferentiated carcinomas of salivary glands in the University of Hamburg's Salivary Gland Register, Takata et al. (600) concluded that 8 were metastatic tumors and 10 could be classified as other specific types of salivary gland carcinoma, although their criteria for reclassification of some of these tumors were questionable. The AFIP's experience is in agreement with the findings of several investigations from the United States,

Japan, Europe, and China that undifferentiated carcinoma is a rare primary salivary gland tumor that accounts for about 1 percent of epithelial salivary gland neoplasms (583,593,595, 596,598,602,606). Batsakis and Luna and Nagao et al. (593) included both small cell and large cell types in their data. In the study of Hui et al., small cell carcinoma was three times more frequent than large cell undifferentiated carcinoma, and Nagao et al. found a ratio of 2 to 1. Recent data at the AFIP show that large cell undifferentiated carcinoma is more common than small cell carcinoma, but in a discussion of such uncommon neoplasms these differences are not significant.

The majority of undifferentiated carcinomas have occurred in the parotid gland (583,588, 593), but at the AFIP about 25 percent of the large cell type have been from the submandibular gland. None of the AFIP cases were from the minor salivary glands, but such cases have been occasionally reported (585,591,599,603,604).

These tumors develop in adults. At the AFIP, patients ranged in age from 40 to 96 years, with a peak incidence in the seventh and eight decades of life; however, four of the six patients in the study of Nagao et al. (593) were under 50 years old. Men and women were equally affected when the male bias of military patients was eliminated from the AFIP data. In Nagao et al.'s report, five of six patients were women in contrast to the male predominance among their patients with small cell carcinoma. In Hui et al.'s data (588), which combined small cell and large cell undifferentiated carcinomas, there was a 3 to 1 male to female ratio. Unlike the lymphoepithelial type of undifferentiated carcinoma, no racial predilection has been identified.

Also, unlike lymphoepithelial carcinoma, a specific association of Epstein-Barr virus infection with large cell undifferentiated carcinoma has not been established.

Clinical Features. Information on the clinical signs and symptoms associated with large cell undifferentiated carcinoma, separate from those of small cell carcinoma, is limited, but parotid gland swelling of short duration and rapid growth is a common clinical presentation (588). The tumors are firm and fixed. Many patients have cervical lymphadenopathy at the time of diagnosis of their primary salivary gland carcinoma.

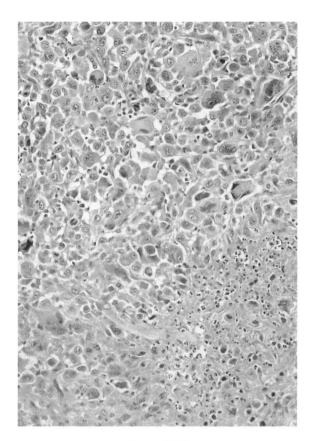

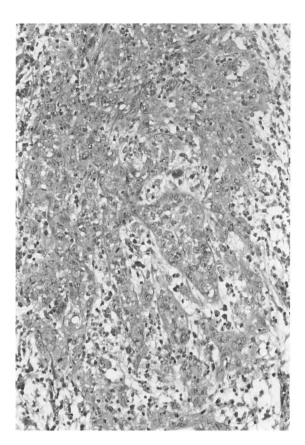

Figure 5-231
LARGE CELL UNDIFFERENTIATED CARCINOMA
A sheet of closely apposed but loosely attached, pleomorphic tumor cells has a large amount of amphophilic to eosinophilic cytoplasm, and some cells are multinucleated. The cell boundaries are relatively distinct. An area of necrosis is evident at the lower right.

Figure 5-232
LARGE CELL UNDIFFERENTIATED CARCINOMA
Branching, irregular trabeculae of large, eosinophilic tumor cells with indistinct cell boundaries are supported by loose fibrous connective tissue. While there are a number of plasma cells and lymphocytes in the stroma, their number is considerably less than that in lymphoepithelial carcinoma.

Gross Findings. Cut section of the gross specimen usually reveals solid, gray-white to yellow-tan, unencapsulated and poorly circumscribed tumor tissue that has invaded parotid gland parenchyma and often has extended into adjacent tissues such as muscle, fat, dermis, and bone. The tumors have ranged from 2 to 10 cm in diameter and most have been larger than 3 cm. Areas of necrosis and hemorrhage are common, but cystic structures are absent.

Microscopic Findings. At the light microscopic level, features of acinar, ductal, epidermoid, or myoepithelial differentiation are absent in undifferentiated carcinomas although occasional poorly formed duct-like structures can be found. Tumor cells are arranged in sheets, nests, and trabecular cords separated by fibrous connective tissue stroma (figs. 5-231–5-233). These features are similar to those of poorly differentiated epidermoid carcinoma, but no keratinization, partial or complete, is evident in large cell undifferentiated carcinoma.

The tumors are unencapsulated and infiltrative (fig. 5-234). They extend into adjacent lobules of salivary gland tissue and frequently invade fat, skeletal muscle, and dermis and even involve facial and cranial bones. Lymphatic and blood vessel invasion are frequently evident. Neural invasion is common, but it is not the conspicuous feature that often characterizes adenoid cystic carcinoma. The fibrous connective stroma that accompanies the neoplastic epithelial proliferation often contains variable numbers of inflammatory cells, principally lymphocytes and plasma

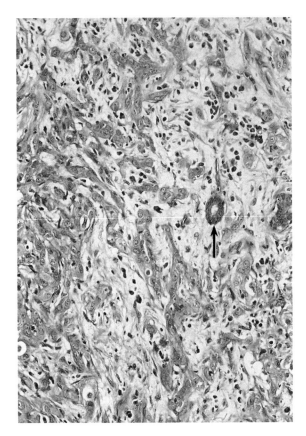

Figure 5-233
LARGE CELL UNDIFFERENTIATED CARCINOMA
Thin cords of tumor cells, often only one cell thick, are within a loose, collagenous stroma. A residual salivary gland duct is evident (arrow).

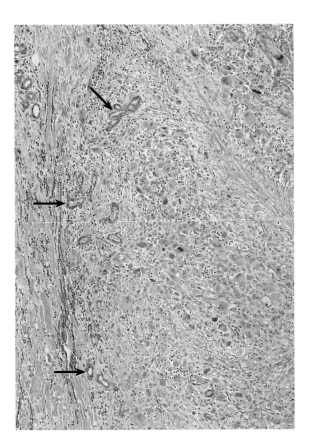

Figure 5-234
LARGE CELL UNDIFFERENTIATED CARCINOMA
Large, pleomorphic cells have infiltrated and replaced lobules of parotid gland parenchyma. Several residual ducts are still evident along the left portion of the field (arrows). A dense, collagenous stroma accompanies the tumor cells.

cells, but the diffuse, dense lymphocytic infiltrates that are associated with the lymphoepithelial type of undifferentiated carcinoma are absent (figs. 5-232, 5-235).

The tumor cells are mostly polygonal shaped, but some spindled forms occur as well. They have abundant amphophilic to eosinophilic cytoplasm, which is sometimes partially clear or vacuolated, and large, round, vesicular nuclei, which frequently contain one or more nucleoli (fig. 5-236). Most cells are two or more times the size of those of small cell carcinoma, but smaller forms are frequently scattered among the large cells. Tumor cells vary from relatively uniform to anaplastic (fig. 5-237). Mitotic figure counts are variable from tumor to tumor and within areas of any one tumor, but mitoses are common. In some tumors cells are closely apposed to one another

while in others they are more loosely arranged and separated (figs. 5-235, 5-236). Balogh et al. (582) and Hayashi and Aoki (587) described undifferentiated carcinomas of the parotid gland with osteoclast-like and bizarre giant cells; two anaplastic large cell undifferentiated carcinomas with multinucleated giant cells from the parotid gland have been reviewed at the AFIP (fig. 5-238). In four other cases undifferentiated carcinomas occurred in close association with acinic cell adenocarcinomas that contained numerous well-differentiated acinar cells (see Acinic Cell Adenocarcinoma). It is uncertain whether these represented dedifferentiation of acinic cell adenocarcinoma or concomitant proliferation of two separate neoplastic clones.

Occasionally, intracytoplasmic glycogen is evident in some cells stained with PAS before and

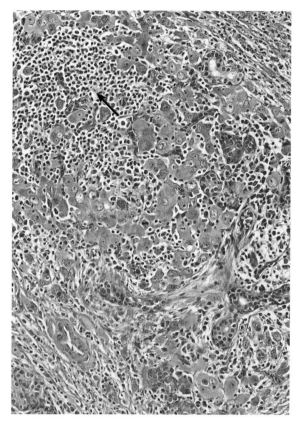

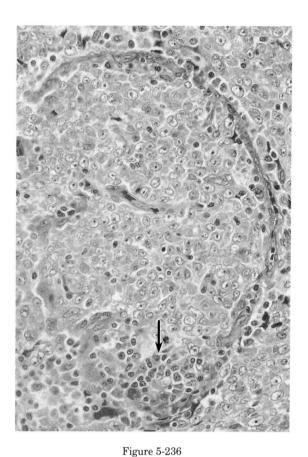

Figure 5-235
LARGE CELL UNDIFFERENTIATED CARCINOMA
The lymphocytic inflammatory infiltrate associated with this undifferentiated carcinoma of the parotid is focally dense (arrow) but otherwise sparse to moderate.

Figure 5-236
LARGE CELL UNDIFFERENTIATED CARCINOMA
This sheet of tumor cells is composed of relatively uniform, large, polygonal cells with pale, eosinophilic cytoplasm and round, vesicular nuclei that contain prominent nucleoli. A few smaller cells are present (arrow) that are difficult to distinguish from inflammatory cells.

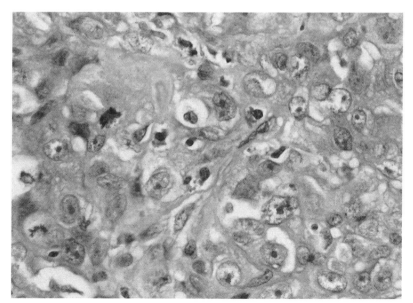

Figure 5-237
LARGE CELL
UNDIFFERENTIATED
CARCINOMA
These tumor cells are more pleomorphic than those in figure 5-236. They have indistinct cell borders and large, pleomorphic, vesicular nuclei with prominent nucleoli. The pale, eosinophilic cytoplasm is clear or partially vacuolated in some cells. Two mitotic figures are evident (left).

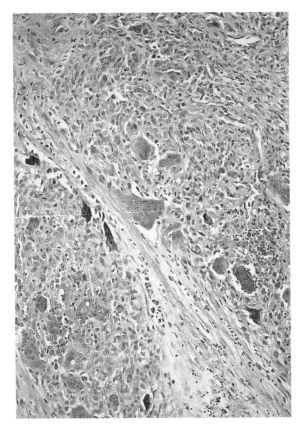

Figure 5-238
OSTEOCLASTIC-LIKE CELLS IN LARGE CELL
UNDIFFERENTIATED CARCINOMA
Several large, multinucleated, osteoclast-like giant cells are seen in this undifferentiated carcinoma of the parotid gland.

after tissue digestion with diastase. Although Yaku et al. (605) found some secretory granules with electron microscopic examination of a large cell undifferentiated carcinoma, manifestation of acinar cell differentiation is lacking at the light microscopic level. Mucicarmine staining fails to reveal mucous cell differentiation or salivary mucin.

Although not evident with light microscopy, ultrastructural examination reveals adenomatous, epidermoid, and neuroendocrine features among undifferentiated tumor cells (582,588, 605). Yaku et al. (605) found secretory granules in some cells in one of two large cell undifferentiated carcinomas they examined, and Hui et al. (588) found neuroendocrine granules in one large cell undifferentiated carcinoma. Desmosomal attachments are common, but microvilli and tonofilaments are less frequent findings.

Differential Diagnosis. Primary poorly differentiated squamous cell carcinoma and adenocarcinoma, large cell and anaplastic types of malignant lymphoma, and metastatic carcinoma and melanoma are the principal considerations in the differential diagnosis of large cell undifferentiated carcinoma of salivary glands.

Even poorly differentiated primary and metastatic adenocarcinomas have focal ductal, organoid, papillary, or cystic architectural features that distinguish them from undifferentiated carcinoma. Metastatic poorly differentiated squamous cell carcinoma and undifferentiated carcinomas that are not confined to periparotid lymph nodes can often only be differentiated from primary undifferentiated carcinoma by clinical evaluation and identification of another primary tumor site. Face and scalp are common sites of epidermal and skin adnexal carcinomas that metastasize to the parotid gland. Evidence of keratinization rules out undifferentiated carcinoma.

Large cell and anaplastic lymphomas and metastatic malignant melanoma are sometimes difficult to distinguish from undifferentiated carcinoma on the basis of light microscopic features alone. Immunohistochemistry can be helpful. Undifferentiated carcinomas are typically reactive for cytokeratins but little else (figs. 5-239, 5-240). Malignant lymphoma can be identified by one or more of several lymphoid markers that include CD45, CD20, CD45RO, CD3, and CD30 (Ki-1). In the absence of melanin pigment, metastatic melanoma can frequently be identified by immunoreactivity for S-100 protein and HMB45 antigen.

Prognosis and Treatment. Undifferentiated carcinomas are high-grade, aggressive neoplasms that frequently metastasize and have a poor prognosis. In a study of 87 patients with salivary gland carcinomas at Johns Hopkins Hospital, North et al. (594) found that none of 5 patients with undifferentiated carcinoma survived 10 years while Theriault and Fitzpatrick (601) reported a 35 percent 10-year survival rate. The mean number of silver staining nucleolar organizer regions (AgNORs) in cell nuclei has been correlated with the aggressiveness of some tumors. One undifferentiated carcinoma among 43 salivary gland tumors was found to have a higher mean AgNOR count (603). Soini et al. (597) found increased p53 protein expression in 5 of 51

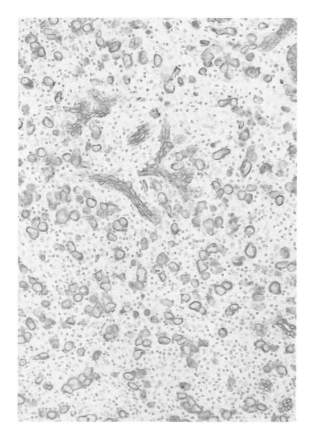

Figure 5-239
LARGE CELL UNDIFFERENTIATED CARCINOMA:
IMMUNOHISTOCHEMISTRY
Immunohistochemical staining with a cocktail of monoclonal anti-cytokeratin antibodies highlights the noncohesive individual tumor cells. (Avidin-biotin peroxidase stain)

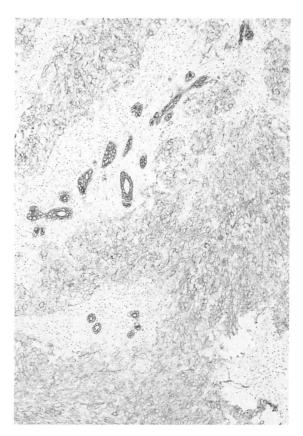

Figure 5-240
LARGE CELL UNDIFFERENTIATED CARCINOMA:
IMMUNOHISTOCHEMISTRY
In contrast to figure 5-239, anti-cytokeratin immunohistochemical staining shows sheets and trabeculae of epithelial cells that have infiltrated parotid gland parenchyma. Intensely stained residual ducts are conspicuous. (Avidin-biotin peroxidase stain)

salivary gland tumors: 3 of 12 mucoepidermoid carcinomas and 2 of 3 undifferentiated carcinomas. Little distinction has been made for prognosis and therapy among the various subtypes of undifferentiated carcinoma, and they are essentially the same for large cell undifferentiated carcinoma as for small cell carcinoma.

Hui et al. (588) and Batsakis and Luna (583) found that cell size (large cell versus small cell) or any other histopathologic feature of undifferentiated carcinomas had no prognostic importance; however, tumor size was the single most important prognostic factor. Neoplasms 4 cm or larger had a particularly poor outcome. Combined radical surgery and postoperative radiation therapy offer the best chance of survival for affected patients (586,592,594,601).

Lymphoepithelial Carcinoma

Definition. Lymphoepithelial carcinomas are essentially undifferentiated carcinomas that are associated with a dense lymphoid stroma. Because of histologic similarity to and, in some cases, origin within benign lymphoepithelial lesions (more recently called myoepithelial sialadenitis), these tumors have frequently been referred to as malignant lymphoepithelial lesions. Since lymphoepithelial lesions have both epithelial and lymphoid components, either of which may manifest malignant neoplasia, there is an inherent ambiguity about the malignant component in the term malignant lymphoepithelial lesion. Although traditionally the term has referred to a malignant epithelial neoplasm, less ambiguous terminology has been sought. The WHO and others have used the phrase *undifferentiated carcinoma with lymphoid stroma* (616,633). Still other investigators have referred to these tumors as *carcinoma ex lymphoepithelial lesion* (611,615) or simply as *undifferentiated carcinomas* without distinction from undifferentiated carcinomas without lymphoid stroma (618). Kott et al. (623) used the term *lymphoepithelial carcinoma*, which is used in this Fascicle for its brevity and clarity.

General Features. Most reported surveys of salivary gland neoplasias do not include a category for lymphoepithelial carcinoma; however, despite its relative rarity among salivary gland carcinomas, this neoplasm has received considerable attention in the literature since its initial description by Hilderman et al. (620) in 1962. A survey of the English language literature by Borg et al. (613) found 108 reported cases. While we found 133 reported cases, several were surveys of cases from the same geographic region, and it is impossible to determine how much, if any, duplication exists in some of these reports (609,618,624,626,629).

Lymphoepithelial carcinoma comprises only about 0.4 percent of the salivary gland neoplasms accessioned into the files of the AFIP since 1985. Yet, this rarity is relative because lymphoepithelial carcinoma manifests a racial preference that is unknown for any other salivary gland neoplasm. Approximately 75 percent of affected patients are of Mongolian ancestry: about three quarters of these are arctic native people (Eskimo, Inuit) from Greenland, Canada, and Alaska, and one quarter are Southern Chinese. The incidence of salivary gland cancer in the Eskimo population is the highest in the world, 10 times the expected rate, and most of these cancers are lymphoepithelial carcinomas (607,613,616,624,627,629). Less than 15 percent of affected patients are Caucasians, mostly North Americans, and the remainder are Japanese, blacks, Indians, and others (613,616). The female to male ratio is 1.5 to 1. Patients range in age from 10 to 86 years, with a median of about 40 years (613). Familial clustering of affected patients has been reported (607,610,627).

The parotid gland is the site of primary occurrence in 82 percent of tumors, and the submandibular gland in the remainder. Some carcinomas occur in association with, or subsequent to, biopsy-proven benign lymphoepithelial lesions (myo-epithelial sialadenitis) in the same gland, which implies malignant transformation of the epithelial elements of a benign lymphoepithelial lesion (608,612,613,615,617,619,621,623,624). On the other hand, most lymphoepithelial carcinomas are not diagnosed within a milieu of benign lymphoepithelial lesion and probably develop de novo.

There is marked histologic similarity between lymphoepithelial carcinoma of salivary gland and the lymphoepithelioma type of undifferentiated nasopharyngeal carcinoma. Likewise, similar to nasopharyngeal carcinoma, an association between Epstein-Barr virus (EBV) infection and lymphoepithelial carcinoma has been documented (607,613, 618,624,625,630,631). More than 50 percent of patients have elevated titers of serum IgA against EBV capsid antigen or IgG against EBV nuclear antigen (607,613). Hamilton-Dutoit et al. (618) reported that EBV genomes have been detected with nucleic acid hybridization in malignant epithelial cells but not in lymphoid stromal cells or adjacent salivary gland tissue in all 18 lymphoepithelial carcinomas from Greenlandic and Alaskan Eskimos they studied (618,624,625,630). However, two lymphoepithelial carcinomas from Caucasian patients were negative for EBV by in situ hybridization (618). Thus far, the association of EBV infection and lymphoepithelial carcinoma has only been established in patients of Mongoloid race (613).

Clinical Features. Lymphoepithelial carcinomas present as parotid or submandibular masses of variable duration, usually months but extending up to 10 years (631). Associated pain or discomfort is frequent, and facial nerve palsy occurs in up to 20 percent of patients (613). Cervical lymphadenopathy is present in 40 percent of patients at presentation (631).

Pathologic Findings. Macroscopically, these tumors are lobulated, firm, and tan. Some tumors are circumscribed but unencapsulated, but most are clearly infiltrative into adjacent salivary gland, fat, muscle, or skin. In their primary occurrence they have varied from 1 to 10 cm in largest dimension.

Low magnification microscopy reveals circumscribed or irregular infiltrates of densely aggregated lymphoid cells. Lymphoid germinal centers can often be recognized (fig. 5-241), but the epithelial component is frequently inconspicuous at low magnification. With higher magnification, irregular shaped islands of eosinophilic epithelioid cells

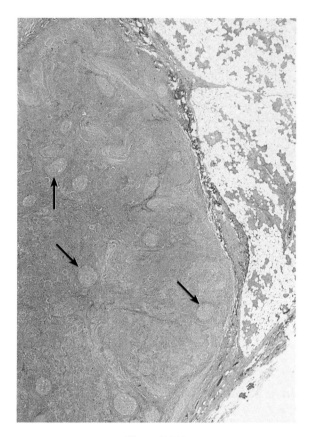

Figure 5-241
LYMPHOEPITHELIAL CARCINOMA

This low-magnification micrograph shows a deeply baso-philic, circumscribed mass within the parotid parenchyma. Paler, round structures (arrows) within the basophilic mass represent germinal centers of lymphoid follicles. Carcinoma-tous epithelial nests within the basophilic area are not easily recognizable at this magnification.

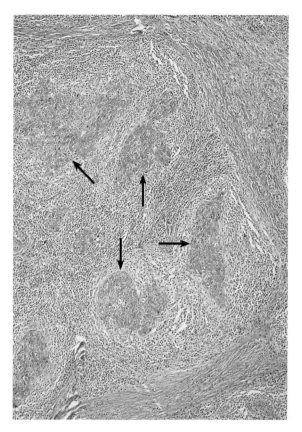

Figure 5-242
LYMPHOEPITHELIAL CARCINOMA

Irregularly shaped nests of epithelium (arrows) are sep-arated from one another by a dense lymphocytic infiltrate in a fibrous tissue stroma.

within a lymphocyte-rich stroma are evident (fig. 5-242). The architectural growth pattern of these epithelioid cells are small islands, syncytial masses, cords, trabeculae, or isolated cells (figs. 5-243–5-245). Epithelial islands are frequently widely sepa-rated by the lymphoid-rich stroma (fig. 5-242).

Cytologically, the malignant epithelial cells are similar to those described for large cell undifferen-tiated carcinoma. They vary in shape from polyg-onal to slightly spindled. They have abundant amphophilic to eosinophilic cytoplasm with large, round to oval, lightly basophilic to vesicular nuclei that usually contain one or more prominent nucle-oli. Cell boundaries are often indistinct (fig. 5-245). A few cells have cytoplasmic vacuoles or clear cytoplasm (fig. 5-246). Mitotic figures are usually evident but vary in number from 1 to 10 or more

per 10 high-power fields (fig. 5-245). The cells are typically fairly uniform, but anaplasia can be marked in some tumors. Although epidermoid fea-tures are occasionally manifest, the overall appear-ance is that of undifferentiated carcinoma.

Dense lymphocytic infiltrates surround and permeate the nodules of carcinomatous cells (fig. 5-246). Small lymphocytes and plasma cells com-prise most of the lymphoid component, but single or small groups of histiocytes are often inter-spersed. Lymphoid follicles with germinal cen-ters vary from none to many (figs. 5-241, 5-244). A variable amount of collagenous tissue is usu-ally present within the lymphoid component.

In some tumors, so-called epimyoepithelial islands that are characteristic of benign lympho-epithelial lesions are present in addition to the aggregates of undifferentiated carcinoma cells (fig. 5-247). These nests of epithelial cells are

Figure 5-243
LYMPHOEPITHELIAL
CARCINOMA

Thin cords and small nests of carcinomatous cells are surrounded by lymphoid
cells. On the basis of this field alone, the
epithelial character of the tumor cells
may be difficult to recognize.

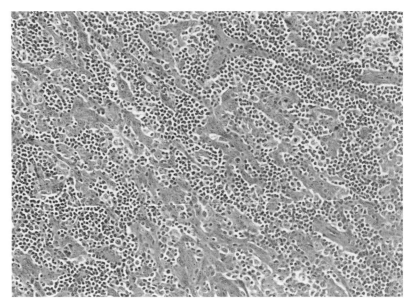

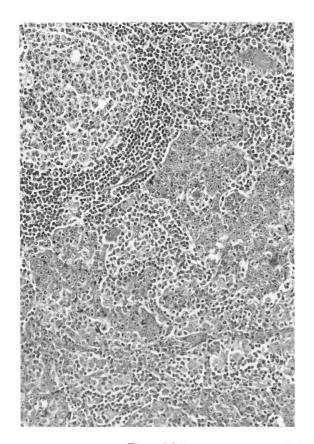

Figure 5-244
LYMPHOEPITHELIAL CARCINOMA

Asymmetric and jagged nests of undifferentiated epithelial cells lie in a lymphoid stroma in which a lymphoid follicle
is evident (upper left).

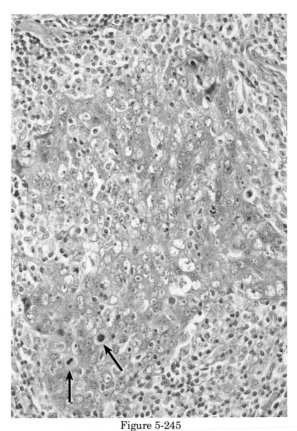

Figure 5-245
LYMPHOEPITHELIAL CARCINOMA

A syncytial mass of undifferentiated epithelial cells is
within a lymphoid stroma. The cells have indistinct cell boundaries, round vesicular nuclei, and prominent nucleoli. Several
mitotic figures are present in this field (arrows).

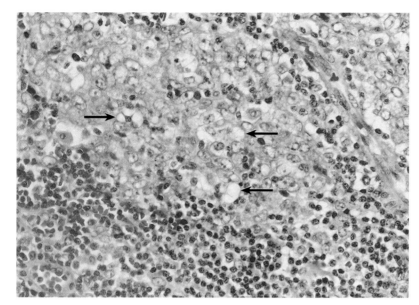

Figure 5-246
LYMPHOEPITHELIAL CARCINOMA
This nest of undifferentiated epithelial cells is enveloped and permeated by lymphocytes so that the boundary between carcinoma and stroma is vague. Some of the epithelial cells have clear vacuoles in their cytoplasm (arrows).

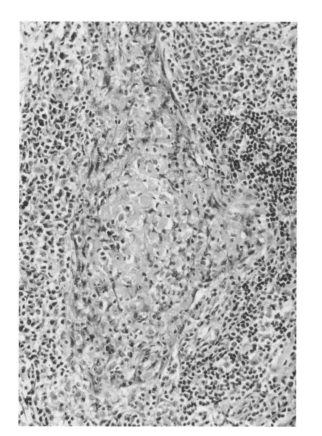

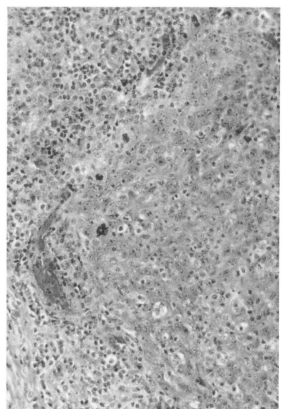

Figure 5-247
LYMPHOEPITHELIAL CARCINOMA ARISING IN BENIGN LYMPHOEPITHELIAL LESION
Left: This so-called epimyoepithelial island in a lymphoid infiltrate is characteristic of benign lymphoepithelial lesion of the parotid gland. It is a roughly triangular-shaped nest of poorly defined epithelial cells with small, basophilic nuclei and without cytoplasmic or nuclear atypia. Intercellular, eosinophilic hyaline material that is often seen in these epithelial islands, is evident.
Right: Within the same parotid gland, islands of atypical epithelial cells with vesicular nuclei, nucleoli, and mitotic figures are also present in the lymphoid stroma.

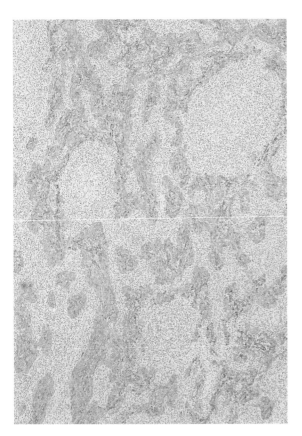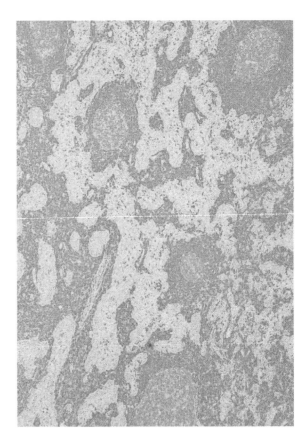

Figure 5-248
LYMPHOEPITHELIAL CARCINOMA: IMMUNOHISTOCHEMISTRY
Left: Low-magnification examination of anti-cytokeratin stained lymphoepithelial carcinoma highlights the trabeculae of carcinoma in the lymphoid stroma.
Right: A comparable field immunostained with anti-leukocyte common antigen highlights the lymphoid stroma with lymphoid follicles. (Avidin-biotin peroxidase stain)

typically irregular shaped, are surrounded and infiltrated by lymphocytes, and have poorly defined borders. Eosinophilic hyaline material is frequently present as intercellular deposits. These islands differ from the carcinomatous islands in their cytologic features: their cells lack mitotic figures, cellular and nuclear pleomorphism, vesicular nuclei, and prominent nucleoli.

The histochemical, immunohistochemical, and electron microscopic features of the carcinomatous cells are similar to those of large cell undifferentiated carcinomas. Electron microscopic studies have generally described epidermoid type features such as desmosomal cell attachments and conspicuous cytoplasmic microfilaments and tonofilaments. Viral particles are usually not found (621–623,628,632,634). Anti-cytokeratin and anti-leukocyte common antigen immunoreactiv-

ity demonstrate the intimate relationship between the epithelial and lymphoid components (figs. 5-248, 5-249).

Differential Diagnosis. Many investigators have noted the marked histopathologic similarity between lymphoepithelial carcinoma of the salivary gland and undifferentiated nasopharyngeal carcinoma of the so-called lymphoepithelioma type (607,613,616,618,622,631,632). The association with EBV infection and the predilection for people of Mongoloid ancestry that these two carcinomas have in common suggests the possibility of a common pathogenesis. Metastatic nasopharyngeal carcinoma is the principal consideration in the differential diagnosis of lymphoepithelial carcinoma. Histologic, histochemical, immunohistochemical, and ultrastructural studies cannot reliably distinguish between

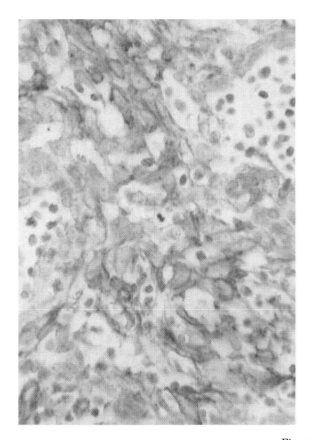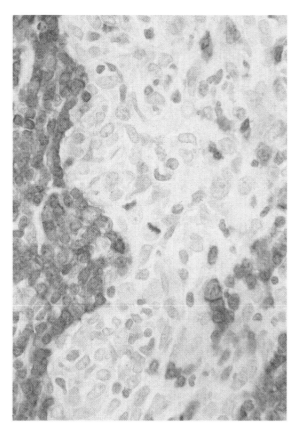

Figure 5-249
LYMPHOEPITHELIAL CARCINOMA: IMMUNOHISTOCHEMISTRY
High-magnification microscopy with anti-cytokeratin (left) and anti-leukocyte common antigen (CD45) (right) stained lymphoepithelial carcinoma demonstrates the intimate, intermingled relationship of lymphocytes and malignant epithelial cells. (Avidin-biotin peroxidase stain)

these two carcinomas. Careful clinical evaluation, possibly including biopsies, of the nasopharynx and Waldeyer's ring region and close patient follow-up are necessary. Fortunately, the parotid gland, which is the predominant site of occurrence for lymphoepithelial carcinoma, is an infrequent site of metastasis for nasopharyngeal carcinoma, which more typically metastasizes to the cervical or submandibular lymph nodes.

Metastatic amelanotic melanoma of the face or scalp can be distinguished from lymphoepithelial carcinoma with anti-cytokeratin, anti-S-100 protein, and HMB45 immunohistochemistry. Lymphocytic and histiocytic immunohistochemical markers, such as antibodies to CD20, CD45RO, CD68, Leu-M1, and Ki-1, along with epithelial markers, help differentiate large cell lymphocytic and histiocytic neoplasms from lymphoepithelial carcinoma. It should be noted

that epimyoepithelial islands do not rule out malignant lymphoma.

Benign lymphoepithelial lesion (BLEL) has a similar histopathologic architectural structure to lymphoepithelial carcinoma. BLEL is distinguished on the basis of the cytologic features of the epithelial structures as well as an absence of invasion into adjacent tissues, such as skin, skeletal muscle, fat, and bone.

Prognosis and Treatment. For some reason, lymphoepithelial carcinoma seems to have a better prognosis than large cell undifferentiated carcinoma of the salivary glands, which it resembles cytologically, although reported survival rates vary considerably. Perhaps the lymphoid stroma has a role in limiting the aggressiveness of this carcinoma. Over 40 percent of patients have metastases to cervical lymph nodes at initial presentation, 20 percent develop local recurrences or lymph node metastases, and 20 percent experience distant metastases within 3 years following therapy (613,614,616,631). Distant metastases usually involve the lung, but also the liver, bone, and brain (613,614).

Survival ranges from 17 to 86 percent, but 5-year survival rates of over 60 percent have been reported (631). Factors cited as indicators of poor prognosis include high mitotic rate, anaplasia, and necrosis (616). Histologic features of benign lymphoepithelial lesion correlated with a good prognosis in one study (624). The clinical stage of disease has a significant impact on outcome. Advanced disease in the form of large size or lymph node metastasis corresponds to poor survival (616). The better survival rates reported in the more recent literature result from combined surgery, often including neck dissection, and radiation therapy rather than surgery alone (613,614).

ONCOCYTIC CARCINOMA

Definition. Oncocytic carcinoma is a rare, predominantly oncocytic neoplasm whose malignant nature is reflected by both its abnormal morphologic features and infiltrative growth. The oncocytic nature of the tumor cells is confirmed with either histochemical or electron microscopic studies.

The terms *oncocytic carcinoma* and *oncocytic adenocarcinoma* are synonymous. The terms *malignant oncocytoma* and *malignant oxyphilic adenoma* have also been used synonymously with oncocytic carcinoma. However, some investigators have suggested that the malignant nature of these neoplasms is not manifest until the tumor unexpectedly metastasizes, and they use the latter terms to imply the tumors are oncocytomas that are malignant by behavior (639,640,661). More succinctly, these terms suggest that malignant oncocytoma and benign oncocytoma do not have sufficient histologic differences to permit easy separation (637). Review of published cases and experience at the AFIP indicate that oncocytic carcinoma can usually be recognized at the time of initial diagnosis. Exceptions are those such as the large, multinodular but well-circumscribed tumor reported by Sugimoto et al. (661) that recurred and metastasized. In this case, nuclear abnormalities were reported as minimal and the mitotic rate less than 1 in 10 high-power fields.

Another term, *oncocytoid carcinoma,* has been used for tumors that are composed of cells that have abundant, granular, eosinophilic cytoplasm but in which there is no evidence of increased numbers of mitochondria (636,653). While descriptively accurate, this term is not consistent with current classification schemes for salivary gland tumors (659). Such tumors that lack histochemical or electron microscopic evidence of oncocytic features should be designated adenocarcinoma, not otherwise specified.

General Features. Malignant oncocytic tumors occur in sites other than the salivary glands, including the thyroid and parathyroid glands, kidney, ovary, nasal cavity, superior mediastinum, lung, and breast (643,650). Many of these and other sites are also affected by oncocytosis or benign oncocytic neoplasms. Although oncocytosis frequently occurs in the major salivary glands of adults and focal oncocytic features occur in a wide variety of salivary neoplasms, both benign and malignant oncocytic neoplasms are extremely rare. This rarity is shown by the absence of oncocytic carcinoma in many large published series of salivary gland neoplasms (647, 648,658,662,664,665).

Oncocytic carcinoma represents less than 1 percent of nearly 3,100 salivary gland tumors accessioned to the AFIP files since 1985. Benign oncocytomas are five times more frequent. About 20 percent of patients with oncocytomas have received direct or indirect radiation exposure to the affected gland (640), but no such association has been noted in patients with oncocytic carcinoma. Transformation from a benign tumor, however, is suggested by the development of oncocytic carcinoma in the site of a longstanding glandular mass (646). In one report, the histologic diagnosis of a subtotal parotidectomy specimen was oncocytoma; residual or recurrent tumor in the resected specimen the following year showed atypical oncocytic cells, frequent mitoses, and invasion into bone and soft tissues (651).

Most cases of oncocytic carcinoma occur in the parotid glands, but recent reports have included tumors that involved the submandibular gland (640,650,666) and minor glands of the palate (641) and buccal mucosa (650). The average age of patients at the AFIP is about 63 years, similar to the collective average of patients in other series (635,639,640,649,653–656,661,663). The

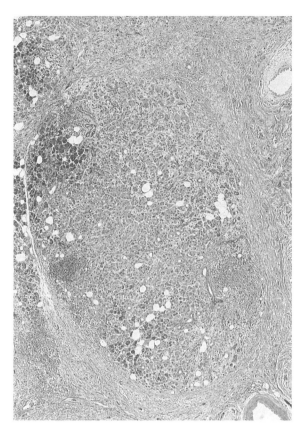

Figure 5-250
ONCOCYTIC CARCINOMA
Tumor has replaced the salivary gland lobule in the center of the illustration, leaving only a few acini and ducts. Individual cells have infiltrated the connective tissue (top).

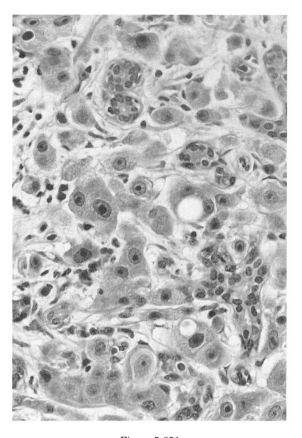

Figure 5-251
ONCOCYTIC CARCINOMA
The shape and size of the tumor cells are variable, the nuclei are large, and prominent nucleoli are evident. A few small residual ducts are present.

youngest patient was 29 and the oldest 91 years. There is a male predominance in reported cases.

Clinical Features. Patients typically develop parotid masses that cause pain or paralysis one third of the time (661). The skin overlying the gland occasionally is discolored or wrinkled (635). The rate of growth may be rapid, but a 1- or 2-year duration is usual prior to diagnosis. Clinical evidence of nodal involvement has been observed at the time of presentation.

Gross and Microscopic Findings. Typically, oncocytic carcinoma appears grossly as a single or multinodular, firm, unencapsulated gray to gray-brown mass that in some cases is focally necrotic (653,655,656,661).

Microscopically, the tumor is predominantly composed of large, round or polyhedral cells that are arranged in solid sheets, islands, and cords, or as scattered individual cells (fig. 5-250). The

cells have abundant, finely granular eosinophilic cytoplasm (fig. 5-251) that largely represents excessive numbers of mitochondria. Histochemical or ultrastructural confirmation of the oncocytic (mitochondrial) nature of the cytoplasm is necessary because cytoplasmic accumulation of smooth endoplasmic reticula, lysosomes, or secretory granules may cause a similar appearance. Phosphotungstic acid–hematoxylin (PTAH) stains mitochondria-rich cytoplasm dark blue (fig. 5-252). This stain can sometimes help reveal the extent of infiltration of tumor cells better than hematoxylin and eosin, which stains the cells pale and eosinophilic like collagenous tissue. However, PTAH may be falsely negative, possibly because of delayed fixation (654), and this necessitates electron microscopy to confirm the oncocytic nature of the tumor cells. Normal striated ducts serve as a dependable

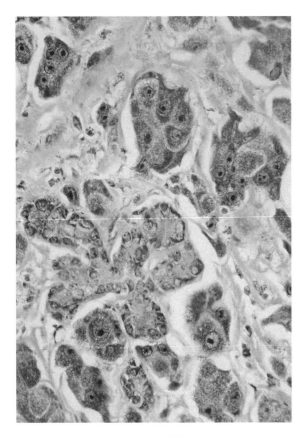

Figure 5-252
PHOSPHOTUNGSTIC ACID–
HEMATOXYLIN (PTAH) STAIN
The cytoplasm of individual and clustered tumor cells stains dark blue and its granularity is emphasized. This contrasts with the orange-pink residual acinar cells seen in the center of the field. (PTAH stain)

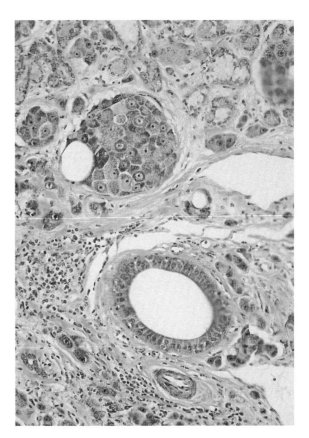

Figure 5-253
ONCOCYTIC CARCINOMA: PTAH STAIN
The striated duct seen just below center serves as a valuable internal positive control. Fortunately, these ducts are present in most parotid or submandibular specimens. As shown here, the staining intensity of the ductal cells is similar to the tumor cells. (PTAH stain)

internal positive control for PTAH staining (fig. 5-253). The staining intensity of PTAH often varies from cell to cell and within different areas of the tumor. The presence of glycogen and mucin is variable (636).

Many of the neoplastic oncocytic cells have moderately pleomorphic, medium-sized or large nuclei that are often located centrally within the cytoplasm. Nucleoli are often large and irregular (fig. 5-251). Goode and Corio (650) reported that the degree of pleomorphism varies and in a minority of cases may be altogether lacking. This variation occurs within tumors as well as among tumors. Pleomorphic and nonpleomorphic areas in a tumor suggest that the carcinoma arose from a preexisting oncocytoma, especially if a long-standing tumor recently demonstrated rapid

growth clinically. Most cell borders are distinct but cells in small clusters often overlap with one another. The tumor cells may focally form small pseudoluminal spaces (fig. 5-251), and in some cases ductal differentiation is evident (fig. 5-254). Scattered mitotic figures are usually evident and focally numerous in some cases and atypical mitoses are occasionally evident (fig. 5-255).

Oncocytic carcinomas frequently compress connective tissue and form pseudocapsules, but tumors usually demonstrate unequivocal evidence of infiltrative growth. Individual cells and clusters of cells invade salivary gland parenchyma and surrounding connective tissue (fig. 5-256). Perineural (fig. 5-257) and perivascular infiltration (fig. 5-258) are often evident, and necrosis (fig. 5-259) is present in some cases.

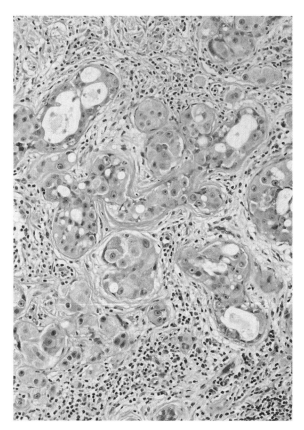

Figure 5-254
ONCOCYTIC CARCINOMA
Although ductal differentiation is rarely prominent, it may
be present in some areas of the tumor, as shown in this example.

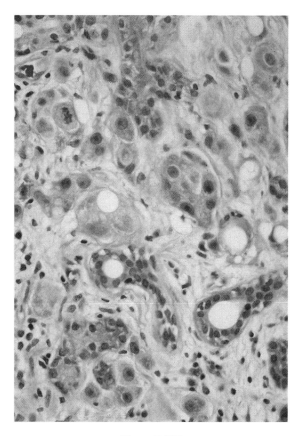

Figure 5-255
ONCOCYTIC CARCINOMA
Mitotic figures are increased and may be atypical, as shown
in the top portion of this field.

Ultrastructural Findings. Electron microscopy confirms that the abundant and granular cytoplasm of the tumor cells represents numerous mitochondria. The cytoplasm is typically packed with mitochondria. A quantitative study of the neoplastic cells of benign oncocytoma demonstrated that between 45 and 73 percent of the cytoplasm was occupied by these organelles (642), and a similar proportion probably occurs in oncocytic carcinomas. The mitochondria in oncocytic carcinoma vary in size and shape and exhibit an electron-lucent matrix (636,655,661). The space between mitochondria is occupied by free ribosomes, lysosomes, and endoplasmic reticulum. The cells are attached to each other by desmosomes. Ultrastructural distinction between benign and malignant oncocytic neoplasms is not possible, although unlike most oncocytomas some oncocytic carcinomas have prominent intercellular spaces and basal lamina (654,655).

Differential Diagnosis. All types of benign or malignant salivary gland tumors can have foci of oncocytic cells, but the oncocytic component usually comprises such a small portion that it is unlikely to be confused with oncocytic carcinoma.

Multifocal oncocytosis occurs as variably sized foci of oncocytic cells within salivary gland lobules without altering the normal architecture. These foci ordinarily have no surrounding connective tissue and appear to "infiltrate" into parenchyma. Individual acinar and ductal cells show similar metaplastic oncocytic changes. Because this process is usually seen in older patients, nests and individual oncocytes admixed with normal acinar cells may be embedded within fat.

Oncocytomas are frequently unencapsulated and some have atypical nuclear changes, which complicates distinction from oncocytic carcinoma. Secondary hemorrhage and necrosis from previous

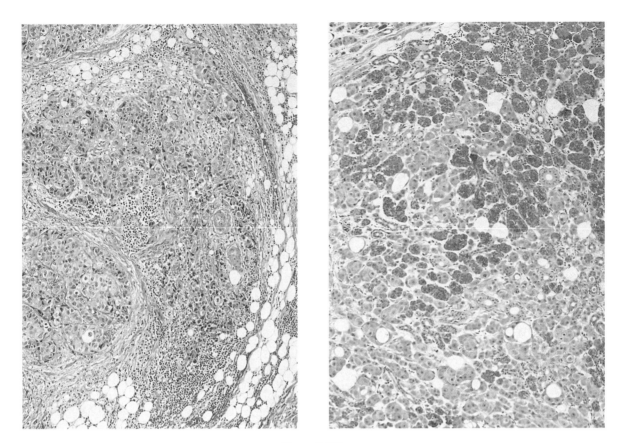

Figure 5-256
INFILTRATIVE GROWTH

In addition to the nearly constant nuclear morphologic abnormalities, unquestionable infiltration into periglandular connective tissue and salivary parenchyma is evident.

Figure 5-257
PERINEURAL INFILTRATION
IN ONCOCYTIC CARCINOMA

Tumor cells surround this peripheral nerve, a feature not acceptable in oncocytomas.

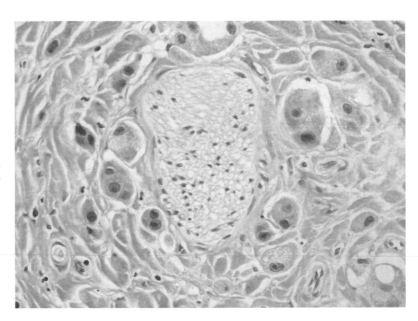

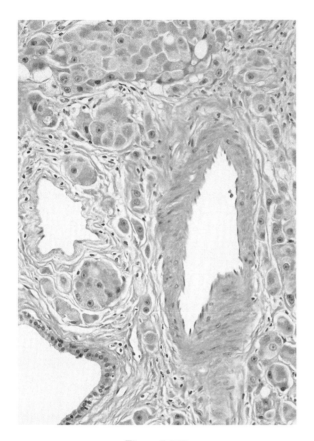

Figure 5-258
PERIVASCULAR GROWTH
Islands of tumor cells completely surround these two blood vessels and contact their walls in several areas. The presence of numerous individual and small clusters of tumor cells and their arrangement around the vessels supports a malignant interpretation despite the lack of intravascular invasion.

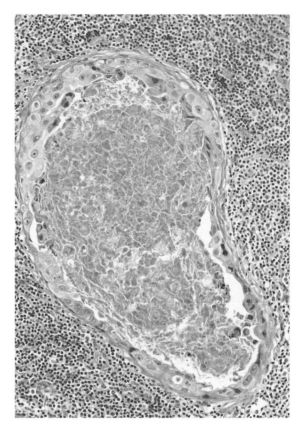

Figure 5-259
METASTATIC ONCOCYTIC CARCINOMA
Metastatic tumor seen in a cervical lymph node is largely necrotic. The small amount of viable tumor maintains its oncocytic appearance.

surgical manipulation or fine-needle aspiration further complicate interpretation. Compared to oncocytomas, oncocytic carcinomas usually show considerably greater mitotic activity, cellular pleomorphism, and unequivocal evidence of infiltration into surrounding tissues; the nuclei are not usually pyknotic and they often have enlarged nucleoli; and necrosis in the absence of prior manipulation occurs. Although encapsulation of oncocytomas is often incomplete or absent they are clearly demarcated from adjacent tissues, whereas oncocytic carcinomas have small clusters and individual cells that surround nerves and blood vessels and form an irregular interface with normal tissues. We disagree with those investigators who suggest perineural invasion is an acceptable feature of oncocytomas (640).

Other salivary gland tumors composed of large cells with abundant granular cytoplasm that may resemble oncocytes include acinic cell adenocarcinoma and salivary duct carcinoma. The granules in the tumor cells of acinic cell adenocarcinoma are usually amphophilic or basophilic and are periodic acid–Schiff positive before and after diastase digestion. Small quantities of glycogen in oncocytic carcinomas can complicate interpretation if diastase digestion is not performed. Microcystic or papillary cystic patterns and an acinar arrangement of tumor cells are features that support acinic cell adenocarcinoma. Salivary duct carcinoma often has pleomorphic cells that infiltrate individually or in small clusters, and these areas can resemble oncocytic carcinoma. However, the tumor cells in salivary duct carcinoma form cysts and duct-like spaces, show papillary and cribriform growth, and often demonstrate

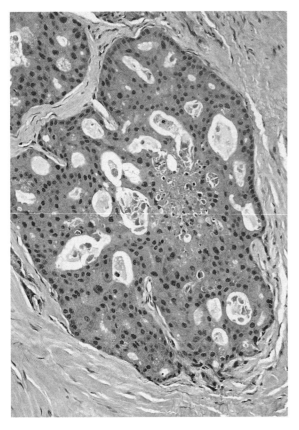

Figure 5-260
SALIVARY DUCT CARCINOMA

The neoplastic cells of salivary duct carcinoma may have an oncocytic appearance. Unlike oncocytic carcinoma, cribriform growth may be evident in the walls of the neoplastic cysts or within solid tumor islands. Comedonecrosis is much more often seen in salivary duct carcinoma than oncocytic carcinoma.

comedonecrosis (fig. 5-260). The granular cytoplasm of the large cells in either acinic cell adenocarcinoma or salivary duct carcinoma are unreactive with PTAH stain (644,652,654).

Prognosis and Treatment. Despite the rarity of oncocytic carcinoma, there is evidence for considering it a high-grade neoplasm. In the largest series reviewed thus far, Goode and Corio (650) reported that five of their nine patients had recurrences; metastases occurred in four of these five, three of whom died of disease and the other was alive with disease. A number of other studies have reported multiple recurrences (638,650, 651,657) and distant metastases (650,651, 654,655). Metastatic sites include lungs, kidney, liver, thyroid, mediastinum, and bone; cervical lymph nodes are also frequently involved. Tu-

mors less than 2 cm appear to have a noticeably better prognosis than larger tumors (650).

Of the four patients who died of disease in the review by Goode and Corio, three did so less than 2 years after initial diagnosis and the other after 7 years. The average reported survival for patients with metastasizing tumors was 3.8 years (640).

As with other high-grade salivary gland neoplasms, aggressive surgical intervention seems warranted. Goode and Corio observed that patients who had total parotidectomy rather than excision of the tumor had a significantly better outcome. Radiotherapy has been used in too few cases to reach any meaningful conclusions, but in at least one case its use was followed by rapid and widespread dissemination of disease (650).

SALIVARY DUCT CARCINOMA

Definition. Salivary duct carcinoma is a rare, high-grade malignant epithelial neoplasm composed of structures that resemble expanded salivary gland ducts. Comedonecrosis of these structures is a frequent feature. There is some histologic but not behavioral similarity to intraductal carcinoma of the breast.

Kleinsasser et al. (684) first used the term salivary duct carcinoma in 1968; however, it is now recognized that two of the five cases they reported are more appropriately classified as epithelial-myoepithelial carcinoma. This lack of distinction between salivary duct carcinoma and epithelial-myoepithelial carcinoma persisted in some descriptions in the literature (679,689,692), including the previous Atlas of Tumor Pathology Fascicle on salivary gland tumors (693). Separation of these two entities is critical because it is now recognized that they have markedly different biologic behavior.

Since most salivary gland carcinomas of various types are derived from the duct system and exhibit ductal differentiation, salivary duct carcinoma may not be the best term for a specific category of salivary gland neoplasm. There is potential for confusion if terms such as "ductal" or "duct carcinoma" are used descriptively. To avoid such confusion Brandwein et al. (671) suggested the term cribriform salivary carcinoma of excretory ducts; however, salivary duct carcinoma has become the established terminology (667,669,671,672,675, 676,678,680–682,686–688) and is recognized as a specific clinicopathologic entity. Although this tumor was not identified in the WHO classification of 1972 (694), it is included in the recent WHO classification (690). The terms *salivary duct adenocarcinoma* and *intraductal carcinoma* have been used synonymously for salivary duct carcinoma (668,673,683,691). We believe that intraductal carcinoma is an inappropriate term since it implies a noninvasive tumor with little potential to metastasize, similar to breast tumors of the same name. Quite to the contrary, salivary duct carcinomas are very aggressive neoplasms with a poor prognosis. Chen and Hafez (674) suggested calling these tumors *infiltrating salivary duct carcinoma*.

General Features. Because of its rarity and recent acceptance as a specific entity, salivary duct carcinoma of salivary glands generally has not been identified among investigations of large series of salivary gland neoplasms. On the basis of limited reports in the literature and experience at the AFIP, salivary duct carcinoma is an uncommon neoplasm. About 100 cases have been reported (668,672,675–680,691) and 9 cases have been added to AFIP files since 1985. Colmenero Ruiz et al. (675) found that it represented 3.4 percent of salivary gland malignancies reviewed in one hospital in Bolivia, and Garland et al. (682) reported an incidence of 3.9 percent among salivary gland carcinomas in the tumor registry of the University of Virginia. Simpson et al. (691) reported an incidence of 2 percent among all salivary gland tumors at one institution in England. The 9 salivary duct carcinomas in the AFIP files represent only 0.2 percent, 0.5 percent, and 1.1 percent of all epithelial salivary gland neoplasms, salivary gland carcinomas, and parotid gland carcinomas, respectively, accessioned since 1985.

All the AFIP cases and 86 percent of those in the literature have involved the parotid gland, 7 percent of reported tumors occurred in the submandibular gland, and 5 percent occurred in intraoral minor salivary glands. The sublingual gland and extraparotid Stensen's duct were the sites of one case each.

Seventy-six percent of patients have been men. Two of the cases of salivary gland tumors in children reported by Lack and Upton (685) may have been salivary duct carcinomas, but otherwise patients have ranged in age from 22 to 91 years. The peak incidence is in the sixth and seventh decades of life.

Clinical Features. Parotid swelling is the most frequent sign, but facial nerve dysfunction or paralysis occur in over one fourth of patients and may be the initial manifestation of disease. Many patients report rapid growth of their tumors, and most patients seek medical evaluation of their signs and symptoms within 2 years of onset. Cervical lymphadenopathy is evident in over a third of patients.

Gross Findings. Salivary duct carcinomas are unencapsulated and usually poorly circumscribed, grayish white to yellowish white, multinodular tumors. The cut surface often reveals several small but variably sized cysts and foci of necrosis. Fibrosis is usually prominent. Average size is about 3.0 cm, with a range of 1.0 cm to over 6.0 cm in largest dimension.

Microscopic Findings. The most characteristic feature is variably sized, rounded nodules of tumor cells that in some ways resemble intraductal carcinoma of the breast (fig. 5-261). Small nodules, which are about one to two times the diameter of interlobular salivary gland ducts, are solid or cystic, but larger nodules are almost invariably cystic (fig. 5-262). Large cystic nodules are often irregularly shaped (fig. 5-262). The cystic nodules frequently demonstrate central comedonecrosis (fig. 5-263). Comedonecrosis was a diagnostic requisite for Garland et al. (682), but most investigators consider comedonecrosis to be characteristic but not requisite for diagnosis. The epithelium of the cystic tumor nodules are in band-like, papillary, and cribriform patterns, and all three configurations are usually evident in most tumors (figs. 5-263–5-267). The cribriform pattern has been likened to "Roman bridge" architecture because thin bands of neoplastic epithelium appear to be arched over small luminal spaces (fig. 5-268) (672).

In addition to the intraductal-like nodules, small aggregates of neoplastic epithelium, which resemble infiltrating ductal carcinoma of the breast, are often observed between or adjacent to the cystic tumor nodules (fig. 5-269). Perineural infiltration and intralymphatic infiltration are frequent findings (fig. 5-270). Dense fibrosis is a conspicuous component of salivary duct carcinoma and is associated with both the intraductal-like and infiltrating ductal-like epithelia (figs. 5-261, 5-262,5-269). Focal hyalinization of the stroma is sometimes evident (fig. 5-271). A

325

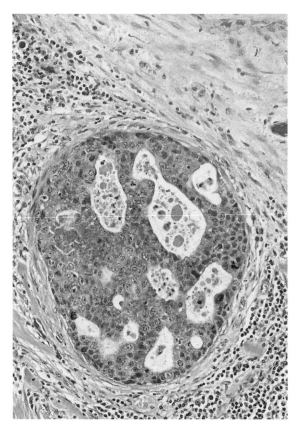

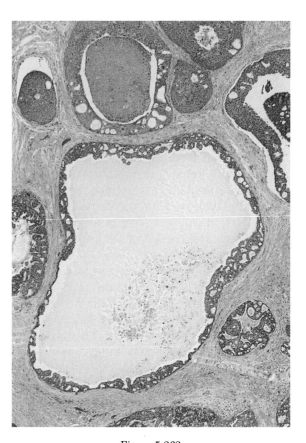

Figure 5-261
SALIVARY DUCT CARCINOMA

A round, well-circumscribed nodule of neoplastic ductal epithelium has a cribriform architecture that is similar to intraductal carcinoma of the breast. Cell necrosis is evident, but comedonecrosis is not present. The tumor nodule is in a fibrous tissue stroma with a lymphoplasmacytic infiltrate.

Figure 5-262
SALIVARY DUCT CARCINOMA

Among the several circumscribed nodules of tumor, some are composed of solid tumor cells (top) while others are cystic.

Figure 5-263
SALIVARY DUCT CARCINOMA

Comedonecrosis is evident in the central area of this cystic nodule of tumor. The necrotic material has slightly retracted from the surrounding epithelium during fixation of the tissue. Two mitotic figures (arrows) as well as moderate cytologic atypia are apparent. The epithelium of the left half of the cyst is a solid sheet while the epithelium on the right half has microcysts and a cribriform pattern.

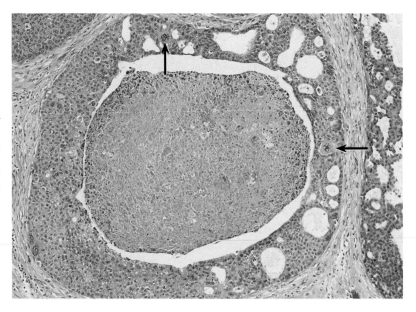

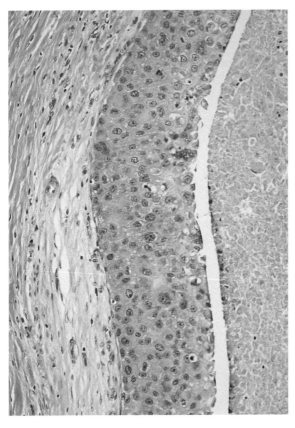

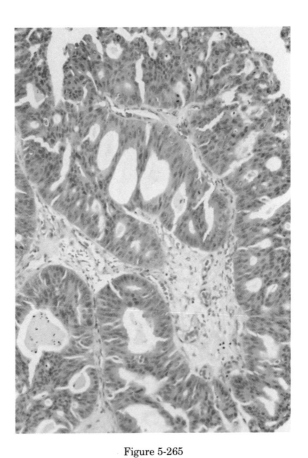

Figure 5-264
SALIVARY DUCT CARCINOMA

A 10- to 12-cell thick, solid layer of neoplastic epithelium lines this cystic tumor nodule. Comedo-type necrotic material fills the luminal space.

Figure 5-265
SALIVARY DUCT CARCINOMA

Numerous microcysts within the epithelium that lines a large cystic structure produce a cribriform configuration.

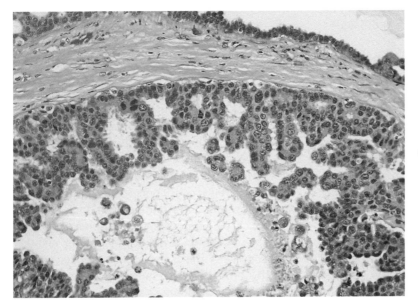

Figure 5-266
SALIVARY DUCT CARCINOMA

Small papillary projections of ductal epithelium line a cystic nodule of tumor.

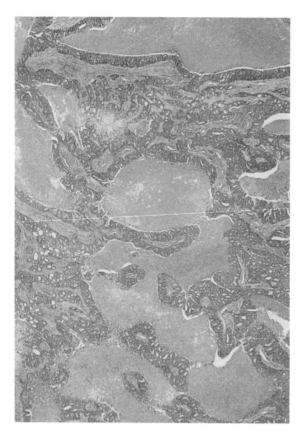

Figure 5-267
SALIVARY DUCT CARCINOMA
At lower magnification than that of figure 5-266, multiple large, irregularly shaped cystic tumor nodules with a papillary-cystic conformation are seen.

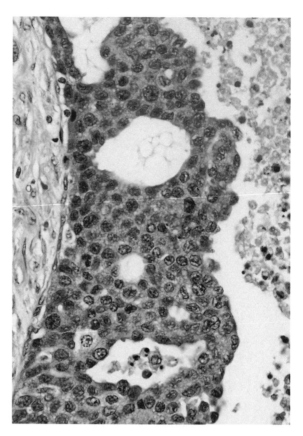

Figure 5-268
SALIVARY DUCT CARCINOMA
The epithelial tumor cells that line this cystic nodule of tumor form arches over microcystic spaces, creating a pattern that has been likened to a "Roman bridge." The eosinophilic tumor cells are fairly uniform in this field.

lymphoplasmacytic infiltrate is usually present within the fibrous tissue and is often quite dense in focal areas (fig. 5-261).

Consistent with the macroscopic features, salivary duct carcinomas are microscopically unencapsulated and infiltrate salivary gland lobules and periglandular tissues such as fat, skeletal muscle, and dermis.

The cuboidal and polygonal epithelial tumor cells have moderately abundant eosinophilic cytoplasm, and the nuclei are typically round to oval but are occasionally slightly irregular (fig. 5-272). Some nuclei contain a single nucleolus, but this is an inconsistent finding. Some investigators have ascribed apocrine-like features to cyst-lining cells that have apical globules of eosinophilic cytoplasm and are arranged in small papillary projections (fig. 5-273) (675,682,683,686). Cytologic pleomor-

phism varies from slight to marked, even within different areas of the same neoplasm. Likewise, the number of mitotic figures is quite variable but is as high as one per high-power field in some tumors (figs. 5-261, 5-274).

Rounded tumor nodules were described above as intraductal-like, which infers that these foci do not represent actual in situ neoplasia of salivary gland ducts. Other investigators have interpreted these structures to be true intraductal neoplasia as occurs in intraductal carcinoma of the breast (667,668,678). Their observation of foci of transition from normal-appearing ductal epithelium to carcinomatous epithelium lends support to this view. While some of the smaller nodules may represent in situ ductal carcinogenesis, most nodules probably are a morphologic variation of infiltrating carcinoma. Factors that favor this

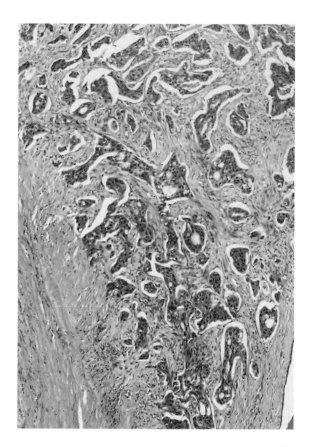
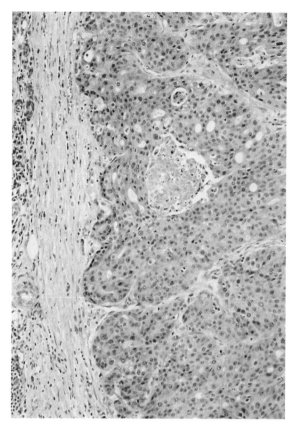

Figure 5-269
SALIVARY DUCT CARCINOMA

Left: Small nests and cords of carcinomatous ductal epithelium within a fibrous tissue stroma are histologically similar to infiltrating ductal carcinoma of the breast.

Right: The neoplastic ductal epithelium has a cribriform pattern and is more densely aggregated as irregular nests than those on the left. A small focus of necrosis is present in the center of one nest.

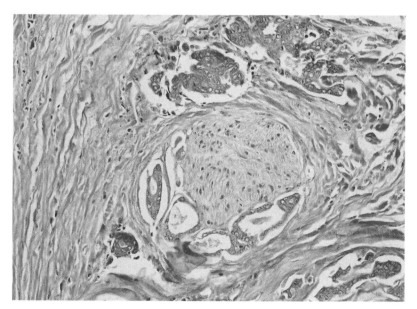

Figure 5-270
SALIVARY DUCT CARCINOMA
Several small neoplastic ductal structures have infiltrated a perineural space.

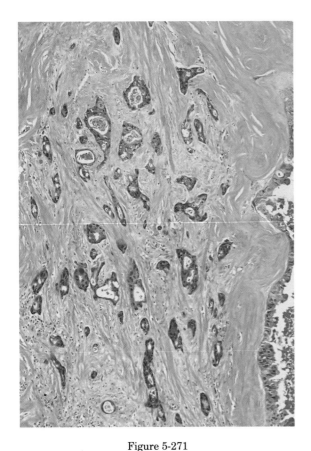

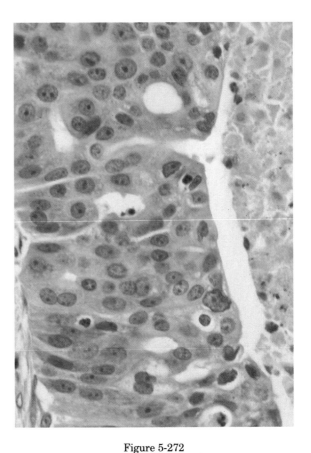

Figure 5-271
SALIVARY DUCT CARCINOMA
Dense, hyalinized fibrous stroma gives a scirrhous appearance to this focus of salivary duct carcinoma.

Figure 5-272
SALIVARY DUCT CARCINOMA
Eosinophilic cytoplasm and uniform, round, lightly stained nuclei characterize the neoplastic ductal epithelium in this field. Most nuclei in this field have small, basophilic nucleoli, but this is an inconsistent finding.

Figure 5-273
SALIVARY DUCT CARCINOMA
The epithelial cells are arranged in small papillary projections and are uniform, with eosinophilic cytoplasm and round nuclei. Comedonecrosis is present at the top of the illustration.

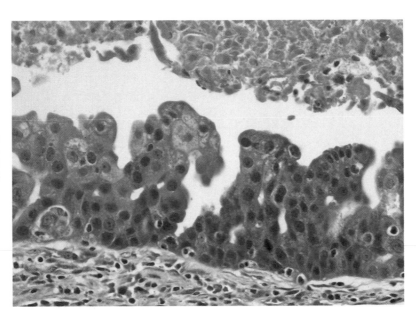

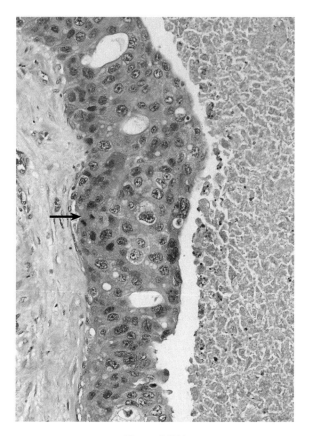

Figure 5-274
SALIVARY DUCT CARCINOMA
Some nuclei of the neoplastic ductal cells in this field are vesicular and variable in size and shape, and several have prominent nucleoli. A mitotic figure (arrow) is evident.

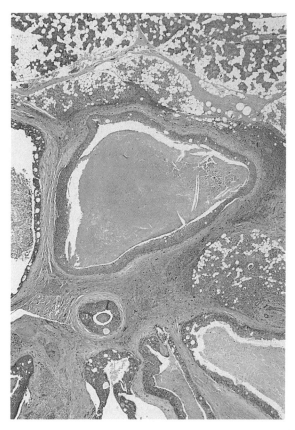

Figure 5-275
SALIVARY DUCT CARCINOMA
This cystic tumor nodule is as large or larger than some normal parotid gland lobules, which are present on the top and right center of the field.

interpretation are: 1) large size and irregular shape of some of the cystic nodules, which may be 15 to 20 times larger than normal interlobular ducts and 50 times larger than intralobular ducts (fig. 5-275); 2) marked fibrosis and absence of non-neoplastic glandular parenchyma that surrounds even small tumor nodules; 3) occurrence of intraductal-like patterns in metastatic foci (678); and 4) poor prognosis of salivary duct carcinoma compared to the good prognosis of intraductal carcinoma of the breast.

Histochemical studies provide little useful information. Mucicarmine and Alcian blue stains sometimes demonstrate some luminal or interstitial reactivity, but the tumor cells are generally unreactive, although Simpson et al. (691) and Hui et al. (683) reported occasional intracellular mucin. Phosphotungstic acid–hematoxylin stain is unreactive but helps rule out oncocytic differ-

entiation. Immunohistochemically, the tumor cells are reactive for epithelial antigens such as cytokeratin, epithelial membrane antigen, and carcinoembryonic antigen (671,672,678,686, 691). Many investigators have found the tumors to be unreactive for S-100 protein, myosin, and smooth muscle actin (672,678,686,691), but Brandwein et al. (671) reported that all nine tumors they examined were reactive for S-100 protein. Most salivary duct carcinomas are immunoreactive with one or more antibodies raised against breast carcinoma (671,678), but unreactive for estrogen receptor (678) and prostatic carcinoma markers (691).

Ultrastructurally, salivary duct carcinomas have features of ductal cells with basal lamina, luminal cells with microvilli, desmosomes, tight junctions, a rough endoplasmic reticulum, a moderate number of mitochondria, and some glycogen (676,678,683). Delgado et al. (678) described occasional basally located, non-neoplastic myoepithelial cells. It is uncertain how they were able to distinguish neoplastic from non-neoplastic cells on the basis of ultrastructural features. Hui et al. (683) found no evidence of myoepithelial cells.

Differential Diagnosis. Although the "intraductal" appearance is characteristic of salivary duct carcinoma, tumors with eosinophilic cells or cystic, papillary, or cribriform morphologic growth patterns are considered in the differential diagnosis and include oncocytic carcinoma, mucoepidermoid carcinoma, acinic cell adenocarcinoma, cystadenocarcinoma, adenoid cystic carcinoma, and polymorphous low-grade adenocarcinoma.

Electron microscopy readily identifies the mitochondria-rich cells of oncocytic carcinoma, but at the light microscopic level phosphotungstic acid–hematoxylin stain helps distinguish oncocytic cells from other eosinophilic cells in salivary gland neoplasms. In addition, the oncocytes in oncocytic carcinomas are usually larger and have more abundant granular eosinophilic cytoplasm than the cells in salivary duct carcinomas. Oncocytic carcinoma typically lacks comedonecrosis and papillary, cystic, and cribriform growth patterns.

Mucocytes that are demonstrable with mucicarmine stain, epidermoid cells, and an absence of papillary-cystic and cribriform growth patterns discriminates high-grade mucoepidermoid carcinoma from salivary duct carcinoma.

Acinic cell adenocarcinomas contain acinar cells, which react with periodic acid–Schiff stain after tissue digestion with diastase, as well as vacuolated and clear cells that are not components of the essentially isocellular salivary duct carcinomas. In addition to an absence of comedonecrosis, acinic cell adenocarcinomas generally have fewer mitotic figures and less cytologic pleomorphism than salivary duct carcinomas.

Similar to salivary duct carcinoma, cystadenocarcinomas have a papillary and cystic microscopic architecture. Unlike salivary duct carcinoma, however, cystadenocarcinomas lack comedonecrosis, only rarely have a cribriform growth pattern, lack cytologic pleomorphism, and often have a population of columnar cells, some of which are mucinous.

A cribriform growth pattern is characteristic of adenoid cystic carcinoma. Dissimilar to salivary duct carcinoma, the cribriform type of adenoid cystic carcinoma is not cystic, lacks comedonecrosis, and has pseudolumens that contain a basophilic or eosinophilic hyalinized product. Also, the tumor cells are less eosinophilic and have more irregular, angular-shaped nuclei than those of salivary duct carcinoma.

Polymorphous low-grade adenocarcinoma is primarily a tumor that involves intraoral minor salivary glands while salivary duct carcinoma occurs principally in the parotid gland. There are few, if any, mitotic figures and no comedonecrosis and cytologic pleomorphism. This tumor often manifests several morphologic patterns, even within the same neoplasm, unlike the rather uniform morphology of salivary duct carcinomas.

Prognosis and Treatment. Salivary duct carcinoma is one of the most aggressive types of salivary gland carcinoma and is characterized by local invasion, lymphatic and hematogenous metastasis, and poor prognosis. Given the poor prognosis of this tumor, Garland et al. (682) comment that it is immaterial whether the epithelium is confined within preexisting ducts or is a larger circumscribed nest of tumor no longer within a duct. The concern is that a term like "intraductal carcinoma" suggests a less aggressive biologic course and a need for less aggressive therapy than is warranted.

Reported survival rates for salivary duct carcinoma have ranged from 100 percent to 17 percent, but an overall assessment of reported cases shows that about 60 percent of patients die of their tumors and another 16 percent are alive with tumor at the time of their last follow-up (668,670,672,675, 678,686,691). While survival has been as long as 12 years after diagnosis, most patients die within 5 years and many within 3 years. Over 40 percent of patients have regional lymph node metastases, and a similar number of patients have distant metastases to lung, bone, liver, spleen, adrenal gland, kidney, and brain. Hui et al. (683) and Brandwein et al. (671) found a correlation between prognosis and tumor size (less than 3.0 cm indicated a better prognosis). In addition, Delgado et al. (678) suggested that gross circumscription of the tumor, a higher proportion of "intraductal" than "extraductal" growth (unclear distinction), and absence of comedonecrosis indicated a more favorable prognosis. On the other hand, Colmenero Ruiz et al. (675) found no relationship between prognosis and size of tumor or tumor free surgical margins. Hui et al. (683) studied two salivary duct carcinomas with flow cytometry and found both to be aneuploid with high proliferative activity.

The poor prognosis and aggressiveness of salivary duct carcinomas dictates aggressive therapy. This includes combination therapy of wide surgical excision, radical neck dissection, and radiation. Colmenero Ruiz et al. (675) found that even aggressive treatment did not ensure cure even for small tumors, but all patients that were still alive had received such therapy.

SEBACEOUS ADENOCARCINOMA AND SEBACEOUS LYMPHADENOCARCINOMA

Sebaceous Adenocarcinoma

Definition. Sebaceous adenocarcinoma is a rare malignant epithelial tumor composed of islands and sheets of cells that have morphologically atypical nuclei, an infiltrative growth pattern, and focal sebaceous differentiation.

General Features. A previous review of this tumor noted that 23 cases had been reported in the literature (695) and there are three cases in the AFIP registry accessioned since 1985. Two cases have been reported to have arisen in minor salivary gland sites. Because sebaceous glands are so common in oral mucosa (Fordyce granules) and are not usually associated with minor salivary glands, origin from minor salivary gland is doubtful. With this caveat in mind, all cases of sebaceous carcinoma of salivary gland origin have occurred in the parotid gland. The age range of affected patients is 17 to 93 years, with an average of 69 years (695). The incidence in men and women is essentially equal. Patients often present with a painless, slow-growing, asymptomatic swelling, but an equal number experience pain and, a few, facial paralysis.

Gross and Microscopic Findings. The tumors range from 0.6 to 8.5 cm in greatest dimension (695). They vary in color from tan-white to yellow. Partial encapsulation and focal circumscription in some areas is typical of these tumors. The neoplastic cells may form numerous islands that coalesce into large, solid sheets (fig. 5-276). The tumor cells also grow as narrow cords and small islands that individually or in groups infil-

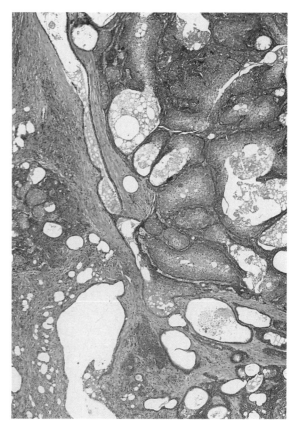

Figure 5-276
SEBACEOUS ADENOCARCINOMA
This tumor has predominantly sheet-like growth with scattered, variably sized cystic spaces.

trate adjacent connective tissue and salivary gland parenchyma (fig. 5-277). Well-formed ductal structures are often numerous and occasionally become cystic. Most tumor cells are characterized as either basaloid, squamous, or sebaceous. Rarely, small groups of mucous cells are seen. The degree of sebaceous differentiation is variable. In some tumors, large islands of sebaceous cells develop that are associated with equal proportions of basaloid or squamous cells (fig. 5-278). In other cases, individual or small clusters of sebaceous cells are so few that they could easily be overlooked.

The basaloid and squamous cells demonstrate atypical cytomorphology. Their nuclei are large, hyperchromatic, and moderately to severely pleomorphic (fig. 5-279). Nucleoli are prominent and often multiple, and mitoses frequent in some

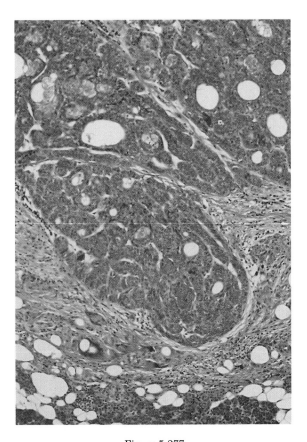

Figure 5-277
SEBACEOUS ADENOCARCINOMA
Irregular cords, islands, and neoplastic ducts extend into fibrous and parenchymal tissue.

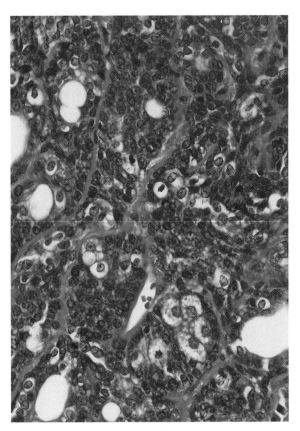

Figure 5-278
SEBACEOUS ADENOCARCINOMA
At high magnification it is evident that this focus is comprised of approximately equal proportions of basaloid and sebaceous cells. Ductal structures are evident. In other areas of this tumor sebaceous differentiation was much more limited.

tumors. The cytoplasm is usually poorly delineated in these cells. Cellular necrosis is present in some cases. Perineural invasion occurs in 20 percent of cases (695). The cells that line the ductal structures or small cysts are usually cuboidal to low columnar, have abundant eosinophilic cytoplasm, and have nuclei that lack the marked abnormalities of the other cell types.

Treatment and Prognosis. As with other extremely rare neoplasms, limited data precludes meaningful conclusions regarding optimal therapy. Most sebaceous adenocarcinomas are probably intermediate-grade malignancies. In these cases, superficial parotidectomy and possibly postoperative radiotherapy are appropriate if this procedure ensures complete removal. For tumors that have marked cytologic atypia or involve the facial nerve, radical parotidectomy and

elective neck dissection should be considered. Chemotherapy has been used with uncertain efficacy (695,696). Tumor recurs in about one third of the cases (696,697). Of 19 patients with parotid tumors treated with various but generally aggressive modalities, and in which follow-up information is available, 5 died as a result of their tumor, all within 5 years of diagnosis; 2 are alive with disease; 1 died of unrelated causes with no evidence of disease more than 5 years after diagnosis; and 11 are free of disease. Metastases to both regional and distant sites may occur.

Sebaceous Lymphadenocarcinoma

Definition. Sebaceous lymphadenocarcinoma is an extremely rare malignant tumor that represents carcinomatous transformation of sebaceous lymphadenoma. The carcinomatous

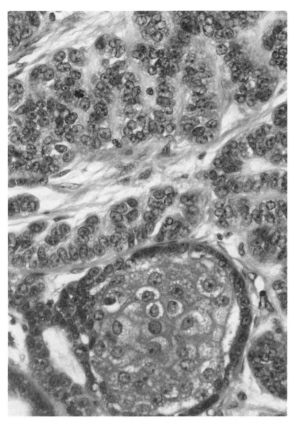

Figure 5-279
SEBACEOUS ADENOCARCINOMA

The nuclear abnormalities and frequent mitoses attest to the malignant nature of this tumor. A large island of sebaceous cells is surrounded by smaller but hyperchromatic cuboidal cells.

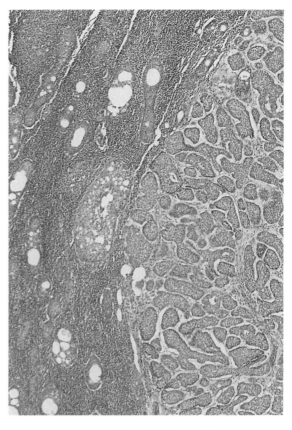

Figure 5-280
SEBACEOUS LYMPHADENOCARCINOMA

The left half of this illustration reveals sebaceous lymphadenoma except for the single, pale-staining island of carcinoma in the center. Separation from the carcinoma to the right is sharply outlined by the lymphoid element.

element may be sebaceous carcinoma or some other specific or nonspecific form of salivary gland carcinoma.

General Features. Only three cases have been reported (696,698): two occurred in the parotid gland and one in a periparotid lymph node. All patients were in their seventh decade of life. There were two men and one woman. The masses were present for 20 years, 2.5 years, and 1 month before diagnosis. Two patients were asymptomatic, but one had pain on palpation and during movement of the head.

Gross and Microscopic Findings. The tumors are yellow-tan to gray and partially encapsulated but locally invasive. Areas of typical sebaceous lymphadenoma in which the lymphoid element usually has lymphoid follicles are

present (figs. 5-280, 5-281). These areas are sharply demarcated from the adjacent carcinoma that lacks lymphoid stroma and infiltrates surrounding tissues. The carcinomas consist of sebaceous carcinoma with ductal differentiation or with other forms of salivary carcinoma focally, such as undifferentiated carcinoma, adenoid cystic carcinoma, or epithelial-myoepithelial carcinoma (fig. 5-282) (696,697). Mitotic figures are numerous and atypical.

Treatment and Prognosis. Of the three reported patients, one died of unrelated causes and the other two were free of disease at 6 and 14 years (697,698). Treatment was superficial parotidectomy, "total extirpation," and an unspecified surgical procedure with adjunctive postoperative irradiation.

Figure 5-281
ASSOCIATED SEBACEOUS
LYMPHADENOMA
As in other sebaceous lymph-
adenomas, a complete lack of cyto-
morphologic abnormalities is evident.

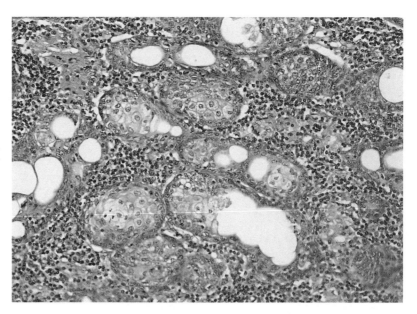

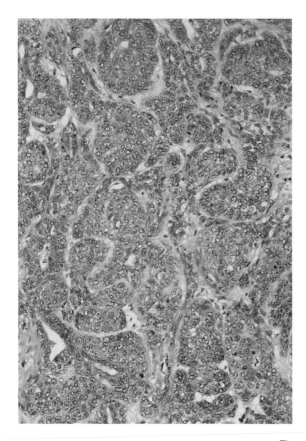
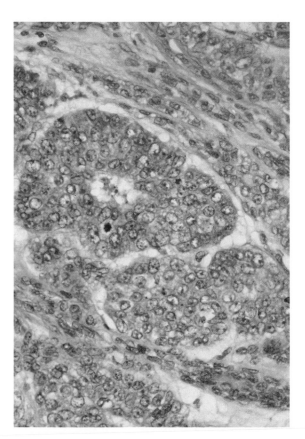

Figure 5-282
SEBACEOUS LYMPHADENOCARCINOMA
Left: Irregular islands and ductal structures in this case represent undifferentiated carcinoma.
Right: The infiltrative growth and abnormal nuclear features contrast with those in the sebaceous lymphadenoma.

MYOEPITHELIAL CARCINOMA

Definition. Myoepithelial carcinomas are rare, malignant salivary gland neoplasms in which the tumor cells almost exclusively manifest myoepithelial differentiation. These neoplasms represent the malignant counterpart of benign myoepithelioma. Myoepithelial carcinoma (malignant myoepithelioma) is one of several new entities added to the updated classification of salivary gland tumors by the WHO in 1991 (719).

Two requirements need to be fulfilled to establish a diagnosis of myoepithelial carcinoma: the neoplastic cells must be characterized as myoepithelial, and the tumor must be identified as malignant. Although these requirements seem obvious, they are often difficult to assess. Although myoepithelial differentiation is common in many different types of salivary gland neoplasm, both myoepitheliomas and myoepithelial carcinomas are uncommon neoplasms. It is perhaps the fact that myoepithelial differentiation manifests in many different neoplasms that makes it difficult to identify purely myoepithelial neoplasms. The problems associated with defining neoplastic myoepithelial cells and myoepithelioma are equally applicable to myoepithelial carcinoma (see Myoepithelioma). Most investigators use a combination of morphologic, ultrastructural, and immunohistochemical criteria to ascribe myoepithelial differentiation to these tumors, while cytologic abnormalities and infiltrative growth are the histopathologic features that are used to impute malignant potential (see Pathologic Findings).

General Features. Myoepithelial carcinomas are rare neoplasms of salivary glands. About 35 cases have been reported in the English language literature (700–703,708,710,712,713,717,720–724,726,727), but some of these provide very limited clinical data or histopathologic illustrations or descriptions (710,720,722,726). The largest series is 10 cases reported by Di Palma and Guzzo (708). Eight cases have been added to the AFIP files over the past decade, which constitutes only about 0.2 percent of all epithelial neoplasms of salivary glands accessioned during this period. This neoplasm has not been distinguished in most general surveys of salivary gland neoplasia or carcinoma, but Spiro et al. (722) classified 1 neoplasm among 204 adenocarcinomas of salivary gland as malignant myoepithelioma. No details were reported. Sheldon (720) may have been the first to classify tumors as myoepitheliomas when he categorized 3 tumors as such in a review of 54 mixed tumors of salivary gland in 1943. On the basis of mitotic figures and pleomorphism he considered 1 of the 3 tumors to be cancerous. In a survey of reported cases of myoepithelioma until 1985, Barnes et al. (699) found 3 malignant myoepitheliomas among 42 myoepitheliomas. Sciubba and Brannon (718) did not ascribe malignancy to any of the 23 myoepitheliomas they reported. Tortoledo et al. (726) reported that the carcinomatous component in 3 of 37 carcinomas ex mixed tumor in their study was myoepithelial carcinoma. No specific demographic data was given for these three patients, but two patients died as a consequence of their neoplasms. The AFIP and others (708,709,721) have also observed myoepithelial carcinoma as the malignant element in carcinoma ex mixed tumor. Saxe et al. (717) described a 15-year-old girl who developed myoepithelial carcinoma in the right parotid gland 14 years after being treated with radiation for retinoblastoma of her right eye. The patient died with disseminated myoepithelial carcinoma a year after diagnosis.

Among a group of 35 cases from the literature (700–703,708,712,713,717,720,721,723,724,727) and the AFIP in which demographic information could be ascertained, the parotid gland was the primary site of occurrence in 23 cases (66 percent), the minor salivary glands in 9 cases (26 percent), and the submandibular gland in 3 cases (9 percent). Similar to benign myoepitheliomas, the palate was the most common intraoral site of involvement. Patients ranged in age from 14 to 86 years, and the mean age was 51 years. No significant sex predilection was evident: 19 patients were men and 15 were women (1 unknown).

Clinical Features. Other than descriptions of asymptomatic masses, very little information on the clinical signs and symptoms associated with myoepithelial carcinoma has been reported. The duration of the primary tumor before initial treatment has ranged from 1 month to 15 years (708). Hoarseness, dysphagia, and weight loss were associated with a laryngeal myoepithelial carcinoma (713). Similar to many other cases of carcinoma ex mixed tumor, the patient with myoepithelial carcinoma ex mixed tumor

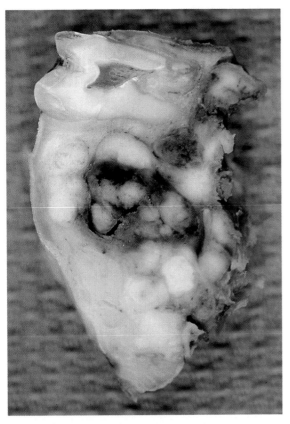

Figure 5-283
MYOEPITHELIAL CARCINOMA
A section of the palate and maxilla, which includes a second molar tooth, shows infiltration by multinodular tumor tissue with focal necrosis and cystic degeneration.

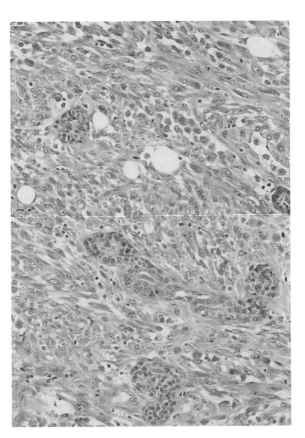

Figure 5-284
MYOEPITHELIAL CARCINOMA
Foci of glandular structures represent residual normal ducts within a lobule of parotid gland tissue that has been infiltrated by spindled and plasmacytoid neoplastic myoepithelial cells.

reported by Singh and Cawson (721) experienced a sudden rapid increase in size of a parotid gland mass that had been present for 15 years. Skin ulceration occurred with the 20-cm parotid tumor reported by Crissman et al. (702). Radiographic evidence of bone destruction has been associated with some intraoral neoplasms.

Pathologic Findings. Myoepithelial carcinomas range from 2 to 20 cm in largest dimension. Macroscopically, they are usually unencapsulated, and the cut surfaces are gray-white, sometimes with areas of necrosis or cystic degeneration (fig. 5-283). Microscopically, myoepithelial carcinoma is distinguished from benign myoepithelioma on the basis of cytologic abnormalities, infiltrative growth, or both.

The neoplastic cell population in myoepithelial carcinoma should nearly exclusively manifest myoepithelial differentiation. Although ductal and acinar differentiation are generally absent, a rare ductal structure is acceptable (figs. 5-284, 5-285). Squamous differentiation is one of the manifestations of neoplastic myoepithelial cells and is acceptable as a minor component in myoepithelial carcinoma. Of course, in myoepithelial carcinomas that develop in benign mixed tumors (carcinomas ex mixed tumor), the benign mixed tumor portion of the neoplasm manifests ductal differentiation. The cellular configurations in myoepithelial carcinomas are the same as those in benign myoepitheliomas and include spindle, plasmacytoid, clear, and epithelioid types (figs. 5-284–5-286) (see Myoepithelioma and Mixed Tumor). Although Franquemont and Mills (711) have argued that the plasmacytoid cell does not demonstrate myoepithelial differentiation, others (704,706) dispute this, and most investigators accept plasmacytoid morphology as one of

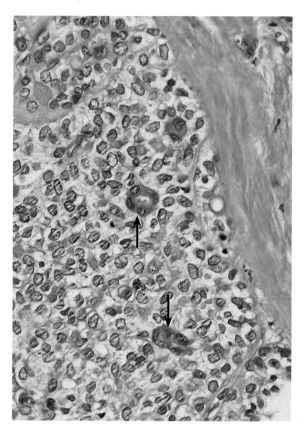

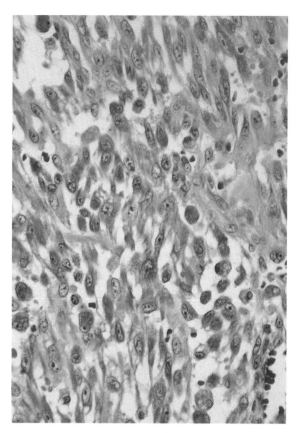

Figure 5-285
MYOEPITHELIAL CARCINOMA
These two small ducts (arrows) represented the only foci of ductal differentiation within a large, infiltrative parotid tumor mass that was composed of epithelioid and clear myoepithelial cells. This focus was considered insufficient to reject a diagnosis of myoepithelial carcinoma in favor of epithelial-myoepithelial carcinoma.

Figure 5-286
MYOEPITHELIAL CARCINOMA
High magnification shows elongated, spindled, and round cells with eosinophilic cytoplasm. The cells demonstrate a lack of cohesion, and many have vesicular nuclei with prominent nucleoli.

the variants of neoplastic myoepithelial cells. The spindle cell type is the most common and most easily recognized as myoepithelial with light microscopy, but many myoepithelial carcinomas manifest more than one type of cell morphology. Cellular and nuclear pleomorphism vary from slight to severe (figs. 5-285, 5-287). Marked pleomorphism, high number of mitotic figures, and necrosis indicate malignancy in the few myoepithelial carcinomas that do not manifest invasive growth. On the other hand, some infiltrative, destructive myoepithelial carcinomas that resulted in patient death have had only slight cellular atypia, a low mitotic figure count (2 or less per 10 high-power fields), and absence of necrosis.

The cellular density varies from moderate to high. Highly cellular carcinomas generally ap-

pear to have little intercellular stroma, but fibrous tissue is often present at the periphery of the infiltrative nodules of tumor. Less cellular tumors frequently have mucoid or myxoid stroma, but cartilaginous tissue, like that in the myoepithelial regions of mixed tumors, is usually not present (fig. 5-288). As already alluded to, invasive growth is an important diagnostic feature that distinguishes malignant from benign myoepithelial neoplasms, and it has characterized most myoepithelial carcinomas, even in the absence of severe cytologic abnormalities (fig. 5-289).

Immunohistochemical Findings. Neoplastic myoepithelial cells have expressed reactivity with antibodies to cytokeratin, S-100 protein, smooth muscle actin, muscle-specific actin, vimentin, and glial fibrillary acidic protein

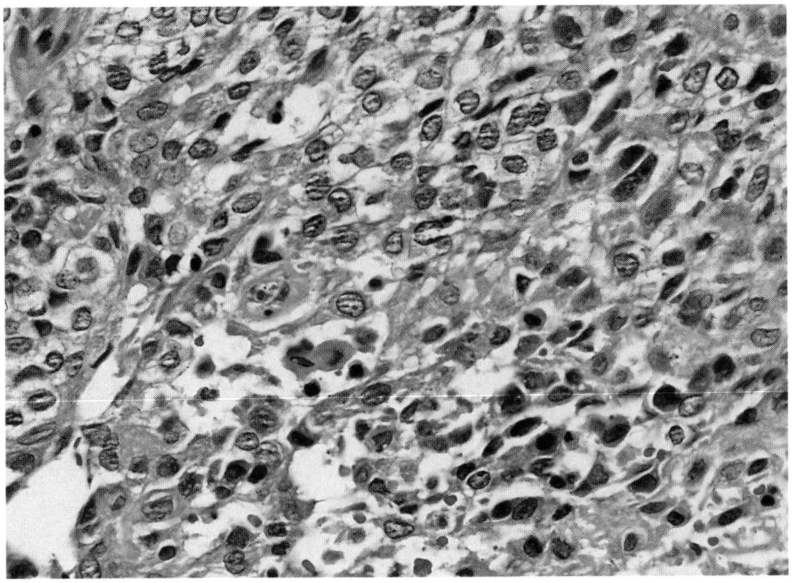

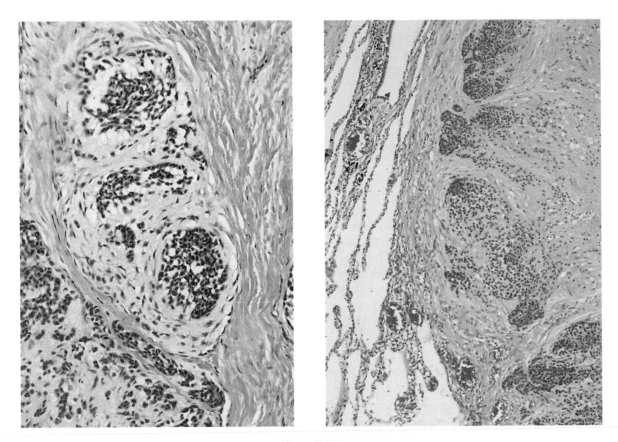

Figure 5-287
MYOEPITHELIAL CARCINOMA
Cellular and nuclear pleomorphism, nuclear hyperchromatism, and focal cell necrosis are evident in these epithelioid myoepithelial cells.

Figure 5-288
MYOEPITHELIAL CARCINOMA
Pale-staining mucoid material surrounds small nodules and individual cells of this myoepithelial carcinoma of the submandibular gland (left) that recurred twice and metastasized to the lung 4 years after the initial excision (right).

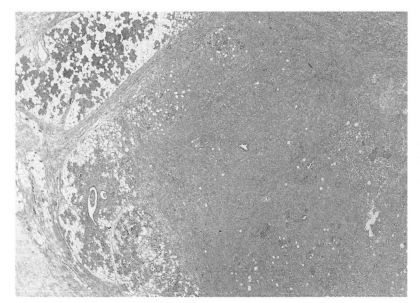

Figure 5-289
MYOEPITHELIAL CARCINOMA
Low magnification of the spindled type myoepithelial carcinoma seen in figure 5-284. The tumor is unencapsulated and has infiltrated adjacent parotid gland parenchyma.

(GFAP) (fig. 5-290) (716). Reactivity for S-100 protein has been considered by some investigators as diagnostic of myoepithelial differentiation in the context of salivary gland neoplasms (715). While nearly all myoepithelial carcinomas are immunoreactive for S-100 protein, this protein immunoreactivity can be detected in neoplastic and non-neoplastic duct cells as well, and by itself is not pathognomonic of myoepithelial differentiation; combinations of antigen reactivity from the immunohistochemical profile listed above are more specific (704,707,708,712,717,721,724). Reactivity for actin is not requisite for myoepithelial differentiation (704,705,708,714), and reactivity for carcinoembryonic antigen and epithelial membrane antigen has been negative (713,724).

Each of the 10 myoepithelial carcinomas reported by Di Palma and Guzzo (708) were reactive for S-100 protein, high or low molecular weight cytokeratin, and vimentin. Anti-actin and anti-GFAP reacted focally with 4 tumors each. Others have reported negative reactions for cytokeratin but positive reactions for S-100 protein, vimentin, and actin (703,721,724).

Ultrastructural Findings. Longitudinally oriented 6- to 8-nm fine filaments with focal dense bodies, pinocytotic vesicles, desmosomes, and basal lamina are features of myoepithelial differentiated cells. In neoplastic myoepithelial cells, including those in myoepithelial carcinomas, the fine filaments inconsistently manifest

as characteristic parallel arrays with focal dense bodies (699,702,703,705,712,721,723–725). Spindle-shaped cells are more likely to demonstrate parallel microfilaments than plasmacytoid or epithelioid myoepithelial cells. Aggregates of fine filaments without dense bodies, occasional desmosomes, and basal lamina, however, seem to be minimal features of modified myoepithelial cells (702,703,705,712,721,723,724). Intermediate filaments are prominent in some cells (703). Dardick et al. (705) found no correlation between the cytoplasmic accumulation of fine filaments and immunoreactivity for actin. Glycogen is sometimes conspicuous (702,713,723).

Differential Diagnosis. Spindled and often loosely cohesive tumor cells and absence of glandular features often give myoepithelial carcinoma a sarcomatous appearance. Leiomyosarcoma, fibrosarcoma, malignant schwannoma, synovial sarcoma, and malignant fibrous histiocytoma are considered in the differential diagnosis. The immunohistochemical profile of neoplastic myoepithelial cells given above is often helpful for distinguishing myoepithelial from mesenchymal differentiation. Leiomyosarcoma and fibrosarcoma do not demonstrate immunoreactivity for S-100 protein, cytokeratin, and GFAP. Although cytokeratin reactivity has been present in rare malignant fibrous histiocytomas, cytokeratin, S-100 protein, and GFAP reactivities favor myoepithelial carcinoma. Malignant

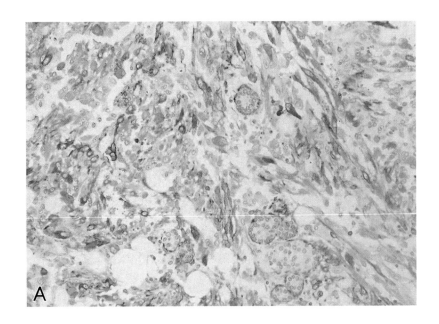

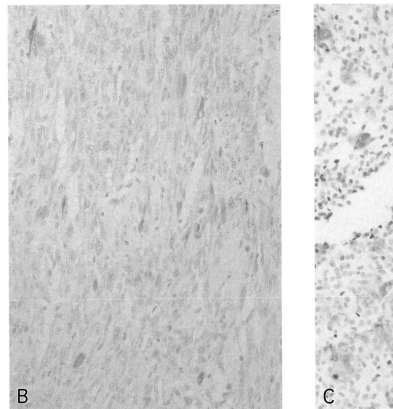

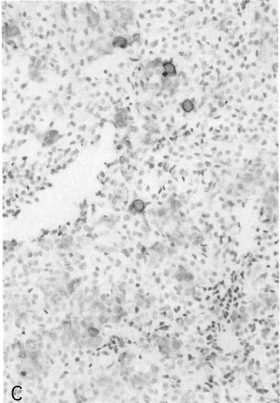

Figure 5-290

MYOEPITHELIAL CARCINOMA: IMMUNOHISTOCHEMISTRY

This spindled type myoepithelial carcinoma demonstrates strong reactivity for smooth muscle actin (A) and scattered, focal reactivity for S-100 protein (B). Scattered rounded cells in a myoepithelial carcinoma are reactive with a cocktail of monoclonal antibodies for low and high molecular weight keratins (C). (Avidin-biotin peroxidase stain)

schwannomas and synovial sarcoma may be the most difficult sarcomas to rule out on the basis of immunohistochemistry. GFAP and S-100 protein reactivity indicate myoepithelial carcinoma rather than synovial sarcoma. Paradoxically, the glandular-like structures of synovial sarcoma are not present in myoepithelial carcinoma, and myoepithelial carcinoma usually lacks the densely cellular intersecting fascicles of monophasic synovial sarcoma. Malignant schwannomas usually lack cytokeratin and smooth muscle actin reactivities and ultrastructurally demonstrate complex interdigitation and entanglement of cytoplasmic processes. Evidence of ductal differentiation in conjunction with a sarcomatous component indicates that carcinosarcoma (true malignant mixed tumor) is a preferable diagnosis.

Metastatic amelanotic malignant melanomas are unreactive for cytokeratin, smooth muscle actin, and GFAP while myoepithelial carcinomas are unreactive for the HMB45 antigen. Characteristic ultrastructural melanosomes are absent in myoepithelial carcinoma.

Prognosis and Treatment. In the one AFIP case and the 20 reported cases of myoepithelial carcinoma with follow-up information, 6 patients (29 percent) died as a result of their disease, 1 patient died of unrelated causes, 7 patients (33 percent) were living with disease at last follow-up, and 7 patients (33 percent) were free of disease (701–703,708,713,717,721,723,724). The follow-up interval ranged from a few weeks to 43 years. The interval to death ranged from 3 months to 35 years. Two thirds of tumors recurred, often multiple times, and 7 patients developed distant metastases, which were most often to lung but also involved liver, vertebra, and inguinal lymph node. Two patients with pulmonary metastasis were living with disease, but their follow-up had not extended beyond discovery of the metastases. The high incidence of patients who died or were living with disease indicate that myoepithelial carcinoma should be considered an intermediate- to high-grade carcinoma. Di Palma and Guzzo (708) considered malignant myoepithelioma to be low grade when it arose in a mixed tumor (pleomorphic adenoma) and high grade when it arose de novo, but Tortoledo et al. (726) reported that two of three patients with myoepithelial carcinoma ex mixed tumor died of their disease. Carrillo et al. (701) found no correlation between the average number

of silver stained nucleolar organizer regions (AgNORs) per cell and the clinical outcome. In an earlier study on similar or identical cases, el-Naggar et al. (710) found that a high S-phase fraction as determined by flow cytometric studies appeared to be a better indicator of aggressiveness than DNA content (aneuploidy).

Total parotidectomy, submandibular glandectomy, or wide excision of minor salivary gland tumors is recommended. Seven of the eight parotid tumors reported by Di Palma and Guzzo (708) were initially treated with resections or partial parotidectomies and had to be retreated with total parotidectomies after recurrences. Carrillo et al. (701) noted that increased morbidity was associated with tumor involvement of surgical margins. Chemotherapy was unsuccessful in controlling extensive disease in two cases (713,717) but may have been helpful in another (710). The limited experience with radiation therapy has had mixed results but for the most part has not been encouraging (702,709,713,723,724).

ADENOSQUAMOUS CARCINOMA

Definition. Adenosquamous carcinoma is a rare malignant neoplasm that simultaneously arises from mucosal surface epithelium and salivary gland ductal epithelium and manifests histopathologic features of both squamous cell carcinoma and adenocarcinoma.

Adenosquamous carcinoma is not listed in the updated classification of salivary gland tumors of the WHO (738) but is mentioned in the discussion of "other carcinomas." The term adenosquamous carcinoma is used to categorize certain epithelial malignancies in many tissues throughout the body, including intestine, cervix, vagina, esophagus, nose, larynx, skin, lung, gallbladder, ovary, liver, prostate, stomach, kidney, uterus, urethra, fallopian tube, pancreas, and thyroid gland (730). For many of these sites the term simply defines carcinomas that demonstrate stratified squamous and adenomatous differentiation. In the context of salivary gland neoplasia, however, that definition is insufficient to segregate adenosquamous carcinoma from other tumor categories without further elaboration since several types of benign and malignant neoplasms manifest both ductal and squamous differentiation, including mixed tumors, Warthin tumors, basal cell adenomas, papillomas, basal cell adenocarcinomas, and, especially, mucoepidermoid carcinomas. It is the carcinomatous changes in the mucosal surface epithelium, combined with distinct adenocarcinomatous areas, that characterize adenosquamous carcinoma of the upper aerodigestive tract (see differential diagnosis section below). Adenocarcinomas with foci of squamous differentiation should not be classified as adenosquamous carcinoma. The recently described basaloid squamous carcinoma of mucosal epithelium resembles adenosquamous carcinoma and is considered in the differential diagnosis.

General Features. Adenosquamous carcinoma is a rare neoplasm of the oral cavity, and there is controversy over whether it is a distinct entity (736). Only a handful of reports have discussed this neoplasm (730–732,736,737,739): Gerughty et al. (732) reported 10 cases in the oral cavity, nasal cavity, and larynx; Siar and Ng (739) reported a tumor in the floor of the mouth; Martinez-Madrigal et al. (736) reported four tumors in the oral cavity and pharynx; and the AFIP has identified eight cases that involved the oral cavity during the past decade. Bombi et al. (729) reported an esophageal adenosquamous carcinoma and reviewed 30 such cases reported in the literature; they pointed out that several of these tumors had been diagnosed as mucoepidermoid carcinoma.

As indicated by the definition, adenosquamous carcinoma is an epithelial neoplasm of the mucosa and minor salivary glands. In the oral cavity, the posterior tongue, tonsillar pillars, and floor of mouth have been the sites of 85 percent of the tumors. Male patients have outnumbered female patients 3 to 1. All of the patients have been over 45 years old, and the peak incidence was in the sixth decade of life.

Clinical Features. Like most other salivary gland tumors adenosquamous carcinomas produce swelling, but unlike most others, adenosquamous carcinomas produce visible changes in the mucosa. These mucosal features vary from erythema to ulceration and induration. Pain frequently accompanies ulceration.

Pathologic Findings. Adenosquamous carcinoma is the manifestation of malignant transformation of both the mucosal surface epithelium and ductal epithelium of the minor salivary glands. It is characterized by squamous cell carcinoma and adenocarcinoma. The epidermoid and ductal elements intermix, but squamous cell carcinoma usually comprises most of the superficial portion of the tumor while adenocarcinoma is located in the deeper portion (fig. 5-291). The squamous carcinoma component is usually moderately well to poorly differentiated. Moderately well-differentiated tumors display intercellular bridges, keratinization, and cellular and nuclear pleomorphism while poorly differentiated tumors have a more basaloid appearance, more mitotic figures, and sparse keratinization (fig. 5-292). The adenomatous component is typically a simple ductal adenocarcinoma without features that identify it as any other specific type of salivary gland adenocarcinoma, such as adenoid cystic carcinoma or acinic cell adenocarcinoma. Ductal and tubular structures are formed by one to several layers of cuboidal or basaloid cells around varying sized lumens. Moderate cellular and nuclear pleomorphism are usually evident (fig. 5-293). Intraluminal mucinous material is sometimes present (fig. 5-294), and intracellular mucin is visible with mucicarmine or Alcian blue stains in some tumors. Mucin production is not required for the diagnosis of adenosquamous carcinoma. Zones of transition from squamous carcinoma to adenocarcinoma are usually evident (figs. 5-291, 5-295).

Carcinomatous changes in the mucosal surface epithelium are an important component of this neoplasm. These changes manifest in the overlying or adjacent mucosa as severe epithelial dysplasia, carcinoma in situ, or invasive squamous cell carcinoma (fig. 5-296). Similar changes are often evident in the superficial portion of salivary gland excretory ducts. Gerughty et al. (732) speculated that the carcinomatous transformation begins in a salivary gland duct and later spreads to the surface mucosal epithelium. The opposite may be more likely. Squamous carcinoma in situ as an isolated phenomenon in salivary gland ducts has not been observed. On the other hand, squamous carcinoma of the mucosa is the most common malignancy in the head and neck, and mucosal carcinomatous transformation associated with squamous metaplasia and dysplasia of contiguous salivary duct epithelium is common. These observations suggest that on rare occasions this dysplastic ductal epithelium transforms to adenocarcinoma.

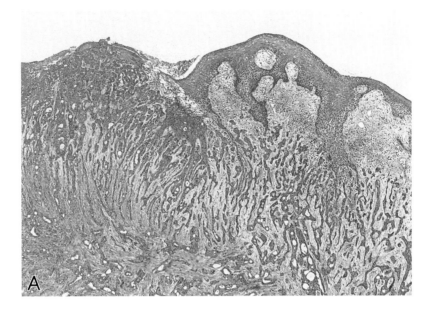

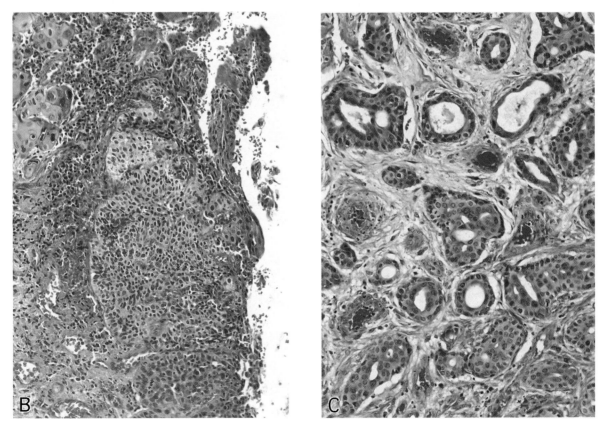

Figure 5-291
ADENOSQUAMOUS CARCINOMA

In A, there is a transition from epidermoid carcinoma in the upper half (toward the mucosal surface) (higher magnification in B) of this field to adenocarcinoma in the lower half (higher magnification in C) in a tumor from the floor of the mouth.

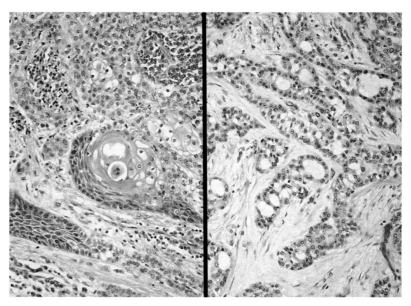

Figure 5-292
ADENOSQUAMOUS CARCINOMA
Left: Foci of moderately differentiated squamous cell carcinoma display keratinization in an adenosquamous carcinoma from the floor of the mouth.

Right: In deeper portions of the same neoplasm glandular differentiation is evident.

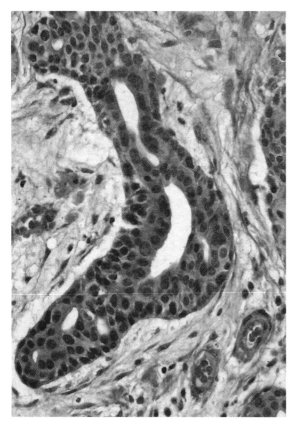

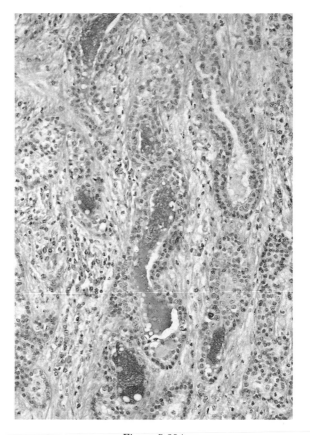

Figure 5-293
ADENOSQUAMOUS CARCINOMA

High magnification of a tubular structure shows ductal cells with moderate nuclear pleomorphism and hyperchromatism.

Figure 5-294
ADENOSQUAMOUS CARCINOMA

PAS stain highlights intraluminal mucin in the adenocarcinomatous portion of an adenosquamous carcinoma from the floor of the mouth.

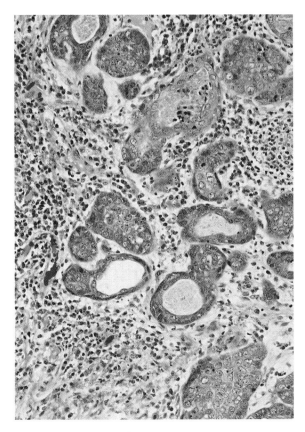

Figure 5-295
ADENOSQUAMOUS CARCINOMA
This section shows a mixture of nests of poorly differentiated squamous carcinoma and ductal structures with intraluminal mucin.

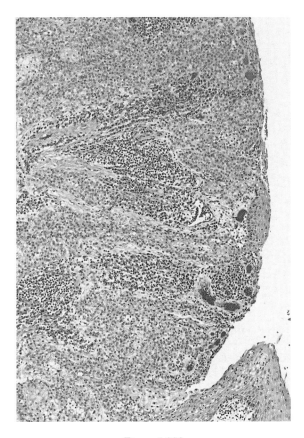

Figure 5-296
ADENOSQUAMOUS CARCINOMA
Infiltrating trabeculae of squamous carcinoma are contiguous with dysplastic mucosal epithelium from the same tumor represented in figures 5-292 and 5-294.

Adenosquamous carcinomas are distinctly infiltrative and invade adjacent tissues, such as salivary gland, muscle, fat, connective tissue, blood vessel, and nerve (fig. 5-297). A fibrous stroma frequently has a lymphocytic inflammatory infiltrate.

Immunohistochemical studies by Martinez-Madrigal et al. (736) showed the epidermoid component of adenosquamous carcinomas to be diffusely reactive for high molecular weight cytokeratin and unreactive or only focally reactive for low molecular weight cytokeratin and carcinoembryonic antigen. The adenocarcinoma portion of the tumor was diffusely reactive for high and low molecular weight cytokeratins and carcinoembryonic antigen.

Differential Diagnosis. Three entities are the principal considerations in the differential diagnosis of adenosquamous carcinoma: mucoepidermoid carcinoma, adenoid (acantholytic) squamous carcinoma, and basaloid squamous carcinoma.

Distinction of adenosquamous carcinoma from mucoepidermoid carcinoma is the most controversial of the differential diagnoses. Hyams et al. (733) considered mucoepidermoid carcinoma and adenosquamous carcinoma of the upper respiratory tract to be equivalent. However, they stated that there is support for considering these tumors to develop from mucosa rather than from mucoserous glands, and they suggested that adenosquamous carcinoma might be the better term because these tumors were histopathologically different from mucoepidermoid carcinoma of salivary glands. In mucoepidermoid carcinoma the glandular and epidermoid components are inseparable. Even when origin from excretory ductal epithelium is obvious, the two components are intimately associated with

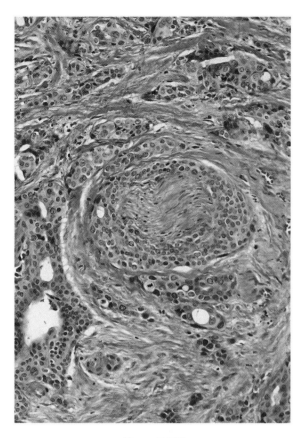

Figure 5-297
ADENOSQUAMOUS CARCINOMA
Perineural invasion is manifest in the carcinoma of the tongue seen in figures 5-291 and 5-293.

one another (see Mucoepidermoid Carcinoma). Glandular features and cyst formation are usually dominant in low-grade mucoepidermoid carcinomas, and solid sheets of epidermoid and other cells are typically prominent in high-grade mucoepidermoid carcinomas. Keratinization is an uncommon feature. Although the mucosa can be ulcerated due to subjacent tumor growth, carcinomatous changes along the mucosal epithelium are not evident. Conversely, much of the neoplastic ductal elements in adenosquamous carcinoma appear to have proliferated independently. Keratinization within the epidermoid component is common, and cytologic features of malignancy are present in the mucosal epithelium.

Adenoid squamous carcinoma of the oral mucosa primarily occurs on the vermilion surface of the lips although rarely it has been reported at other intraoral sites (734). These carcinomas arise from malignant transformation of mucosal epithe-lium. Histologically, pseudoglandular structures are formed within the carcinoma due to acantholysis of cells. No mucin production is evident within the neoplasm, and many of the pseudoglandular spaces contain acantholytic, dyskeratotic epithelial cells. Immunohistochem-ically, the tumor cells are reactive for cytokeratin but are unreactive for carcinoembryonic antigen. The adenocarcinoma component of adenosquam-ous carcinoma does not contain acantholytic cells, often contains sialomucin, occasionally demon-strates intracytoplasmic mucin, and is usually immunoreactive for carcinoembryonic antigen.

Basaloid squamous carcinoma is a recently described variant of squamous cell carcinoma of the upper aerodigestive tract that has features that resemble adenosquamous carcinoma (728, 735,740). Similar to adenosquamous carcinoma, basaloid squamous carcinoma has a predilection for the hypopharynx, base of tongue, and supra-glottic larynx. This tumor is composed of small, hyperchromatic cells that form solid lobules, ad-enomatoid arrangements, and cords. The basaloid cells resemble solid adenoid cystic carci-noma. The tumor aggregates are often associated with eosinophilic hyaline material and comedo-necrosis. Basaloid squamous carcinoma involves the mucosal epithelium in the form of epithelial dysplasia, carcinoma in situ, and invasive squa-mous cell carcinoma, and foci of epidermoid cells also occur in the basaloid lobules (see section on Adenoid Cystic Carcinoma for illustrations of basaloid squamous cell carcinoma). In contrast to adenosquamous carcinoma, the tumor cells are predominantly basaloid, and the duct-like struc-tures are an integral part of the basaloid and epidermoid proliferation and do not occur as a separate adenocarcinomatous component. Immu-nohistochemically, basaloid squamous cell carci-noma is reported to be reactive for carcino-embryonic antigen but reactivity occurs in the epidermoid cells rather than the ductal cells (728).

Prognosis and Treatment. Eighty percent of patients develop regional lymph node metasta-ses, which are often evident at the time of diagnosis of the primary tumors. Only one patient has been followed for more than 5 years (732,736,739). Nev-ertheless, 6 of 15 patients with any follow-up infor-mation died of disease, and 7 other patients were alive with disease following an average follow-up interval of 1.5 years. One patient survived for 15 years before dying of tumor, but the other patients died within 3 years of diagnosis. This limited data indicates that adenosquamous carcinoma is a highly aggressive neoplasm with a poor prognosis. Gerughty et al. (732) recommended radical surgery but found that radiation therapy had little benefit. Still, not enough data are available for conclusions, and multimodality therapy may be appropriate for such an aggressive tumor.

MUCINOUS ADENOCARCINOMA

Definition. Mucinous adenocarcinoma is a rare malignant neoplasm characterized by large amounts of extracellular epithelial mucin that contains cords, nests, and solitary epithelial cells. This tumor is analogous and histologically nearly identical to the mucinous eccrine carcinoma of skin and mucinous carcinoma of breast as defined in the corresponding Fascicles in the third series of the Atlas of Tumor Pathology (751,753); those latter tumors in turn resemble the colloid type of colonic adenocarcinoma (745).

The classification, mucinous adenocarcinoma of salivary glands, is controversial. This category was included in the recent classification of salivary gland tumors by the WHO (754), but the information provided in that monograph was insufficient to adequately define a distinct neoplasm. The WHO monograph refers to epithelial-lined, mucin-filled cysts. The two photomicrographs of mucinous adenocarcinoma in the WHO publication illustrate tumors that would be classified as cystadenocarcinoma in this Fascicle, and are similar to the photomicrographs of cystadenocarcinoma in the WHO monograph as well. There have been a few other attempts to classify a group of salivary gland neoplasms on the basis of abundant mucin formation (741,742,744, 755). Since several different types and architectural patterns of salivary gland neoplasms produce epithelial mucins, most of these reports have described a heterogenous group of neoplasms that today would include variants of mucoepidermoid carcinoma, acinic cell adenocarcinoma, cystadenocarcinoma, and polymorphous low-grade adenocarcinoma, as well as sinonasal carcinomas. To date, no clearly independent prognostic significance has been ascribed to the presence or absence of mucins in salivary gland neoplasms.

General Features. The actual incidence is unknown, but mucinous adenocarcinoma is certainly rare. Few studies have mentioned this entity, and only two reports have adequately described mucinous adenocarcinomas of salivary gland that were analogous to the tumors of skin and breast of the same name (743,752). Kitamura et al. (748) reported a mucinous carcinoma of the external auditory canal that involved the parotid gland and invaded the temporal bone. The authors believed that the tumor in the parotid gland represented metastatic disease. Other reports are less specific. Spiro et al. (755) counted 25 "mucinous (mucin-producing or mucous cell) adenocarcinomas" among 204 adenocarcinomas they studied; however, they stated that there was a "wide histologic structural range and grade of malignancy." Most of the tumors in their study occurred in the nasal cavity or paranasal sinuses. Many probably represented papillary and colonic type adenocarcinomas of nasal and paranasal sinuses as described by Moran et al. (750) and Hyams et al. (747); most adenomatous neoplasms in these sites probably arise from surface mucosal epithelium (746). Main et al. (749) compared salivary gland tumors from Toronto and Edinburgh and listed six mucinous adenocarcinomas in the Toronto group without any histologic description or definition. Blanck et al. (742) reported 47 "mucus-producing adenopapillary (nonepidermoid) carcinomas" of the parotid gland among 1,678 tumors. Their description and illustrations revealed a heterogeneous group of tumors. They noted that many were very similar to mucoepidermoid carcinoma except for lack of epidermoid cells.

Five mucinous adenocarcinomas of salivary glands have been reviewed at the AFIP during the last decade. In conjunction with the information provided in the report by Osaki et al. (752), two tumors occurred in the parotid gland and four occurred in the submandibular gland. The patients, two women, three men, and one of unknown sex, ranged in age from 41 to 83 years. The tumor reported by Osaki et al. (752) and one in the AFIP files, both submandibular tumors, were associated with dull pain and tenderness.

Pathologic Findings. Mucinous adenocarcinomas are 2.5 to 4.0 cm in their largest dimension. Due to the large amount of mucin, these

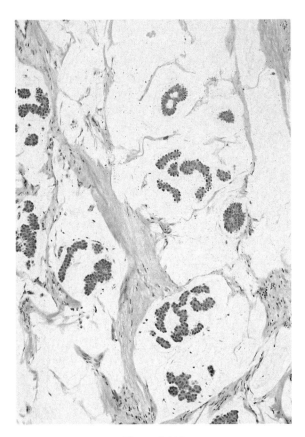

Figure 5-298
MUCINOUS ADENOCARCINOMA
Very pale-staining mucinous material appears partitioned by septa of fibrous connective tissue of varying thickness. A few small islands of epithelium lie dispersed within the mucin.

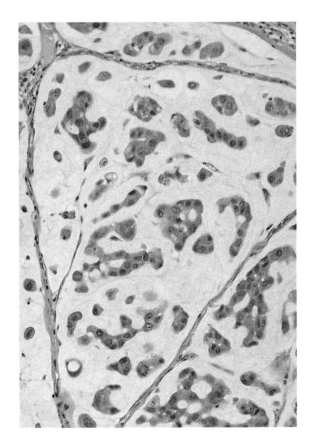

Figure 5-299
MUCINOUS ADENOCARCINOMA
Round and irregular-shaped nests of epithelial cells appear to be detached and "floating" in pools of mucin. In this section some of the epithelial islands contain as few as one or two cells.

tumors are soft, and the cut surface is gelatinous with a glistening appearance.

Microscopically, pools of pale basophilic mucin are separated by fibrous connective tissue bands of variable thickness that appear to compartmentalize the tumor (fig. 5-298). Within the mucin pools lie nests, cords, and sheets of epithelial cells, which often seem to be "floating" in the mucin (fig. 5-299). The epithelium appears as isolated islands, branching cords or papillae, small ducts, epithelial-lined cysts, and cribriform configurations. The epithelial cells vary from cuboidal to polygonal. Their cytoplasm is eosinophilic to clear, and intracellular mucin is demonstrable in some tumors with mucicarmine or other stains for mucin. Cytologic atypia varies from minimal to moderate, and mitotic figures have not been a conspicuous feature (figs. 5-300, 5-301). The quantity of epithelium varies from sparse, widely separated foci to prominent aggregates that are about equal in area to the extracellular mucinous material (figs. 5-298, 5-302). Although the tumors are compartmentalized by fibrous tissue, they are not encapsulated (fig. 5-302).

The mucinous material stains with PAS, mucicarmine, and Alcian blue at pH 2.5 (fig. 5-303).

Differential Diagnosis. Since mucin production is a feature frequently observed in many types of salivary gland neoplasm, such as mucoepidermoid carcinoma; acinic cell adenocarcinoma; cystadenocarcinoma; adenocarcinoma, not otherwise specified (NOS); polymorphous low-grade adenocarcinoma; and mixed tumor, mucin production alone does not segregate mucinous adenocarcinoma from the others. Specific features of other neoplasms, such as epidermoid and intermediate cells for mucoepidermoid carcinoma and acinar cells for acinic cell adenocarcinoma, are

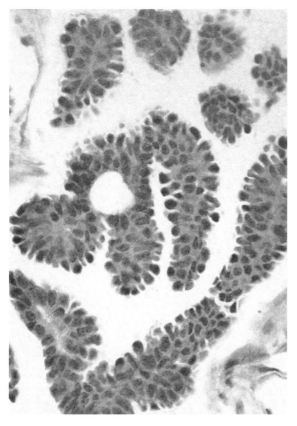

Figure 5-300
MUCINOUS ADENOCARCINOMA
Small nests and branching trabecular cords of uniform epithelial cells have eosinophilic cytoplasm and round to ovoid, fairly homogeneously stained nuclei. In the center of the field the epithelial cells have produced a small lumen-like structure.

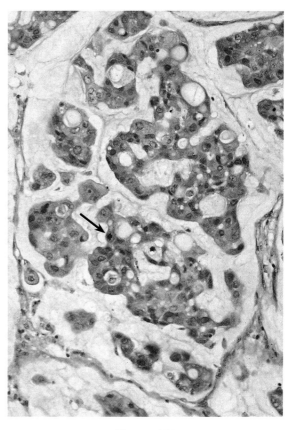

Figure 5-301
MUCINOUS ADENOCARCINOMA
The epithelial cells in this parotid gland tumor almost have a cribriform architecture, and small lumen-like structures are evident within the epithelial cords. Moderate cytologic atypia is present as is a mitotic figure (arrow).

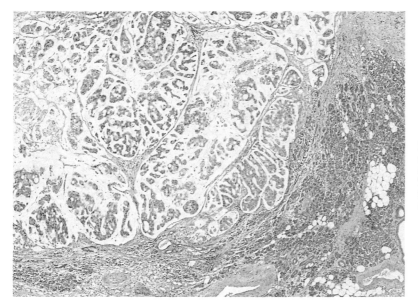

Figure 5-302
MUCINOUS ADENOCARCINOMA
This carcinoma is associated with fibrosis at the periphery, but it is unencapsulated and infiltrates the parenchyma of the submandibular gland. The areas occupied by neoplastic epithelium and extracellular mucin are about equal.

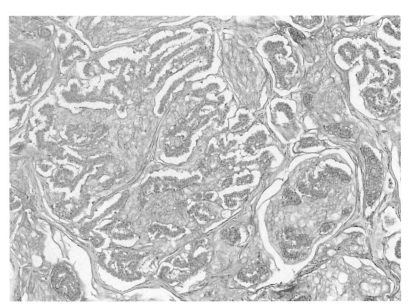

Figure 5-303
MUCINOUS ADENOCARCINOMA
Mucicarmine stain highlights the mucinous material that surrounds the cords of epithelium, but there is little or no intracellular mucin in this parotid carcinoma.

absent, but the most distinguishing feature is the relationship of the extracellular mucin to the epithelium. In most other types of salivary gland neoplasms the mucin is confined and bounded by epithelium within cystic or papillary-cystic structures. Pools of mucin that are occasionally present in mucoepidermoid carcinomas contain isolated epithelial structures that are usually papillary. The intramucinous epithelial cells in mucoepidermoid carcinoma are much less numerous than those in mucinous adenocarcinoma, and evidence of mucus spillage from a ruptured cyst is nearly always present (see Mucoepidermoid Carcinoma). In mucinous adenocarcinoma the extracellular mucin surrounds and contains the epithelium.

Differentiation of mucinous adenocarcinoma of salivary gland from mucinous carcinoma of skin is based on site of occurrence rather than histologic features. The face or head is a common site for mucinous eccrine carcinomas (751), and extension or metastasis to the parotid gland has

been reported (748). Metastasis of mucinous carcinoma of the breast to salivary glands is unlikely, and clinical evaluation shows a breast primary tumor.

Prognosis and Treatment. The mucinous adenocarcinoma of the submandibular gland reported by Osaki et al. (752) invaded the mandibular bone and metastasized to cervical lymph nodes. Six years after excision and neck dissection there had been no recurrence at the primary site, but additional cervical lymph node metastases appeared. The patient was being treated with chemotherapy at the time of the report; other follow-up information is not available. Extrapolation from data on skin and breast tumors suggests a low-grade behavior pattern for mucinous adenocarcinoma of salivary gland. Mucinous eccrine carcinomas frequently recur but uncommonly metastasize (748), and mucinous carcinoma of breast has a relatively favorable prognosis (753). Complete surgical eradication is the preferred primary therapy for low-grade salivary gland carcinomas.

REFERENCES

Mucoepidermoid Carcinoma

1. Accetta PA, Gray GF Jr, Hunter RM, Rosenfeld L. Mucoepidermoid carcinoma of salivary glands. Arch Pathol Lab Med 1984;108:321–5.

2. Adkins GF, Hinckley DM. Primary muco-epidermoid carcinoma arising in a parotid lymph node. Aust N Z J Surg 1989;59:433–5.

3. Armstrong JG, Harrison LB, Spiro RH, Fass DE, Strong EW, Fuks ZY. Malignant tumors of major salivary gland origin. A matched-pair analysis of the role of combined surgery and postoperative radiotherapy. Arch Otolaryngol Head Neck Surg 1990;116:290–3.

4. Auclair PL. Tumor-associated lymphoid proliferation in the parotid gland: a potential diagnostic pitfall. Oral Surg Oral Med Oral Pathol 1994;77:19–26.

5. Auclair PL, Ellis GL. Mucoepidermoid carcinoma. In: Ellis GL, Auclair PL, Gnepp DR, eds. Surgical pathology of the salivary glands. Philadelphia: WB Saunders, 1991:269–98.

6. Auclair PL, Ellis GL, Gnepp DR, Wenig BM, Janney CG. Salivary gland neoplasms: general considerations. In: Ellis GL, Auclair PL, Gnepp DR, eds. Surgical pathology of the salivary glands. Philadelphia: WB Saunders, 1991:135–64.

7. Auclair PL, Goode RK, Ellis GL. Mucoepidermoid carcinoma of intraoral salivary glands. Evaluation and application of grading criteria in 143 cases. Cancer 1992;69:2021–30.

8. Beahrs OH, Henson DE, Hutter RV, Myers MH. Manual for staging of cancer. 3rd ed. Philadelphia: JB Lippincott, 1988:51–6.

9. Belani CP, Eisenberger MA, Gray WC. Preliminary experience with chemotherapy in advanced salivary gland neoplasms. Med Pediatr Oncol 1988;16:197–202.

10. Bhargava S, Sant MS, Arora MM. Histomorphologic spectrum of tumours of minor salivary glands. Indian J Cancer 1982;19:134–40.

11. Breitenecker G, Wepner F. A pleomorphic adenoma (so-called mixed tumor) in the wall of a dentigerous cyst. Oral Surg Oral Med Oral Pathol 1973;36:63–71.

12. Brookstone MS, Huvos AG. Central salivary gland tumors of the maxilla and mandible: a clinicopathologic study of 11 cases with an analysis of the literature. J Oral Maxillofac Surg 1992;50:229–36.

13. Brookstone MS, Huvos AG, Spiro RH. Central adenoid cystic carcinoma of the mandible. J Oral Maxillofac Surg 1990;48:1329–33.

14. Browand BC, Waldron CA. Central mucoepidermoid tumors of the jaws. Report of nine cases and review of the literature. Oral Surg Oral Med Oral Pathol 1975;40:631–43.

15. Bruner JM, Batsakis JG. Salivary neoplasms of the jaw bones with particular reference to central mucoepidermoid carcinomas. Ann Otol Rhinol Laryngol 1991;100:954–5.

16. Caselitz J, Schmitt P, Seifert G, Wustrow J, Schuppan D. Basal membrane associated substances in human salivary glands and salivary gland tumours. Pathol Res Pract 1988;183:386–94.

17. Chaudhry AP, Cutler LS, Leifer C, Labay G, Satchidanand S, Yamane GM. Ultrastructural study of the histogenesis of salivary gland mucoepidermoid carcinoma. J Oral Pathol Med 1989;18:400–9.

18. Chomette G, Auriol M, Tereau Y, Vaillant JM. Les tumeurs mucoepidermoides des glandes salivaires accessoires. Denombrement. Etude clinico-pathologique, histoenzymologique et ultrastructurale. Ann Pathol 1982;2:29–40.

19. Chomette G, Auriol MM, Labrousse F, Vaillant JM. Mucoepidermoid tumors of salivary glands: histoprognostic value of NORs stained with AgNOR technique. J Oral Pathol Med 1991;20:130–2.

20. Chung CT, Sagerman RH, Ryoo MC, King GA, Yu WS, Dalal PS. The changing role of external-beam irradiation in the management of malignant tumors of the major salivary glands. Radiology 1982;145:175–7.

21. Dardick I, Gliniecki MR, Heathcote JG, Burford-Mason A. Comparative histogenesis and morphogenesis of mucoepidermoid carcinoma and pleomorphic adenoma. An ultrastructural study. Virchows Arch [A] 1990;417:405–17.

22. De MN, Tribedi BP. A mixed epidermoid and mucus-secreting carcinoma of the parotid gland. J Pathol Bact 1939;49:432–3.

23. Dhawan IK, Bhargava S, Nayak NC, Gupta RK. Central salivary gland tumors of jaws. Cancer 1970;26:211–7.

24. Eneroth CM, Hjertman L, Moberger G. Muco-epidermoid carcinoma of the palate. Acta Otolaryngol (Stockh) 1970;70:408–18.

25. Eneroth CM, Hjertman L, Moberger G, Sderberg G. Muco-epidermoid carcinomas of the salivary glands with special reference to the possible existence of a benign variety. Acta Otolaryngol (Stockh) 1972;73:68–74.

26. Evans HL. Mucoepidermoid carcinoma of salivary glands: a study of 69 cases with special attention to histologic grading. Am J Clin Pathol 1984;81:696–701.

27. Eversole LR. Glycoprotein heterogeneity in mucoepidermoid carcinoma. A histochemical evaluation. Arch Otolaryngol Head Neck Surg 1972;96:426–32.

28. Eversole LR, Rovin S, Sabes WR. Mucoepidermoid carcinoma of minor salivary glands: report of 17 cases with follow-up. J Oral Surg 1972;30:107–12.

29. Eversole LR, Sabes WR, Rovin S. Aggressive growth and neoplastic potential of odontogenic cysts. With special reference to central epidermoid and mucoepidermoid carcinomas. Cancer 1975;35:270–82.

30. Eveson JW, Cawson RA. Salivary gland tumours. A review of 2410 cases with particular reference to histological types, site, age and sex distribution. J Pathol 1985;146:51–8.

31. Fitzpatrick PJ, Theriault C. Malignant salivary gland tumors. Int J Radiat Oncol Biol Phys 1986;12:1743–7.

32. Frable WJ, Elzay RP. Tumors of minor salivary glands. A report of 73 cases. Cancer 1970;25:932–41.

33. Freedman SI, van de Velde RL, Kagan AR, Perzik SL. Primary malignant mixed tumor of the mandible. Cancer 1972;30:167–73.

34. Fujita S, Takahashi H, Okabe H. Nucleolar organizer regions in malignant salivary gland tumors. Acta Pathol Jpn 1992;42:727–33.

35. Gingell JC, Beckerman T, Levy BA, Snider LS. Central mucoepidermoid carcinoma. Review of the literature and report of a case associated with an apical periodontal cyst. Oral Surg Oral Med Oral Pathol 1984;57:436–40.

353

36. Gnepp DR, Schroeder W, Heffner D. Synchronous tumors arising in a single major salivary gland. Cancer 1989;63:1219–24.
37. Hamed G, Shmookler BM, Ellis GL, Punja U, Feldman D. Oncocytic mucoepidermoid carcinoma of the parotid gland. Arch Pathol Lab Med 1994;118:313–4.
38. Hamper K, Schimmelpenning H, Caselitz J, et al. Mucoepidermoid tumors of the salivary glands. Correlation of cytophotometrical data and prognosis. Cancer 1989;63:708–17.
39. Hamper K, Schmitz-Watjen W, Mausch HE, Caselitz J, Seifert G. Multiple expression of tissue markers in mucoepidermoid carcinomas and acinic cell carcinomas of the salivary glands. Virchows Arch [A] 1989;414:407–13.
40. Hanna DC, Clairmont AA. Submandibular gland tumors. Plast Reconstr Surg 1978;61:198–203.
41. Hassanin MB, Ghosh L, Das AK, Waterhouse JP. Immunohistochemical and fluorescent microscopic study of histogenesis of salivary mucoepidermoid carcinoma. J Oral Pathol Med 1989;18:291–8.
42. Healey WV, Perzin KH, Smith L. Mucoepidermoid carcinoma of salivary gland origin. Classification, clinical-pathologic correlation, and results of treatment. Cancer 1970;26:368–88.
43. Hickman RE, Cawson RA, Duffy SW. The prognosis of specific types of salivary gland tumors. Cancer 1984;54:1620–4.
44. Huang JW, Mori M, Yamada K, et al. Mucoepidermoid carcinoma of the salivary glands: immunohistochemical distribution of intermediate filament proteins, involucrin and secretory proteins. Anticancer Res 1992;12:811–20.
45. Isacsson G, Shear M. Intraoral salivary gland tumors: a retrospective study of 201 cases. J Oral Pathol 1983;12:57–62.
46. Ishige T, Kaneko T, Konno A, Naitoh J, Hayasaki K. TNM classification system in cancer of the submandibular gland—a comprehensive retrospective study of 271 primary cases. Nippon Jibiinkoka Gakkai Kaiho 1992;95:32–40.
47. Ito H, Soda T, Asakura A, Nakajima T, Kobayashi Y, Miyazawa M. Central acinic cell tumor of the mandible. Bull Tokyo Med Dent Univ 1970;17:239–47.
48. Jakobsson PA, Blanck C, Eneroth CM. Mucoepidermoid carcinoma of the parotid gland. Cancer 1968;22:111–24.
49. Jensen OJ, Poulsen T, Schidt T. Mucoepidermoid tumors of salivary glands. A long term follow-up study. APMIS 1988;96:421–7.
50. Kaplan MJ, Johns ME, Cantrell RW. Chemotherapy for salivary gland cancer. Otolaryngol Head Neck Surg 1986;95:165–70.
51. Kaste SC, Hedlund G, Pratt CB. Malignant parotid tumors in patients previously treated for childhood cancer: clinical and imaging findings in eight cases. AJR Am J Roentgenol 1994;162:655–9.
52. King JJ, Fletcher GH. Malignant tumors of the major salivary glands. Radiology 1971;100:381–4.
53. Kumasa S, Yuba R, Sagara S, Okutomi T, Okada Y, Mori M. Mucoepidermoid carcinomas: immunohistochemical studies on keratin, S-100 protein, lactoferrin, lysozyme and amylase. Basic Appl Histochem 1988;32:429–41.
54. Ma DQ, Yu GY. Tumours of the minor salivary glands. A clinicopathologic study of 243 cases. Acta Otolaryngol (Stockh) 1987;103:325–31.
55. Matsumura K, Sasaki K, Tsuji T, Shinozaki F. The nucleolar organizer regions associated protein (AgNORs) in salivary gland tumors. Int J Oral Maxillofac Surg 1989;18:76–8.
56. McNaney D, McNeese MD, Guillamondegui OM, Fletcher GH, Oswald MJ. Postoperative irradiation in malignant epithelial tumors of the parotid. Int J Radiat Oncol Biol Phys 1983;9:1289–95.
57. Melrose RJ, Abrams AM, Howell FV. Mucoepidermoid tumors of the intraoral minor salivary glands: a clinicopathologic study of 54 cases. J Oral Pathol 1973;2:314–25.
58. Nascimento AG, Amaral LP, Prado LA, Kligerman J, Silveira TR. Mucoepidermoid carcinoma of salivary glands: a clinicopathologic study of 46 cases. Head Neck Surg 1986;8:409–17.
59. Neville BW, Damm DD, Weir JC, Fantasia JE. Labial salivary gland tumors. Cancer 1988;61:2113–6.
60. Olsen KD, Devine KD, Weiland LH. Mucoepidermoid carcinoma of the oral cavity. Otolaryngol Head Neck Surg 1981;89:783–91.
61. Posner MR, Ervin TJ, Weichselbaum RR, Fabian RL, Miller D. Chemotherapy of advanced salivary gland neoplasms. Cancer 1982;50:2261–4.
62. Regezi JA, Zarbo RJ, Batsakis JG. Immunoprofile of mucoepidermoid carcinomas of minor salivary glands. Oral Surg Oral Med Oral Pathol 1991;71:189–92.
63. Roa RA, Hruban RH, McKenzie P, Richtsmeier W. Tumor-associated glycoprotein expression in salivary gland mucoepidermoid carcinomas: an immunohistochemical study using the monoclonal antibody B72.3. Laryngoscope 1994;104:304–8.
64. Sadeghi A, Tran LM, Mark R, Sidrys J, Parker RG. Minor salivary gland tumors of the head and neck: treatment strategies and prognosis. Am J Clin Oncol 1993;16:3–8.
65. Seifert G, Rieb H, Donath K. Classification of the tumours of the minor salivary glands. Pathohistologic analysis of 160 cases. Laryngol Rhinol Otol 1980;59:379–400.
66. Sikorowa L. Mucoepidermoid carcinomas of salivary glands. Pol Med J 1964;3:1345–67.
67. Slavin F, Mitchell RM. Adenoid cystic carcinoma of the mandible. Br J Surg 1971;58:546–8.
68. Smith A, Winkler B, Perzin KH, Wazen J, Blitzer A. Mucoepidermoid carcinoma arising in an intraparotid lymph node. Cancer 1985;55:400–3.
69. Soini Y, Kamel D, Nuorva K, Lane DP, Vähäkangas K, Pääkkö P. Low p53 protein expression in salivary gland tumours compared with lung carcinomas. Virchows Arch [A] 1992;421:415–20.
70. Spiro RH. The management of salivary neoplasms: an overview. Auris Nasus Larynx 1985;12(Suppl 2):S122–7.
71. Spiro RH. Salivary neoplasms: overview of a 35-year experience with 2,807 patients. Head Neck Surg 1986; 8:177–84.
72. Spiro RH, Hajdu SI, Strong EW. Tumors of the submaxillary gland. Am J Surg 1976;132:463–8.
73. Spiro RH, Huvos AG, Berk R, Strong EW. Mucoepidermoid carcinoma of salivary gland origin. A clinicopathologic study of 367 cases. Am J Surg 1978;136:461–8.
74. Spiro RH, Thaler HT, Hicks WF, Kher UA, Huvos AH, Strong EW. The importance of clinical staging of minor salivary gland carcinoma. Am J Surg 1991;162:330–6.
75. Spitz MR, Batsakis JG. Major salivary gland carcinoma. Descriptive epidemiology and survival of 498 patients. Arch Otolaryngol Head Neck Surg 1984;110:45–9.

76. Stewart FW, Foote FW, Becker WF. Mucoepidermoid tumors of salivary glands. Ann Surg 1945;122:820–44.

77. Suen JY, Johns ME. Chemotherapy for salivary gland cancer. Laryngoscope 1982;92:235–9.

78. Takahashi H, Fujita S, Tsuda N, Tezuka F, Okabe H. Intraoral minor salivary gland tumors: a demographic and histologic study of 200 cases. Tohoku J Exp Med 1990;161:111–28.

79. Tateishi A, Nodai T, Fukuyama H, Yamada N. Primary mucoepidermoid carcinoma of an intraparotid lymph node. J Oral Maxillofac Surg 1992;50:535–8.

80. Taxy JB. Necrotizing squamous/mucinous metaplasia in oncocytic salivary gland tumors. A potential diagnostic problem. Am J Clin Pathol 1992;97:40–5.

81. Therkildsen MH, Mandel U, Christensen M, Dabelsteen E. Simple mucin-type Tn and sialosyl-Tn carbohydrate antigens in salivary gland carcinomas. Cancer 1993;72:1147–54.

82. Thorvaldsson SE, Beahrs OH, Woolner LB, Simons JN. Mucoepidermoid tumors of the major salivary glands. Am J Surg 1970;120:432–8.

83. Tran L, Sadeghi A, Hanson D, Ellerbroek N, Calcaterra TC, Parker RG. Salivary gland tumors of the palate: the UCLA experience. Laryngoscope 1987;97:1343–5.

84. Tran L, Sadeghi A, Hanson D, et al. Major salivary gland tumors: treatment results and prognostic factors. Laryngoscope 1986;96:1139–44.

85. van Heerden WF, Raubenheimer EJ. Evaluation of the nucleolar organizer region associated proteins in minor salivary gland tumors. J Oral Pathol Med 1991;20: 291–5.

86. van Heerden WF, Raubenheimer EJ, Turner ML. Glandular odontogenic cyst. Head Neck 1992;14:316–20.

87. Venook AP, Tseng AJ Jr, Meyers FJ, et al. Cisplatin, doxorubicin, and 5-fluorouracil chemotherapy for salivary gland malignancies: a pilot study of the Northern California Oncology Group. J Clin Oncol 1987;5:951–5.

88. Waldron CA, Koh ML. Central mucoepidermoid carcinoma of the jaws: report of four cases with analysis of the literature and discussion of the relationship to mucoepidermoid, sialodontogenic, and glandular odontogenic cysts. J Oral Maxillofac Surg 1990;48:871–7.

89. Waldron CA, Mustoe TA. Primary intraosseous carcinoma of the mandible with probable origin in an odontogenic cyst. Oral Surg Oral Med Oral Pathol 1989;67:716–24.

90. Wang SZ. Quantitative study on nucleolar organizer regions in salivary gland tumours. (Article in Chinese, English abstract.) Chung Hua Kou Chiang Hsueh Tsa Chih 1992;27:74–6, 127.

91. Yu GY, Ma DQ. Carcinoma of the salivary gland: a clinicopathologic study of 405 cases. Semin Surg Oncol 1987;3:240–4.

Adenocarcinoma, Not Otherwise Specified

92. Allen MS Jr, Fitz-Hugh GS, Marsh WL Jr. Low-grade papillary adenocarcinoma of the palate. Cancer 1974;33:153–8.

93. Auclair PL, Ellis GL. Adenocarcinoma, not otherwise specified. In: Ellis GL, Auclair PL, Gnepp DR, eds. Surgical pathology of the salivary glands. Philadelphia: WB Saunders, 1991:318–32.

94. Bauer WH, Bauer JD. Classification of glandular tumors of salivary glands. Arch Pathol 1953;55:328–46.

95. Foote FW Jr, Frazell EL. Tumors of the major salivary glands. Cancer 1953;6:1065–133.

96. Hrebinko R, Taylor SR, Bahnson RR. Carcinoma of prostate metastatic to parotid gland. Urology 1993;41:272–3.

97. Main JH, Orr JA, McGurk FM, McComb RJ, Mock D. Salivary gland tumors: review of 643 cases. J Oral Pathol 1976;5:88–102.

98. Matsuba HM, Mauney M, Simpson JR, Thawley SE, Pikul FJ. Adenocarcinomas of major and minor salivary gland origin: a histopathologic review of treatment failure patterns. Laryngoscope 1988;98:784–8.

99. Mills SE, Garland TA, Allen MS Jr. Low-grade papillary adenocarcinoma of palatal salivary gland origin. Am J Surg Pathol 1984;8:367–74.

100. Nagao K, Matsuzaki O, Saiga H, et al. Histopathologic studies on adenocarcinoma of the parotid gland. Acta Pathol Jpn 1986;36:337–47.

101. Nishijima W, Tokita N, Takooda S, Tsuchiya S, Watanabe I. Adenocarcinoma of the sublingual gland: case report and 50 year review of the literature. Laryngoscope 1984;94:96–101.

102. Seifert G, Schulz JP. Das adenocarinoma der speicheldrusen. Pathohistologie und subklassifikation von 77 fallen. HNO 1985;33:433–42.

103. Seifert G, Sobin LH. Histological classification of salivary gland tumours. World Health Organization. International histological classification of tumours. 2nd ed. Berlin: Springer-Verlag, 1991:28.

104. Spiro RH, Huvos AG, Strong EW. Adenocarcinoma of salivary origin. Clinicopathologic study of 204 patients. Am J Surg 1982;144:423–31.

105. Spitz MR, Batsakis JG. Major salivary gland carcinoma. Descriptive epidemiology and survival of 498 patients. Arch Otolaryngol Head Neck Surg 1984;110:45–9.

106. Stene T, Koppang HS. Intraoral adenocarcinomas. J Oral Pathol 1981;10:216–25.

107. Thackray AC, Lucas RB. Tumors of the major salivary glands. Atlas of Tumor Pathology, 2nd Series, Fascicle 10. Washington, D.C.: Armed Forces Institute of Pathology, 1974:100–1.

108. Thackrey AC, Sobin LH. Histological typing of salivary gland tumours. World Health Organization. International histological classification of tumours. Geneva: World Health Organization, 1972.

109. van Krieken JH. Prostate marker immunoreactivity in salivary gland neoplasms. A rare pitfall in immunohistochemistry. Am J Surg Pathol 1993;17:410–4.

110. Whittaker JS, Turner EP. Papillary tumours of the minor salivary glands. J Clin Pathol 1976;29:795–805.

111. Woods JE, Chong GC, Beahrs OH. Experience with 1,360 primary parotid tumors. Am J Surg 1975; 130:460–2.

Acinic Cell Adenocarcinoma

112. Abrams AM, Cornyn J, Scofield HH, Hansen LS. Acinic cell adenocarcinoma of the major salivary glands: a clinico-pathologic study of 77 cases. Cancer 1965;18:1145–62.

113. Abrams AM, Melrose RJ. Acinic cell tumors of minor salivary gland origin. Oral Surg Oral Med Oral Pathol 1978;46:220–33.

114. Auclair PL. Tumor-associated lymphoid proliferation in the parotid gland: a potential diagnostic pitfall. Oral Surg Oral Med Oral Pathol 1994;77:19–26.

115. Batsakis JG, Chinn E, Regezi JA, Repola DA. The pathology of head and neck tumors: salivary glands, part 2. Head Neck Surg 1978;1:167–80.

116. Batsakis JG, Chinn EK, Weimert TA, Work WP, Krause CJ. Acinic cell carcinoma: a clinicopathologic study of thirty-five cases. J Laryngol Otol 1979;93:325–40.

117. Batsakis JG, Luna MA, el-Naggar AK. Histopathologic grading of salivary gland neoplasms: II. Acinic cell carci-nomas. Ann Otol Rhinol Laryngol 1990;99:929–33.

118. Bloom GD, Carlsöö B, Henriksson R. Some ultrastruc-tural features of acinic cell carcinoma. J Laryngol Otol 1977;91:947–58.

119. Buxton RW, Maxwell JH, French AJ. Surgical treat-ment of epithelial tumors of the parotid gland. Surg Gynecol Obstet 1953;97:401–16.

120. Callender DL, Frankenthaler RA, Luna MA, Lee SS, Goepfert H. Salivary gland neoplasms in children. Arch Otolaryngol Head Neck Surg 1992;118:472–6.

121. Caselitz J, Seifert G, Grenner G, Schmidtberger R. Amylase as an additional marker of salivary gland neoplasms. An immunoperoxidase study. Pathol Res Pract 1983;176:276–83.

122. Castellanos JL, Lally ET. Acinic cell tumor of the minor salivary glands. J Oral Maxillofac Surg 1982;40:428–31.

123. Chau MN, Radden BG. Intra-oral salivary gland neo-plasms: a retrospective study of 98 cases. J Oral Pathol 1986;15:339–42.

124. Chaudhry AP, Cutler LS, Leifer C, Satchidanand S, Labay G, Yamane G. Histogenesis of acinic cell carci-noma of the major and minor salivary glands. An ultrastructural study. J Pathol 1986;148:307–20.

125. Chen SY, Brannon RB, Miller AS, White DK, Hooker SP. Acinic cell adenocarcinoma of minor salivary glands. Cancer 1978;42:678–85.

126. Chomette G, Auriol M, Vaillant JM. Acinic cell tumors of salivary glands. Frequency and morphological study. J Biol Buccale 1984;12:157–69.

127. Chomette G, Auriol M, Wann A, Guilbert F. Acinic cell carcinomas of salivary glands histoprognosis. Value of NORs stained with AgNOR technique and examined with semi-automatic image analysis. J Biol Buccale 1991;19:205–10.

128. Chong GC, Beahrs OH, Woolner LB. Surgical manage-ment of acinic cell carcinoma of the parotid gland. Surg Gynecol Obstet 1974;138:65–8.

129. Clemis JD, Bland J, Fung C. Acinic cell tumors of salivary gland origin. Laryngoscope 1977;87:1500–8.

130. Colmenero C, Patron M, Sierra I. Acinic cell carcinoma of the salivary glands. A review of 20 new cases. J Craniomaxillofac Surg 1991;19:260–6.

131. Dardick I, George D, Jeans MT, et al. Ultrastructural morphology and cellular differentiation in acinic cell carci-noma. Oral Surg Oral Med Oral Pathol 1987;63:325–34.

132. Deguchi H, Hamano H, Haneji N, Takahashi M, Hayashi Y. Immunopathology of phenotypic change on human par-otid gland adenocarcinoma. Pathobiology 1993;61:83–8.

133. Echevarria RA. Ultrastructure of the acinic cell carci-noma and clear cell carcinoma of the parotid gland. Cancer 1967;20:563–71.

134. Egan M, Crocker J, Nar P. Localization of salivary amylase and epithelial membrane antigen in salivary gland tu-mours by means of immunoperoxidase and immunogold-silver techniques. J Laryngol Otol 1988;102:242–7.

135. el-Naggar AK, Batsakis JG, Luna MA, McLemore D, Byers RM. DNA flow cytometry of acinic cell carcinomas of major salivary glands. J Laryngol Otol 1990;104:410–6.

136. Ellis GL, Auclair PL. Acinic cell adenocarcinoma. In: Ellis GL, Auclair PL, Gnepp DR, eds. Surgical pathol-ogy of the salivary glands. Philadelphia: WB Saunders, 1991:299–317.

137. Ellis GL, Corio RL. Acinic cell adenocarcinoma. A clin-icopathologic analysis of 294 cases. Cancer 1983; 52:542–9.

138. Eneroth CM, Jakobsson PA, Blanck C. Acinic cell car-cinoma of the parotid gland. Cancer 1966;19:1761–72.

139. Evans RW, Cruickshank AH. Epithelial tumours of the salivary glands. Philadelphia: WB Saunders, 1970:98–119.

140. Eveson JW, Cawson RA. Salivary gland tumours. A review of 2410 cases with particular reference to histological types, site, age and sex distribution. J Pathol 1985;146:51–8.

141. Ferlito A. Acinic cell carcinoma of minor salivary glands. Histopathology 1980;4:331–43.

142. Fitzpatrick PJ, Theriault C. Malignant salivary gland tumors. Int J Radiat Oncol Biol Phys 1986;12:1743–7.

143. Foote FW Jr, Frazell EL. Tumors of the major salivary glands. Cancer 1953;6:1065–133.

144. Fox NM, ReMine WH, Woolner LB. Acinic cell carcinoma of the major salivary glands. Am J Surg 1963;106:860–7.

145. Fujita S, Takahashi H, Okabe H. Nucleolar organizer regions in malignant salivary gland tumors. Acta Pathol Jpn 1992;42:727–33.

146. Gardner DG, Bell ME, Wesley RK, Wysocki GP. Acinic cell tumors of minor salivary glands. Oral Surg Oral Med Oral Pathol 1980;50:545–51.

147. Gnepp DR, Schroeder W, Heffner D. Synchronous tu-mors arising in a single major salivary gland. Cancer 1989;63:1219–24.

148. Godwin JT, Foote FW Jr, Frazell EL. Acinic cell adeno-carcinoma of the parotid gland: report of twenty-seven cases. Am J Pathol 1954;30:465–77.

149. Gorlin RJ, Chaudhry A. Acinic cell tumor of the major and minor salivary glands. J Oral Surg 1957;15:304–6.

150. Guimaraes DS, Amaral AP, Prado LF, Nascimento AG. Acinic cell carcinoma of salivary glands: 16 cases with clinicopathologic correlation. J Oral Pathol Med 1989;18:396–9.

151. Gustafsson H, Carlsöö B, Henriksson R. Ultrastruc-tural morphometry and secretory behavior of acinic cell carcinoma. Cancer 1985;55:1706–10.

152. Gustafsson H, Lindholm C, Carlsöö B. DNA cytopho-tometry of acinic cell carcinoma and its relation to prognosis. Acta Otolaryngol (Stockh) 1987;104:370–6.

153. Gustafsson H, Virtanen I, Thornell LE. Expression of cytokeratins and vimentin in salivary gland carcino-mas as revealed with monoclonal antibodies. Virchows Arch [A] 1988;412:515–24.

154. Hamper K, Caselitz J, Arps H, Askensten U, Auer G, Seifert G. The relationship between nuclear DNA content in salivary gland tumors and prognosis. Comparison of mucoepidermoid tumors and acinic cell tumors. Arch Otorhinolaryngol 1989;246:328–32.

155. Hamper K, Mausch HE, Caselitz J, et al. Acinic cell carcinoma of the salivary glands: the prognostic relevance of DNA cytophotometry in a retrospective study of long duration (1965-1987). Oral Surg Oral Med Oral Pathol 1990;69:68–75.

156. Hamper K, Schmitz-Watjen W, Mausch HE, Caselitz J, Seifert G. Multiple expression of tissue markers in mucoepidermoid carcinomas and acinic cell carcinomas of the salivary glands. Virchows Arch [A] 1989;414:407–13.

157. Hayashi Y, Nishida T, Yoshida H, Yanagawa T, Yura Y, Sato M. Immunoreactive vasoactive intestinal polypeptide in acinic cell carcinoma of the parotid gland. Cancer 1987;60:962–8.

158. Hickman RE, Cawson RA, Duffy SW. The prognosis of specific types of salivary gland tumors. Cancer 1984;54:1620–4.

159. Hunter RM, Davis BW, Gray GF Jr, Rosenfeld L. Primary malignant tumors of salivary gland origin. A 52-year review. Am Surg 1983;49:82–9.

160. Inoue T, Shimono M, Yamamura T, Saito I, Watanabe O, Kawahara H. Acinic cell carcinoma arising in the glossopalatine glands: a report of two cases with electron microscopic observations. Oral Surg Oral Med Oral Pathol 1984;57:398–407.

161. Isacsson G, Shear M. Intraoral salivary gland tumors: a retrospective study of 201 cases. J Oral Pathol 1983;12:57–62.

162. Kay S, Schatzki PF. Ultrastructure of acinic cell carcinoma of the parotid salivary gland. Cancer 1972;29:235–44.

163. Lack EE, Upton MP. Histopathologic review of salivary gland tumors in childhood. Arch Otolaryngol Head Neck Surg 1988;114:898–906.

164. Lewis JE, Olsen KD, Weiland LH. Acinic cell carcinoma. Clinicopathologic review. Cancer 1991;67:172–9.

165. Lidang Jensen M, Kiaer H. Acinic cell carcinoma with primary presentation in an intraparotid lymph node [Discussion]. Pathol Res Pract 1992;188:226–31.

166. Luna MA, Batsakis JG, el-Naggar AK. Salivary gland tumors in children. Ann Otol Rhinol Laryngol 1991;100:869–71.

167. Minic AJ. Acinic cell carcinoma arising in a parotid lymph node. Int J Oral Maxillofac Surg 1993;22:289–91.

168. Morley DJ, Hodes JE, Calland J, Hodes ME. Immunohistochemical demonstration of ribonuclease and amylase in normal and neoplastic parotid glands. Hum Pathol 1983;14:969–73.

169. Murakami M, Ohtani I, Hojo H, Wakasa H. Immunohistochemical evaluation with Ki-67: an application to salivary gland tumours. J Laryngol Otol 1992;106:35–8.

170. Nelson DW, Nichols RD, Fine G. Bilateral acinous cell tumors of the parotid gland. Laryngoscope 1978;88:1935–41.

171. Nuutinen J, Kansanen M, Syrjanen K. View from beneath: pathology in focus bilateral acinic cell tumours of the parotid gland. J Laryngol Otol 1991;105:796–8.

172. O'Brien CJ, Soong SJ, Herrera GA, Urist MM, Maddox WA. Malignant salivary tumors—analysis of prognostic factors and survival. Head Neck Surg 1986;9:82–92.

173. Oliveira P, Fonseca I, Soares J. Acinic cell carcinoma of the salivary glands. A long term follow-up study of 15 cases. Eur J Surg Oncol 1992;18:7–15.

174. Perzin KH, LiVolsi VA. Acinic cell carcinomas arising in salivary glands: a clinicopathologic study. Cancer 1979;44:1434–57.

175. Seifert G. Histopathology of malignant salivary gland tumours. Eur J Cancer B Oral Oncol 1992;28B:49–56.

176. Seifert G, Caselitz J. Tumor markers in parotid gland carcinomas: immunohistochemical investigations. Cancer Detect Prev 1983;6:119–30.

177. Seifert G, Miehlke A, Haubrich J, Chilla R. Diseases of the salivary glands: pathology, diagnosis, treatment, facial nerve surgery. New York: Georg Thieme Verlag, 1986:171.

178. Seifert G, Miehlke A, Haubrich J, Chilla R. Diseases of the salivary glands: pathology, diagnosis, treatment, facial nerve surgery. New York: Georg Thieme Verlag, 1986:224–30.

179. Seifert G, Okabe H, Caselitz J. Epithelial salivary gland tumors in children and adolescents. Analysis of 80 cases (Salivary Gland Register 1965-1984). ORL J Otorhinolaryngol Relat Spec 1986;48:137–49.

180. Seifert G, Sobin LH. Histological typing of salivary gland tumours. World Health Organization international histological classification of tumours. 2nd ed. New York: Springer-Verlag, 1991.

181. Sharkey FE. Systematic evaluation of the World Health Organization classification of salivary gland tumors: a clinicopathologic study of 366 cases. Am J Clin Pathol 1977;67:272–8.

182. Spafford PD, Mintz DR, Hay J. Acinic cell carcinoma of the parotid gland: review and management. J Otolaryngol 1991;20:262–6.

183. Spiro RH. Salivary neoplasms: overview of a 35-year experience with 2,807 patients. Head Neck Surg 1986;8:177–84.

184. Spiro RH, Huvos AG, Strong EW. Acinic cell carcinoma of salivary origin. A clinicopathologic study of 67 cases. Cancer 1978;41:924–35.

185. Spitz MR, Batsakis JG. Major salivary gland carcinoma. Descriptive epidemiology and survival of 498 patients. Arch Otolaryngol 1984;110:45–9.

186. Stanley RJ, Weiland LH, Olsen KD, Pearson BW. Dedifferentiated acinic cell (acinous) carcinoma of the parotid gland. Otolaryngol Head Neck Surg 1988;98:155–61.

187. Takahashi H, Fujita S, Okabe H, Tsuda N, Tezuka F. Distribution of tissue markers in acinic cell carcinomas of salivary gland. Pathol Res Pract 1992;188:692–700.

188. Takahashi H, Fujita S, Tsuda N, Tezuka F, Okabe H. Intraoral minor salivary gland tumors: a demographic and histologic study of 200 cases. Tohoku J Exp Med 1990;161:111–28.

189. Thackray AC, Lucas RB. Tumors of the major salivary glands. Atlas of Tumor Pathology, 2nd Series, Fascicle 10. Washington, D.C.: Armed Forces Institute of Pathology, 1974:81–90.

190. Thackray AC, Sobin LH. Histological typing of salivary gland tumours. International histological classification of tumours No. 7. Geneva: World Health Organization, 1972.

191. Theron EJ, Middlecote BD. Tumours of the salivary glands. The Bloemfontein experience. S Afr J Surg 1984;22:237–42.

192. Thomas KM, Hutt MS, Borgstein J. Salivary gland tumors in Malawi. Cancer 1980;46:2328–34.

193. Timon CI, Dardick I, Panzarella T, et al. Acinic cell carcinoma of salivary glands: prognostic relevance of DNA flow cytometry and nucleolar organizer regions. Arch Otolaryngol Head Neck Surg 1994;120:727–33.

194. van Heerden WF, Raubenheimer EJ. Intraoral salivary gland neoplasms: a retrospective study of seventy cases in an African population. Oral Surg Oral Med Oral Pathol 1991;71:579–82.

195. Waldron CA, el-Mofty SK, Gnepp DR. Tumors of the intraoral minor salivary glands: a demographic and histologic study of 426 cases. Oral Surg Oral Med Oral Pathol 1988;66:323–33.

196. Yu GY, Ma DQ. Carcinoma of the salivary gland: a clinicopathologic study of 405 cases. Semin Surg Oncol 1987;3:240–4.

197. Zbaeren P, Lehmann W, Widgren S. Acinic cell carcinoma of minor salivary gland origin. J Laryngol Otol 1991;105:782–5.

Adenoid Cystic Carcinoma

198. Abiose BO, Oyejide O, Ogunniyi J. Salivary gland tumours in Ibadan, Nigeria: a study of 295 cases. Afr J Med Med Sci 1990;19:195–9.

199. Ampil FL, Misra RP. Factors influencing survival of patients with adenoid cystic carcinoma of the salivary glands. J Oral Maxillofac Surg 1987;45:1005–10.

200. Azumi N, Battifora H. The cellular composition of adenoid cystic carcinoma. An immunohistochemical study. Cancer 1987;60:1589–98.

201. Banks ER, Frierson HF Jr, Mills SE, George E, Zarbo RJ, Swanson PE. Basaloid squamous cell carcinoma of the head and neck. A clinicopathologic and immunohistochemical study of 40 cases. Am J Surg Pathol 1992;16:939–46.

202. Batsakis JG, Luna MA, el-Naggar A. Histopathologic grading of salivary gland neoplasms: III. Adenoid cystic carcinomas. Ann Otol Rhinol Laryngol 1990;99:1007–9.

203. Batsakis JG, Pinkston GR, Luna MA, Byers RM, Sciubba JJ, Tillery GW. Adenocarcinomas of the oral cavity: a clinicopathologic study of terminal duct carcinomas. J Laryngol Otol 1983;97:825–35.

204. Caselitz J, Becker J, Seifert G, Weber K, Osborn M. Coexpression of keratin and vimentin filaments in adenoid cystic carcinomas of salivary glands. Virchows Arch [A] 1984;403:337–44.

205. Caselitz J, Schulze I, Seifert G. Adenoid cystic carcinoma of the salivary glands: an immunohistochemical study. J Oral Pathol 1986;15:308–18.

206. Casler JD, Conley JJ. Surgical management of adenoid cystic carcinoma in the parotid gland. Otolaryngol Head Neck Surg 1992;106:332–8.

207. Chau MN, Radden BG. Intra-oral salivary gland neoplasms: a retrospective study of 98 cases. J Oral Pathol 1986;15:339–42.

208. Chaudhry AP, Leifer C, Cutler LS, Satchidanand S, Labay GR, Yamane GM. Histogenesis of adenoid cystic carcinoma of the salivary glands. Light and electron microscopic study. Cancer 1986;58:72–82.

209. Chen JC, Gnepp DR, Bedrossian CW. Adenoid cystic carcinoma of the salivary glands: an immunohistochemical analysis. Oral Surg Oral Med Oral Pathol 1988;65:316–26.

210. Chomette G, Auriol M, Vaillant JM, Kasai T, Niwa M, Mori M. An immunohistochemical study of the distribution of lysozyme, lactoferrin, alpha 1-antitrypsin and alpha 1-antichymotrypsin in salivary adenoid cystic carcinoma. Pathol Res Pract 1991;187:1001–8.

211. Chomette G, Auriol M, Vaillant JM, Kasai T, Okada Y, Mori M. Heterogeneity and co-expression of intermediate filament proteins in adenoid cystic carcinoma of salivary glands. Pathol Biol (Paris) 1991;39:110–6.

212. Cowie VJ, Pointon RC. Adenoid cystic carcinoma of the salivary glands. Clin Radiol 1984;35:331–3.

213. Crocker J, Jenkins R, Campbell J, Fuggle WJ, Shah VM. Immunohistochemical demonstration of S-100 protein in salivary gland neoplasms. J Pathol 1985;146:115–21.

214. d'Ardenne AJ, Kirkpatrick P, Wells CA, Davies JD. Laminin and fibronectin in adenoid cystic carcinoma. J Clin Pathol 1986;39:138–44.

215. Dal Maso M, Lippi L. Adenoid cystic carcinoma of the head and neck: a clinical study of 37 cases. Laryngoscope 1985;95:177–81.

216. Eibling DE, Johnson JT, McCoy JP Jr, et al. Flow cytometric evaluation of adenoid cystic carcinoma: correlation with histologic subtype and survival. Am J Surg 1991;162:367–72.

217. Eveson JW, Cawson RA. Tumours of the minor (oropharyngeal) salivary glands: a demographic study of 336 cases. J Oral Pathol 1985;14:500–9.

218. Fonseca I, Soares J. Adenoid cystic carcinoma: a study of nucleolar organizer regions (AgNOR) counts and their relation to prognosis. J Pathol 1993;169:255–8.

219. Franzén G, Klausen OG, Grenko RT, Carstensen J, Nordenskjld B. Adenoid cystic carcinoma: DNA as a prognostic indicator. Laryngoscope 1991;101:669–73.

220. Freedman PD, Lumerman H. Lobular carcinoma of intraoral minor salivary gland origin. Report of twelve cases. Oral Surg Oral Med Oral Pathol 1983;56:157–66.

221. Fujita S, Takahashi H, Okabe H. Nucleolar organizer regions in malignant salivary gland tumors. Acta Pathol Jpn 1992;42:727–33.

222. Gnepp DR, Chen JC, Warren C. Polymorphous low-grade adenocarcinoma of minor salivary gland. An immunohistochemical and clinicopathologic study. Am J Surg Pathol 1988;12:461–8.

223. Greiner TC, Robinson RA, Maves MD. Adenoid cystic carcinoma. A clinicopathologic study with flow cytometric analysis. Am J Clin Pathol 1989;92:711–20.

224. Gunhan O, Evren G, Demiriz M, Can C, Celasun B, Finci R. Expression of S-100 protein, epithelial membrane antigen, carcinoembryonic antigen and alpha fetoprotein in normal salivary glands and primary salivary gland tumors. J Nihon Univ Sch Dent 1992;34:240–8.

225. Gustafsson H, Carlsöö B, Kjrell U, Thornell LE. Immunohistochemical and ultrastructural observations on adenoid cystic carcinoma of salivary glands. With special reference to intermediate filaments and proteoglycan particles. Acta Otolaryngol (Stockh) 1986;102:152–60.

226. Gustafsson H, Virtanen I, Thornell LE. Glial fibrillary acidic protein and desmin in salivary neoplasms. Expression of four different types of intermediate filament proteins within the same cell type. Virchows Arch [Cell Pathol] 1989;57:303–13.

227. Hamper K, Lazar F, Dietel M, et al. Prognostic factors for adenoid cystic carcinoma of the head and neck: a retrospective evaluation of 96 cases. J Oral Pathol Med 1990;19:101–7.

228. Higashi K, Jin Y, Johansson M, et al. Rearrangement of 9p13 as the primary chromosomal aberration in adenoid cystic carcinoma of the respiratory tract. Genes Chromosom Cancer 1991;3:21–3.

229. Hirano T, Gluckman JL, deVries EJ. The expression of alpha vascular smooth-muscle actin in salivary gland tumors. Arch Otolaryngol Head Neck Surg 1990;116:692–6.

230. Horiuchi J, Shibuya H, Suzuki S, Takeda M, Takagi M. The role of radiotherapy in the management of adenoid cystic carcinoma of the head and neck. Int J Radiat Oncol Biol Phys 1987;13:1135–41.

231. Hosokawa Y, Ohmori K, Kaneko M, et al. Analysis of adenoid cystic carcinoma treated by radiotherapy. Oral Surg Oral Med Oral Pathol 1992;74:251–5.

232. Isacsson G, Shear M. Intraoral salivary gland tumors: a retrospective study of 201 cases. J Oral Pathol 1983; 12:57–62.

233. Koka VN, Tiwari RM, van der Waal I, et al. Adenoid cystic carcinoma of the salivary glands: clinicopathological survey of 51 patients. J Laryngol Otol 1989;103:675–9.

234. Luna MA, el Naggar A, Batsakis JG, Weber RS, Garnsey LA, Goepfert H. Flow cytometric DNA content of adenoid cystic carcinoma of submandibular gland. Correlation of histologic features and prognosis. Arch Otolaryngol Head Neck Surg 1990;116:1291–6.

235. Luna MA, el-Naggar A, Parichatikanond P, Weber RS, Batsakis JG. Basaloid squamous carcinoma of the upper aerodigestive tract. Clinicopathologic and DNA flow cytometric analysis. Cancer 1990;66:537–42.

236. Ma DQ, Yu GY. Tumours of the minor salivary glands. A clinicopathologic study of 243 cases. Acta Otolaryngol (Stockh) 1987;103:325–31.

237. Matsuba HM, Spector GJ, Thawley SE, Simpson JR, Mauney M, Pikul FJ. Adenoid cystic salivary gland carcinoma. A histopathologic review of treatment failure patterns. Cancer 1986;57:519–24.

238. Matsuba HM, Thawley SE, Simpson JR, Levine LA, Mauney M. Adenoid cystic carcinoma of major and minor salivary gland origin. Laryngoscope 1984;94:1316–8.

239. Matsumura K, Sasaki K, Tsuji T, Shinozaki F. The nucleolar organizer regions associated protein (AgNORs) in salivary gland tumors. Int J Oral Maxillofac Surg 1989;18:76–8.

240. Miller AS, Hartman GG, Chen SY, Edmonds PR, Brightman SA, Harwick RD. Estrogen receptor assay in polymorphous low-grade adenocarcinoma and adenoid cystic carcinoma of salivary gland origin. An immunohistochemical study. Oral Surg Oral Med Oral Pathol 1994;77:36–40.

241. Morgan DW, Crocker J, Watts A, Shenoi PM. Salivary gland tumours studied by means of the AgNOR technique. Histopathology 1988;13:553–9.

242. Mori M, Kasai T, Yuba R, Chomette G, Auriol M, Vaillant JM. Immunohistochemical studies of S-100 protein alpha and beta subunits in adenoid cystic carcinoma of salivary glands. Virchows Arch [Cell Pathol] 1990;59:115–23.

243. Morinaga S, Nakajima T, Shimosato Y. Normal and neoplastic myoepithelial cells in salivary glands: an immunohistochemical study. Hum Pathol 1987;18:1218–26.

244. Nakanishi K, Kawai T, Suzuki M, Shinmei M. Glycosaminoglycans in pleomorphic adenoma and adenoid cystic carcinoma of the salivary gland. Arch Pathol Lab Med 1990;114:1227–31.

245. Nakazato Y, Ishida Y, Takahashi K, Suzuki K. Immunohistochemical distribution of S-100 protein and glial fibrillary acidic protein in normal and neoplastic salivary glands. Virchows Arch [A] 1985;405:299–310.

246. Nara Y, Takeuchi J, Yoshida K, et al. Immunohistochemical characterisation of extracellular matrix components of salivary gland tumours. Br J Cancer 1991;64:307–14.

247. Nascimento AG, Amaral AL, Prado LA, Kligerman J, Silveira TR. Adenoid cystic carcinoma of salivary glands. A study of 61 cases with clinicopathologic correlation. Cancer 1986;57:312–9.

248. Orenstein JM, Dardick I, van Nostrand AW. Ultrastructural similarities of adenoid cystic carcinoma and pleomorphic adenoma. Histopathology 1985;9:623–38.

249. Ozono S, Onozuka M, Sato K, Ito Y. Immunohistochemical localization of estradiol, progesterone, and progesterone receptor in human salivary glands and salivary adenoid cystic carcinomas. Cell Struct Funct 1992;17:169–75.

250. Regezi JA, Lloyd RV, Zarbo RJ, McClatchey KD. Minor salivary gland tumors. A histologic and immunohistochemical study. Cancer 1985;55:108–15.

251. Regezi JA, Zarbo RJ, Stewart JC, Courtney RM. Polymorphous low-grade adenocarcinoma of minor salivary gland. A comparative histologic and immunohistochemical study. Oral Surg Oral Med Oral Pathol 1991;71:469–75.

252. Saka T, Yamamoto Y, Takahashi H. Comparative cytofluorometric DNA analysis of pleomorphic adenoma and adenoid cystic carcinoma of the salivary glands. Virchows Arch [Cell Pathol] 1991;61:255–61.

253. Saku T, Okabe H, Yagi Y, Sato E, Tsuda N. A comparative study on the immunolocalization of keratin and myosin in salivary gland tumors. Acta Pathol Jpn 1984;34:1031–40.

254. Santucci M, Bondi R. Histologic-prognostic correlations in adenoid cystic carcinoma of major and minor salivary glands of the oral cavity. Tumori 1986;72:293–300.

255. Santucci M, Bondi R. New prognostic criterion in adenoid cystic carcinoma of salivary gland origin. Am J Clin Pathol 1989;91:132–6.

256. Schramm VL Jr, Srodes C, Myers EN. Cisplatin therapy for adenoid cystic carcinoma. Arch Otolaryngol 1981;107:739–41.

257. Seifert G, Miehlke A, Haubrich J, Chilla R. Diseases of the salivary glands: pathology, diagnosis, treatment, facial nerve surgery. New York: Georg Thieme Verlag, 1986:239–47.

258. Sessions RB, Lehane DE, Smith RJ, Bryan RN, Suen JY. Intra-arterial cisplatin treatment of adenoid cystic carcinoma. Arch Otolaryngol 1982;108:221–4.

259. Shingaki S, Saito R, Kawasaki T, Nakajima T. Adenoid cystic carcinoma of the major and minor salivary glands. A clinicopathological study of 17 cases. J Maxillofac Surg 1986;14:53–6.

260. Shirasuna K, Watatani K, Furusawa H, et al. Biological characterization of pseudocyst-forming cell lines from human adenoid cystic carcinomas of minor salivary gland origin. Cancer Res 1990;50:4139–45.

261. Simpson JR, Thawley SE, Matsuba HM. Adenoid cystic salivary gland carcinoma: treatment with irradiation and surgery. Radiology 1984;151:509–12.

262. Simpson RH, Clarke TJ, Sarsfield PT, Gluckman PG, Babajews AV. Polymorphous low-grade adenocarcinoma of the salivary glands: a clinicopathological comparison with adenoid cystic carcinoma. Histopathology 1991;19:121–9.

263. Slichenmyer WJ, LeMaistre CF, Von Hoff DD. Response of metastatic adenoid cystic carcinoma and Merkel cell tumor to high-dose melphalan with autologous bone marrow transplantation. Invest New Drugs 1992;10:45–8.

264. Spiro RH. Salivary neoplasms: overview of a 35-year experience with 2,807 patients. Head Neck Surg 1986;8:177–84.

265. Spiro RH, Huvos AG. Stage means more than grade in adenoid cystic carcinoma. Am J Surg 1992;164:623–8.

266. Stell PM, Cruikshank AH, Stoney PJ, Canter R, McCormick MS. Adenoid cystic carcinoma: the results of radical surgery. Clin Otolaryngol 1985;10:205–8.

267. Stenman G, Sandros J, Dahlenfors R, Juberg-Ode M, Mark J. 6q- and loss of the Y chromosome—two common deviations in malignant human salivary gland tumors. Cancer Genet Cytogenet 1986;22:283–93.

268. Szanto PA, Luna MA, Tortoledo ME, White RA. Histologic grading of adenoid cystic carcinoma of the salivary glands. Cancer 1984;54:1062–9.

269. Takahashi H, Fujita S, Tsuda N, Tezuka F, Okabe H. Intraoral minor salivary gland tumors: a demographic and histologic study of 200 cases. Tohoku J Exp Med 1990;161:111–28.

270. Takahashi H, Fujita S, Tsuda N, Tezuka F, Okabe H. Iron-binding proteins in adenoid cystic carcinoma of salivary glands: an immunohistochemical study. Tohoku J Exp Med 1991;163:1–16.

271. Takahashi H, Tsuda N, Fujita S, Tezuka F, Okabe H. Immunohistochemical investigation of vimentin, neuron-specific enolase, alpha 1-antichymotrypsin and alpha 1-antitrypsin in adenoid cystic carcinoma of the salivary gland. Acta Pathol Jpn 1990;40:655–64.

272. Teshima T, Inoue T, Ikeda H, et al. Radiation therapy for carcinoma of the major salivary glands. Results of conventional irradiation technique. Strahlenther Onkol 1993;169:486–91.

273. Toida M, Takeuchi J, Sobue M, et al. Histochemical studies on pseudocysts in adenoid cystic carcinoma of the human salivary gland. Histochem J 1985;17:913–24.

274. Tomasino RM, Nuara R, Morello V, Florena AM, Daniele E. Pleomorphic adenoma and adenoid-cystic carcinoma of the salivary glands: comparative immunohistochemical patterns. Int J Biol Markers 1987;2:1–8.

275. Tran L, Sidrys J, Sadeghi A, Ellerbroek N, Hanson D, Parker RG. Salivary gland tumors of the oral cavity. Int J Radiat Oncol Biol Phys 1990;18:413–7.

276. van der Wal JE, Snow GB, Karim AB, van der Waal I. Intraoral adenoid cystic carcinoma: the role of postoperative radiotherapy in local control. Head Neck 1989;11:497–9.

277. van der Wal JE, Snow GB, van der Waal I. Intraoral adenoid cystic carcinoma. The presence of perineural spread in relation to site, size, local extension, and metastatic spread in 22 cases. Cancer 1990;66:2031–3.

278. van Heerden WF, Raubenheimer EJ. Evaluation of the nucleolar organizer region associated proteins in minor salivary gland tumors. J Oral Pathol Med 1991;20:291–5.

279. Vikram B, Strong EW, Shah JP, Spiro RH. Radiation therapy in adenoid-cystic carcinoma. Int J Radiat Oncol Biol Phys 1984;10:221–3.

280. Vrielinck LJ, Ostyn F, van Damme B, van den Bogaert W, Fossion E. The significance of perineural spread in adenoid cystic carcinoma of the major and minor salivary glands. Int J Oral Maxillofac Surg 1988;17:190–3.

281. Wain SL, Kier R, Vollmer RT, Bossen EH. Basaloid-squamous carcinoma of the tongue, hypopharynx, and larynx: report of 10 cases. Hum Pathol 1986;17:1158–66.

282. Waldron CA, el-Mofty SK, Gnepp DR. Tumors of the intraoral minor salivary glands: a demographic and histologic study of 426 cases. Oral Surg Oral Med Oral Pathol 1988;66:323–33.

283. Yamamoto Y, Saka T, Makimoto K, Takahashi H. Histological changes during progression of adenoid cystic carcinoma. J Laryngol Otol 1992;106:1016–20.

Polymorphous Low-Grade Adenocarcinoma

284. Aberle AM, Abrams AM, Bowe R, Melrose RJ, Handlers JP. Lobular (polymorphous low-grade) carcinoma of minor salivary glands. A clinicopathologic study of twenty cases. Oral Surg Oral Med Oral Pathol 1985;60:387–95.

285. Anderson C, Krutchkoff D, Pedersen C, Cartun R, Berman M. Polymorphous low grade adenocarcinoma of minor salivary gland: a clinicopathologic and comparative immunohistochemical study. Mod Pathol 1990;3:76–82.

286. Batsakis JG, Pinkston GR, Luna MA, Byers RM, Sciubba JJ, Tillery GW. Adenocarcinomas of the oral cavity: a clinicopathologic study of terminal duct carcinomas. J Laryngol Otol 1983;97:825–35.

287. Brocheriou C. Adénocarcinome polymorphe de faible malignité des glands salivaires accessoires. Sept observations. Arch Anat Cytol Pathol 1992;40:66–72.

288. Cleveland DB, Cosgrove MM, Martin SE. Tyrosine-rich crystalloids in a fine needle aspirate of a polymorphous low grade adenocarcinoma of a minor salivary gland. A case report. Acta Cytol 1994;38:247–51.

289. Dardick I, van Nostrand AW. Polymorphous low-grade adenocarcinoma: a case report with ultrastructural findings. Oral Surg Oral Med Oral Pathol 1988;66:459–65.

290. Evans HL, Batsakis JG. Polymorphous low-grade adenocarcinoma of minor salivary glands. A study of 14 cases of a distinctive neoplasm. Cancer 1984;53:935–42.

291. Fliss DM, Zirkin H, Puterman M, Tovi F. Low-grade papillary adenocarcinoma of buccal mucosa salivary gland origin. Head Neck 1989;11:237–41.

292. Freedman PD, Lumerman H. Lobular carcinoma of intraoral minor salivary gland origin. Report of twelve cases. Oral Surg Oral Med Oral Pathol 1983;56:157–65.

293. Frierson HF Jr. Pathologic quiz case 1, Polymorphous low-grade adenocarcinoma of minor salivary gland. Arch Otolaryngol Head Neck Surg 1986;112:568–70.

294. Frierson HF Jr, Mills SE, Garland TA. Terminal duct carcinoma of minor salivary glands. A nonpapillary subtype of polymorphous low-grade adenocarcinoma. Am J Clin Pathol 1985;84:8–14.

295. George MK, Mansour P, Pahor AL. Terminal parotid duct carcinoma. J Laryngol Otol 1991;105:780–1.

296. Gnepp DR, Chen JC, Warren C. Polymorphous low-grade adenocarcinoma of minor salivary gland. An immunohistochemical and clinicopathologic study. Am J Surg Pathol 1988;12:461–8.

297. Haba R, Kobayashi S, Miki H, et al. Polymorphous low-grade adenocarcinoma of submandibular gland origin. Acta Pathol Jpn 1993;43:774–8.

298. Iwasaki K, Ono I, Ebihara S: Clinicopathologic study of salivary gland adenocarcinomas. Nippon Jibiinkoka Gakka Kaiho 1989;92:2047–54.

299. Katoh T, Yoshihara T, Naitoh J, et al. A case of polymorphous adenocarcinoma in the right parotid gland. Gan No Rinsho 1985;31:861–4.

300. Luna MA, Batsakis JG, Ordóñez NG, Mackay B, Tortoledo ME. Salivary gland adenocarcinomas: a clinicopathologic analysis of three distinctive types. Semin Diagn Pathol 1987;4:117–35.

301. Miliauskas JR. Polymorphous low-grade (terminal duct) adenocarcinoma of the parotid gland. Histopathology 1991;19:555–7.

302. Mills SE, Garland TA, Allen MS Jr. Low-grade papillary adenocarcinoma of palatal salivary gland origin. Am J Surg Pathol 1984;8:367–74.

303. Nicolatou O, Kakarantza-Angelopoulou E, Angelopoulos AP, Anagnostopoulou S. Polymorphous low-grade adenocarcinoma of the palate: report of a case with electron microscopy. J Oral Maxillofac Surg 1988;46:1008–13.

304. Norberg LE, Burford-Mason AP, Dardick I. Cellular differentiation and morphologic heterogeneity in polymorphous low-grade adenocarcinoma of minor salivary gland. J Oral Pathol Med 1991;20:373–9.

305. Raubenheimer EJ, van Heerden WF, Thein T. Tyrosine-rich crystalloids in a polymorphous low-grade adenocarcinoma. Oral Surg Oral Med Oral Pathol 1990;70:480–2.

306. Regezi JA, Zarbo RJ, Stewart JC, Courtney RM. Polymorphous low-grade adenocarcinoma of minor salivary gland. A comparative histologic and immunohistochemical study. Oral Surg Oral Med Oral Pathol 1991;71:469–75.

307. Ritland F, Lubensky I, LiVolsi VA. Polymorphous low-grade adenocarcinoma of the parotid salivary gland. Arch Pathol Lab Med 1993;117:1261–3.

308. Seifert G, Sobin LH. Histological classification of salivary gland tumours. World Health Organization. International histological classification of tumours. 2nd ed. Berlin: Springer-Verlag, 1991:28.

309. Simpson RH, Clarke TJ, Sarsfield PT, Gluckman PG, Babajews AV. Polymorphous low-grade adenocarcinoma of the salivary glands: a clinicopathological comparison with adenoid cystic carcinoma. Histopathology 1991;19:121–9.

310. Slootweg PJ. Low-grade adenocarcinoma of the oral cavity: polymorphous or papillary? J Oral Pathol Med 1993;22:327–30.

311. Slootweg PJ, Muller H. Low-grade adenocarcinoma of the oral cavity. A comparison between the terminal duct and the papillary type. J Craniomaxillofac Surg 1987;15:359–64.

312. Tortoledo ME, Luna MA, Batsakis JG. Carcinomas ex pleomorphic adenoma and malignant mixed tumors. Histomorphologic indexes. Arch Otolaryngol Head Neck Surg 1984;110:172–6.

313. van Heerden WF, Raubenheimer EJ. Intraoral salivary gland neoplasms: a retrospective study of seventy cases in an African population. Oral Surg Oral Med Oral Pathol 1991;71:579–82.

314. Vincent SD, Hammond HL, Finkelstein MW. Clinical and therapeutic features of polymorphous low-grade adenocarcinoma. Oral Surg Oral Med Oral Pathol 1994;77:41–7.

315. Waldron CA, el-Mofty SK, Gnepp DR. Tumors of the intraoral minor salivary glands: a demographic and histologic study of 426 cases. Oral Surg Oral Med Oral Pathol 1988;66:323–33.

316. Wenig BM, Gnepp DR. Polymorphous low-grade adenocarcinoma of minor salivary glands. In: Ellis GL, Auclair PL, Gnepp DR, eds. Surgical pathology of the salivary glands. Philadelphia: WB Saunders, 1991:390–411.

317. Wenig BM, Harpaz N, DelBridge C. Polymorphous low-grade adenocarcinoma of seromucous glands of the nasopharynx. A report of a case and a discussion of the morphologic and immunohistochemical features. Am J Clin Pathol 1989;92:104–9.

Carcinoma Ex Mixed Tumor

318. Boles R, Raines J, Lebovits M, Fu KK. Malignant tumors of salivary glands. A university experience. Laryngoscope 1980;90:729–36.

319. Dardick I, Hardie J, Thomas MJ, van Nostrand AW. Ultrastructural contributions to the study of morphological differentiation in malignant mixed (pleomorphic) tumors of salivary gland. Head Neck 1989;11:5–21.

320. Duck SW, McConnel FM. Malignant degeneration of pleomorphic adenoma—clinical implications. Am J Otolaryngol 1993;14:175–8.

321. Eneroth CM. Die klinik der kopfspeicheldrüsentumoren. Arch Otorhinolaryngol 1976;213:61–110.

322. Eneroth CM, Blanck C, Jakobsson PA. Carcinoma in pleomorphic adenoma of the parotid gland. Acta Otolaryngol (Stockh) 1968;66:477–92.

323. Eneroth CM, Zetterberg A. Malignancy in pleomorphic adenoma. A clinical and microspectrophotometric study. Acta Otolaryngol (Stockh) 1974;77:426–32.

324. Eneroth CM, Zetterberg A. Microspectrophotometric DNA analysis of malignant salivary gland tumours. Acta Otolaryngol (Stockh) 1974;77:289–94.

325. Gerughty RM, Scofield HH, Brown FM, Hennigar GR. Malignant mixed tumors of salivary gland origin. Cancer 1969;24:471–86.

326. Gnepp DR. Malignant mixed tumors of the salivary glands: a review. Pathol Annu 1993;28 (Pt 1):279–328.

327. Hickman RE, Cawson RA, Duffy SW. The prognosis of specific types of salivary gland tumors. Cancer 1984;54:1620–4.

328. Jacobs JC. Low grade mucoepidermoid carcinoma ex pleomorphic adenoma. A diagnostic problem in fine needle aspiration biopsy. Acta Cytol 1994;38:93–7.

329. Krolls SO, Trodahl JN, Boyers RC. Salivary gland lesions in children. A survey of 430 cases. Cancer 1972;30:459–69.

330. Lack EE, Upton MP. Histopathologic review of salivary gland tumors in childhood. Arch Otolaryngol Head Neck Surg 1988;114:898–906.

331. Littman CD, Alguacil-Garcia A. Clear cell carcinoma arising in pleomorphic adenoma of the salivary gland. Am J Clin Pathol 1987;88:239–43.

332. LiVolsi VA, Perzin KH. Malignant mixed tumors arising in salivary glands. I. Carcinomas arising in benign mixed tumors: a clinicopathologic study. Cancer 1977;39:2209–30.

333. Luna MA, Stimson PG, Bardwil JM. Minor salivary gland tumors of the oral cavity. A review of sixty-eight cases. Oral Surg Oral Med Oral Pathol 1968;25:71–86.

334. Moberger JG, Eneroth CM. Malignant mixed tumors of the major salivary glands. Special reference to the histologic structure in metastases. Cancer 1968;21:1198–211.

335. Nagao K, Matsuzaki O, Saiga H, et al. Histopathologic studies on carcinoma in pleomorphic adenoma of the parotid gland. Cancer 1981;48:113–21.

336. Seifert G, Miehlke A, Haubrich J, Chilla R. Diseases of the salivary glands: diagnosis, pathology, treament, facial nerve surgery. Stuttgart: Georg Thieme Verlag, 1986:222–81.

337. Seifert G, Sobin LH. Histological classification of salivary gland tumours. World Health Organization. International histological classification of tumours. 2nd ed. Berlin: Springer-Verlag, 1991:29.

338. Shrikhande SS, Talvalkar GV. Malignant mixed salivary gland tumors—a clinico-pathological study of 48 cases. Indian J Cancer 1979;16:9–12.

339. Spiro RH. Salivary neoplasms: overview of a 35-year experience with 2,807 patients. Head Neck Surg 1986;8:177–84.

340. Spiro RH, Huvos AG, Strong EW. Malignant mixed tumor of salivary origin: a clinicopathologic study of 146 cases. Cancer 1977;39:388–96.

341. Spitz MR, Batsakis JG. Major salivary gland carcinoma. Descriptive epidemiology and survival of 498 patients. Arch Otolaryngol Head Neck Surg 1984;110:45-9.

342. Tortoledo ME, Luna MA, Batsakis JG. Carcinomas ex pleomorphic adenoma and malignant mixed tumors. Histomorphologic indexes. Arch Otolaryngol Head Neck Surg 1984;110:172–6.

Carcinosarcoma

343. Auclair PL, Ellis GL. Nonlymphoid sarcomas of the major salivary glands. In: Ellis GL, Auclair PL, Gnepp DR, eds. Surgical pathology of the salivary glands. Philadelphia: WB Saunders, 1991:514–27.

344. Auclair PL, Langloss JM, Weiss SW, Corio RL. Sarcomas and sarcomatoid neoplasms of the major salivary gland regions. A clinicopathologic and immunohistochemical study of 67 cases and review of the literature. Cancer 1986;58:1305–15.

345. Bleiweiss IJ, Huvos AG, Lara J, Strong EW. Carcinosarcoma of the submandibular salivary gland. Immunohistochemical findings. Cancer 1992;69:2031–5.

346. Chen KT, Weinberg RA, Moseley D. Carcinosarcoma of the salivary gland. Am J Otolaryngol 1984;5:415–7.

347. Dardick I, Hardie J, Thomas MJ, van Nostrand AW. Ultrastructural contributions to the study of morphological differentiation in malignant mixed (pleomorphic) tumors of salivary gland. Head Neck 1989;11:5–21.

348. Ellis GL, Corio RL. Spindle cell carcinoma of the oral cavity. A clinicopathologic assessment of fifty-nine cases. Oral Surg Oral Med Oral Pathol 1980;50:523–33.

349. Eusebi V, Martin SA, Govoni E, Rosai J. Giant cell tumor of major salivary glands: report of three cases, one occurring in association with a malignant mixed tumor. Am J Clin Pathol 1984;81:666–75.

350. Garner SL, Robinson RA, Maves MD, Barnes CH. Salivary gland carcinosarcoma: true malignant mixed tumor. Ann Otol Rhinol Laryngol 1989;98:611–4.

351. Granger JK, Houn HY. Malignant mixed tumor (carcinosarcoma) of parotid gland diagnosed by fine-needle aspiration biopsy. Diagn Cytopathol 1991;7:427–32.

352. Grenko RT, Tytor M, Boeryd B. Giant-cell tumour of the salivary gland with associated carcinosarcoma. Histopathology 1993;23:594–5.

353. Hellquist H, Michaels L. Malignant mixed tumour. A salivary gland tumour showing both carcinomatous and sarcomatous features. Virchows Arch [A] 1986;409:93–103.

354. Huntington HW, Dardick I. Intracranial metastasis from a malignant mixed tumor of parotid salivary gland. Ultrastruct Pathol 1985;9:169–73.

355. King OH, Jr. Carcinosarcoma of accessory salivary gland. First report of a case. Oral Surg Oral Med Oral Pathol 1967;23:651–9.

356. Kirklin JW, McDonald JR, Harrington SW, New GB. Parotid tumors: histopathology, clinical behavior and end results. Surg Gynecol Obstet 1951;92:721–33.

357. Rumnong V, Banerjee AK, Joshi K, Kataria RN. Carcinosarcoma of parotid gland having osteosarcoma as sarcomatous component: a case report. Indian J Pathol Microbiol 1993;36:492–4.

358. Seifert G, Sobin LH. Histological typing of salivary gland tumours. World Health Organization international histological classification of tumours. 2nd ed. New York: Springer-Verlag, 1991.

359. Stephen J, Batsakis JG, Luna MA, von der Heyden U, Byers RM. True malignant mixed tumors (carcinosarcoma) of salivary glands. Oral Surg Oral Med Oral Pathol 1986;61:597–602.

360. Suzuki J, Takagi M, Okada N, Hatakeyama S, Yamamoto H. Carcinosarcoma of the submandibular gland. An autopsy case. Acta Pathol Jpn 1990;40:827–31.

361. Takata T, Nikai H, Ogawa I, Ijuhin N. Ultrastructural and immunohistochemical observations of a true malignant mixed tumor (carcinosarcoma) of the tongue. J Oral Pathol Med 1990;19:261–5.

362. Tortoledo ME, Luna MA, Batsakis JG. Carcinomas ex pleomorphic adenoma and malignant mixed tumors. Histomorphologic indexes. Arch Otolaryngol 1984; 110:172–6.

363. Toynton SC, Wilkins MJ, Cook HT, Stafford ND. True malignant mixed tumour of a minor salivary gland. J Laryngol Otol 1994;108:76–9.

364. Yamashita T, Kameda N, Katayama K, Hiruta N, Nakada M, Takeda Y. True malignant mixed tumor of the submandibular gland. Acta Pathol Jpn 1990; 40:137–42.

Metastasizing Mixed Tumor

365. Chen KT. Metastasizing pleomorphic adenoma of the salivary gland. Cancer 1978;42:2407–11.

366. Collina G, Eusebi V, Carasoli PT. Pleomorphic adenoma with lymph-node metastases report of two cases. Pathol Res Pract 1989;184:188–93.

367. Cresson DH, Goldsmith M, Askin FB, Reddick RL, Postma DS, Siegal GP. Metastatic pleomorphic adenoma with myoepithelial cell predominance [Discussion]. Pathol Res Pract 1990;186:795–800.

368. el-Naggar A, Batsakis JG, Kessler S. Benign metastatic mixed tumours or unrecognized salivary carcinomas? J Laryngol Otol 1988;102:810–2.

369. Freeman SB, Kennedy KS, Parker GS, Tatum SA. Metastasizing pleomorphic adenoma of the nasal septum. Arch Otolaryngol Head Neck Surg 1990;116:1331–3.

370. Gnepp DR, Wenig BM. Malignant mixed tumors. In: Ellis GL, Auclair PL, Gnepp DR, eds. Surgical pathology of the salivary glands. Philadelphia: WB Saunders, 1991:350–68.

371. Hellquist H, Michaels L. Malignant mixed tumour. A salivary gland tumour showing both carcinomatous and sarcomatous features. Virchows Arch [A] 1986;409:93–103.

372. Minic AJ. Unusual variant of a metastasizing malignant mixed tumor of the parotid gland. Oral Surg Oral Med Oral Pathol 1993;76:330–2.

373. Moberger JG, Eneroth CM. Malignant mixed tumors of the major salivary glands. Special reference to the histologic structure in metastases. Cancer 1968;21:1198–211.

374. Morrison PD, McMullin JP. A case of metastasizing benign pleomorphic adenoma of the parotid. Clin Oncol 1984;10:173–6.

375. Pitman MB, Thor AD, Goodman ML, Rosenberg AE. Benign metastasizing pleomorphic adenoma of salivary gland: diagnosis of bone lesions by fine-needle aspiration biopsy. Diagn Cytopathol 1992;8:384–7.

376. Seifert G, Miehlke A, Haubrich J, Chilla R. Diseases of the salivary glands: pathology, diagnosis, treatment, facial nerve surgery. New York: Georg Thieme Verlag, 1986:182–94.

377. Sim DW, Maran AG, Harris D. Metastatic salivary pleomorphic adenoma. J Laryngol Otol 1990;104:45–7.

378. Wenig BM, Hitchcock CL, Ellis GL, Gnepp DR. Metastasizing mixed tumor of salivary glands. A clinicopathologic and flow cytometric analysis. Am J Surg Pathol 1992;16:845–58.

379. Wermuth DJ, Mann CH, Odere F. Metastasizing pleomorphic adenoma arising in the soft palate. Otolaryngol Head Neck Surg 1988;99:505–8.

380. Youngs GR, Scheuer PJ. Histologically benign mixed parotid tumour with hepatic metastasis. J Pathol 1973;109:171–2.

Primary Squamous Cell Carcinoma

381. Baker SR, Malone B. Salivary gland malignancies in children. Cancer 1985;55:1730–6.

382. Batsakis JG, McClatchey KD, Johns M, Regazi J. Primary squamous cell carcinoma of the parotid gland. Arch Otolaryngol Head Neck Surg 1976;102:355–7.

383. Bissett RJ, Fitzpatrick PJ. Malignant submandibular gland tumors. A review of 91 patients [published erratum appears in Am J Clin Oncol 1988 Aug;11(4):514]. Am J Clin Oncol 1988;11:46–51.

384. Brauneis J, Laskawi R, Schrder M, Eilts M. Plattenepithelkarcinome im bereich der glandula parotis gland. Metastase oder primärtumor? HNO 1990;38:292–4.

385. Chau MN, Radden BG. Intra-oral salivary gland neoplasms: a retrospective study of 98 cases. J Oral Pathol 1986;15:339–42.

386. Conley J, Hamaker RC. Prognosis of malignant tumors of the parotid gland with facial paralysis. Arch Otolaryngol Head Neck Surg 1975;101:39–41.

387. Eneroth CM, Hjertman L, Moberger G. Malignant tumours of the submandibular gland. Acta Otolaryngol (Stockh) 1967;64:514–36.

388. Eveson JW, Cawson RA. Salivary gland tumours. A review of 2410 cases with particular reference to histological types, site, age and sex distribution. J Pathol 1985;146:51–8.

389. Friedman M, Levin B, Grybauskas V, et al. Malignant tumors of the major salivary glands. Otolaryngol Clin North Am 1986;19:625–36.

390. Gaughan RK, Olsen KD, Lewis JE. Primary squamous cell carcinoma of the parotid gland. Arch Otolaryngol Head Neck Surg 1992;118:798–801.

391. Isacsson G, Shear M. Intraoral salivary gland tumors: a retrospective study of 201 cases. J Oral Pathol 1983;12:57–62.

392. Ju DM. Salivary gland tumors occurring after radiation of the head and neck area. Am J Surg 1968;116:518–23.

393. Katsantonis GP, Friedman WH, Rosenblum BN. The surgical management of advanced malignancies of the parotid gland. Otolaryngol Head Neck Surg 1989;101:633–40.

394. Leader M, Jass JR. In-situ neoplasia in squamous cell carcinoma of the parotid. A case report. Histopathology 1985;9:325–9.

395. Lee K, McKean ME, McGregor IA. Metastatic patterns of squamous carcinoma in the parotid lymph nodes. Br J Plast Surg 1985;38:6–10.

396. Marks MW, Ryan RF, Litwin MS, Sonntag BV. Squamous cell carcinoma of the parotid gland. Plast Reconstr Surg 1987;79:550–4.

397. Rasp G, Permanetter W. Malignant salivary gland tumors: squamous cell carcinoma of the submandibular gland in a child. Am J Otolaryngol 1992;13:109–12.

398. Reddy SP, Marks JE. Treatment of locally advanced, high-grade, malignant tumors of major salivary glands. Laryngoscope 1988;98:450–4.

399. Ridenhour CE, Spratt JS Jr. Epidermoid carcinoma of the skin involving the parotid gland. Am J Surg 1966;112:504–7.

400. Schneider AB, Favus MJ, Stachura ME, Arnold MJ, Frohman LA. Salivary gland neoplasms as a late consequence of head and neck irradiation. Ann Intern Med 1977;87:160–4.

401. Seifert G, Miehlke A, Haubrich J, Chilla R. Diseases of the salivary glands: diagnosis, pathology, treament, facial nerve surgery. Stuttgart: Georg Thieme Verlag, 1986:222–81.

402. Shemen LJ, Huvos AG, Spiro RH. Squamous cell carcinoma of salivary gland origin. Head Neck Surg 1987;9:235–40.

403. Spiro RH. Salivary neoplasms: overview of a 35-year experience with 2,807 patients. Head Neck Surg 1986;8:177–84.
404. Spiro RH, Hajdu SI, Strong EW. Tumors of the submaxillary gland. Am J Surg 1976;132:463–8.
405. Spitz MR, Batsakis JG. Major salivary gland carcinoma. Descriptive epidemiology and survival of 498 patients. Arch Otolaryngol Head Neck Surg 1984;110:45–9.
406. Sterman BM, Kraus DH, Sebek BA, Tucker HM. Primary squamous cell carcinoma of the parotid gland. Laryngoscope 1990;100:146–8.
407. Takata T, Caselitz J, Seifert G. Undifferentiated tumours of salivary glands. Immunocytochemical investigations and differential diagnosis of 22 cases. Pathol Res Pract 1987;182:161–8.
408. Teshima T, Inoue T, Ikeda H, et al. Radiation therapy for carcinoma of the major salivary glands. Results of

409. Thackray AC, Lucas RB. Tumors of the major salivary glands. Atlas of Tumor Pathology, 2nd Series, Fascicle 10. Washington, D.C.: Armed Forces Institute of Pathology, 1974:100–1.
410. Tran L, Sadeghi A, Hanson D, et al. Major salivary gland tumors: treatment results and prognostic factors. Laryngoscope 1986;96:1139–44.
411. Tu G, Hu Y, Jiang P, Qin D. The superiority of combined therapy (surgery and postoperative irradiation) in parotid cancer. Arch Otolaryngol Head Neck Surg 1982;108:710–3.
412. Vigorita VJ, Huvos AG, Gerold F. Squamous-cell carcinoma of Stensen's duct. Head Neck Surg 1980;2:513–7.
413. Woods JE, Chong GC, Beahrs OH. Experience with 1,360 primary parotid tumors. Am J Surg 1975;130:460–2.

conventional irradiation technique. Strahlenther Onkol 1993;169:486–91.

Basal Cell Adenocarcinoma

414. Adkins GF. Low grade basaloid adenocarcinoma of salivary gland in childhood—the so-called hybrid basal cell adenoma—adenoid cystic carcinoma. Pathology 1990;22:187–90.
415. Atula T, Klemi PJ, Donath K, Happonen RP, Joensuu H, Grenman R. Basal cell adenocarcinoma of the parotid gland: a case report and review of the literature. J Laryngol Otol 1993;107:862–4.
416. Banks ER, Frierson HF Jr, Mills SE, George E, Zarbo RJ, Swanson PE. Basaloid squamous cell carcinoma of the head and neck. A clinicopathologic and immunohistochemical study of 40 cases. Am J Surg Pathol 1992;16:939–46.
417. Batsakis JG, Brannon RB, Sciubba JJ. Monomorphic adenomas of major salivary glands: a histologic study of 96 tumours. Clin Otolaryngol 1981;6:129–43.
418. Batsakis JG, Luna MA. Basaloid salivary carcinoma. Ann Otol Rhinol Laryngol 1991;100:785–7.
419. Bernacki EG, Batsakis JG, Johns ME. Basal cell adenoma. Distinctive tumor of salivary glands. Arch Otolaryngol 1974;99:84–7.
420. Cadier MA, Kelly SA, Parkhouse N, Brough MD. Basaloid squamous carcinoma of the buccal cavity. Head Neck 1992;14:387–91.
421. Chen KT. Carcinoma arising in monomorphic adenoma of the salivary gland. Am J Otolaryngol 1985;6:39–41.
422. Chomette G, Auriol M, Vaillant JM, Kasai T, Okada Y, Mori M. Basaloid carcinoma of salivary glands, a variety of undifferentiated adenocarcinoma. Immunohistochemical study of intermediate filament proteins in 24 cases. J Pathol 1991;163:39–45.
423. Ellis GL, Wiscovitch JG. Basal cell adenocarcinomas of the major salivary glands. Oral Surg Oral Med Oral Pathol 1990;69:461–9.
424. Evans RW, Cruickshank AH. Epithelial tumours of the salivary glands. Philadelphia: WB Saunders, 1970:254.
425. Evans RW, Cruickshank AH. Epithelial tumours of the salivary glands. Philadelphia: WB Saunders, 1970:58–76.
426. Hyma BA, Scheithauer BW, Weiland LH, Irons GB. Membranous basal cell adenoma of the parotid gland. Malignant transformation in a patient with multiple dermal cylindromas. Arch Pathol Lab Med 1988;112:209–11.
427. Klima M, Wolfe K, Johnson PE. Basal cell tumors of the parotid gland. Arch Otolaryngol 1978;104:111–6.

428. Lo AK, Topf JS, Jackson IT, Silberberg B. Minor salivary gland basal cell adenocarcinoma of the palate. J Oral Maxillofac Surg 1992;50:531–4.
429. Luna MA, Batsakis JG, Tortoledo ME, del Junco GW. Carcinomas ex monomorphic adenoma of salivary glands. J Laryngol Otol 1989;103:756–9.
430. Luna MA, el Naggar A, Parichatikanond P, Weber RS, Batsakis JG. Basaloid squamous carcinoma of the upper aerodigestive tract. Clinicopathologic and DNA flow cytometric analysis. Cancer 1990;66:537–42.
431. Luna MA, Tortoledo ME, Allen M. Salivary dermal analogue tumors arising in lymph nodes. Cancer 1987;59:1165–9.
432. Murty GE, Welch AR, Soames JV. Basal cell adenocarcinoma of the parotid gland. J Laryngol Otol 1990;104:150–1.
433. Pingitore R, Campani D. Salivary gland involvement in a case of dermal eccrine cylindroma of the scalp (turban tumor). Report of a case with lung metastases. Tumori 1984;70:385–8.
434. Seifert G, Miehlke A, Haubrich J, Chilla R. Diseases of the salivary glands: pathology, diagnosis, treatment, facial nerve surgery. New York: Georg Thieme Verlag, 1986:273.
435. Seifert G, Sobin LH. Histological typing of salivary gland tumours. World Health Organization international histological classification of tumours. 2nd ed. New York: Springer-Verlag, 1991.
436. Simpson PR, Rutledge JC, Schaefer SD, Anderson RC. Congenital hybrid basal cell adenoma—adenoid cystic carcinoma of the salivary gland. Pediatr Pathol 1986;6:199–208.
437. Strauss M, Abt A, Mahataphongse VP, Conner GH. Basal cell adenoma of the major salivary glands. Report of a case with facial nerve encroachment. Arch Otolaryngol 1981;107:120–4.
438. Wain SL, Kier R, Vollmer RT, Bossen EH. Basaloid-squamous carcinoma of the tongue, hypopharynx, and larynx: report of 10 cases. Hum Pathol 1986;17:1158–66.
439. Warnock GR, Jensen JL, Kratochvil FJ. Developmental diseases. In: Ellis GL, Auclair PL, Gnepp DR, eds. Surgical pathology of the salivary glands. Philadelphia: WB Saunders, 1991:10–25.
440. Williams SB, Ellis GL, Auclair PL. Immunohistochemical analysis of basal cell adenocarcinoma. Oral Surg Oral Med Oral Pathol 1993;75:64–9.

Epithelial-Myoepithelial Carcinoma

441. Adlam DM. The monomorphic clear cell tumor: a report of two cases. Br J Oral Maxillofac Surg 1986;24:130–6.
442. Batsakis JG, el-Naggar AK, Luna MA. Epithelial-myoepithelial carcinoma of salivary glands. Ann Otol Rhinol Laryngol 1992;101:540–2.
443. Bauer WH, Fox RA. Adenomyoepithelioma (cylindroma) of palatal mucous glands. Arch Pathol 1945;39:96–102.
444. Chaudhry AP, Cutler LS, Satchidanand S, Labay G, Raj MS, Lin CC. Glycogen-rich tumor of the oral minor salivary glands. A histochemical and ultrastructural study. Cancer 1983;52:105–11.
445. Chen KT. Clear cell carcinoma of the salivary gland. Hum Pathol 1983;14:91–3.
446. Collina G, Gale N, Visona A, Betts CM, Cenacchi V, Eusebi V. Epithelial-myoepithelial carcinoma of the parotid gland: a clinico-pathologic and immunohistochemical study of seven cases. Tumori 1991;77:257–63.
447. Corio RL, Sciubba JJ, Brannon RB, Batsakis JG. Epithelial-myoepithelial carcinoma of intercalated duct origin. A clinicopathologic and ultrastructural assessment of sixteen cases. Oral Surg Oral Med Oral Pathol 1982;53:280–7.
448. Corridan M. Glycogen-rich clear-cell adenoma of the parotid gland. J Pathol Bacteriol 1956;72:623–6.
449. Daley TD, Wysocki GP, Smout MS, Slinger RP. Epithelial-myoepithelial carcinoma of salivary glands. Oral Surg Oral Med Oral Pathol 1984;57:512–9.
450. de Araújo VC, de Araújo NS. Vimentin as a marker of myoepithelial cells in salivary gland tumors. Eur Arch Otorhinolaryngol 1990;247:252–5.
451. Donath K, Seifert G, Schmitz R. Diagnose und ultrastruktur des tubulären speichelgangcarcinoms. Epithelial-myoepitheliales schaltstüstuckcarcinom. Virchows Arch [A] 1972;356:16–31.
452. Feyrter F. Cher das solide (tubular-solide) adenom de schlerm und speicheldrusen. Frankfurt Z Pathol 1964;71:300–26.
453. Fonseca I, Soares J. Epithelial-myoepithelial carcinoma of the salivary glands. A study of 22 cases. Virchows Arch [A] 1993;422:389–96.
454. Goldman RL, Klein HZ. Glycogen-rich adenoma of the parotid gland. An uncommon benign clear-cell tumor resembling certain clear-cell carcinomas of salivary origin. Cancer 1972;30:749–54.
455. Hamper K, Brügmann M, Koppermann R, et al. Epithelial-myoepithelial duct carcinoma of salivary glands: a follow-up and cytophotometric study of 21 cases. J Oral Pathol Med 1989;18:299–304.
456. Kleinsasser O, Klein HJ, Hbner G. Speichelgangearcinom. Ein den milchgangcarcinomen der brustdräse analoge gruppe von speichldräsentumoren. Arch Klin Exp Ohren Nasen Kehlkopfheilkd 1968;192:100–5.
457. Lattanzi DA, Polverini P, Chin DC. Glycogen-rich adenocarcinoma of a minor salivary gland. J Oral Maxillofac Surg 1985;43:122–4.
458. Luna MA, Batsakis JG, Ordóñez NG, Mackay B, Tortoledo ME. Salivary gland adenocarcinomas: a clinicopathologic analysis of three distinctive types. Semin Diagn Pathol 1987;4:117–35.
459. Luna MA, Ordóñez NG, Mackay B, Batsakis JG, Guillamondegui O. Salivary epithelial-myoepithelial carcinomas of intercalated ducts: a clinical, electron microscopic, and immunocytochemical study. Oral Surg Oral Med Oral Pathol 1985;59:482–90.
460. Mohamed AH, Cherrick HM. Glycogen-rich adenocarcinoma of minor salivary glands. A light and electron microscopic study. Cancer 1975;36:1057–66.
461. Morinaga S, Hashimoto S, Tezuka F. Epithelial-myoepithelial carcinoma of the parotid gland in a child. Acta Pathol Jpn 1992;42:358–63.
462. Murphy GF, Elder DE. Non-melanocytic tumors of the skin. Atlas of Tumor Pathology, 3rd series, Fascicle 1. Washington, D.C.: Armed Forces Institute of Pathology, 1991:83–6.
463. Noel S, Brozna JP. Epithelial-myoepithelial carcinoma of salivary gland with metastasis to lung: report of a case and review of the literature. Head Neck 1992;14:401–6.
464. Palmer RM. Epithelial-myoepithelial carcinoma: an immunocytochemical study. Oral Surg Oral Med Oral Pathol 1985;59:511–5.
465. Rosen PP, Oberman HA. Tumors of the mammary gland. Atlas of Tumor Pathology, 3rd Series, Fascicle 7. Washington, D.C.: Armed Forces Institute of Pathology, 1993:91–6.
466. Saksela E, Tarkkanen J, Wartiovaara J. Parotid clear-cell adenoma of possible myoepithelial origin. Cancer 1972;30:742–8.
467. Seifert G, Miehlke A, Haubrich J, Chilla R. Diseases of the salivary glands: pathology, diagnosis, treatment, facial nerve surgery. New York: Georg Thieme Verlag, 1986:265–7.
468. Seifert G, Sobin LH. Histological typing of salivary gland tumours. World Health Organization international histological classification of tumours. 2nd ed. New York: Springer-Verlag, 1991.
469. Simpson RH, Clarke TJ, Sarsfield PT, Gluckman PG. Epithelial-myoepithelial carcinoma of salivary glands. J Clin Pathol 1991;44:419–23.
470. Simpson RH, Sarsfield PT, Clarke T, Babajews AV. Clear cell carcinoma of minor salivary glands. Histopathology 1990;17:433–8.
471. Thackray AC, Lucas RB. Tumors of the major salivary glands. Atlas of Tumor Pathology, 2nd Series, Fascicle 10. Washington, D.C.: Armed Forces Institute of Pathology, 1974:62–3.
472. Thackray AC, Sobin LH. Histological typing of salivary gland tumours. International histological classification of tumours No. 7. Geneva: World Health Organization, 1972.

Clear Cell Adenocarcinoma

473. Bedrosian SA, Goldman RL, Dekelboum AM. Renal carcinoma presenting as a primary submandibular gland tumor. Oral Surg Oral Med Oral Pathol 1984;58:699–701.
474. Chaudhry AP, Cutler LS, Satchidanand S, Labay G, Raj MS, Lin CC. Glycogen-rich tumor of the oral minor salivary glands. A histochemical and ultrastructural study. Cancer 1983;52:105–11.
475. Chen KT. Clear cell carcinoma of the salivary gland. Hum Pathol 1983;14:91–3.
476. Coppa GF, Oszczakiewicz M. Parotid gland metastasis from renal carcinoma. Int Surg 1990;75:198–202.

477. Eversole LR. On the differential diagnosis of clear cell tumours of the head and neck. Eur J Cancer B Oral Oncol 1993;29B:173–9.

478. Hayashi K, Ohtsuki Y, Sonobe H, et al. Glycogen-rich clear cell carcinoma arising from minor salivary glands of the uvula. A case report. Acta Pathol Jpn 1988;38:1227–34.

479. Lattanzi DA, Polverini P, Chin DC. Glycogen-rich adenocarcinoma of a minor salivary gland. J Oral Maxillofac Surg 1985;43:122–4.

480. Melnick SJ, Amazon K, Dembrow V. Metastatic renal cell carcinoma presenting as a parotid tumor: a case report with immunohistochemical findings and a review of the literature. Hum Pathol 1989;20:195–7.

481. Milchgrub S, Gnepp DR, Vuitch F, Delgado R, Albores-Saavedra J. Hyalinizing clear cell carcinoma of salivary gland. Am J Surg Pathol 1994;18:74–82.

482. Milles M, Doyle JL, Mesa M, Raz S. Clear cell odontogenic carcinoma with lymph node metastasis. Oral Surg Oral Med Oral Pathol 1993;76:82–9.

483. Mohamed AH, Cherrick HM. Glycogen-rich adenocarcinoma of minor salivary glands. A light and electron microscopic study. Cancer 1975;36:1057–66.

484. Ogawa I, Nikai H, Takata T, et al. Clear cell tumors of minor salivary gland origin. An immunohistochemical and ultrastructural analysis. Oral Surg Oral Med Oral Pathol 1991;72:200–7.

485. Owens RM, Friedman CD, Becker SP. Renal cell carcinoma with metastasis to the parotid gland: case reports and review of the literature. Head Neck 1989;11:174–8.

486. Ravi R, Tongaonkar HB, Kulkarni JN, Kamat MR. Synchronous bilateral parotid metastases from renal cell carcinoma. A case report. Indian J Cancer 1992;29:40–2.

487. Seifert G, Sobin LH. Histological typing of salivary gland tumours. World Health Organization international histological classification of tumours. 2nd ed. New York: Springer-Verlag, 1991.

488. Simpson RH, Clarke TJ, Sarsfield PT, Gluckman PG. Epithelial-myoepithelial carcinoma of salivary glands. J Clin Pathol 1991;44:419–23.

489. Simpson RH, Sarsfield PT, Clarke T, Babajews AV. Clear cell carcinoma of minor salivary glands. Histopathology 1990;17:433–8.

490. Sist TC Jr, Marchetta FC, Milley PC. Renal cell carcinoma presenting as a primary parotid gland tumor. Oral Surg Oral Med Oral Pathol 1982;53:499–502.

491. Smits JG, Slootweg PJ. Renal cell carcinoma with metastasis to the submandibular and parotid glands. A case report. J Maxillofac Surg 1984;12:235–6.

492. Spiro RH, Huvos AG, Strong EW. Adenocarcinoma of salivary origin. Clinicopathologic study of 204 patients. Am J Surg 1982;144:423–31.

493. Thomas KM, Hutt MS, Borgstein J. Salivary gland tumors in Malawi. Cancer 1980;46:2328–34.

494. Uri AK, Wetmore RF, Iozzo RV. Glycogen-rich clear cell carcinoma in the tongue. A cytochemical and ultrastructural study. Cancer 1986;57:1803–9.

495. Waldron CA, el-Mofty SK, Gnepp DR. Tumors of the intraoral minor salivary glands: a demographic and histologic study of 426 cases. Oral Surg Oral Med Oral Pathol 1988;66:323–33.

Cystadenocarcinoma

496. Allen MS Jr, Fitz-Hugh GS, Marsh WL Jr. Low-grade papillary adneocarcinoma of the palate. Cancer 1974;33:153–8.

497. Attar A, Scheffer P, Roucayrol AM, Blanchard P. Papillary cystadenocarcinoma of the submaxillary gland. A rare diagnosis. Rev Stomatol Chir Maxillofac 1989;90:330–3.

498. Auclair PL, Ellis GL, Gnepp DR, Wenig BM, Janney CG. Salivary gland neoplasms: general considerations. In: Ellis GL, Auclair PL, Gnepp DR, eds. Surgical pathology of the salivary glands. Philadelphia: WB Saunders, 1991:135–64.

499. Blanck C, Eneroth CM, Jakobsson PA. Mucus-producing adenopapillary (non-epidermoid) carcinoma of the parotid gland. Cancer 1971;28:676–85.

500. Caselitz J, Jaup T, Seifert G. Immunohistochemical detection of carcinoembryonic antigen (CEA) in parotid gland carcinomas. Analysis of 52 cases. Virchows Arch [A] 1981;394:49–60.

501. Caselitz J, Jaup T, Seifert G. Lactoferrin and lysozyme in carcinomas of the parotid gland. A comparative immunocytochemical study with the occurrence in normal and inflamed tissue. Virchows Arch [A] 1981;394:61–73.

502. Caselitz J, Seifert G, Jaup T. Tumor antigens in neoplasms of the human parotid gland. J Oral Pathol 1982;11:374–86.

503. Chaudhry AP, Vickers RA, Gorlin RJ. Intraoral minor salivary gland tumors: An analysis of 1,414 cases. Oral Surg Oral Med Oral Pathol 1961;14:1194–226.

504. Chen XM. Papillary cystadenocarcinoma of the salivary glands: clinicopathologic analysis of 22 cases. Chung Hua Kou Chiang Hsueh Tsa Chih 1990;25:102–4, 126.

505. Danford M, Eveson JW, Flood TR. Papillary cystadenocarcinoma of the sublingual gland presenting as a ranula. Br J Oral Maxillofac Surg 1992;30:270–2.

506. Dong SZ. Papillary cystadenocarcinoma of the salivary glands. Chinese language article, English abstract. Chung Hua Kou Chiang Hsueh Tsa Chih 1988;23:8–10, 62.

507. Ellis GL, Auclair PL. Classification of salivary gland neoplasms. In: Ellis GL, Auclair PL, Gnepp DR, eds. Surgical pathology of the salivary glands. Philadelphia: WB Saunders, 1991:129–34.

508. Ellis GL, Corio RL. Acinic cell adenocarcinoma. A clinicopathologic analysis of 294 cases. Cancer 1983;52:542–9.

509. Eneroth CM. Salivary gland tumors in the parotid gland, submandibular gland, and the palate region. Cancer 1971;27:1415–8.

510. Evans RW, Cruickshank AH. Epithelial tumours of the salivary glands. Philadelphia: WB Saunders, 1970.

511. Goldblatt LI, Ellis GL. Salivary gland tumors of the tongue. Analysis of 55 new cases and review of the literature. Cancer 1987;60:74–81.

512. Ma DQ, Yu GY. Tumours of the minor salivary glands. A clinicopathologic study of 243 cases. Acta Otolaryngol (Stockh) 1987;103:325–31.

513. Main JH, Orr JA, McGurk FM, McComb RJ, Mock D. Salivary gland tumors: review of 643 cases. J Oral Pathol 1976;5:88–102.

514. Mills SE, Garland TA, Allen MS Jr. Low-grade papillary adenocarcinoma of palatal salivary gland origin. Am J Surg Pathol 1984;8:367–74.

515. Mostofi R, Wood RS, Christison W, Talerman A. Low-grade papillary adenocarcinoma of minor salivary glands. Case report and literature review. Oral Surg Oral Med Oral Pathol 1992;73:591–5.

516. Rawson AJ, Howard JM, Royster HP, Horn RC Jr. Tumors of the salivary glands: a clinicopathologic study of 160 cases. Cancer 1950;3:445–58.

517. Schenk P, Konrad K. Merkel cell carcinoma of the head and neck associated with Bowen's disease. Eur Arch Otorhinolaryngol 1991;248:436–41.

518. Seifert G, Miehlke A, Haubrich J, Chilla R. Diseases of the salivary glands: diagnosis, pathology, treament, facial nerve surgery. Stuttgart: Georg Thieme Verlag, 1986:248–52.

519. Seifert G, Sobin LH. Histological classification of salivary gland tumours. World Health Organization. International histological classification of tumours. 2nd ed. Berlin: Springer-Verlag, 1991:28.

520. Shteyer A, Fundoianu-Dayan D. Papillary cystic adenocarcinoma of minor salivary glands. Int J Oral Maxillofac Surg 1986;15:361–4.

521. Slootweg PJ. Low-grade adenocarcinoma of the oral cavity: polymorphous or papillary? J Oral Pathol Med 1993;22:327–30.

522. Spiro RH. Salivary neoplasms: overview of a 35-year experience with 2,807 patients. Head Neck Surg 1986;8:177–84.

523. Spiro RH, Huvos AG, Strong EW. Adenocarcinoma of salivary origin. Clinicopathologic study of 204 patients. Am J Surg 1982;144:423–31.

524. Spiro RH, Koss LG, Hajdu SI, Strong EW. Tumors of minor salivary origin. A clinicopathologic study of 492 cases. Cancer 1973;31:117–29.

525. Tanaka N, Hsieh KJ, Kino J, et al. A case report of papillary adenocarcinoma in the sublingual region—ultrastructural and histochemical study. Bull Tokyo Med Dent Univ 1989;36:41–8.

526. Thackray AC, Lucas RB. Tumors of the major salivary glands. Atlas of Tumor Pathology, 2nd Series, Fascicle 10. Washington, D.C.: Armed Forces Institute of Pathology, 1974.

527. Thackray AC, Sobin LH. Histological typing of salivary gland tumours. World Health Organization. International histological classification of tumours. Geneva: World Health Organization, 1972.

528. Whittaker JS, Turner EP. Papillary tumours of the minor salivary glands. J Clin Pathol 1976;29:795–805.

529. Yu GY, Ma DQ. Carcinoma of the salivary gland: a clinicopathologic study of 405 cases. Semin Surg Oncol 1987;3:240–4.

Undifferentiated Carcinomas

530. Batsakis JG, Luna MA. Undifferentiated carcinomas of salivary glands. Ann Otol Rhinol Laryngol 1991;100:82–4.

531. Cleary KR, Batsakis JG. Undifferentiated carcinoma with lymphoid stroma of the major salivary glands. Ann Otol Rhinol Laryngol 1990;99:236–8.

532. Gnepp DR, Corio RL, Brannon RB. Small cell carcinoma of the major salivary glands. Cancer 1986;58:705–14.

533. Gnepp DR, Wick MR. Small cell carcinoma of the major salivary glands. An immunohistochemical study. Cancer 1990;66:185–92.

534. Hamilton-Dutoit SJ, Therkildsen MH, Neilsen NH, Jensen H, Hansen JP, Pallesen G. Undifferentiated carcinoma of the salivary gland in Greenlandic Eskimos: demonstration of Epstein-Barr virus DNA by in situ nucleic acid hybridization. Hum Pathol 1991;22:811–5.

535. Hui KK, Luna MA, Batsakis JG, Ordóñez NG, Weber R. Undifferentiated carcinomas of the major salivary glands. Oral Surg Oral Med Oral Pathol 1990;69:76–83.

536. Kraemer BB, Mackay B, Batsakis JG. Small cell carcinomas of the parotid gland. A clinicopathologic study of three cases. Cancer 1983;52:2115–21.

537. Nagao K, Matsuzaki O, Saiga H, et al. Histopathologic studies of undifferentiated carcinoma of the parotid gland. Cancer 1982;50:1572–9.

538. Seifert G, Sobin LH. Histological typing of salivary gland tumours. World Health Organization international histological classification of tumours. 2nd ed. New York: Springer-Verlag, 1991.

Small Cell Carcinoma

539. Battifora H, Silva EG. The use of antikeratin antibodies in the immunohistochemical distinction between neuroendocrine (Merkel cell) carcinoma of the skin, lymphoma, and oat cell carcinoma. Cancer 1986;58:1040–6.

540. Baugh RF, Wolf GT, McClatchey KD. Small cell carcinoma of the head and neck. Head Neck Surg 1986;8:343–54.

541. Brodsky G, Rabson AB. Metastasis to the submandibular gland as the initial presentation of small cell (oat cell) lung carcinoma. Oral Surg Oral Med Oral Pathol 1984;58:76–80.

542. Cameron WR, Johansson L, Tennvall J. Small cell carcinoma of the parotid. Fine needle aspiration and immunochemical findings in a case. Acta Cytol 1990;34:837–41.

543. Cantera JM, Hernandez AV. Bilateral parotid gland metastasis as the initial presentation of a small cell lung carcinoma. J Oral Maxillofac Surg 1989;47:1199–201.

544. Carlsöö B, Ostberg Y. On the occurrence of argyrophil cells in salivary glands. Cell Tiss Res 1976;167:341–50.

545. Carter D. Small-cell carcinoma of the lung. Am J Surg Pathol 1983;7:787–95.

546. Eusebi V, Pileri S, Usellini L, Grassigli A, Capella C. Primary endocrine carcinoma of the parotid salivary gland associated with a lung carcinoid: a possible new association. J Clin Pathol 1982;35:611–6.

547. Eversole LR, Gnepp DR, Eversole GM. Undifferentiated carcinoma. In: Ellis GL, Auclair PL, Gnepp DR, eds. Surgical pathology of the salivary glands. Philadelphia: WB Saunders, 1991:422–40.

548. Gnepp DR. Metastatic disease to the major salivary glands. In: Ellis GL, Auclair PL, Gnepp DR, eds. Surgical pathology of the salivary glands. Philadelphia: WB Saunders, 1991:560–9.

549. Gnepp DR, Corio RL, Brannon RB. Small cell carcinoma of the major salivary glands. Cancer 1986;58:705–14.

550. Gnepp DR, Ferlito A, Hyams VJ. Primay anaplastic small cell (oat cell) carcinoma of the larynx: Review of the literature and report of 18 cases. Cancer 1983;51:1731–45.

551. Gnepp DR, Wick MR. Small cell carcinoma of the major salivary glands. An immunohistochemical study. Cancer 1990;66:185–92.

552. Gould VE, Lee I, Wiedenmann B, et al. Synaptophysin: a novel marker for neurons, certain neuroendocrine cells, and their neoplasms. Hum Pathol 1986;17:979–83.

553. Haneke E, Schulze HJ, Mahrle G. Immunohistochemical and immunoelectron microscopic demonstration of chromogranin A in formalin-fixed tissue of Merkel cell carcinoma. J Am Acad Dermatol 1993;28:222–6.

554. Hayashi Y, Nagamine S, Yanagawa T, et al. Small cell undifferentiated carcinoma of the minor salivary gland containing exocrine, neuroendocrine, and squamous cells. Cancer 1987;60:1583–8.

555. Hui KK, Luna MA, Batsakis JG, Ordez NG, Weber R. Undifferentiated carcinomas of the major salivary glands. Oral Surg Oral Med Oral Pathol 1990;69:76–83.

556. Huntrakoon M. Neuroendocrine carcinoma of the parotid gland: a report of two cases with ultrastructural and immunohistochemical studies. Hum Pathol 1987;18:1212–7.

557. Ibrahim NB, Briggs JC, Corbishley CM. Extrapulmonary oat cell carcinoma. Cancer 1984;54:1645–61.

558. Islas Andrade SA, Frati Munari AC, Gonzalez Angulo J, Iturralde P, Llanos Vega LM. Aumento de los de secrecion neuroendocrina en grandulas submaxilares y parotidas en pacientes con diabetes mellitus no dependiente de insulina. Gac Med Mex 1992;128:411–4.

559. Koss LG, Spiro RH, Hajdu S. Small cell (oat cell) carcinoma of minor salivary gland origin. Cancer 1972;30:737–41.

560. Kraemer BB, Mackay B, Batsakis JG. Small cell carcinomas of the parotid gland. A clinicopathologic study of three cases. Cancer 1983;52:2115–21.

561. Leader M, Collins M, Patel J, Henry K. Antineuron specific enolase staining reactions in sarcomas and carcinomas: its lack of neuroendocrine specificity. J Clin Pathol 1986;39:1186–92.

562. Leipzig B, Gonzales-Vitale JC. Small cell epidermoid carcinoma of salivary glands. 'Pseudo'-oat cell carcinoma. Arch Otolaryngol Head Neck Surg 1982;108:511–4.

563. Mair S, Phillips JI, Cohen R. Small cell undifferentiated carcinoma of the parotid gland. Cytologic, histologic, immunohistochemical and ultrastructural features of a neuroendocrine variant. Acta Cytol 1989;33:164–8.

564. Michels S, Swanson PE, Robbs JA, Wick MR. Leu-7 in small cell neoplasms. Cancer 1987;60:2958–64.

565. Nagao K, Matsuzaki O, Saiga H, et al. Histopathologic studies of undifferentiated carcinoma of the parotid gland. Cancer 1982;50:1572–9.

566. Nolan JA, Trojanowski JQ, Hogue-Angeletti R. Neurons and neuroendocrine cells contain chromogranin: detection of the molecule in normal bovine tissues by immunochemical and immunohistochemical methods. J Histochem Cytochem 1985;33:791–8.

567. Patterson SD. Oat-cell carcinoma, primary in parotid gland. Ultrastruct Pathol 1985;9:77–82.

568. Pinkus GS, Kurtin PJ. Epithelial membrane antigen—a diagnostic discriminant in surgical pathology: immunohistochemical profile in epithelial, mesenchymal, and hematopoietic neoplasms using paraffin sections and monoclonal antibodies. Hum Pathol 1985;16:929–40.

569. Richardson RL, Weiland LH. Undifferentiated small cell carcinomas in extrapulmonary sites. Semin Oncol 1982;9:484–96.

570. Scher RL, Feldman PS, Levine PA. Small-cell carcinoma of the parotid gland with neuroendocrine features. Arch Otolaryngol Head Neck Surg 1988;114:319–21.

571. Seifert G, Miehlke A, Haubrich J, Chilla R. Diseases of the salivary glands: diagnosis, pathology, treament, facial nerve surgery. Stuttgart: Georg Thieme Verlag, 1986:19.

572. Seifert G, Sobin LH. Histological classification of salivary gland tumours. World Health Organization. International histological classification of tumours. 2nd ed. Berlin: Springer-Verlag, 1991:28.

573. Shalowitz JI, Cassidy C, Anders CB. Parotid metastasis of small cell carcinoma of the lung causing facial nerve paralysis. J Oral Maxillofac Surg 1988;46:404–6.

574. Sibley RK, Dahl D. Primary neuroendocrine (Merkel cell?) carcinoma of the skin: II. An immunocytochemical study of 21 cases. Am J Surg Pathol 1985;9:109–16.

575. Takata T, Caselitz J, Seifert G. Undifferentiated tumours of salivary glands. Immunocytochemical investigations and differential diagnosis of 22 cases. Pathol Res Pract 1987;182:161–8.

576. Tischler AS, Mobtaker H, Mann K, et al. Anti-lymphocyte antibody Leu-7 (HNK-1) recognizes a constituent of neuroendocrine granule matrix. J Histochem Cytochem 1986;34:1213–6.

577. Weiler R, Fischer-Colbrie R, Schmid KW, et al. Immunological studies on the occurrence and properties of chromogranin A and B and secretogranin II in endocrine tumors. Am J Surg Pathol 1988;12:877–84.

578. Wirman JA, Battifora HA. Small cell undifferentiated carcinoma of salivary gland origin: an ultrastructural study. Cancer 1976;37:1840–8.

579. World Health Organization. The World Health Organization histological typing of lung tumours. 2nd ed. Am J Clin Pathol 1982;77:123–36.

580. Yesner R. Small cell tumors of the lung. Am J Surg Pathol 1983;7:775–85.

Large Cell Undifferentiated Carcinoma

581. Abiose BO, Oyejide O, Ogunniyi J. Salivary gland tumours in Ibadan, Nigeria: a study of 295 cases. Afr J Med Med Sci 1990;19:195–9.

582. Balogh K, Wolbarsht RL, Federman M, O'Hara CJ. Carcinoma of the parotid gland with osteoclastlike giant cells. Immunohistochemical and ultrastructural observations. Arch Pathol Lab Med 1985;109:756–61.

583. Batsakis JG, Luna MA. Undifferentiated carcinomas of salivary glands. Ann Otol Rhinol Laryngol 1991;100:82–4.

584. Eveson JW, Cawson RA. Salivary gland tumours. A review of 2410 cases with particular reference to histological types, site, age and sex distribution. J Pathol 1985;146:51–8.

585. Eveson JW, Cawson RA. Tumours of the minor (oropharyngeal) salivary glands: a demographic study of 336 cases. J Oral Pathol 1985;14:500–9.

586. Fitzpatrick PJ, Theriault C. Malignant salivary gland tumors. Int J Radiat Oncol Biol Phys 1986;12:1743–7.

587. Hayashi Y, Aoki N. Undifferentiated carcinoma of the parotid gland with bizarre giant cells. Clinicopathologic report with ultrastructural study. Acta Pathol Jpn 1983;33:169–76.

588. Hui KK, Luna MA, Batsakis JG, Ordóñez NG, Weber R. Undifferentiated carcinomas of the major salivary glands. Oral Surg Oral Med Oral Pathol 1990;69:76–83.

589. Humberstone DA, Levestrom M, Shaw JH. Parotid cancer in Auckland 1970-1986—too little, too late. N Z Med J 1987;100:703–5.

590. Hunter RM, Davis BW, Gray GF Jr, Rosenfeld L. Primary malignant tumors of salivary gland origin. A 52-year review. Am Surg 1983;49:82–9.

591. Ma DQ, Yu GY. Tumours of the minor salivary glands. A clinicopathologic study of 243 cases. Acta Otolaryngol (Stockh) 1987;103:325–31.

592. Matsuba HM, Thawley SE, Devineni VR, Levine LA, Smith PG. High-grade malignancies of the parotid gland: effective use of planned combined surgery and irradiation. Laryngoscope 1985;95:1059–63.

593. Nagao K, Matsuzaki O, Saiga H, et al. Histopathologic studies of undifferentiated carcinoma of the parotid gland. Cancer 1982;50:1572–9.

594. North CA, Lee DJ, Piantadosi S, Zahurak M, Johns ME. Carcinoma of the major salivary glands treated by surgery or surgery plus postoperative radiotherapy. Int J Radiat Oncol Biol Phys 1990;18:1319–26.

595. O'Brien CJ, Soong SJ, Herrera GA, Urist MM, Maddox WA. Malignant salivary tumors—analysis of prognostic factors and survival. Head Neck Surg 1986;9:82–92.

596. Seifert G, Miehlke A, Haubrich J, Chilla R. Diseases of the salivary glands: pathology, diagnosis, treatment, facial nerve surgery. New York: Georg Thieme Verlag, 1986:171.

597. Soini Y, Kamel D, Nuorva K, Lane DP, Vähäkangas K, Pääkkö P. Low p53 protein expression in salivary gland tumours compared with lung carcinomas. Virchows Arch [A] 1992;421:415–20.

588. Spiro RH. Salivary neoplasms: overview of a 35-year experience with 2,807 patients. Head Neck Surg 1986;8:177–84.

599. Takahashi H, Fujita S, Tsuda N, Tezuka F, Okabe H. Intraoral minor salivary gland tumors: a demographic and histologic study of 200 cases. Tohoku J Exp Med 1990;161:111–28.

600. Takata T, Caselitz J, Seifert G. Undifferentiated tumours of salivary glands. Immunocytochemical investigations and differential diagnosis of 22 cases. Pathol Res Pract 1987;182:161–8.

601. Theriault C, Fitzpatrick PJ. Malignant parotid tumors. Prognostic factors and optimum treatment. Am J Clin Oncol 1986;9:510–6.

602. Tu G, Hu Y, Jiang P, Qin D. The superiority of combined therapy (surgery and postoperative irradiation) in parotid cancer. Arch Otolaryngol 1982;108:710–3.

603. van Heerden WF, Raubenheimer EJ. Evaluation of the nucleolar organizer region associated proteins in minor salivary gland tumors. J Oral Pathol Med 1991;20:291–5.

604. Waldron CA, el-Mofty SK, Gnepp DR. Tumors of the intraoral minor salivary glands: a demographic and histologic study of 426 cases. Oral Surg Oral Med Oral Pathol 1988;66:323–33.

605. Yaku Y, Kanda T, Yoshihara T, Kaneko T, Nagao K. Undifferentiated carcinoma of the parotid gland. Case report with electron microscopic findings. Virchows Arch [A] 1983;401:89–97.

606. Yu GY, Ma DQ. Carcinoma of the salivary gland: a clinicopathologic study of 405 cases. Semin Surg Oncol 1987;3:240–4.

Lymphoepithelial Carcinoma

607. Albeck H, Nielsen NH, Hansen HE, et al. Epidemiology of nasopharyngeal and salivary gland carcinoma in Greenland. Arctic Med Res 1992;51:189–95.

608. Amaral AL, Nascimento AG. Malignant lymphoepithelial lesion of the submandibular gland. Oral Surg Oral Med Oral Pathol 1984;58:184–90.

609. Arthaud JB. Anaplastic parotid carcinoma ("malignant lymphoepithelial lesion") in seven Alaskan natives. Am J Clin Pathol 1972;57:275–86.

610. Autio-Harmainen H, Pääkkö P, Alavaikko M, Karvonen J, Leisti J. Familial occurrence of malignant lymphoepithelial lesion of the parotid gland in a Finnish family with dominantly inherited trichoepithelioma. Cancer 1988;61:161–6.

611. Batsakis JG. Pathology consultation. Carcinoma ex lymphoepithelial lesion. Ann Otol Rhinol Laryngol 1983;92:657–8.

612. Batsakis JG, Bernacki EG, Rice DH, Stebler ME. Malignancy and the benign lymphoepithelial lesion. Laryngoscope 1975;85:389–99.

613. Borg MF, Benjamin CS, Morton RP, Llewellyn HR. Malignant lympho-epithelial lesion of the salivary gland: a case report and review of the literature. Australas Radiol 1993;37:288–91.

614. Bosch JD, Kudryk WH, Johnson GH. The malignant lymphoepithelial lesion of the salivary glands. J Otolaryngol 1988;17:187–90.

615. Chen KT. Carcinoma arising in a benign lymphoepithelial lesion. Arch Otolaryngol 1983;109:619–21.

616. Cleary KR, Batsakis JG. Undifferentiated carcinoma with lymphoid stroma of the major salivary glands. Ann Otol Rhinol Laryngol 1990;99:236–8.

617. Gleeson MJ, Cawson RA, Bennett MH. Benign lymphoepithelial lesion: a less than benign disease. Clin Otolaryngol 1986;11:47–51.

618. Hamilton-Dutoit SJ, Therkildsen MH, Neilsen NH, Jensen H, Hansen JP, Pallesen G. Undifferentiated carcinoma of the salivary gland in Greenlandic Eskimos: demonstration of Epstein-Barr virus DNA by in situ nucleic acid hybridization. Hum Pathol 1991;22:811–5.

619. Hanji D, Gohao L. Malignant lymphoepithelial lesions of the salivary glands with anaplastic carcinomatous change. Report of nine cases and review of literature. Cancer 1983;52:2245–52.

620. Hilderman WC, Gordon JS, Large HL Jr, Carroll CF Jr. Malignant lymphoepithelial lesion with carcinomatous component apparently arising in parotid gland: a malignant counterpart of benign lymphoepithelial lesion? Cancer 1962;15:606–10.

621. James PD, Ellis IO. Malignant epithelial tumours associated with autoimmune sialadenitis. J Clin Pathol 1986;39:497–502.

622. Kitazawa M, Ohnishi Y, Nonomura N, Kobayashi E. Malignant lymphoepithelial lesion. Acta Pathol Jpn 1987;37:515–26.

623. Kott ET, Goepfert H, Ayala AG, Ordóñez NG. Lymphoepithelial carcinoma (malignant lymphoepithelial lesion) of the salivary glands. Arch Otolaryngol 1984;110:50–3.

624. Krishnamurthy S, Lanier AP, Dohan P, Lanier JF, Henle W. Salivary gland cancer in Alaskan natives, 1966-1980 [published erratum appears in Hum Pathol 1988 Mar;19(3):328]. Hum Pathol 1987;18:986–96.

625. Lanier AP, Clift SR, Bornkamm G, Henle W, Goepfert H, Raab-Traub N. Epstein-Barr virus and malignant lymphoepithelial lesions of the salivary gland. Arctic Med Res 1991;50:55–61.

626. Manoukian JJ, Attia EL, Baxter JD, Viloria JB, Daou RA. Undifferentiated carcinoma with lymphoid stroma of the parotid gland. J Otolaryngol 1984;13:147–52.

627. Merrick Y, Albeck H, Nielsen NH, Hansen HS. Familial clustering of salivary gland carcinoma in Greenland. Cancer 1986;57:2097–102.

628. Nagao K, Matsuzaki O, Saiga H, et al. A histopathologic study of benign and malignant lymphoepithelial lesions of the parotid gland. Cancer 1983;52:1044–52.

629. Nielsen NH, Mikkelsen F, Hansen JP. Incidence of salivary gland neoplasms in Greenland with special reference to an anaplastic carcinoma. Acta Pathol Microbiol Scand [A] 1978;86:185–93.

630. Saemundsen AK, Albeck H, Hansen JP, et al. Epstein-Barr virus in nasopharyngeal and salivary gland carcinomas of Greenland Eskimos. Br J Cancer 1982;46:721–8.

631. Saw D, Lau WH, Ho JH, Chan JK, Ng CS. Malignant lymphoepithelial lesion of the salivary gland. Hum Pathol 1986;17:914–23.

632. Sehested M, Hainau B, Albeck H, Nielsen NH, Hart Hansen JP. Ultrastructural investigation of anaplastic salivary gland carcinomas in Eskimos. Cancer 1985;55:2732–6.

633. Seifert G, Sobin LH. Histological typing of salivary gland tumours. World Health Organization international histological classification of tumours. 2nd ed. New York: Springer-Verlag, 1991.

634. Yazdi HM, Hogg GR. Malignant lymphoepithelial lesion of the submandibular salivary gland. Am J Clin Pathol 1984;82:344–8.

Oncocytic Carcinoma

635. Abioye AA. Malignant oncocytoma (oxyphilic granular-cell tumour) of the parotid gland. Case report. East Afr Med J 1972;49:235–8.

636. Austin MB, Frierson HF Jr, Feldman PS. Oncocytoid adenocarcinoma of the parotid gland. Cytologic, histologic and ultrastructural findings. Acta Cytol 1987;31:351–6.

637. Batsakis JG. Tumors of the head and neck. Clinical and pathological considerations. 2nd ed. Baltimore: Williams & Wilkins, 1979:61.

638. Bauer WH, Bauer JD. Classification of glandular tumors of salivary glands. Study of one-hundred forty-three cases. Arch Pathol 1953;55:328–46.

639. Bazaz-Malik G, Gupta DN. Metastasizing (malignant) oncocytoma of the parotid gland. Z Krebsforsch Klin Onkol Cancer Res Clin Oncol 1968;70:193–7.

640. Brandwein MS, Huvos AG. Oncocytic tumors of major salivary glands. A study of 68 cases with follow-up of 44 patients. Am J Surg Pathol 1991;15:514–28.

641. Briggs J, Evans JN. Malignant oxyphilic granular-cell tumor (oncocytoma) of the palate. Review of the recent literature and report of a case. Oral Surg Oral Med Oral Pathol 1967;23:796–802.

642. Carlsöö B, Domeij S, Helander HF. A quantitative ultrastructural study of a parotid oncocytoma. Arch Pathol Lab Med 1979;103:471–4.

643. Chang A, Harawi SJ. Oncocytes, oncocytosis, and oncocytic tumors. Pathol Annu 1992;27 (Pt. 1):263–304.

644. de Araújo VC, de Souza SO, Sesso A, Sotto MN, de Arajo NS. Salivary duct carcinoma: ultrastructural and histogenetic considerations. Oral Surg Oral Med Oral Pathol 1987;63:592–6.

645. Delgado R, Vuitch F, Albores-Saavedra J. Salivary duct carcinoma. Cancer 1993;72:1503–12.

646. Eneroth CM. Oncocytoma of major salivary glands. J Laryngol 1965;79:1064–72.

647. Evans RW, Cruickshank AH. Epithelial tumours of the salivary glands. Philadelphia: WB Saunders, 1970.

648. Eveson JW, Cawson RA. Salivary gland tumours. A review of 2410 cases with particular reference to histological types, site, age and sex distribution. J Pathol 1985;146:51–8.

649. Fayemi AO, Toker C. Malignant oncocytoma of the parotid gland. Arch Otolaryngol Head Neck Surg 1974;99:375–6.

650. Goode RK, Corio RL. Oncocytic adenocarcinoma of salivary glands. Oral Surg Oral Med Oral Pathol 1988;65:61–6.

651. Gray SR, Cornog JL Jr, Seo IS. Oncocytic neoplasms of salivary glands: a report of fifteen cases including two malignant oncocytomas. Cancer 1976;38:1306–17.

652. Hui KK, Batsakis JG, Luna MA, Mackay B, Byers RM. Salivary duct adenocarcinoma: a high grade malignancy. J Laryngol Otol 1986;100:105–14.

653. Johns ME, Batsakis JG, Short CD. Oncocytic and oncocytoid tumors of the salivary glands. Laryngoscope 1973;83:1940–52.

654. Johns ME, Regezi JA, Batsakis JG. Oncocytic neoplasms of salivary glands: an ultrastructural study. Laryngoscope 1977;87:862–71.

655. Lee SC, Roth LM. Malignant oncocytoma of the parotid gland. A light and electron microscopic study. Cancer 1976;37:1606–14.

656. Ramakrishna B, Perakath B, Chandi SM. Malignant multinodular oncocytoma of parotid gland—a case report and literature review. Indian J Cancer 1992;29:230–3.

657. Ross CF. Malignant oncocytoma ("oxyphilic granular-cell tumour") of parotid gland. Clin Oncol 1976;2:253–60.

658. Seifert G, Miehlke A, Haubrich J, Chilla R. Diseases of the salivary glands: diagnosis, pathology, treament, facial nerve surgery. Stuttgart: Georg Thieme Verlag, 1986.

659. Seifert G, Sobin LH. Histological classification of salivary gland tumours. World Health Organization. International histological classification of tumours. 2nd ed. Berlin: Springer-Verlag, 1991:28.

660. Spiro RH. Salivary neoplasms: overview of a 35-year experience with 2,807 patients. Head Neck Surg 1986;8:177–84.

661. Sugimoto T, Wakizono S, Uemura T, Tsuneyoshi M, Enjoji M. Malignant oncocytoma of the parotid gland: a case report with an immunohistochemical and ultrastructural study. J Laryngol Otol 1993;107:69–74.

662. Thackray AC, Lucas RB. Tumors of the major salivary glands. Atlas of Tumor Pathology, 2nd Series, Fascicle 10. Washington, D.C.: Armed Forces Institute of Pathology, 1974.

663. Whittam DE, Bose B. Malignant oncocytoma of the parotid gland. Br J Surg 1971;58:851–3.

664. Woods JE, Chong GC, Beahrs OH. Experience with 1,360 primary parotid tumors. Am J Surg 1975;130:460–2.

665. Yu GY, Ma DQ. Carcinoma of the salivary gland: a clinicopathologic study of 405 cases. Semin Surg Oncol 1987;3:240–4.

666. Ziegler M, Maibach EA, Ussmuller J. Malignes Onkozytom der Glandula submandibularis. Laryngol Rhinol Otol 1992;71:423–5.

Salivary Duct Carcinoma

667. Afzelius LE, Cameron WR, Svensson C. Salivary duct carcinoma—a clinicopathologic study of 12 cases. Head Neck Surg 1987;9:151–6.

668. Anderson C, Muller R, Piorkowski R, Knibbs DR, Vignoti P. Intraductal carcinoma of major salivary gland. Cancer 1992;69:609–14.

669. Batsakis JG, Luna MA. Low-grade and high-grade adenocarcinomas of the salivary duct system. Ann Otol Rhinol Laryngol 1989;98:162–3.

670. Brandwein M, Biller H. Intraductal carcinoma of major salivary gland [Letter]. Cancer 1992;70:1202.

671. Brandwein MS, Jagirdar J, Patil J, Biller H, Kaneko M. Salivary duct carcinoma (cribriform salivary carcinoma of excretory ducts). A clinicopathologic and immunohistochemical study of 12 cases. Cancer 1990;65:2307–14.

672. Butterworth DM, Jones AW, Kotecha B. Salivary duct carcinoma: report of a case and review of the literature. Virchows Arch [A] 1992;420:371–4.

673. Chen KT. Intraductal carcinoma of the minor salivary gland. J Laryngol Otol 1983;97:189–91.

674. Chen KT, Hafez GR. Infiltrating salivary duct carcinoma. A clinicopathologic study of five cases. Arch Otolaryngol 1981;107:37–9.

675. Colmenero Ruiz C, Patrön Romero M, Martin P. Salivary duct carcinoma: a report of nine cases. J Oral Maxillofac Surg 1993;51:641–6.

676. de Araújo VC, de Souza SO, Sesso A, Sotto MN, de Araújo NS. Salivary duct carcinoma: ultrastructural and histogenetic considerations. Oral Surg Oral Med Oral Pathol 1987;63:592–6.

677. Dee S, Masood S, Issacs JH Jr., Hardy NM. Cytomorphologic features of salivary duct carcinoma on fine needle aspiration biopsy. A case report. Acta Cytol 1993;37:539–42.

678. Delgado R, Vuitch F, Albores-Saavedra J. Salivary duct carcinoma. Cancer 1993;72:1503–12.

679. Evans RW, Cruickshank AH. Epithelial tumours of the salivary glands. Philadelphia: WB Saunders, 1970:265–6.

680. Fayemi AO, Toker C. Salivary duct carcinoma. Arch Otolaryngol 1974;99:366–8.

681. Gal R, Strauss M, Zohar Y, Kessler E. Salivary duct carcinoma of the parotid gland. Cytologic and histopathologic study. Acta Cytol 1985;29:454–6.

682. Garland TA, Innes DJ Jr, Fechner RE. Salivary duct carcinoma: an analysis of four cases with review of literature. Am J Clin Pathol 1984;81:436–41.

683. Hui KK, Batsakis JG, Luna MA, Mackay B, Byers RM. Salivary duct adenocarcinoma: a high grade malignancy. J Laryngol Otol 1986;100:105–14.

684. Kleinsasser O, Klein HJ, Hübner G. Speichelgangearcarcinom: ein den Milchgangcarcinomen der Brustdrse Analoge Gruppe von Speichldrsentumoren. Arch Klin Exp Ohren Nasen Kehlkopfheilkd 1968;192:100–5.

685. Lack EE, Upton MP. Histopathologic review of salivary gland tumors in childhood. Arch Otolaryngol Head Neck Surg 1988;114:898–906.

686. Luna MA, Batsakis JG, Ordez NG, Mackay B, Tortoledo ME. Salivary gland adenocarcinomas: a clinicopathologic analysis of three distinctive types. Semin Diagn Pathol 1987;4:117–35.

687. Murrah VA, Batsakis JG. Salivary duct carcinoma. Ann Otol Rhinol Laryngol 1994;103:244–7.

688. Pesce C, Colacino R, Buffa P. Duct carcinoma of the minor salivary glands: a case report. J Laryngol Otol 1986;100:611–3.

689. Seifert G, Miehlke A, Haubrich J, Chilla R. Diseases of the salivary glands: pathology, diagnosis, treatment, facial nerve surgery. New York: Georg Thieme Verlag, 1986:265–7.

690. Seifert G, Sobin LH. Histological typing of salivary gland tumours. World Health Organization international histological classification of tumours. 2nd ed. New York: Springer-Verlag, 1991.

691. Simpson RH, Clarke TJ, Sarsfield PT, Babajews AV. Salivary duct adenocarcinoma. Histopathology 1991;18:229–35.

692. Takata T, Caselitz J, Seifert G. Undifferentiated tumours of salivary glands. Immunocytochemical investigations and differential diagnosis of 22 cases. Pathol Res Pract 1987;182:161–8.

693. Thackray AC, Lucas RB. Tumors of the major salivary glands. Atlas of Tumor Pathology, 2nd Series, Fascicle 10. Washington, D.C.: Armed Forces Institute of Pathology, 1974:102.

694. Thackray AC, Sobin LH. Histological typing of salivary gland tumours. International histological classification of tumours No. 7. Geneva: World Health Organization, 1972.

Sebaceous Adenocarcinoma and Sebaceous Lymphadenocarcinoma

695. Ellis GL, Auclair PL, Gnepp DR, Goode RK. Other malignant epithelial neoplasms. In: Ellis GL, Auclair PL, Gnepp DR, eds. Surgical pathology of the salivary glands. Philadelphia: WB Saunders, 1991:455–88.

696. Gnepp DR. Sebaceous neoplasms of salivary gland origin: a review. Pathol Annu 1983;18 (Pt. 1):71–102.

697. Gnepp DR, Brannon R. Sebaceous neoplasms of salivary gland origin. Report of 21 cases. Cancer 1984;53:2155–70.

698. Linhartová A. Sebaceous glands in salivary gland tissue. Arch Pathol 1974;98:320–4.

Myoepithelial Carcinoma

699. Barnes L, Appel BN, Perez H, El-Attar AM. Myoepithelioma of the head and neck: case report and review. J Surg Oncol 1985;28:21–8.

700. Batsakis JG, Ordóñez NG, Ro J, Meis JM, Bruner JM. S-100 protein and myoepithelial neoplasms. J Laryngol Otol 1986;100:687–98.

701. Carrillo R, el-Naggar AK, Luna MA, Rodriguez-Peralto JL, Batsakis JG. Nucleolar organizer regions (NORs) and myoepitheliomas: a comparison with DNA content and clinical course. J Laryngol Otol 1992;106:616–20.

702. Crissman JD, Wirman JA, Harris A. Malignant myoepithelioma of the parotid gland. Cancer 1977;40:3042–9.

703. Dardick I. Malignant myoepithelioma of parotid salivary gland. Ultrastruct Pathol 1985;9:163–8.

704. Dardick I, Cavell S, Boivin M, et al. Salivary gland myoepithelioma variants. Histological, ultrastructural, and immunocytological features. Virchows Arch [A] 1989;416:25–42.

705. Dardick I, Ostrynski VL, Ekem JK, Leung R, Burford-Mason AP. Immunohistochemical and ultrastructural correlates of muscle-actin expression in pleomorphic adenomas and myoepitheliomas based on comparison of formalin and methanol fixation. Virchows Arch [A] 1992;421:95–104.

706. Dardick I, Thomas MJ, van Nostrand AW. Myoepithelioma—new concepts of histology and classification: a light and electron microscopic study. Ultrastruct Pathol 1989;13:187–224.

707. de Araújo VC, de Araújo NS. Vimentin as a marker of myoepithelial cells in salivary gland tumors. Eur Arch Otorhinolaryngol 1990;247:252–5.

708. Di Palma S, Guzzo M. Malignant myoepithelioma of salivary glands: clinicopathological features of ten cases. Virchows Arch [A] 1993;423:389–96.

709. Di Palma S, Pilotti S, Rilke F. Malignant myoepithelioma of the parotid gland arising in a pleomorphic adenoma. Histopathology 1991;19:273–5.

710. el-Naggar A, Batsakis JG, Luna MA, Goepfert H, Tortoledo ME. DNA content and proliferative activity of myoepitheliomas. J Laryngol Otol 1989;103:1192–7.

711. Franquemont DW, Mills SE. Plasmacytoid monomorphic adenoma of salivary glands. Absence of myogenous differentiation and comparison to spindle cell myoepithelioma. Am J Surg Pathol 1993;17:146–53.

712. Herrera GA. Light microscopic, ultrastructural and immunocytochemical spectrum of malignant lacrimal and salivary gland tumors, including malignant mixed tumors [published erratum appears in Pathobiology 1991;59(1):56]. Pathobiology 1990;58:312–22.

713. Ibrahim R, Bird DJ, Sieler MW. Malignant myoepithelioma of the larynx with massive metastatic spread to the liver: an ultrastructural and immunocytochemical study. Ultrastruct Pathol 1991;15:69–76.

714. Jones H, Moshtael F, Simpson RH. Immunoreactivity of alpha smooth muscle actin in salivary gland tumours: a comparison with S100 protein. J Clin Pathol 1992;45:938–40.

715. Mori M, Tsukitani K, Ninomiya T, Okada Y. Various expressions of modified myoepithelial cells in salivary pleomorphic adenoma. Immunohistochemical studies. Pathol Res Pract 1987;182:632–46.

716. Mori M, Yamada K, Tanaka T, Okada Y. Multiple expression of keratins, vimentin, and S-100 protein in pleomorphic salivary adenomas. Virchows Arch [Cell Pathol] 1990;58:435–44.

717. Saxe SJ, Grossniklaus HE, Someren AO. Malignant myoepithelioma after radiation for retinoblastoma [Letter]. Am J Ophthalmol 1992;114:512–3.

718. Sciubba JJ, Brannon RB. Myoepithelioma of salivary glands: report of 23 cases. Cancer 1982;49:562–72.

719. Seifert G, Sobin LH. Histological typing of salivary gland tumours. World Health Organization international histological classification of tumours. 2nd ed. New York: Springer-Verlag, 1991.

720. Sheldon WH. So-called mixed tumors of the salivary glands. Arch Pathol 1943;35:1–20.

721. Singh R, Cawson RA. Malignant myoepithelial carcinoma (myoepithelioma) arising in a pleomorphic adenoma of the parotid gland. An immunohistochemical study and review of the literature. Oral Surg Oral Med Oral Pathol 1988;66:65–70.

722. Spiro RH, Huvos AG, Strong EW. Adenocarcinoma of salivary origin. Clinicopathologic study of 204 patients. Am J Surg 1982;144:423–31.

723. Stromeyer FW, Haggitt RC, Nelson JF, Hardman JM. Myoepithelioma of minor salivary gland origin. Light and electron microscopical study. Arch Pathol 1975;99:242–5.

724. Takeda Y. Malignant myoepithelioma of minor salivary gland origin. Acta Pathol Jpn 1992;42:518–22.

725. Thompson SH, Bender S, Richards A. Plasmacytoid myoepithelioma of a minor salivary gland. J Oral Maxillofac Surg 1985;43:285–8.

726. Tortoledo ME, Luna MA, Batsakis JG. Carcinomas ex pleomorphic adenoma and malignant mixed tumors. Histomorphologic indexes. Arch Otolaryngol 1984;110:172–6.

727. Toto PD, Hsu DJ. Product definition in a case of myoepithelioma. Oral Surg Oral Med Oral Pathol 1986;62:169–74.

Adenosquamous Carcinoma

728. Banks ER, Frierson HF Jr, Mills SE, George E, Zarbo RJ, Swanson PE. Basaloid squamous cell carcinoma of the head and neck. A clinicopathologic and immunohistochemical study of 40 cases. Am J Surg Pathol 1992;16:939–46.

729. Bombi JA, Riverola A, Bordas JM, Cardesa A. Adenosquamous carcinoma of the esophagus. A case report. Pathol Res Pract 1991;187:514–9; discussion 519–21.

730. Ellis GL, Auclair PL, Gnepp DR, Goode RK. Other malignant epithelial neoplasms. In: Ellis GL, Auclair PL, Gnepp DR, eds. Surgical pathology of the salivary glands. Philadelphia: WB Saunders, 1991:455–88.

731. Ellis GL, Gnepp DR. Unusual salivary gland tumors. In: Gnepp DR, ed. Pathology of the head and neck. New York: Churchill Livingstone, 1988:585–661.

732. Gerughty RM, Hennigar GR, Brown FM. Adenosquamous carcinoma of the nasal, oral and laryngeal cavities. A clinicopathologic survey of ten cases. Cancer 1968;22:1140–55.

733. Hyams VJ, Batsakis JG, Michaels L. Tumors of the upper respiratory tract and ear. Atlas of Tumor Pathology, 2nd Series, Fascicle 25. Washington, D.C.: Armed Forces Institute of Pathology, 1986:104–7.

734. Jones AC, Freedman PD, Kerpel SM. Oral adenoid squamous cell carcinoma: a report of three cases and review of the literature. J Oral Maxillofac Surg 1993;51:676–81.

735. Luna MA, el Naggar A, Parichatikanond P, Weber RS, Batsakis JG. Basaloid squamous carcinoma of the upper aerodigestive tract. Clinicopathologic and DNA flow cytometric analysis. Cancer 1990;66:537–42.

736. Martinez-Madrigal F, Baden E, Casiraghi O, Micheau C. Oral and pharyngeal adenosquamous carcinoma. A report of four cases with immunohistochemical studies. Eur Arch Otorhinolaryngol 1991;248:255–8.

737. Peel RL, Gnepp DR. Diseases of the salivary glands. In: Barnes L, ed. Surgical pathology of the head and neck. New York: Marcel Dekker, 1985:533–645.

738. Seifert G, Sobin LH. Histological typing of salivary gland tumours. World Health Organization international histological classification of tumours. 2nd ed. New York: Springer-Verlag, 1991.

739. Siar CH, Ng KH. Adenosquamous carcinoma of the floor of the mouth and lower alveolus: a radiation-induced lesion? Oral Surg Oral Med Oral Pathol 1987;63:216–20.

740. Wain SL, Kier R, Vollmer RT, Bossen EH. Basaloid-squamous carcinoma of the tongue, hypopharynx, and larynx: report of 10 cases. Hum Pathol 1986;17:1158–66.

Mucinous Adenocarcinoma

741. Angell DC, Ousterhout D, Hendrix RC, French AJ. Epithelial neoplasms of salivary gland: acinic-cell, mucous-cell, and duct-cell tumors. Oral Surg Oral Med Oral Pathol 1967;23:362–70.

742. Blanck C, Eneroth CM, Jakobsson PA. Mucus-producing adenopapillary (non-epidermoid) carcinoma of the parotid gland. Cancer 1971;28:676–85.

743. Ellis GL, Auclair PL, Gnepp DR, Goode RK. Other malignant epithelial neoplasms. In: Ellis GL, Auclair PL, Gnepp DR, eds. Surgical pathology of the salivary glands. Philadelphia: WB Saunders, 1991:455–88.

744. Eneroth CM. Salivary gland tumors in the parotid gland, submandibular gland, and the palate region. Cancer 1971;27:1415–8.

745. Fenoglio-Preiser CM, Pascal RR, Perzin KH. Tumors of the intestines. Atlas of Tumor Pathology, 2nd Series, Fascicle 27. Washington, D.C.: Armed Forces Institute of Pathology, 1990:209–22.

746. Gnepp DR, Heffner DK. Mucosal origin of sinonasal tract adenomatous neoplasms. Mod Pathol 1989;2:365–71.

747. Hyams VJ, Batsakis JG, Michaels L. Tumors of the upper respiratory tract and ear. Atlas of Tumor Pathology, 2nd Series, Fascicle 25. Washington, D.C.: Armed Forces Institute of Pathology, 1986:95–100.

748. Kitamura K, Asai M, Kubo T, Harii K, Hasegawa A. Mucinous carcinoma of the external auditory canal: case report. Head Neck 1990;12:417–20.

749. Main JH, Orr JA, McGurk FM, McComb RJ, Mock D. Salivary gland tumors: review of 643 cases. J Oral Pathol 1976;5:88–102.

750. Moran CA, Wenig BM, Mullick FG. Primary adenocarcinoma of the nasal cavity and paranasal sinuses. Ear Nose Throat J 1991;70:821–8.

751. Murphy GF, Elder DE. Non-melanocytic tumors of the skin. Atlas of Tumor Pathology, 3rd Series, Fascicle 1. Washington, D.C.: Armed Forces Institute of Pathology, 1991;102–5.

752. Osaki T, Hirota J, Ohno A, Tatemoto Y. Mucinous adenocarcinoma of the submandibular gland. Cancer 1990;66:1796–801.

753. Rosen PP, Oberman HA. Tumors of the mammary gland. Atlas of Tumor Pathology, 3rd Series, Fascicle 7. Washington, D.C.: Armed Forces Institute of Pathology, 1993:187–93.

754. Seifert G, Sobin LH. Histological typing of salivary gland tumours. World Health Organization international histological classification of tumours. 2nd ed. New York: Springer-Verlag, 1991.

755. Spiro RH, Huvos AG, Strong EW. Adenocarcinoma of salivary origin. Clinicopathologic study of 204 patients. Am J Surg 1982;144:423–31.

✧✧✧

6
NONLYMPHOID MESENCHYMAL NEOPLASMS

Benign and malignant nonlymphoid mesenchymal neoplasms account for only 1.9 to 5 percent of all neoplasms that occur within the major salivary glands (3,49). In patients younger than 19 years of age, however, benign vascular tumors of the parotid glands may comprise a large proportion of all tumors and, in some series, have outnumbered tumors of epithelial derivation (3,18,25,37,38,61,63). Furthermore, some mesenchymal proliferations that occasionally occur in the major glands, such as nodular fasciitis or epithelioid malignant schwannoma, may histologically mimic epithelial neoplastic disease. This discussion is limited to involvement of the major salivary glands. Since minor salivary glands are small and embedded within fibrous connective tissue, fat, and skeletal muscle, it is not possible to determine origin of a mesenchymal neoplasm from the stroma. A brief discussion of some of the more common benign and malignant mesenchymal tumors follows. A comprehensive review of these and other mesenchymal neoplasms is available elsewhere (12).

BENIGN MESENCHYMAL TUMORS

Hemangioma

General Features. Capillary and cavernous hemangiomas occur in many sites including the major salivary glands (32). The immature form of capillary hemangioma known as *juvenile hemangioma* (14), is occasionally associated with extensive and life-threatening growth (47). In the past these immature cellular hemangiomas of the salivary glands were often designated *benign infantile hemangioendothelioma,* a term still preferred today for similar tumors that occur in the liver (11,23,38). In the liver and deep soft tissues they are frequently complicated by the development of consumptive coagulopathy (Kasabach-Merritt syndrome) (11,47,66), but only one such case (which lacked a biopsy diagnosis) has been associated with a parotid tumor (53).

Juvenile hemangiomas occur principally in patients less than 1 year of age whereas the typical capillary and cavernous forms are usually seen in adolescents or adults (10,25,32,37, 38,41,64). The cellular type has a predilection for females. While several reports have noted a decided left-sided laterality, this finding has not been universal (19,25,32,37). Most occur in the parotid glands. The cavernous form does not show a gender predilection (10,37).

Clinical Features. The cellular form often manifests as a small swelling at birth. A mass is nearly always detected by 6 months of age and occasionally shows rapid enlargement, a feature that clinically could suggest malignancy (19,25,37). Extension into the hypopharynx and intracranial areas occurs (32). A bluish discoloration of the overlying skin is usually evident and is accentuated when the infant cries (19). Pain and tenderness are not typically experienced.

Gross and Microscopic Findings. Grossly, hemangiomas appear to expand rather than destroy the salivary gland lobules. A distinctive tumor mass is usually not apparent (19,25). Microscopically, the juvenile form shows closely packed sheets of cells that are confined by the salivary lobules (fig. 6-1). In many areas evidence of vascular differentiation is limited to small inconspicuous lumens. As these areas mature, small capillary channels and larger thin-walled vessels (fig. 6-2), similar to those seen in adult forms, are evident, often most prominently at the periphery of the tumors. Residual ducts and acinar elements are more numerous than expected with such an extensive intraglandular proliferation (fig. 6-3). High magnification reveals proliferating plump, round to ovoid endothelial cells (fig. 6-4). Moderate numbers of mitotic figures may be seen but the nuclei are not frankly atypical. Enzinger and Weiss (14) report that regression is accompanied by progressive diffuse interstitial fibrosis and have noted infarction of some tumors. Histochemical staining for reticulin highlights the small fibers that encircle the primitive vessels.

Treatment and Prognosis. In the past many juvenile hemangiomas were treated with parotidectomy, embolization, injection of alcohol, steroid therapy, laser cautery or thermocautery,

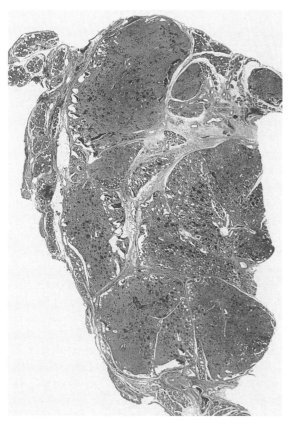

Figure 6-1
JUVENILE HEMANGIOMA
Despite extensive involvement the lobular architecture of the parotid gland is maintained.

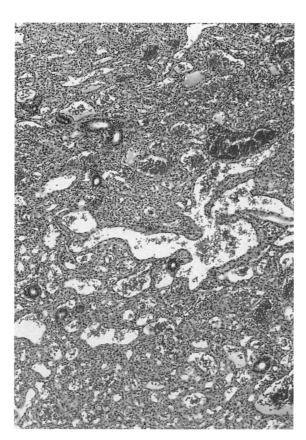

Figure 6-2
JUVENILE HEMANGIOMA
Several vascular spaces lined by flattened endothelial cells have formed within the otherwise solid, hypercellular proliferation of less mature cells. Several residual ducts are also evident.

and radiotherapy. Some cases treated surgically persisted or recurred while others were complicated by facial nerve paralysis (32). The current recommendation is to delay treatment when possible in the hope of spontaneous regression (18, 25,27,32,57,61,63). Compression therapy may assist in this process (56). It has been estimated that by the age of 7 years, 75 to 90 percent of the lesions will have involuted (14). Surgery is recommended when the lesion is disfiguring or growing rapidly, and preoperative chemotherapy and radiation may be indicated in rare life-threatening cases (9,47,53,63). Cavernous hemangiomas lack the tendency to regress and usually require surgical intervention (14,41).

Lipoma

General Features. Lipomas of major salivary glands have only been described in relation to the parotid gland. Baker et al. (5) described

three lipomas of the parotid gland and conducted an extensive literature review. They found that lipomas comprised 1.2 percent of parotid gland neoplasms. In recent experience at the Armed Forces Institute of Pathology (AFIP), lipomas represented slightly less than 0.5 percent of parotid gland tumors. The report of Walts et al. (60) of 32 lipomatous lesions of the parotid gland is the largest published series of lipomas of salivary gland. Twenty of the lipomas in their series were described as intraparotid while the others were periparotid. Other series have been described by Layfield et al. (26), Korentager et al. (24), and Janecka et al. (21).

There is a striking male sex predilection of about 10 to 1. Most patients are over 30 years of age. Reilly et al. (45) reported an angiolipoma of the parotid gland in a 6-month-old female, Calhoun et al. (8) described a lipoblastoma of the

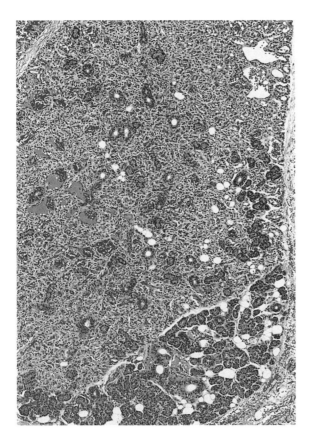

Figure 6-3
JUVENILE HEMANGIOMA
Other than the small amount of normal glandular tissue remaining at the bottom, the rest of this salivary lobule is involved by hemangioma. Many ducts and a few acinar structures of the involved gland persist. While the lobule is enlarged, the lesion characteristically does not violate the interlobular septa.

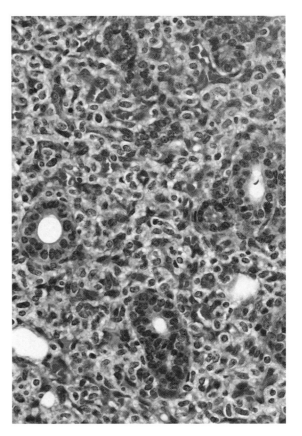

Figure 6-4
JUVENILE HEMANGIOMA
A proliferation of plump spindle cells contains small, irregular luminal spaces filled with red blood cells that serve as evidence of vascular differentiation.

parotid in a 7-month-old male, and Adams et al. (1) described lipomatosis of the parotid in a 2-month-old.

Clinical Features. Slow growth and a preoperative duration of several years are common for lipomas of the parotid gland although occasionally more rapid enlargement and shorter duration have been noted (5). The tumors are usually described as soft or rubbery, and most patients report no symptoms other than swelling.

Gross Findings. Parotid gland lipomas have ranged from 1 to 8 cm in largest dimension, but the average size is about 3 cm. They are typically well circumscribed and usually encapsulated. Like most lipomas, the cut surfaces are yellow to white with a smooth greasy texture (fig. 6-5).

Microscopic Findings. Most lipomas of the parotid are composed of mature adipose tissue without myxoid, spindle cell, pleomorphic, or angiomatous features. Reilly et al. (45) reported an angiolipoma, and the AFIP has a spindle cell lipoma from the parotid gland on file. Vinayak and Reddy (58) reported a hibernoma in the parotid region, but this tumor was actually extraglandular and superficial to the gland itself. Lipomas are usually separated from the parotid parenchyma by thin fibrous capsules (fig. 6-6), but in a few cases the adipose tissue is unencapsulated and incorporates foci of glandular parenchyma within the tumor (fig. 6-7). These latter cases need to be distinguished from fatty replacement that manifests in old age or chronic sialadenosis, which is sometimes associated with long-term diabetes mellitus and chronic alcoholism. In fatty replacement there are foci of

377

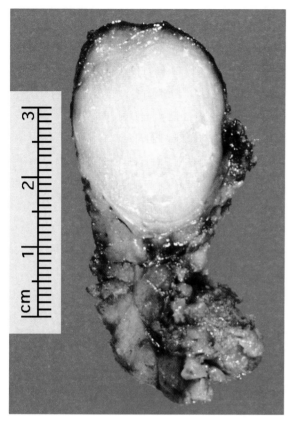

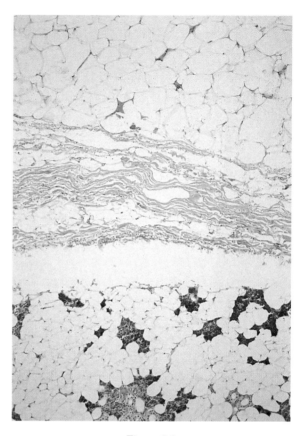

Figure 6-5
LIPOMA OF THE PAROTID GLAND

The well-demarcated nodule of yellowish white adipose tissue is distinct from the adjacent parotid tissue. (Courtesy of Drs. Glen Houston and Robert Brannon, Wilford Hall Medical Center, San Antonio, TX, and Armed Forces Institute of Pathology, Washington, DC.)

Figure 6-6
LIPOMA OF THE PAROTID GLAND

The lipoma is composed of large, mature adipocytes (top) and is separated from the parenchyma and fatty stroma of the parotid gland (bottom) by a fibrous connective tissue capsule.

Figure 6-7
LIPOMA OF THE
PAROTID GLAND

No capsule separates this lipoma from the parenchyma of the parotid gland (left).

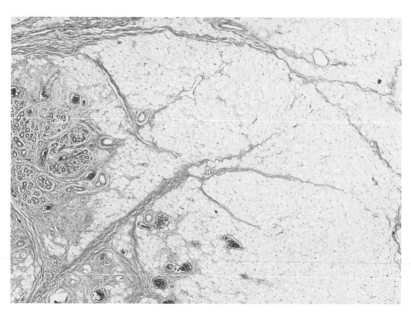

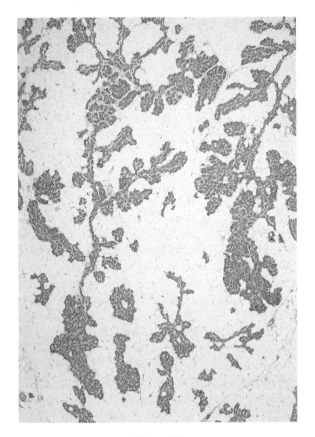

Figure 6-8
FATTY INFILTRATION OF PAROTID GLAND
Multiple foci of atrophic parotid parenchyma are embedded within a fatty stroma.

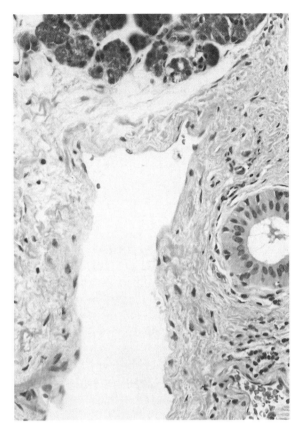

Figure 6-9
LYMPHANGIOMA
A large lymphatic space lined by flattened endothelial cells insinuates between a striated duct and lobule of serous acini in the parotid gland.

residual parotid parenchyma scattered throughout the adipose tissue (fig. 6-8). In lipomas with focal infiltration, the bulk of the mass is adipose tissue without glandular parenchyma, and foci of normal acinar tissue are evident only among the lipocytes along the periphery of the lipoma.

Treatment and Prognosis. Excision is appropriate treatment. These tumors do not recur.

Lymphangioma

In contrast to hemangioma, involvement of the salivary glands by lymphangioma is much less frequent (32,33). Most lymphangiomas manifest during childhood as fluctuant, slow-growing masses in the head and neck. They occasionally occur in the parotid gland or, less often, in the submandibular gland. As in other

sites, histologically variable numbers of medium to large irregular spaces are lined by endothelium. The spaces are supported by walls of loose or dense collagenous tissue (fig. 6-9). Complete surgical excision is usually necessary.

MALIGNANT MESENCHYMAL TUMORS

Primary nonlymphoid sarcomas of the major salivary glands represent about 0.5 percent of all benign and malignant salivary gland tumors and about 1.5 percent of malignant tumors (2,29,49). The criteria for establishing a primary origin are: 1) the patient must not have, or have had, a sarcoma in some other site; 2) patient evaluation has excluded the likelihood of metastatic disease; 3) the gross and microscopic appearances support a primary origin rather than invasion from adjacent soft tissues; and 4) carcinosarcoma has been excluded (4,29). In a study of sarcomas in the AFIP files, it was difficult to establish the exact origin of many of the cases based on surgical, gross, and microscopic information (4).

Nearly all forms of sarcoma present as masses within the major salivary glands: published reports include rhabdomyosarcoma, fibrosarcoma, leiomyosarcoma, malignant fibrous histiocytoma, malignant schwannoma, angiosarcoma, hemangiopericytoma, malignant hemangioendothelioma, Kaposi's sarcoma, osteosarcoma, liposarcoma, alveolar soft part sarcoma, and sarcomas that could not be further classified (4,6,22,29,31, 36,39,42,46,50,52,55,59,62). Of these, the types found most commonly in the salivary glands are rhabdomyosarcoma, malignant schwannoma, malignant fibrous histiocytoma, hemangiopericytoma, and fibrosarcoma (2,4,29,49). Kaposi's sarcoma of the parotid gland also occurs in patients with acquired immunodeficiency syndrome (AIDS), but these more often develop within intraparotid lymph nodes (7,35,44,65).

In a study of 67 cases of sarcomatoid neoplasms of the major salivary gland regions, immunohistochemical analysis showed that 5 sarcomatoid tumors could be reclassified as anaplastic carcinomas and an equal number as conventional or neurotropic melanomas (4). These findings illustrate the need for consideration of a wide differential diagnosis and for performing immunohistochemical studies of sarcomatoid tumors of the salivary glands; however, many types of mesenchymal neoplasms occasionally demonstrate cytokeratin immunoreactivity (17,20,30,34,51,54). Except for synovial sarcoma, epithelioid vascular tumors, and epithelioid sarcoma this reactivity is usually limited to scattered cells.

Most sarcomas of the major salivary glands involve the parotid gland (about 80 percent) and clinically present as a nodule or swelling (2). The average tumor duration prior to diagnosis is about 4 months. Rapid growth is experienced just prior to diagnosis in 10 percent of the patients and about the same proportion develop facial paralysis; pain or tenderness occurs in many of the patients. For the most part, the age of patients with each type of tumor conforms to that of patients with soft tissue tumors.

Malignant Schwannoma

The relatively high frequency of benign and malignant neural tumors in the salivary glands may be attributed to the abundant peripheral nerve supply present, particularly within the parotid gland. As in other sites, most malignant schwannomas occurring in the salivary glands are recognized as spindle cell malignancies of mesenchymal origin. The presence of peculiar morphologic and immunohistochemical features help confirm the neural origin (13). However, the epithelioid variant closely resembles carcinoma and needs to be distinguished from a primary parenchymal neoplasm. Malignant epithelioid schwannomas usually have nodular growth and variably cellular to myxoid areas, and some are entirely epithelioid (28). The cohesive clusters and sheets of tumor cells closely mimic undifferentiated carcinoma (fig. 6-10). Many show focal transition to spindled areas, and origin from a nerve can occasionally be documented. Immunohistochemical study helps confirm the neural origin and lack of epithelial differentiation (fig. 6-11).

Hemangiopericytoma

The propensity for parotid involvement by benign vascular tumors has already been noted, so perhaps it is not surprising that malignant vascular tumors are also numerous. Hemangiopericytoma is one of the most common types, both in the literature and in the AFIP files. Benign, borderline, and malignant subtypes of hemangiopericytoma are recognized (16). Malignant hemangiopericytomas are generally more cellular, demonstrate cellular pleomorphism, and are often associated with hemorrhage and necrosis. Characteristically, numerous thin-walled, branching vessels are surrounded by closely packed cells with ovoid nuclei and ill-defined borders. Examples in the parotid gland that contain large, gaping vessels are easily recognized (fig. 6-12). Problems in recognition arise in tumors in which the rich vascularity is not obvious, such as when the vascular channels are compressed (fig. 6-13). In such instances the lesions may be misconstrued as a myoepithelioma or other mesenchymal neoplasm. As with most other mesenchymal neoplasms occurring in the salivary glands, immunohistochemical analysis may be helpful. For instance,

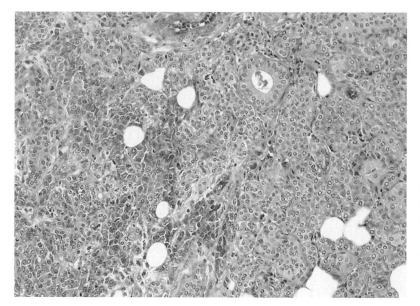

Figure 6-10
MALIGNANT EPITHELIOID
SCHWANNOMA

Most of the left side of this field is occupied by moderately hyperchromatic tumor cells of a malignant epithelioid schwannoma that is infiltrating the parotid tissue on the right. Distinction between this epithelioid infiltrate and a carcinomatous infiltrate is difficult without the help of immunohistochemical analysis.

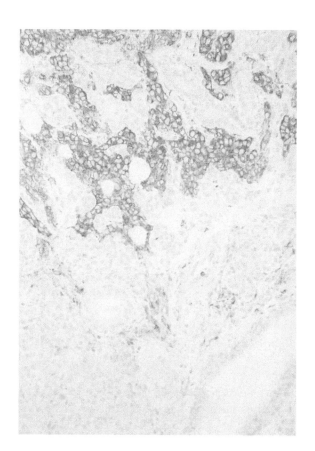 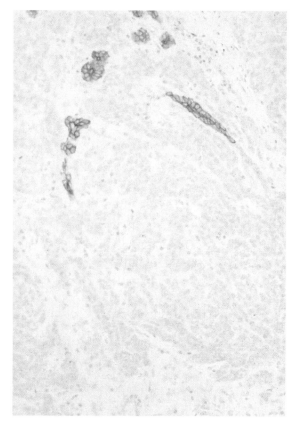

Figure 6-11
MALIGNANT EPITHELIOID SCHWANNOMA
Left: Immunoreactivity of the tumor cells with a neural marker, Leu-7 (top).
Right: Lack of reactivity for cytokeratin (bottom) provides valuable evidence for the diagnosis of sarcoma over carcinoma.
A few residual glandular structures are highlighted by cytokeratin (top).

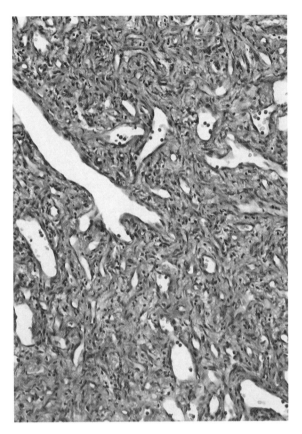

Figure 6-12
HEMANGIOPERICYTOMA
The presence of numerous vascular channels that are lined by flattened endothelial cells and surrounded by haphazardly arranged ovoid or fusiform cells facilitates recognition of this example.

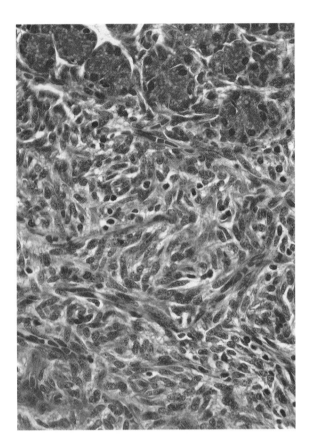

Figure 6-13
HEMANGIOPERICYTOMA
In contrast to the previous tumor, this field is typical of a tumor that lacked the characteristic vascular element and was initially thought to represent a myoepithelioma. A few residual acini are seen at the top.

most tumors that occasionally have a hemangiopericytoma-like growth pattern, such as synovial sarcomas, malignant schwannomas, and leiomyosarcomas, are not immunoreactive with factor XIIIa, unlike hemangiopericytoma (40,43,48).

Malignant Fibrous Histiocytoma

As in other sites, malignant fibrous histiocytomas in the salivary glands have a wide range of histologic appearances (15). Most have storiform and pleomorphic areas (fig. 6-14). Pleomorphic forms are sometimes difficult to distinguish from pleomorphic carcinomas without the help of immunostains for cytokeratin. Those that are well-differentiated occasionally resemble dermatofibrosarcoma protuberans (fig. 6-15), a tumor that only rarely involves the salivary glands.

Treatment and Prognosis of Malignant Mesenchymal Neoplasms

Despite the rarity of these tumors, differences in treatment considerations make distinction between carcinomas and sarcomas important. Although patients with tumors arising within the gland have fewer recurrences and metastases than patients with secondary salivary gland involvement, the improved prognosis is probably related more to stage of disease than tissue origin (4). This is supported by the study of Luna et al. (29) that showed that primary salivary gland sarcomas behaved like their soft tissue counterparts and that prognosis was related to tumor size as well as sarcoma type and histologic grade. Hematogenous rather than lymph node metastasis is more common with sarcomas than carcinomas, so

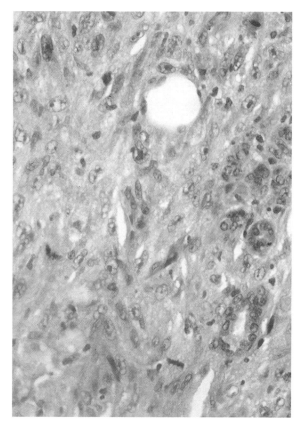

Figure 6-14
MALIGNANT FIBROUS HISTIOCYTOMA

Two residual ducts remain within a sheet of histiocyte-like, mitotically active cells. The cells have large, pleomorphic nuclei, prominent nucleoli, abundant cytoplasm, and indistinct cell borders.

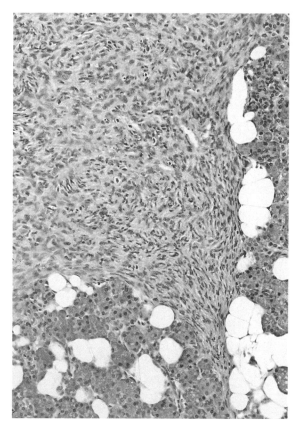

Figure 6-15
DERMATOFIBROSARCOMA PROTUBERANS

As in other sites, this dermatofibrosarcoma protuberans has a scalloped periphery with delicate processes that extend deeply into adjacent glandular tissue. This morphologically uniform tumor lacks the pleomorphism and mitotic activity associated with malignant fibrous histiocytoma.

neck dissection is usually not indicated. Of 42 patients with follow-up who had sarcomas of the major glands, only 3 had metastases to lymph nodes, and 2 of these also had hematogenous dissemination to the lung and brain (4). In a 1991 review of 60

reported cases, 28 percent recurred, most within 1 year after treatment (29); distant metastases were discovered in 40 percent of the patients, and disease-related death in 52 percent.

REFERENCES

1. Adams G, Goycoolea MV, Foster C, Dehner L, Anderson RD. Parotid lipomatosis in a 2-month-old child. Otolaryngol Head Neck Surg 1981;89:402–5.
2. Auclair PL, Ellis GL. Nonlymphoid sarcomas of the major salivary glands. In: Ellis GL, Auclair PL, Gnepp DR, eds. Surgical pathology of the salivary glands. Philadelphia: WB Saunders, 1991:514–27.
3. Auclair PL, Ellis GL, Gnepp DR, Wenig BM, Janney CG. Salivary gland neoplasms: general considerations. In: Ellis GL, Auclair PL, Gnepp DR, eds. Surgical

pathology of the salivary glands. Philadelphia: WB Saunders, 1991:135–64.
4. Auclair PL, Langloss JM, Weiss SW, Corio RL. Sarcomas and sarcomatoid neoplasms of the major salivary gland regions. A clinicopathologic and immunohistochemical study of 67 cases and review of the literature. Cancer 1986;58:1305–15.
5. Baker SE, Jensen JL, Correll RW. Lipomas of the parotid gland. Oral Surg Oral Med Oral Pathol 1981;52:167–71.

6. Bertrand JC, Guilbert F, Vaillant JM, et al. Les hemangiopericytomes de la sphere orofaciale. Ann Otolaryngol Chir Cervicofac 1984;101:607–13.

7. Bonzanini M, Togni R, Barabareschi M, Parenti A, Dalla Palma P. Primary Kaposi's sarcoma of intraparotid lymph node. Histopathology 1992;21:489–91.

8. Calhoun KH, Clark WD, Jones JD. Parotid lipoblastoma in an infant. Int J Pediatr Otorhinolaryngol 1987;14:41–4.

9. Chong GC, Beahrs OH, Chen ML, Hayles AB. Management of parotid gland tumors in infants and children. Mayo Clin Proc 1975;50:279–83.

10. Chuong R, Donoff RB. Intraparotid hemangioma in an adult. Case report and review of the literature. Int J Oral Surg 1984;13:346–51.

11. Dabashi Y, Eisen RN. Infantile hemangioendothelioma of the pelvis associated with Kasabach-Merritt syndrome. Pediatr Pathol 1990;10:407–15.

12. Enzinger FM, Weiss SW. Soft tissue tumors. 2nd ed. St. Louis: CV Mosby, 1988.

13. Enzinger FM, Weiss SW. Soft tissue tumors. 2nd ed. St. Louis: CV Mosby, 1988:781–815.

14. Enzinger FM, Weiss SW. Soft tissue tumors. 2nd ed. St. Louis: CV Mosby, 1988:489–532.

15. Enzinger FM, Weiss SW. Soft tissue tumors. 2nd ed. St. Louis: CV Mosby, 1988:269–300.

16. Enzinger FM, Weiss SW. Soft tissue tumors. 2nd ed. St. Louis: CV Mosby, 1988:596–613.

17. Fletcher CD, Beham A, Bekir S, Clarke AM, Marley NJ. Epithelioid angiosarcoma of deep soft tissue: a distinctive tumor readily mistaken for an epithelial neoplasm. Am J Surg Pathol 1991;15:915–24.

18. George CD, Ng YY, Hall-Craggs MA, Jones BM. Parotid haemangioma in infants: MR imaging at 1.5T. Pediatr Radiol 1991;21:483–5.

19. Goldman RL, Perzik SL. Infantile hemangioma of the parotid gland; a clinicopathological study of 15 cases. Arch Otolaryngol Head Neck Surg 1969;90:605–8.

20. Gray MH, Rosenberg AE, Dickersin GR, Bhan AK. Cytokeratin expression in epithelioid vascular neoplasms. Hum Pathol 1990;21:212–7.

21. Janecka IP, Conley J, Perzin KH, Pitman G. Lipomas presenting as parotid tumors. Laryngoscope 1977;87:1007–10.

22. Katsantonis GP, Friedman WH, Rosenblum BN. The surgical management of advanced malignancies of the parotid gland. Otolaryngol Head Neck Surg 1989;101:633–40.

23. Kauffman SL, Stout AP. Tumors of the major salivary glands in children. Cancer 1963;16:1317–31.

24. Korentager R, Noyek AM, Chapnik JS, Steinhardt M, Luk SC, Cooter N. Lipoma and liposarcoma of the parotid gland: high-resolution preoperative imaging diagnosis. Laryngoscope 1988;98:967–71.

25. Lack EE, Upton MP. Histopathologic review of salivary gland tumors in childhood. Arch Otolaryngol Head Neck Surg 1988;114:898–906.

26. Layfield LJ, Glasgow BJ, Goldstein N, Lufkin R. Lipomatous lesions of the parotid gland. Potential pitfalls in fine needle aspiration biopsy diagnosis. Acta Cytol 1991;35:553–6.

27. Levine E, Wetzel LH, Neff JR. MR imaging and CT of extrahepatic cavernous hemangiomas. Am J Roentgenol 1986;147:1299–304.

28. Lodding P, Kindblom LG, Angervall L. Epithelioid malignant schwannoma. A study of 14 cases. Virchows Arch [A] 1986;409:433–51.

29. Luna MA, Tortoledo ME, Ordóñez NG, Frankenthaler RA, Batsakis JG. Primary sarcomas of the major salivary glands. Arch Otolaryngol Head Neck Surg 1991;117:302–6.

30. Lundgren L, Kindblom LG, Seidal T, Angervall L. Intermediate and fine cytofilaments in cutaneous and subcutaneous leiomyosarcomas. APMIS 1991;99:820–8.

31. Manning JT, Raymond AK, Batsakis JG. Extraosseous osteogenic sarcoma of the parotid gland. J Laryngol Otol 1986;100:239–42.

32. Mantravadi J, Roth LM, Kafrawy AH. Vascular neoplasms of the parotid gland. Parotid vascular tumors. Oral Surg Oral Med Oral Pathol 1993;75:70–5.

33. McDaniel RK. Benign mesenchymal neoplasms. In: Ellis GL, Auclair PL, Gnepp DR, eds. Surgical pathology of the salivary glands. Philadelphia: WB Saunders, 1991:489–513.

34. Miettinen M. Keratin subsets in spindle cell sarcomas. Keratins are widespread but synovial sarcoma contains a distinctive keratin polypeptide pattern and desmoplakins. Am J Pathol 1991;138:505–13.

35. Mongiardo FD, Tewfik TL. Kaposi's sarcoma of the intra-parotid lymph nodes in AIDS. J Otolaryngol 1991;20:243–6.

36. Nagao K, Matsuzaki O, Saiga H, et al. Histopathologic studies of undifferentiated carcinoma of the parotid gland. Cancer 1982;50:1572–9.

37. Nagao K, Matsuzaki O, Saiga H, et al. Histopathological studies on parotid gland tumors in Japanese children. Virchows Arch [A] 1980;388:263–72.

38. Nagao K, Matsuzaki O, Shigematsu H, Kaneko T, Katoh T, Kitamura T. Histopathologic studies of benign infantile hemangioendothelioma of the parotid gland. Cancer 1980;46:2250–6.

39. Neal TF, Starke WR. Hemangiopericytoma of the parotid gland: a case report with autopsy. Laryngoscope 1973;83:1953–8.

40. Nemes Z. Differentiation markers in hemangiopericytoma. Cancer 1992;69:133–40.

41. Nussbaum M, Tan S, Som ML. Hemangiomas of the salivary glands. Laryngoscope 1976;86:1015–9.

42. Piscioli F, Antolini M, Pusiol T, Dalri P, Lo Bello MD, Mair K. Malignant schwannoma of the submandibular gland. A case report. ORL J Otorhinolaryngol Relat Spec 1986;48:156–61.

43. Porter PL, Bigler SA, McNutt M, Gown AM. The immunophenotype of hemangiopericytomas and glomus tumors, with special reference to muscle protein expression: an immunohistochemical study and review of the literature. Mod Pathol 1991;4:46–52.

44. Reath DB, Noone RB, Columbus M, Murphy JB. Primary Kaposi's sarcoma of an intraparotid lymph node with AIDS. Plast Reconstr Surg 1987;80:615–8.

45. Reilly JS, Kelly DR, Royal SA. Angiolipoma of the parotid: case report and review. Laryngoscope 1988;98:818–21.

46. Renick B, Clark RM, Feldman L. Embryonal rhabdomyosarcoma: presentation as a parotid gland mass. Oral Surg Oral Med Oral Pathol 1988;65:575–9.

47. Robertson JS, Wiegand DA, Schaitkin BM. Life-threatening hemangioma arising from the parotid gland. Otolaryngol Head Neck Surg 1991;104:858–62.

48. Schurch W, Skalli O, Lagace R, Seemayer TA, Gabbiani G. Intermediate filament proteins and actin isoforms as markers for soft-tissue tumor differentiation and origin. III Hemangiopericytomas and glomus tumors. Am J Surg Pathol 1990;136:771–86.

49. Seifert G, Oehne H. Die mesenchymalen (nicht-epithelialen) speicheldrusentumorens. Analyse von 167 tumorfallen des speicheldrusen-registers. Laryngol Rhinol Otol (Stuttg) 1986;65:485–91.

50. Stimson PG, Valenzuela-Espinoza A, Tortoledo ME, Luna MA, Ordóñez NG. Primary osteosarcoma of the parotid gland. Oral Surg Oral Med Oral Pathol 1989;68:80–6.

51. Swanson PE. Heffalumps, jagulars, and cheshire cats. A commentary on cytokeratins and soft tissue sarcomas. Am J Clin Pathol 1991;95:S2–7.

52. Taira S, Okuda M, Osato T, Mizuno F. [Detection of Epstein-Barr virus DNA in salivary gland tumors]. Article in Japanese, English abstract. Nippon Jibiinkoka Gakkai Kaiho 1992;95:860–8.

53. Takato T, Komuro Y, Yonehara Y. Giant hemangioma of the parotid gland associated with Kasabach-Merritt syndrome: a case report. J Oral Maxillofac Surg 1993;51:425–8.

54. Tauchi K, Tsutsumi Y, Yoshimura S, Watanabe K. Immunohistochemical and immunoblotting detection of cytokeratin in smooth muscle tumors. Acta Pathol Jpn 1990;40:574–80.

55. Tomec R, Ahmad I, Fu YS, Jaffe S. Malignant hemangioendothelioma (angiosarcoma) of the salivary gland: an ultrastructural study. Cancer 1979;43:1664–71.

56. Totsuka Y, Fukuda H, Tomita K. Compression therapy for parotid haemangioma in infants. A report of three cases. J Craniomaxillofac Surg 1988;16:366–70.

57. Tresserra L, Martinez-Mora J, Boix-Ochoa J. Haemangiomas of the parotid gland in children. J Maxillofac Surg 1977;5:238–41.

58. Vinayak BC, Reddy KT. Hibernoma in the parotid region. J Laryngol Otol 1993;107:257–8.

59. Volpe R, Mazabraud A. Primary sarcomas of the parotid gland. A clinicopathologic report of two cases. Pathologica 1981;73:541-6.

60. Walts AE, Perzik SL. Lipomatous lesions of the parotid area. Arch Otolaryngol Head Neck Surg 1976;102:230–2.

61. Welch KJ, Trump DS. The salivary glands. In: Ravitch MM, Welch KJ, Benson CD, Aberdeen E, Randolph JG, eds. Pediatric surgery. 3rd ed. Chicago: Year Book Medical Publishers, 1979:308–23.

62. Whittam DE, Hellier W. Haemangiopericytoma of the parotid salivary gland: report of a case with literature review. J Laryngol Otol 1993;107:1159–62.

63. Williams HB. Hemangiomas of the parotid gland in children. Plast Reconstr Surg 1975;56:29–34.

64. Winters Z, Mannell A. Parotid haemangioma. A case report. S Afr J Surg 1990;28:105–6.

65. Yeh CK, Fox PC, Fox CH, Travis WD, Lane HC, Baum BJ. Kaposi's sarcoma of the parotid gland in acquired immunodeficiency syndrome. Oral Surg Oral Med Oral Pathol 1989;67:308–12.

66. Zukerberg LR, Nickoloff BJ, Weiss SW. Kaposiform hemangioendothelioma of infancy and childhood. An aggressive neoplasm associated with Kasabach-Merritt syndrome and lymphangiomatosis. Am J Surg Pathol 1993;17:321–8.

7

MALIGNANT LYMPHOMAS OF THE MAJOR SALIVARY GLANDS

Definition. This is a malignant, localized, neoplastic proliferation of lymphoid cells in which major salivary gland involvement is usually the first clinical manifestation of disease. If clinical staging procedures at presentation reveal noncontiguous involvement of more than one site (stage IIIE or IVE) the lymphoma is considered secondary rather than primary. Because the parotid glands normally contain intraparenchymal nodal tissue, it is often difficult to determine whether parotid lymphomas have a nodal or extranodal origin, but distinction is made when possible. As discussed below, non-Hodgkin's malignant lymphoma accounts for a significant proportion of all malignancies of the major salivary glands. Lymphoma may also involve the minor glands of the oral mucosa; however, in these sites it is not usually possible to identify them as primary so they are not included in this discussion. Salivary gland involvement by Hodgkin's disease is rare and probably always secondary to nodal involvement. It is briefly discussed separately at the end of this section.

NON-HODGKIN'S LYMPHOMA

An overview of salivary gland lymphomas would not be complete without a discussion of their relationship to Sjögren's syndrome and to mucosa-associated lymphoid tissue and monocytoid B-cell lymphoma. A brief summary of these two subjects is included.

Relationship to Sjögren's Syndrome. In patients with autoimmune disease, particularly Sjögren's syndrome, the risk of developing lymphoma is markedly increased. Biopsies from these patients often demonstrate replacement of glandular parenchyma by a lymphoreticular infiltrate and disruption and metaplasia of the ductal system that includes the formation of so-called epimyoepithelial islands. This constellation of histologic findings has been labeled *benign lymphoepithelial lesion (BLEL)* or *myoepithelial sialadenitis (MESA)* (18,25,53,61, 62). Because epimyoepithelial complexes in lymphoma are also referred to as lymphoepithelial lesions, MESA is used here instead of BLEL to avoid confusing these overlapping terms. The diagnosis of Sjögren's syndrome requires correlation of the histologic features with serologic, sialographic, oral, and ophthalmologic findings. However, the histologic features of MESA are seen in patients who lack the clinical features of Sjögren's syndrome, and lymphoma also occurs in this setting. Furthermore, lymphoma frequently occurs in the absence of clinical or histologic evidence of either condition (18,26,52).

Kassan and colleagues (37) found the risk of developing lymphoma for female patients with Sjögren's syndrome was about 44 times greater than expected in their control group over an 8-year period. Those patients who manifested clinical symptoms that indicated marked lymphoid proliferation, such as parotid enlargement, splenomegaly, and lymphadenopathy, were at a greater risk than those who did not. Recent studies have shown that about 6 percent of patients with Sjögren's syndrome develop malignant lymphoma, often in extranodal sites that include the salivary and lacrimal glands and lungs, and that many patients develop benign but atypical lymphoproliferative disorders (20,47,54,55).

Because of the suspicion that the initial, morphologically benign lymphoid infiltrates in MESA may slowly but progressively transform to lymphoma, attention has been directed to immunohistochemical and molecular methods to facilitate early recognition of malignancy. Although about 80 percent of the lymphocytes in the salivary glands of patients with Sjögren's syndrome are T cells, most of the lymphomas that develop are phenotypically B-cell type (15,49). It has been shown that areas within the lymphoid infiltrates may contain monotypic cells that have a restricted immunoglobulin pattern (9,25,36,43,60, 61,72,78,79,84). The monotypic cell population is not, however, always associated with local invasion and spread outside the salivary gland tissue and may remain localized for years. Fishleder and colleagues (11) found that the infiltrates in MESA reveal rearrangement of both the heavy and light chain immunoglobulin genes. Their conclusion was that this finding either indicated early development of lymphoma limited to the salivary gland or, alternatively, a more generalized defect in immune surveillance. In the latter case they theorized that subsequent development of lymphoma resulted from neoplastic transformation of the expanded B-cell clone. Falzon and Isaacson (9), however, concluded that monoclonality of the infiltrate in MESA, detected by immunohistochemical or molecular methods, is diagnostic of low-grade B-cell lymphoma. Kossakowska and colleagues (40) stress that in mucosa-associated lymphoid tissue (MALT) lymphomas the results of immunoglobulin heavy chain rearrangement have to be interpreted with caution because of the possible monoclonal proliferation of the inflammatory element.

Some attention has been focused on the possible etiologic role of Epstein-Barr virus (EBV) and human herpes virus-6 in the development of Sjögren's syndrome and lymphoproliferative disease of the salivary glands (12,13,15,58). Viral DNA and increased antibody titers against these viruses have been detected in the lymphomatous tissue of some patients (13).

Mucosa-Associated Lymphoid Tissue. Some salivary gland lymphomas are more difficult to categorize than node-based disease. These are best understood as low-grade B-cell lymphomas that are derived from MALT (21, 22,28,31). Lymphoid tissue associated with mucosa in sites such as the gastrointestinal tract has been designated as MALT. In sites populated by similar lymphoid tissue, including the salivary and thyroid glands, breast, prostate, and thymus, mucosa is not necessarily present but rather it is the glandular epithelium that is the common element. The term *glandular epithelial lymphoid tissue (GELT)* may, therefore, be more accurate than MALT for the lymphoid tissue in these sites (21). The importance of recognizing lymphomas that arise from this tissue, other than for classification, is that as a group they demonstrate indolent clinical behavior. Furthermore, they often have microscopic features that may lead to their inclusion as "benign" extranodal lymphoid infiltrates, which explains why some formerly were designated as "pseudolymphoma."

Although the nature of the relationship of MALT-type lymphomas to monocytoid B-cell lymphomas is not entirely clear, it has been proposed that both MALT and monocytoid B-cell lympho-

mas are derived from post-germinal center marginal zone cells (22,32,50,51,65,66,69,71,81). These cells evolve from memory B cells that occupy the outer follicle mantle zone, known as the marginal zone, where they develop slightly irregular nuclei and pale cytoplasm and, with further enlargement, become monocytoid B cells or plasma cells (22,45,46). This latter capacity explains the morphologic diversity of this group of lymphomas. The marginal zone cells apparently retain the epithelial homing ability of their precursor cells, so they are attracted either to the follicles of lymph nodes or to extranodal sites with glandular epithelium (5). Normal MALT lymphocytes appear to have the ability to home to specific epithelia and their neoplastic counterparts may retain this ability, thereby explaining a tendency to remain localized (5,21). The attraction of the lymphocytes for epithelium may also explain their tendency to infiltrate the epithelial islands and form the lymphoepithelial lesions seen in many salivary gland lymphomas (25,61, 62). Not all MALT-type lymphomas contain typical monocytoid B cells (22). Lennert and Feller (42) proposed using the term monocytoid B-cell lymphoma for neoplasms that occur in lymph nodes and MALT-type lymphoma for those found in extranodal sites such as salivary glands. Harris (22) suggested that in either instance they could be accurately called marginal zone B-cell lymphomas or, alternatively, placed in the most appropriate Working Formulation classification with an accompanying explanatory note (21).

Extranodal non-Hodgkin's lymphomas overall account for about 25 percent of all lymphomas in the United States and as many as 48 percent in other countries (3,4,14,57). Some of the most common sites include the gastrointestinal tract, Waldeyer's ring area, lung, skin, small intestine, orbit, and salivary glands (14,35,57,67). Burke (4) notes that to be categorized as extranodal lymphoma the patient must present with IE or IIE disease; IIIE or IV disease is presumed to represent disseminated lymphoma, even if occult. Relapse of node-based lymphoma to an extranodal site also is excluded.

General Features. Malignant lymphomas represent a significant proportion of the malignant tumors encountered in the major salivary glands. At the Armed Forces Institute of Pathology (AFIP) and elsewhere, the majority of major salivary gland lymphomas arise de novo rather than in patients with clinical or histologic evidence of immune sialadenitis (7,17,26,38). Gleeson and colleagues (17) noted that only 4 of 26 patients had a history suggestive of sicca syndrome. Although the parotid gland normally contains abundant intraglandular lymphoid tissue, because the major salivary glands contain MALT, many of the lymphomas represent extranodal disease. This knowledge helps in their evaluation (10,17).

At the AFIP, lymphoma has accounted for 16.3 percent of all malignant tumors that occurred in the major salivary glands since 1985, and 8.8 percent of all major gland tumors. This latter figure is high compared with the 1.7 to 6 percent range of other studies (7,14,17,26,80). Of recent AFIP cases, only three epithelial malignancies were seen more frequently: mucoepidermoid carcinoma; adenocarcinoma, not otherwise specified; and acinic cell adenocarcinoma. Other investigators have also found the frequency of salivary gland lymphoma higher than typically reported: Mehle et al. (48) found that of 452 patients undergoing parotid gland surgery, 4 percent had lymphoma of the gland (compared to about 3 percent in AFIP files). The AFIP and others have recently noted an increasing proportion of salivary gland lymphomas relative to other tumor types (63,64). The overall incidence of 4 percent in the series of Schusterman and colleagues (63) increased from 1.5 percent initially to 6 percent in the most recent period. Performance of immunohistochemical studies for light chain restriction and other special studies for all suspicious cases has probably influenced the frequency of diagnosing lymphoma.

The recent cases at the AFIP are from patients who presented with salivary gland masses usually thought clinically and surgically to be parenchymal neoplasms. None of the patients were known to have disseminated disease but results of clinical staging are unknown. Some of these cases may represent secondary involvement by systemic disease. Nonetheless, these data indicate the relative likelihood that lesions thought clinically to be epithelial neoplasms are lymphomas. Patients with salivary gland lymphomas should have a thorough staging examination that includes chest radiograph, bilateral pedal lymphangiography or abdominal computerized tomography (CT), and bilateral iliac crest bone marrow biopsy (26,68).

Clinical Features. Patients with Sjögren's syndrome have keratoconjunctivitis sicca and xerostomia or other oral signs. About a third to half have episodic or chronic enlargement of the submandibular or parotid gland (2,7,8,69). The glandular enlargement is usually bilateral, firm, and nontender. Lymphoma is evident in the initial surgical specimen in some patients but in others is discovered following recurrent swelling of one or more years' duration (25). Patients without autoimmune disease usually initially present with a painless mass. Clinical examination in some cases suggests fixation to either superficial or deep structures (17).

Among patients included in published series both with and without autoimmune-associated lymphomas, the parotid gland far outnumbers the submandibular gland as the site of involvement (7,17,26). In AFIP data, the parotid accounts for about 80 percent of all cases. Between 80 to 90 percent of patients with Sjögren's syndrome are women, and the lymphomas that develop in Sjögren's patients have a similar female predilection (7,8,69,82). Studies of patients without autoimmune disease have shown a variable gender predominance (14,26,44,48,60,83). Among the civilian patients with lymphoma in AFIP's files, 64 percent are female. Salivary gland lymphoma is a disease of the elderly. The mean age is about 63 years, with a range of 4 to 96 years (7,14,17,60,63). Only 5 percent of AFIP patients are under 40 years whereas 65 percent are 60 years of age or older.

Gross and Microscopic Findings. Gross examination reveals a firm, solid mass. The cut surface is tan to white and has a homogeneous, slightly gelatinous texture that is similar to that of lymphomas in other sites. The interface of tumor and gland is sometimes circumscribed but is usually at least focally ill-defined and involves surrounding structures.

Microscopically, most tumors are non-Hodgkin's B-cell lymphomas. Many tumors are classified by schemes devised for nodal disease. In this group, the AFIP and others have found that the most frequent types are follicular small cleaved, follicular mixed, and diffuse large cell lymphomas (4,7,17,60). Except in incipient disease, the normal lobular salivary gland architecture is usually altered (fig. 7-1). The infiltrate replaces acini and ducts, surrounds nerves (fig. 7-2), and spills into

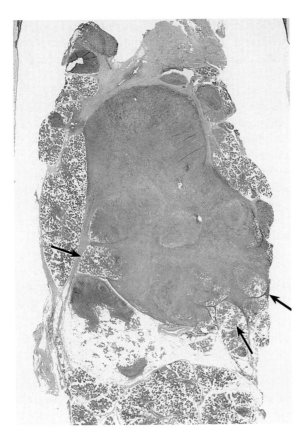

Figure 7-1
MALIGNANT LYMPHOMA

Parotid gland and parenchymal fat have been largely replaced by tumor. In several areas (arrows) remnants of salivary lobules are evident, but in the involved areas most of the gland architecture has been destroyed. Several small satellite extensions are also present.

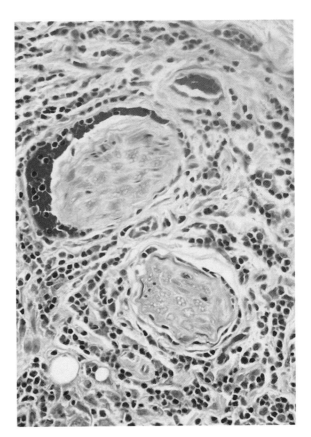

Figure 7-2
PERINEURAL INVOLVEMENT

This follicular, mixed small and large cell lymphoma involves many of the intraparotid peripheral nerves.

fat and interlobular and periglandular connective tissues (fig. 7-3). Dutcher bodies are sometimes evident (fig. 7-4). Periductal fibrosis is often evident (fig. 7-5), and the lymphoid cells frequently demonstrate significant crush artifact. Ductal metaplasia is occasionally present and resembles the epimyoepithelial islands characteristic of myoepithelial sialadenitis.

While many of the same features may be observed in MALT lymphomas (fig. 7-6), additional features are usually seen. The so-called centrocyte-like lymphoma cells are somewhat variable. They are small to medium sized, usually slightly larger than small lymphocytes, and have dense nuclei with irregular outlines (28–31). These cells often have abundant, pale-staining cytoplasm with distinct cell membranes, resembling monocytoid B cells (fig. 7-7). It is these cells

that usually invade the randomly scattered epimyoepithelial islands (fig. 7-8) and form the lymphoepithelial lesions characteristic of this lymphoma (fig. 7-9). Larger "transformed" nucleolated cells are also evident (30). The epithelial complexes are replaced by tumor, and the residual epithelial elements are often eventually obscured by the infiltrate. In some tumors, areas that resemble follicles are present (fig. 7-10). It has been reported that some of the follicular structures have neoplastic cells in the mantle or marginal areas and others have collections of monocytoid cells and neoplastic plasma cells (21, 22). Isaacson et al. (34) have suggested that reactive follicles are colonized by neoplastic centrocyte-like cells. In most areas, however, the diffuse nature of the lymphoma is obvious (74). Like others, the AFIP has observed transformation of low-grade MALT lymphomas to higher grade large cell lymphomas (fig. 7-11) (30,62).

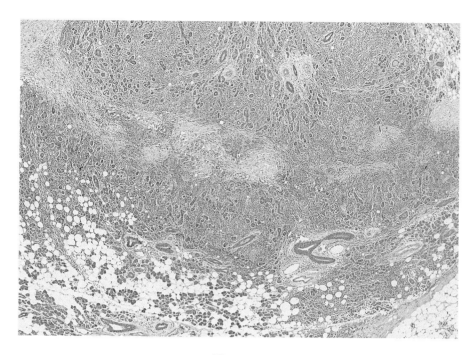

Figure 7-3
MALIGNANT LYMPHOMA

The lymphomatous cells have insinuated through the gland and replaced most acini, but many metaplastic ducts are left. This follicular, mixed lymphoma has focally prominent sclerosis.

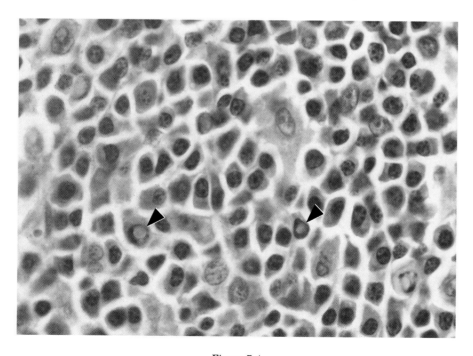

Figure 7-4
MALIGNANT LYMPHOMA

Several plasmacytoid neoplastic cells in this small lymphocytic lymphoma have intranuclear inclusions (Dutcher bodies) (arrowheads). Intracytoplasmic inclusions (Russell bodies) were also evident in this tumor but are not as helpful in distinguishing reactive from neoplastic disease as they typically also occur in inflammatory disease.

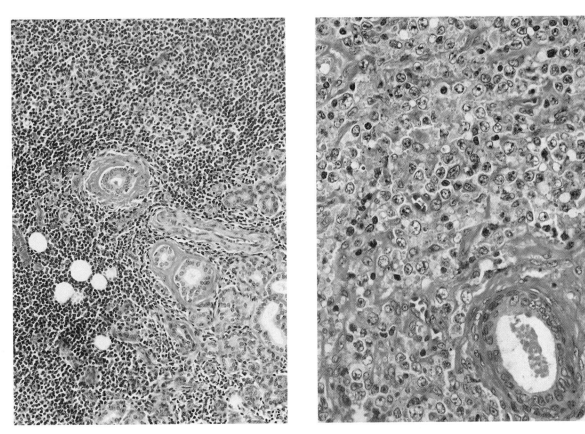

Figure 7-5
MALIGNANT LYMPHOMA
Two different examples of diffuse large cell lymphoma show residual ducts highlighted by thick fibrotic bands. Although this feature is often associated with malignant lymphoma, it also occurs in other conditions.

Figure 7-6
MALT LYMPHOMA
This lesion has multiple distinct and separate foci of lymphoma in regions of the excised gland. In other areas of the surgical specimen, however, confluence of the neoplastic nodules was evident.

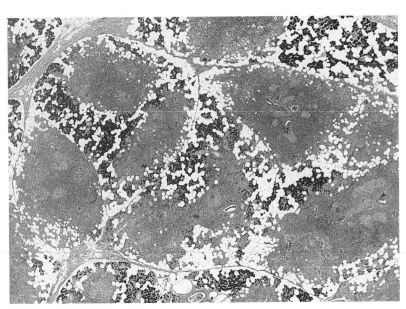

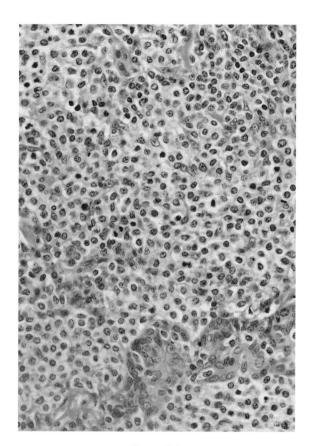

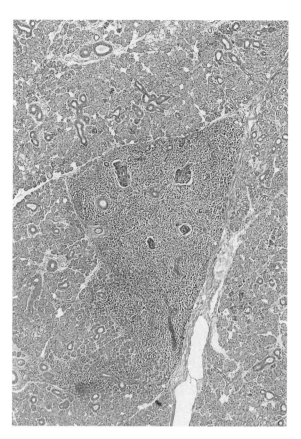

Figure 7-7
MALIGNANT LYMPHOMA
This MALT lymphoma is formed by a solid sheet of monomorphic, centrocyte-like cells that have abundant, partially cleared cytoplasm. The cytoplasmic borders are not well-defined. Strands of epithelium are seen at the bottom.

Figure 7-8
EPIMYOEPITHELIAL ISLANDS
A triangular focus of MALT lymphoma contains several of the characteristic epithelial islands as well as a few residual ducts. While the neoplastic focus is bordered on two sides by interlobular septa (right and top), at the bottom and left lymphoma cells extend into adjacent gland.

Because of the variability of features, MALT-derived low-grade B-cell lymphomas often resemble several types of node-based disease. When composed predominantly of small lymphocytes, they resemble small or intermediate lymphocytic lymphoma, depending on their uniformity (21,31). Those that have a partially follicular pattern mimic follicular lymphoma. In some cases, microscopic distinction of MALT lymphoma from nodal disease is very difficult unless frozen tissue is available for immunohistochemical study (see next section).

Immunohistochemical Findings. Immunohistochemical studies of paraffin-embedded tissue, although not always as useful as frozen tissue, can help confirm the lymphoreticular nature of an infiltrate and distinguish it from benign hyper-

plastic conditions. The demonstration of monotypic immunoglobulin light chains is diagnostic (fig. 7-12) but, unfortunately, with paraffin sections is successful in only about 50 percent of cases or less (22). As with node-based disease, MT-2(CD45RA) and bcl-2 help distinguish follicular hyperplasia from follicular lymphoma (19,77).

Salivary gland lymphomas are immunoreactive for leucocyte common antigen and nearly always for pan-B-cell markers such as L26 (fig. 7-13). They sometimes also express pan-T-cell CD43 antigen (22,83). The myoepithelial complexes in MALT lymphomas are reactive for cytokeratin, and this is especially useful in cases in which these complexes have been largely obscured by tumor cells (fig. 7-14). Recent studies indicate that immunohistochemical distinction

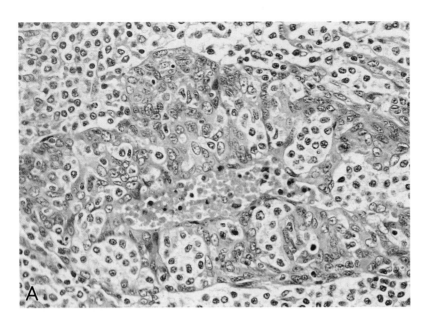

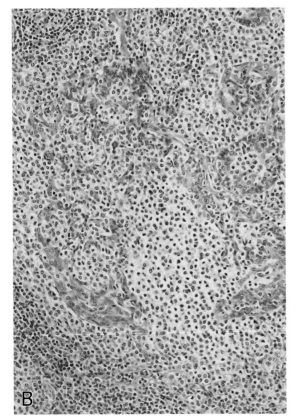
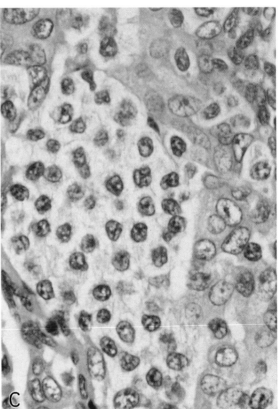

Figure 7-9
MALT LYMPHOMA

A: An epimyoepithelial island is infiltrated by several clusters of large, monocytoid B-cells.

B: With progression the epimyoepithelial island is largely replaced by the lymphoma and eventually would be completely destroyed by tumor.

C: Large cells that have slightly irregular nuclei, abundant pale cytoplasm, and a tendency to cluster are characteristic of MALT lymphomas, but smaller cells that have denser cytoplasm are often seen.

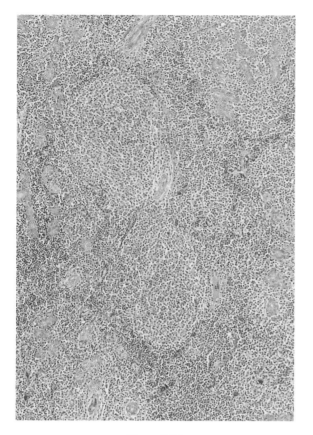

Figure 7-10
MALT LYMPHOMA
Nodular foci of admixed monocytoid B-cells and smaller lymphocytes mimic follicular lymphoma.

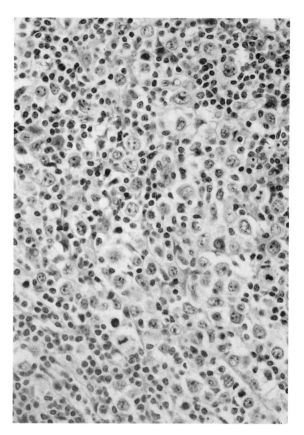

Figure 7-11
TRANSFORMATION OF MALT LYMPHOMA
TO LARGE CELL LYMPHOMA
As shown by this field, MALT lymphoma is largely replaced by large cells that have greater morphologic variation, enlarged and multiple nucleoli, and increased mitotic activity.

between MALT lymphomas and other types of low-grade B-cell lymphoma is possible. Unlike other low-grade B-cell lymphomas, those that arise from marginal zone cells are CD5 and CD10 negative. Currently these markers require frozen unfixed tissue (22,83). The neoplastic cells in patients presenting with exclusively extranodal diffuse B-cell lymphomas do not express CD5, and this feature facilitates their distinction from small lymphocytic lymphoma, chronic lymphocytic leukemia, and mantle zone lymphoma (33,73). Furthermore, it appears that MALT-related lymphomas lack the *bcl*-2 protein (4,39,56).

Differential Diagnosis. The inflammatory infiltrate in nonspecific sialadenitis consists of randomly arranged collections of lymphocytes, plasma cells, and, sometimes, neutrophils. Follicle formation occurs in some infiltrates. The infiltrate initially is often most prominent around

ducts but involves the acini early in the process. Periductal fibrosis occurs in both sialadenitis and lymphoma. Ductal ectasia accompanied by metaplasia of the duct lining is characteristic of obstructive inflammatory disease. Replacement and alteration of the lobular architecture of the gland typically does not occur with inflammatory infiltrates (fig. 7-15) although severe fibrosis, often associated with longstanding sialadenitis, may severely affect the lobular architecture. There are a growing number of reported cases in which the salivary gland lymphocytic infiltrates initially interpreted as myoepithelial sialadenitis are retrospectively interpreted as MALT-related lymphoma based on current knowledge and laboratory techniques not previously available (9,25). This emphasizes the need for extensive study, including immunohistochemical

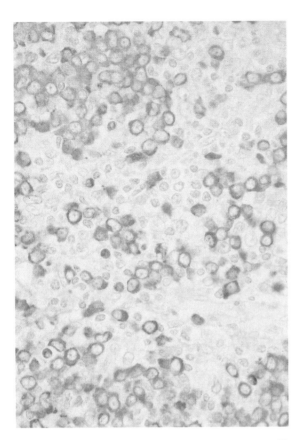
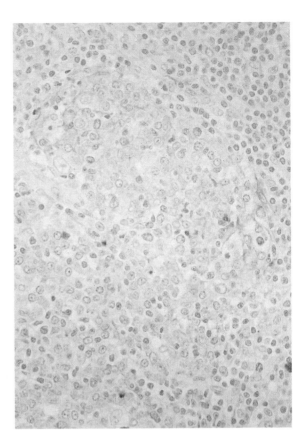

Figure 7-12
LIGHT CHAIN RESTRICTION
Immunohistochemical analysis of this parotid infiltrate shows an overwhelming predominance of kappa (left) over lambda (right) light chain immunoglobulin, helping confirm its neoplastic nature.

analysis (with frozen tissue when possible) of salivary glands that have lymphocytic infiltrates.

The appearance of MESA ranges from focal lymphocytic infiltrates with acinar atrophy to dense confluent infiltrates that form germinal centers. Lymphoma should be suspected anytime sheets of monomorphic, medium-sized lymphoid cells with abundant pale cytoplasm and bland uniform nuclei are seen. Epimyoepithelial complexes are not diagnostic of MESA as they occur in a variety of inflammatory and neoplastic conditions. Infiltration of small collections of monocytoid B cells into epimyoepithelial complexes, and extension of lymphoid infiltrates into paraglandular fibroadipose tissue or into perineural spaces are features favoring a diagnosis of lymphoma.

As with sialadenitis, plasma cells and reactive-appearing follicles are present in MALT lymphomas. Immunohistochemical demonstra-

tion of a B-cell phenotype and light chain restriction are usually diagnostic. If frozen tissue is available, the lack of CD5 in MALT lymphomas separates them from nodal B-cell chronic lymphocytic lymphoma and mantle cell lymphoma, and CD10 negativity distinguishes them from follicular lymphomas (22). Furthermore, MALT lymphoma has been reported to lack the translocation rearrangements of the *bcl*-2 gene (t[14;18]) and the *bcl*-1 gene (t[11;14]) (4,30).

The lymphoid element in patients with human immunodeficiency virus (HIV)-related lymphadenopathy is often atypical and suggestive of lymphoma (24,27,59). Follicular hyperplasia is florid and manifested by follicles with irregular shapes and cells with large irregular nuclei and abundant, sometimes clear cytoplasm that resemble monocytoid cells. Unlike MALT lymphoma, however, the germinal centers contain

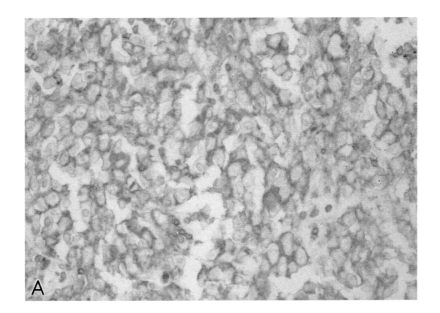

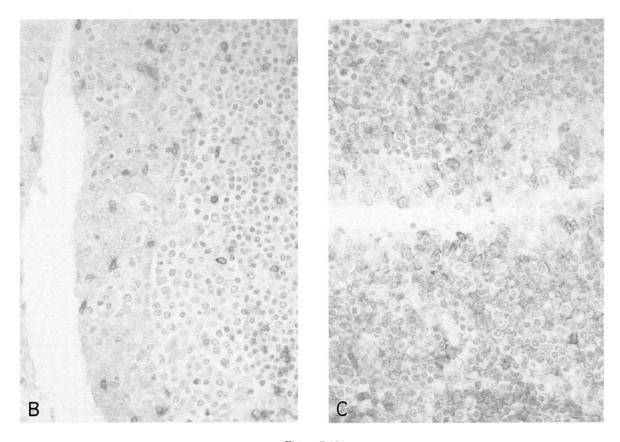

Figure 7-13
IMMUNOHISTOCHEMISTRY OF MALT LYMPHOMA
A: The MALT lymphoma cells contained in this field are diffusely immunoreactive for leucocyte common antigen.
B: The infiltrate and ductal epithelium contain only scattered cells that are reactive with CD3, a T-cell marker.
C: The B-cell phenotype of the lymphoma cells is demonstrated with L26. Only the luminal ductal epithelium has not been densely infiltrated by neoplastic cells.

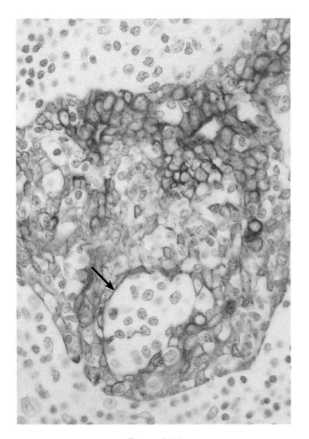

Figure 7-14
LYMPHOEPITHELIAL LESION
With the immunoperoxidase technique the epithelium is clearly defined by its strong immunoreactivity for cytokeratin. The surrounding lymphoma and single cluster of intraepithelial monocytoid B cells (arrow) are nonreactive.

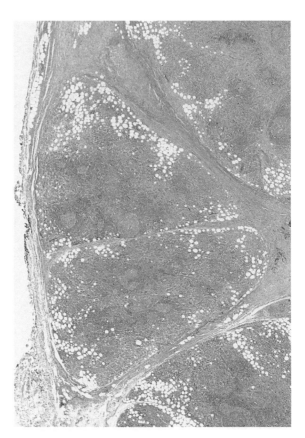

Figure 7-15
CHRONIC SIALADENITIS
In longstanding chronic sialadenitis the lymphocytic infiltrate is sharply confined by the salivary gland lobules. In contradistinction to salivary gland lymphoma, confluence of lobules is not evident nor does the cellular infiltrate spill into surrounding tissues. Several well-defined, pale-staining lymphoid follicles are seen.

macrophages with tingible bodies and neutrophils. Occasional follicle lysis, the disruptive insinuation of mantle lymphocytes into the germinal centers, is evident. Also, the lymphoid element usually contains several squamous-lined cysts and epithelial islands that resemble the epimyoepithelial islands characteristic of myoepithelial sialadenitis (see section, Tumor-Like Conditions). Computerized tomography often shows bilateral disease, although clinically it may appear unilateral, and the images reveal multiple cysts and cervical adenopathy (23,70,75). Parotid swelling may be the first clinical manifestations of HIV disease in asymptomatic patients (16).

Treatment and Prognosis. Non-MALT conventional lymphomas that occur in the salivary glands appear to have a prognosis similar to those in patients who have histologically identical nodal lymphomas (4,7,17,41,57). Treatment has included enucleation or resection, low- and high-dose radiotherapy, chemotherapy, or combinations of these (17,26,60).

MALT-associated lymphomas are relatively indolent, usually remain localized, and may be curable with local therapy (4,21,22,57). Spontaneous regression has been reported (55). In a review of diffuse low-grade B-cell lymphomas, all but one of seven patients with MALT-type lymphomas, defined by the morphologic and immunologic features discussed above, were free of disease and none died in 4 years (83). Survival, at least of patients with tumors occurring in some sites, approximates that of the general population (6).

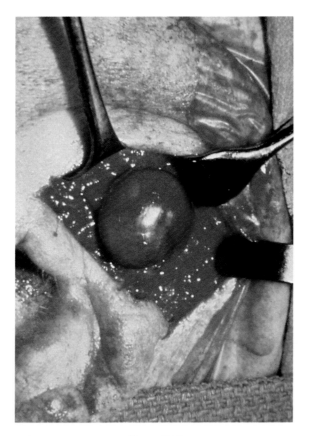

Figure 7-16
HODGKIN'S DISEASE
A parotid gland lymph node has been greatly enlarged by Hodgkin's disease.

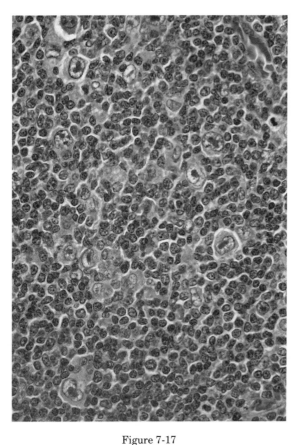

Figure 7-17
HODGKIN'S DISEASE
Characteristic Hodgkin's cells and Reed-Sternberg variants are present and are surrounded by a suitable admixture of background cells.

Isaacson (30) has stated that because MALT lymphoma is slow to disseminate, especially to the bone marrow, local treatment is adequate.

MALT lymphomas, however, sometimes transform to higher grade large cell lymphomas that are more aggressive (4,30,43,51,69). The distinction of high-grade lymphoma of MALT from other high-grade B-cell neoplasms is difficult, but its prognosis is apparently more favorable than comparable nodal disease (30). The presence or absence of synchronous low-grade foci in these cases has no effect on behavior (30).

HODGKIN'S DISEASE

Unlike non-Hodgkin's lymphoma, involvement of the major salivary glands by Hodgkin's disease is rare. Among lymphomas of the salivary glands in the AFIP files since 1985, only 9 are Hodgkin's disease. Most tumors occur in the parotid gland (fig. 7-16), probably because numerous intraglandular and paraglandular lymph nodes are present at this site (17,26,60, 64). Hodgkin's disease associated with Warthin's tumor has been reported (1,76). The clinical features of patients with salivary involvement, similar to those with nodal disease, show a male predominance and a bimodal age distribution.

Microscopically, Hodgkin's lymphoma in the major glands usually appears limited to intraglandular nodes (fig. 7-17) and does not have the extensive parenchymal infiltration characteristic of non-Hodgkin's lymphoma. The most frequent histologic types encountered are the nodular sclerosing and lymphocyte predominant variants (17,60).

REFERENCES

1. Badve S, Evans G, Mady S, Coppen M, Sloane J. A case of Warthin's tumour with coexistent Hodgkin's disease. Histopathology 1993;22:280–1.

2. Bridges AJ, England DM. Benign lymphoepithelial lesion: relationship to Sjögren's syndrome and evolving malignant lymphoma. Semin Arthritis Rheum 1989;19:201–8.

3. Burke JS. Extranodal lymphoid proliferations: general principles and differential diagnosis. In: Knowles DM, ed. Neoplastic hematopathology. Baltimore: Williams & Wilkins, 1992:901–15.

4. Burke JS. Waldeyer's ring, sinonasal region, salivary gland, thyroid gland, central nervous system, and other extranodal lymphomas and lymphoid hyperplasias. In: Knowles DM, ed. Neoplastic hematopathology. Baltimore: Williams & Wilkins, 1992:1047–79.

5. Butcher E. Cellular and molecular mechanisms that direct leukocyte traffic. Am J Pathol 1990;136:3–12.

6. Cogliatti SB, Schmid U, Schumacher U, et al. Primary B-cell gastric lymphoma: a clinicopathological study of 145 patients. Gastroenterology 1991;101:1159–70.

7. Colby TV, Dorfman RF. Malignant lymphomas involving the salivary glands. Pathol Annu 1979;14 (Pt 2):307–24.

8. Daniels TE. Labial salivary gland biopsy in Sjören's syndrome: assessment as a diagnostic criterion in 362 suspected cases. Arthritis Rheum 1984;27:147–56.

9. Falzon M, Isaacson PG. The natural history of benign lymphoepithelial lesion of the salivary gland in which there is a monoclonal population of B cells. A report of two cases. Am J Surg Pathol 1991;15:59–65.

10. Feind CR. The head and neck. In: Haagensen CD, Feind CR, Herter FP, eds. The lymphatics in cancer. 10th ed. Philadelphia: WB Saunders, 1972:63–4.

11. Fishleder A, Tubbs R, Hesse B, Levine H. Uniform detection of immunoglobulin-gene rearrangement in benign lymphoepithelial lesions. N Engl J Med 1987;316:1118–21.

12. Fox RI, Pearson G, Vaughan JH. Detection of Epstein-Barr virus associated antigens and DNA in salivary gland biopsies from patients with Sjögren's syndrome. J Immunol 1986;137:3162–8.

13. Fox RI, Saito I, Chan EK, et al. Viral genomes in lymphomas of patients with Sjögren's syndrome. J Autoimmun 1989;2:449–55

14. Freeman C, Berg JW, Cutler SJ. Occurrence and prognosis of extranodal lymphomas. Cancer 1972;29:252–60.

15. Freimark B, Fantozzi R, Bone R, Bordin G, Fox R. Detection of clonally expanded salivary gland lymphocytes in Sjögren's syndrome. Arthritis Rheum 1989;32:859–69.

16. Galindo LM, Franceschini A, Soltero E, Davila R. Benign cystic lymphoepithelial lesion of the parotid gland an unusual presentation of the acquired immunodeficiency syndrome. Bol Asoc Med P R 1991;83:340–2.

17. Gleeson MJ, Bennett MH, Cawson RA. Lymphomas of salivary glands. Cancer 1986;58:699–704.

18. Gleeson MJ, Cawson RA, Bennett MH. Benign lymphoepithelial lesion: a less than benign disease. Clin Otolaryngol 1986;11:47–51.

19. Griesser H. Applied molecular genetics in the diagnosis of malignant non-Hodgkin's lymphoma. Diagn Mol Pathol 1993;2:177–91.

20. Hansen LA, Prakash UB, Colby TV. Pulmonary lymphoma in Sjögren's syndrome. Mayo Clin Proc 1989;64:920–31.

21. Harris NL. Extranodal lymphoid infiltrates and mucosa-associated lymphoid tissue (MALT). A unifying concept [Editorial]. Am J Surg Pathol 1991;15:879–84.

22. Harris NL. Low-grade B-cell lymphoma of mucosa-associated lymphoid tissue and monocytoid B-cell lymphoma. Related entities that are distinct from other low-grade B-cell lymphomas [Editorial]. Arch Pathol Lab Med 1993;117:771–5.

23. Holliday RA, Cohen WA, Schinella RA, et al. Benign lymphoepithelial parotid cysts and hyperplastic cervical adenopathy in AIDS-risk patients: a new CT appearance. Radiology 1988;168:439–41.

24. Huang RD, Pearlman S, Friedman WH, Loree T. Benign cystic vs. solid lesions of the parotid gland in HIV patients. Head Neck 1991;13:522–7.

25. Hyjek E, Smith WJ, Isaacson PG. Primary B-cell lymphoma of salivary glands and its relationship to myoepithelial sialadenitis. Hum Pathol 1988;19:766–76.

26. Hyman GA, Wolff M. Malignant lymphomas of the salivary glands. Review of the literature and report of 33 new cases, including four cases associated with the lymphoepithelial lesion. Am J Clin Pathol 1976;65:421–38.

27. Ioachim HL, Ryan JR, Blaugrund SM. Salivary gland lymph nodes. The site of lymphadenopathies and lymphomas associated with human immunodeficiency virus infection. Arch Pathol Lab Med 1988;112:1224–8.

28. Isaacson P, Wright DH. Extranodal malignant lymphoma arising from mucosa-associated lymphoid tissue. Cancer 1984;53:2515–24.

29. Isaacson P, Wright DH. Malignant lymphoma of mucosa-associated lymphoid tissue. A distinctive type of B-cell lymphoma. Cancer 1983;52:1410–6.

30. Isaacson PG. Extranodal lymphomas: the MALT concept. Verh Dtsch Ges Pathol 1992;76:14–23.

31. Isaacson PG, Spencer J. Malignant lymphoma of mucosa-associated lymphoid tissue. Histopathology 1987;11:445–62.

32. Isaacson PG, Spencer J. Monocytoid B-cell lymphomas [Comment]. Am J Surg Pathol 1990;14:888–91.

33. Isaacson PG, Spencer J, Finn T. Primary B-cell gastric lymphoma. Hum Pathol 1986;17:72–82.

34. Isaacson PG, Wotherspoon AC, Pan L. Follicular colonization in B-cell lymphoma of mucosa-associated lymphoid tissue. Am J Surg Pathol 1991;15:819–28.

35. Jacobs C, Hoppe RT. Non-Hodgkin's lymphomas of head and neck extranodal sites. Int J Radiat Oncol Biol Phys 1985;11:357–64.

36. Janin A, Morel P, Quiquandon I, et al. Non-Hodgkin's lymphoma and Sjgren's syndrome. An immunopathological study of 113 patients. Clin Exp Rheumatol 1992;10:565–70.

37. Kassan SS, Thomas TL, Moutsopoulos HM, et al. Increased risk of lymphoma in sicca syndrome. Ann Intern Med 1978;89:888–92.

38. Kempf HG. Non-Hodgkin lymphoma of the parotid gland. HNO 1990;38:166–9.

39. Kerrigan DP, Irons J, Chen IM. Bcl-2 gene rearrangement in salivary gland lymphoma. Am J Surg Pathol 1990;14:1133–8.

40. Kossakowska AE, Eyton-Jones S, Urbanski SJ. Immunoglobulin and T-cell receptor gene rearrangements in lesions of mucosa-associated lymphoid tissue. Diagn Mol Pathol 1993;2:233–40.

41. Kuten A, Ben-Shahar M, Epelbaum R, Haim N, Cohen Y, Robinson E. Results of radiotherapy in stage I to II extranodal non-Hodgkin's lymphoma of the head and neck. Strahlenther Onkol 1989;165:578–83.

42. Lennert K, Feller A. Histopathology of non-Hodgkin's lymphomas. 2nd ed. New York: Springer-Verlag, 1992.

43. Lennert K, Schmid U. Prelymphoma, early lymphoma, and manifest lymphoma in immunosialadenitis (Sjögren's syndrome)—a model of lymphomagenesis. Hamatol Bluttransfus 1983;28:418–22.

44. Liang R, Loke SL. Non-Hodgkin's lymphomas involving the parotid gland. Clin Oncol (R Coll Radiol) 1991;3:81–3.

45. Liu Y, Johnson G, Gordon J, MacLennan I. Germinal centres in T-cell-dependent antibody responses. Immunol Today 1992;13:1–39.

46. MacLennan I, Liu Y, Oldfield S, Ahang J, Lane P. The evolution of B-cell clones. Curr Top Microbiol Immunol 1990;159:37–63.

47. McCurley TL, Collins RD, Ball E. Nodal and extranodal lymphoproliferative disorders in Sjgren's syndrome: a clinical and immunopathologic study. Hum Pathol 1990;21:482–92.

48. Mehle ME, Kraus DH, Wood BG, Tubbs R, Tucker HM, Lavertu P. Lymphoma of the parotid gland. Laryngoscope 1993;103:17–21.

49. Moutsopoulos HM, Manoussakis MN. Immunopathogenesis of Sjgren's syndrome: facts and fancy. Autoimmunity 1989;5:17–24.

50. Nathwani BN, Mohrmann RL, Brynes RK, Taylor CR, Hansmann ML, Sheibani K. Monocytoid B-cell lymphomas: an assessment of diagnostic criteria and a perspective on histogenesis. Hum Pathol 1992;23:1061–71.

51. Ngan BY, Warnke RA, Wilson M, Takagi K, Cleary ML, Dorfman RF. Monocytoid B-cell lymphoma: a study of 36 cases. Hum Pathol 1991;22:409–21.

52. Nichols RD, Rebuck JW, Sullivan JC. Lymphoma and the parotid gland. Laryngoscope 1982;92:365–9.

53. Östberg Y. The clinical picture of benign lymphoepithelial lesion. Clin Otolaryngol 1983;8:381–90.

54. Pariente D, Anaya JM, Combe B, et al. Non-Hodgkin's lymphoma associated with primary Sjögren's syndrome. Eur J Med 1992;1:337–42.

55. Pavlidis NA, Drosos AA, Papadimitriou C, Talal N, Moutsopoulos HM. Lymphoma in Sjögren's syndrome. Med Pediatr Oncol 1992;20:279–83.

56. Pisa EK, Pisa P, Kang HI, Fox RI. High frequency of t(14;18) translocation in salivary gland lymphomas from Sjögren's syndrome patients. J Exp Med 1991;174:1245–50.

57. Salhany KE, Pietra GG. Extranodal lymphoid disorders. Am J Clin Pathol 1993;99:472–85.

58. Saw D, Lau WH, Ho JH, Chan JK, Ng CS. Malignant lymphoepithelial lesion of the salivary gland. Hum Pathol 1986;17:914–23.

59. Schiodt M, Dodd CL, Greenspan D, et al. Natural history of HIV-associated salivary gland disease. Oral Surg Oral Med Oral Pathol 1992;74:326–31.

60. Schmid U, Helbron D, Lennert K. Primary malignant lymphomas localized in salivary glands. Histopathology 1982;6:673–87.

61. Schmid U, Helbron D, Lennert K. Development of malignant lymphoma in myoepithelial sialadenitis (Sjögren's syndrome). Virchows Arch [A] 1982;395:11–43.

62. Schmid U, Lennert K, Gloor F. Immunosialadenitis (Sjögren's syndrome) and lymphoproliferation. Clin Exp Rheumatol 1989;7:175–80.

63. Schusterman MA, Granick MS, Erikson ER, Newton ED, Hanna DC, Bragdon RW. Lyphoma presenting as a salivary gland mass. Head Neck Surg 1988;10:411–5.

64. Sciubba JJ, Auclair PL, Ellis GL. Malignant lymphomas. In: Ellis GL, Auclair PL, Gnepp DR, eds. Surgical pathology of the salivary glands. Philadelphia: WB Saunders, 1991:528–43.

65. Sheibani K, Burke JS, Swartz WG, Nademanee A, Winberg CD. Monocytoid B-cell lymphoma. Clinicopathologic study of 21 cases of a unique type of low-grade lymphoma. Cancer 1988;62:1531–8.

66. Sheibani K, Sohn CC, Burke JS, Winberg CD, Wu AM, Rappaport H. Monocytoid B-cell lymphoma. A novel B-cell neoplasm. Am J Pathol 1986;124:310–8.

67. Shidnia H, Hornback NB, Lingeman R, Barlow P. Extranodal lymphoma of the head and neck area. Am J Clin Oncol 1985;8:235–43.

68. Shikhani A, Samara M, Allam C, Salem P, Lenhard R. Primary lymphoma in the salivary glands: report of five cases and review of the literature. Laryngoscope 1987;97:1438–42.

69. Shin SS, Sheibani K, Fishleder A, et al. Monocytoid B-cell lymphoma in patients with Sjögren's syndrome: a clinicopathologic study of 13 patients. Hum Pathol 1991;22:422–30.

70. Shugar JM, Som PM, Jacobson AL, Ryan JR, Bernard PJ, Dickman SH. Multicentric parotid cysts and cervical adenopathy in AIDS patients. A newly recognized entity: CT and MR manifestations. Laryngoscope 1988;98:772–5.

71. Slovak ML, Weiss LM, Nathwani BN, Bernstein L, Levine AM. Cytogenetic studies of composite lymphomas: monocytoid B-cell lymphoma and other B-cell non-Hodgkin's lymphomas. Hum Pathol 1993;24:1086–94.

72. Sugai S, Shimizu S, Konda S. Lymphoproliferative disorders in Japanese patients with Sjögren's syndrome. Scand J Rheumatol Suppl 1986;61:106–10.

73. Sundeen JT, Longo DL, Jaffe ES. CD5 expression in B-cell small lymphocytic malignancies. Am J Surg Pathol 1992;16:130–7.

74. Takahashi H, Cheng J, Fujita S, et al. Primary malignant lymphoma of the salivary gland: a tumor of mucosa-associated lymphoid tissue. J Oral Pathol Med 1992;21:318–25.

75. Terry JH, Loree TR, Thomas MD, Marti JR. Major salivary gland lymphoepithelial lesions and the acquired immunodeficiency syndrome. Am J Surg 1991;162:324–9.

76. Uchinuma E, Abe K, Shioya N. A case of Hodgkin's disease arising from an intraglandular lymph node in the parotid gland. Br J Plast Surg 1988;41:92–4.

77. Utz GL, Swerdlow SH. Distinction of follicular hyperplasia from follicular lymphoma in B5-fixed tissues: comparison of MT2 and bcl-2 antibodies. Hum Pathol 1993;24:1155–8.

78. Walters MT, Stevenson FK, Herbert A, Cawley MI, Smith JL. Lymphoma in Sjögren's syndrome: urinary monoclonal free light chains as a diagnostic aid and a means of tumour monitoring. Scand J Rheumatol Suppl 1986;61:114–7.

79. Walters MT, Stevenson FK, Herbert A, Cawley MI, Smith JL. Urinary monoclonal free light chains in primary Sjögren's syndrome: an aid to the diagnosis of malignant lymphoma. Ann Rheum Dis 1986;45:210–9.

80. Watkin GT, MacLennan KA, Hobsley M. Lymphomas presenting as lumps in the parotid region. Br J Surg 1984;71:701–2.

81. Weiss LM. Monocytoid B-cell lymphoma [Editorial]. Hum Pathol 1991;22:407–8.

82. Yamada K, Shinohara H, Takai Y, Mori M. Monoclonal antibody-detected vimentin distribution in pleomorphic adenomas of salivary glands. J Oral Pathol 1988;17:348–53.

83. Zukerberg LR, Medeiros LJ, Ferry JA, Harris NL. Diffuse low-grade B-cell lymphomas. Four clinically distinct subtypes defined by a combination of morphologic and immunophenotypic features. Am J Clin Pathol 1993;100:373–85.

84. Zulman J, Jaffe R, Talal N. Evidence that the malignant lymphoma in Sjögren's syndrome is a monoclonal B cell neoplasm. N Engl J Med 1978;229:1215–20.

✧✧✧

8
SECONDARY TUMORS

Involvement of major salivary glands by malignant neoplasms whose origins are outside the salivary glands occurs by: 1) direct invasion by tumors that develop in tissues adjacent to the salivary glands; 2) hematogenous metastases from distant primary tumors; and 3) lymphatic metastases to salivary gland lymph nodes from extrasalivary primary tumors. While the minor intraoral salivary glands are often invaded by carcinomas of the oral mucosa, sarcomas of the oral soft tissues, and metastases from distant primary sites, the individual glands are so small that they are not normally considered as the locus for secondary tumors. Other than direct invasion by tumors in the floor of the mouth or tongue, the sublingual gland is not involved as a secondary tumor site either. Therefore, a discussion of secondary tumors is limited to the parotid and submandibular glands.

The intimate relationship of the paraparotid and intraparotid lymph nodes with the parotid parenchyma frequently results in lymphatic migration of extrasalivary gland neoplasms to the parotid region. Conley and Arena (12) assessed the average number of intraparotid lymph nodes as 20 to 30. However, a more definitive assessment of intraparotid lymph nodes of cadavers by McKean et al. (23) found the average to be about 10 per gland, with a range of 3 to 24; most were in the superficial lobe and lateral to the plane of the facial nerve. Differences in reported numbers of intraparotid lymph nodes are probably influenced by each investigator's interpretation of a lymph node since McKean et al. also described scattered aggregates of lymphoid tissue throughout the parotid glands, which they did not count as lymph nodes. They required a definite capsule and sinuses to define lymph nodes, but the structural architecture of parotid lymph nodes is often not as well developed as other lymph nodes. They found germinal centers in only about half of parotid lymph nodes.

Although anatomically the parotid lymph nodes can be segregated into intraglandular and periglandular nodes, they are interconnected by a plexus of lymph vessels and function as a unit (4,39). The drainage area of the parotid lymph nodes covers the anterior frontal region, forehead, anterior temporal region, eyelids and conjunctiva, lacrimal gland, anterior ear, external auditory meatus, eustachian tube, cranial vault, and posterior cheek (18,39). The lymph nodes in the submandibular triangle lie outside the capsule of the submandibular gland, and metastases to these lymph nodes often do not involve the submandibular gland parenchyma. Afferent lymph channels of the submandibular lymph nodes are from the skin and mucous membranes of the nose, anterior face including lips, buccal mucosa, gums, anterolateral tongue, lateral floor of mouth, and anterior tonsillar pillars (33).

Direct extension of nonsalivary gland tumors into the parotid and submandibular glands is primarily from squamous cell and basal cell carcinomas of the skin overlying these glands. The incidence of such invasion is unknown because, unlike metastatic disease, this type of data is not routinely compiled. Due to the higher incidence of solar-induced skin cancer in the preauricular region than the submandibular region, the parotid gland is involved much more often than the submandibular gland. Although the thickness of the subcutaneous adipose tissue is a factor, the close approximation of the superficial surface of the parotid to the dermis and epidermis means that the depth of invasion of skin cancers does not have to be extraordinary for involvement of the parotid gland. Basal cell carcinomas rarely metastasize, so their presence in the parotid gland is nearly always by direct extension (5). Squamous cell carcinomas of the epidermis that extend into the parotid gland are usually clinically obvious. In a study of sarcomas of the major glands, just over 13 percent secondarily invaded the salivary gland from adjacent periglandular tissues, but in over 50 percent of cases it was uncertain whether the sarcoma developed within or outside the salivary glands (2).

In the last decade metastatic tumors constituted about 10 percent of the malignant neoplasms in the major salivary glands reviewed at the Armed Forces Institute of Pathology (AFIP),

403

exclusive of malignant lymphomas. There is a wide range in the reported incidence in the literature, but the average is about 16 percent (15). Both in AFIP's and others' experience approximately 80 percent of metastases to the major salivary glands have been from primary tumors elsewhere in the head and neck, and 20 percent have been from infraclavicular sites (10,15). The parotid gland is the site of 80 to 90 percent of metastases while the remainder involve the submandibular gland (15,32). A higher percentage of metastases from infraclavicular sites are to the submandibular gland. Seifert et al. (32) were able to separate their cases into those with parenchymal metastases and those with glandular lymph node metastases: 47 percent of the metastases were parenchymal and the rest nodal. However, it is frequently difficult to distinguish a lymphoid response to primary tumor from a nodal metastatic tumor once a neoplasm has infiltrated into parotid parenchymal tissue (1). It is presumed that most squamous cell carcinomas and melanomas from head and neck primary sites reach the parotid via the lymphatic system, which is the usual mode of metastasis for these neoplasms, while infraclavicular primary tumors reach the salivary glands by a hematogenous route. Because of the extraglandular location of submandibular lymph nodes, it is usually easier to differentiate parenchymal metastases from lymph node metastases that have extended into the submandibular gland.

The peak incidence for metastatic tumors in the salivary glands is in the seventh decade of life, but a broad age range extends from infants to the elderly. Patient age generally correlates with the types of primary tumors that affect particular age groups. The youngest patient in the AFIP files was a 9-month-old infant with metastatic retinoblastoma, and the oldest was a 98-year-old man with metastatic cutaneous squamous cell carcinoma. Eighty-five percent of patients are over 50 years of age, and men comprise about 70 percent of the patients. For most patients, the primary tumor is known at the time of diagnosis of their salivary gland metastasis, but in some cases, especially melanomas and infraclavicular carcinomas, the salivary gland metastasis is the first manifestation of malignant disease (6,8,10,13,22,24,28,30,36). In other cases, however, there was a lack of communication to the pathologist about a previous diagnosis of malignancy (17,38), perhaps years prior to the appearance of the metastatic tumor in the salivary gland (7,13,25,29).

The majority of metastatic tumors in the parotid and submandibular glands are carcinomas and melanomas, which account for about 80 percent of the metastases to the major salivary glands (5,12,32). In most cases, the primary tumors are cutaneous neoplasms in the area of lymphatic drainage of the parotid lymph nodes; less common are facial, oral, and anterior oropharyngeal carcinomas that metastasize to the submandibular lymph nodes and gland. Metastatic soft tissue sarcomas are rare (fig. 8-1) (15). In their data from the Salivary Gland Register at the University of Hamburg, Seifert et al. (32) reported that squamous cell carcinomas and melanomas accounted for less than 50 percent of metastases; however, their review of the literature found that these two types of neoplasms composed 81 percent of the metastases reported. In data from the AFIP over the past decade, 78 percent of metastases to salivary glands were squamous cell carcinomas and melanomas. Similar to Conley and Arena (12) and Coulthard (14) but in contrast to most other reports (15,32,37), melanomas (fig. 8-2) were more frequent than squamous cell carcinomas (fig. 8-3). One reason that may account for this difference is a very critical exclusion among AFIP cases of metastases to the submandibular region that did not definitely demonstrate parenchymal invasion. Additionally, although melanomas of the head and neck are less common than squamous cell carcinomas, melanomas have a higher relative incidence of metastasis than cutaneous squamous cell carcinomas (19,20,35,39). It has been recommended that patients undergoing regional lymphadenectomy for primary melanomas of the ear, face, and anterior scalp be considered for parotidectomy as well (34,39). Metastases from intraoral, nasal, nasopharyngeal, and laryngeal squamous cell carcinomas; undifferentiated carcinomas; and adenocarcinomas to the parotid and submandibular gland are less frequent (15,27). Retinoblastoma, sebaceous carcinoma, eccrine carcinoma, olfactory neuroblastoma, Merkel's cell carcinoma, and intracranial neoplasms are uncommon head and neck primary tumors that have metastasized to the salivary glands. Although the

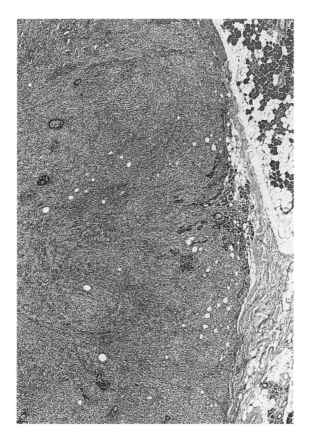 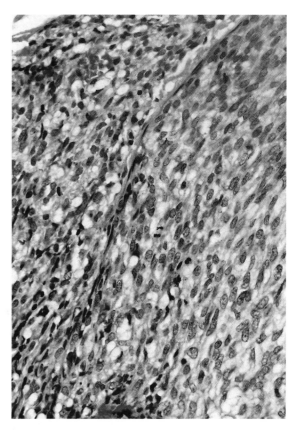

Figure 8-1
METASTATIC LEIOMYOSARCOMA

Left: A leiomyosarcoma of the stomach and a metastasis to the liver were resected 13 years and 3 years, respectively, prior to resection of this parotid gland metastasis in a 71-year-old woman. The patient had a metastasis to the left chest wall synchronous with the parotid metastasis.

Right: High magnification shows cytologic features of leiomyosarcoma that were comparable to the primary tumor of the stomach.

thyroid gland is located inferior to the major salivary glands, the AFIP and others have seen metastases from several thyroid papillary carcinomas (fig. 8-4), and in some cases the metastatic focus preceded the discovery of the primary thyroid carcinoma (22,32).

In descending order of frequency, the most common infraclavicular sites of primary tumors that metastasize to the major salivary glands are lung, kidney, and breast (15). Infrequently, metastases have been from other infraclavicular organs including colon and rectum, prostate, ovary, pancreas, stomach, uterus, and urinary bladder.

Distinguishing metastatic neoplasms from primary salivary gland neoplasms on the basis of histopathologic features can sometimes be difficult. This is especially true for primary squamous cell carcinoma, adenocarcinoma, clear cell carci-

noma, undifferentiated carcinoma, and small cell carcinoma, which have architectural and cytologic features in common with tumors from other sites. The most important and helpful factor in resolving this dilemma is a thorough medical history. Patients occasionally develop more than one primary malignant neoplasm, but histologic similarity between a salivary gland tumor and a previously diagnosed neoplasm in another site is strong evidence in favor of metastasis. Rare primary melanomas of the parotid gland have been reported (3,41), but these interpretations have been based upon the lack of detection of another primary site. Salivary gland melanomas are nearly always best regarded as metastases because: facial and scalp melanomas commonly metastasize to the parotid gland; melanomas, especially of the scalp, are frequently

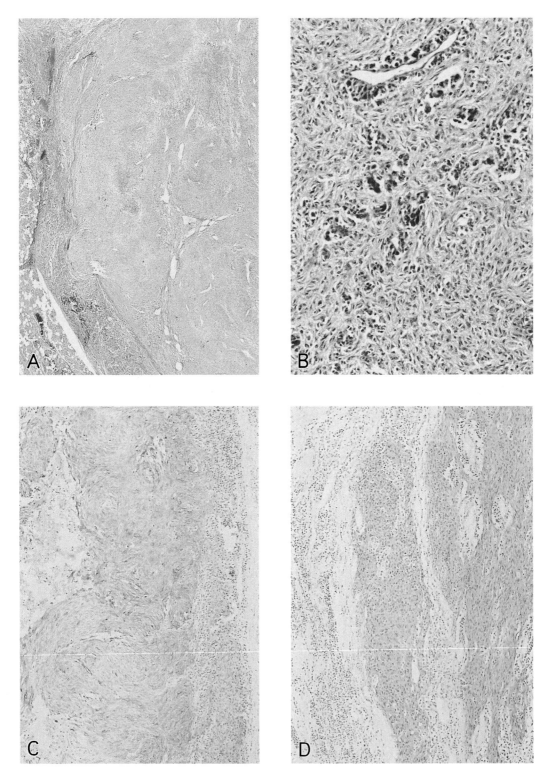

Figure 8-2
METASTATIC MALIGNANT MELANOMA

A: The low-magnification photograph shows the metastatic tumor bounded by a thin rim of lymphoid tissue in the parotid gland.
B: High magnification reveals focal melanin pigment in some tumor cells.
C,D: Immunohistochemical staining was reactive for HMB45 antigen and S-100 protein. (Avidin-biotin peroxidase stain)

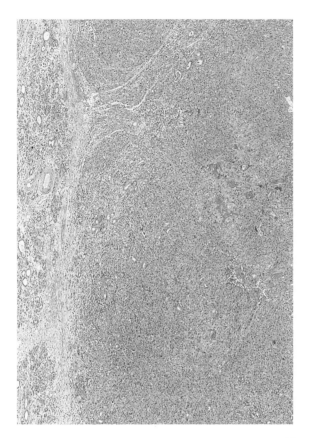 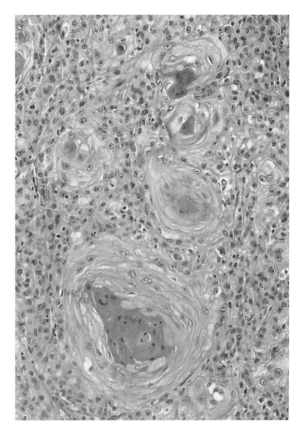

Figure 8-3
METASTATIC SQUAMOUS CELL CARCINOMA
Left: This large nodule of metastatic cutaneous squamous cell carcinoma in the parotid gland shows no evidence of lymph node involvement.
Right: Higher magnification shows focal keratinization within the metastatic carcinoma.

undetected before metastases; and occasionally, primary melanomas undergo regression (5,9,17,30).

Immunohistochemistry can be helpful in some situations. The AFIP has identified or confirmed metastatic papillary carcinomas of the thyroid with anti-thyroglobulin. Anti-HMB45 antigen has been useful for differentiating metastatic melanoma from undifferentiated carcinoma. Anti-prostate-specific antigen has been described as confirmatory of metastatic prostate carcinoma (16,26), but van Krieken (40) reported reactivity for prostate-specific antigen (PSA) and prostate-specific acid phosphatase (PSAP) in 8 of 23 primary salivary gland neoplasms. Therefore, confirmatory evidence of primary prostatic carcinoma, such as elevated serum levels of PSA and PSAP, and clinical and radiographic features of prostatic adenopathy, are needed to de-

finitively establish a diagnosis of metastatic prostate carcinoma. Melnick et al. (24) confirmed a metastatic renal cell carcinoma in the parotid gland by positive immunoreactions for keratin and vimentin and negative immunoreaction for carcinoembryonic antigen (CEA), since they believe that salivary gland carcinomas are CEA positive and vimentin negative. However, this premise is incorrect often enough to make these criteria unreliable. Prominent vascular channels and nuclear and cytoplasmic pleomorphism suggest metastatic renal cell carcinoma over primary clear cell carcinoma (fig. 8-5), but these features are only suggestive. The diagnosis needs to be confirmed by identification of a renal mass or a medical history of renal carcinoma. Differentiation of primary small cell carcinoma from metastatic pulmonary oat cell carcinoma

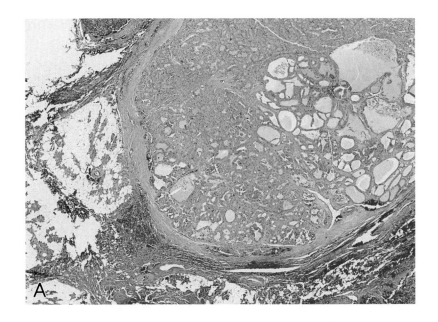

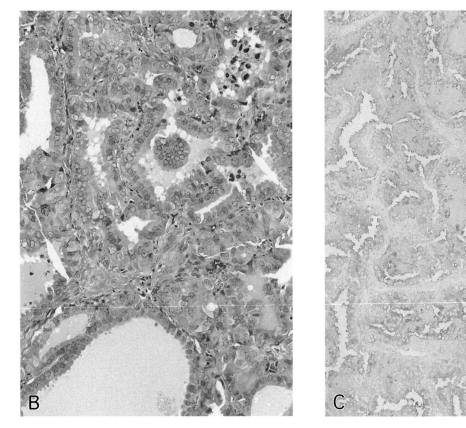

Figure 8-4

METASTATIC PAPILLARY CARCINOMA OF THE THYROID

Low (A) and high (B) magnification of a well-circumscribed nodule of papillary cystic epithelial carcinoma in the parotid gland. The nuclear features suggested thyroid origin, and immunohistochemical staining for thyroglobulin was positive (C). A primary carcinoma in the thyroid gland was discovered. (C: Avidin-biotin peroxidase stain)

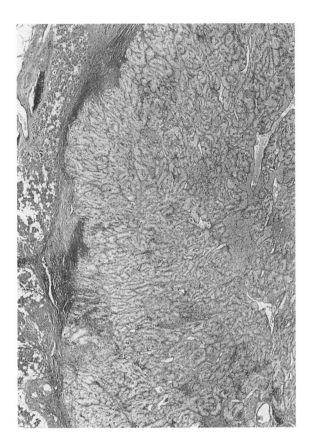 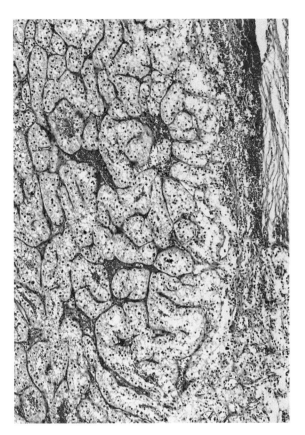

Figure 8-5
METASTATIC RENAL CELL CARCINOMA
Left: This nodule of metastatic clear cell carcinoma appears well demarcated from the parotid gland parenchyma.
Right: Higher magnification reveals several prominent capillaries and dilated vascular spaces within the neoplasm. The
patient had a primary renal cell carcinoma resected several years prior to discovery of the parotid lesion.

and cutaneous Merkel's cell carcinoma is sometimes difficult and may require clinical evaluation and a thorough medical history (see Primary Small Cell Carcinoma).

In general, metastatic disease indicates a poorer prognosis for the specific primary tumor type (21). Salivary gland metastases from infraclavicular primary tumors are frequently only one focus of multifocal metastases, a particularly ominous sign. On the other hand, if the salivary gland is the only focus of metastatic disease, cure may be possible with local control of the primary and metastatic tumor (7,13,29). Patients with melanomas and parotid lymph node metastases have significantly decreased survival at 5 years compared to patients with uninvolved lymph

nodes (9). Of 20 patients with cutaneous squamous cell carcinomas that metastasized to the parotid lymph nodes, 6 died (11). Lee et al. (18) found that the prognosis for patients with metastatic cutaneous squamous cell carcinoma was good if the carcinoma was confined to the parotid region lymph nodes but poor if the metastatic tumor had spread to involve the parotid parenchyma. Likewise, Shimm (35) reported that the size and extent of the parotid metastases were strong predictors of relapse. Since local lymph node metastasis of papillary carcinoma of the thyroid seems to have no prognostic significance (31), it is expected that metastasis to the parotid gland would also have little prognostic importance, but too few cases are available to provide firm data.

REFERENCES

1. Auclair PL. Tumor-associated lymphoid proliferation in the parotid gland: a potential diagnostic pitfall. Oral Surg Oral Med Oral Pathol 1994;77:19–26.

2. Auclair PL, Langloss JM, Weiss SW, Corio RL. Sarcomas and sarcomatoid neoplasms of the major salivary gland regions. A clinicopathologic and immunohistochemical study of 67 cases and review of the literature. Cancer 1986;58:1305–15.

3. Bahar M, Anavi Y, Abraham A, Ben-Bassat M. Primary malignant melanoma in the parotid gland. Oral Surg Oral Med Oral Pathol 1990;70:627–30.

4. Batsakis JG. Pathology consultation. Parotid gland and its lymph nodes as metastatic sites. Ann Otol Rhinol Laryngol 1983;92:209–10.

5. Batsakis JG, Bautina E. Metastases to major salivary glands. Ann Otol Rhinol Laryngol 1990;99:501–3.

6. Bedrosian SA, Goldman RL, Dekelboum AM. Renal carcinoma presenting as a primary submandibular gland tumor. Oral Surg Oral Med Oral Pathol 1984;58:699–701.

7. Bissett D, Bessell EM, Bradley PJ, Morgan DA, McKenzie CG. Parotid metastases from carcinoma of the breast. Clin Radiol 1989;40:309–10.

8. Brodsky G, Rabson AB. Metastasis to the submandibular gland as the initial presentation of small cell (oat cell) lung carcinoma. Oral Surg Oral Med Oral Pathol 1984;58:76–80.

9. Caldwell CB, Spiro RH. The role of parotidectomy in the treatment of cutaneous head and neck melanoma. Am J Surg 1988;156:318–22.

10. Cantera JM, Hernandez AV. Bilateral parotid gland metastasis as the initial presentation of a small cell lung carcinoma. J Oral Maxillofac Surg 1989;47:1199–201.

11. Cassisi NJ, Dickerson DR, Million RR. Squamous cell carcinoma of the skin metastatic to parotid nodes. Arch Otolaryngol 1978;104:336–9.

12. Conley J, Arena S. Parotid gland as a focus of metastasis. Arch Surg 1963;87:757–64.

13. Coppa GF, Oszczakiewicz M. Parotid gland metastasis from renal carcinoma. Int Surg 1990;75:198–202.

14. Coulthard SW. Metastatic disease of the parotid gland. Otolaryngol Clin North Am 1977;10:437–42.

15. Gnepp DR. Metastatic disease to the major salivary glands. In: Ellis GL, Auclair PL, Gnepp DR, eds. Surgical pathology of the salivary glands. Philadelphia: WB Saunders, 1991:560–9.

16. Goldberg JA, Georgiade GS. Accessory parotid glands as a site of metastases from outside the head and neck: case report. Head Neck 1990;12:421–5.

17. Laudadio P, Rinaldi Ceroni A, Cerasoli PT. Metastatic malignant melanoma in the parotid gland. ORL J Otorhinolaryngol Relat Spec 1984;46:42–9.

18. Lee K, McKean ME, McGregor IA. Metastatic patterns of squamous carcinoma in the parotid lymph nodes. Br J Plast Surg 1985;38:6–10.

19. Lever WF, Schaumburg-Lever G. Histopathology of the skin. 7th ed. Philadelphia: JB Lippinocott, 1990:552–6.

20. Lever WF, Schaumburg-Lever G. Histopathology of the skin. 7th ed. Philadelphia: JB Lippinocott, 1990:785–95.

21. Liotta LA, Stetler-Stevenson WG. Principles of molecular cell biology of cancer: cancer metastasis. In: DeVita VT, Hellman S, Rosenberg SA, eds. Cancer: Principles and practice of oncology. 3rd ed. Philadelphia: JB Lippincott, 1989:98–115.

22. Markitziu A, Fisher D, Marmary Y. Thyroid papillary carcinoma presenting as jaw and parotid gland metastases. Int J Oral Maxillofac Surg 1986;15:648–53.

23. McKean ME, Lee K, McGregor IA. The distribution of lymph nodes in and around the parotid gland: an anatomical study. Br J Plast Surg 1985;38:1–5.

24. Melnick SJ, Amazon K, Dembrow V. Metastatic renal cell carcinoma presenting as a parotid tumor: a case report with immunohistochemical findings and a review of the literature. Hum Pathol 1989;20:195–7.

25. Mochimatsu I, Tsukuda M, Furukawa S, Sawaki S. Tumours metastasizing to the head and neck—a report of seven cases. J Laryngol Otol 1993;107:1171–3.

26. Moul JW, Paulson DF, Fuller G, Gottfried MR, Floyd WL. Prostate cancer with solitary parotid metastasis correctly diagnosed with immunohistochemical stains. J Urol 1989;142:1328–9.

27. Ord RA, Ward-Booth RP, Avery BS. Parotid lymph node metastases from primary intra-oral squamous carcinomas. Int J Oral Maxillofac Surg 1989;18:104–6.

28. Owens RM, Friedman CD, Becker SP. Renal cell carcinoma with metastasis to the parotid gland: case reports and review of the literature. Head Neck 1989;11:174–8.

29. Ravi R, Tongaonkar HB, Kulkarni JN, Kamat MR. Synchronous bilateral parotid metastases from renal cell carcinoma. A case report. Indian J Cancer 1992;29:40–2.

30. Roberts C, Jayaramachandran S. Malignant melanoma of the parotid gland. Br J Clin Pract 1992;46:217–8.

31. Rosai J, Carcangiu ML, DeLellis RA. Tumors of the thyroid gland. Atlas of Tumor Pathology, 3rd Series, Fascicle 5. Washington, D.C.: Armed Forces Institute of Pathology, 1992:96.

32. Seifert G, Hennings K, Caselitz J. Metastatic tumors to the parotid and submandibular glands—analysis and differential diagnosis of 108 cases. Pathol Res Pract 1986;181:684–92.

33. Sessions RB, Hudkins CP. Malignant cervical adenopathy. In: Cummings CW, Fredrickson JM, Harker LA, Krause CJ, Schuller DE, eds. Otolaryngology—head and neck surgery. 2nd ed. St. Louis: Mosby Year Book, 1993:1605–15.

34. Shah JP, Kraus DH, Dubner S, Sarkar S. Patterns of regional lymph node metastases from cutaneous melanomas of the head and neck. Am J Surg 1991;162:320–3.

35. Shimm DS. Parotid lymph node metastases from squamous cell carcinoma of the skin. J Surg Oncol 1988;37:56–9.

36. Sist TC Jr, Marchetta FC, Milley PC. Renal cell carcinoma presenting as a primary parotid gland tumor. Oral Surg Oral Med Oral Pathol 1982;53:499–502.

37. Smith RL, Davis TS, Kennedy TJ, Graham WP, Miller SH. Metastatic malignancies of the parotid gland. Am Fam Physician 1977;16:139–40.

38. Smits JG, Slootweg PJ. Renal cell carcinoma with metastasis to the submandibular and parotid glands. A case report. J Maxillofac Surg 1984;12:235–6.

39. Storm FK, Eilber FR, Sparks FC, Morton DL. A prospective study of parotid metastases from head and neck cancer. Am J Surg 1977;134:115–9.

40. van Krieken JH. Prostate marker immunoreactivity in salivary gland neoplasms. A rare pitfall in immunohistochemistry. Am J Surg Pathol 1993;17:410–4.

41. Woodwards RT, Shepherd NA, Hensher R. Malignant melanoma of the parotid gland: a case report and literature review. Br J Oral Maxillofac Surg 1993; 31:313–5.

9

TUMOR-LIKE CONDITIONS

This section presents a heterogeneous group of non-neoplastic disorders of salivary glands that frequently simulate neoplasms clinically and, in some cases, microscopically. These lesions include cysts, inflammatory diseases, and developmental abnormalities.

BENIGN LYMPHOEPITHELIAL LESION

The term benign lymphoepithelial lesion was first used by Godwin (33) for parotid gland lesions that had previously been called *Mikulicz's disease* and other terms. Benign lymphoepithelial lesion is still a popular term among American pathologists while many European pathologists have adopted the term *myoepithelial sialadenitis* for the same histopathologic lesion (37,46,63, 65). Benign lymphoepithelial lesion is a histopathologic disease process that usually manifests in the parotid glands, less frequently in the submandibular glands, and most often in patients with Sjögren's syndrome. It is often equated with Sjögren's syndrome, but that is not entirely accurate: while most patients with Sjögren's syndrome develop lymphoepithelial lesions, these lesions also manifest in patients without the clinical and laboratory signs of Sjögren's syndrome. *Sjögren's syndrome* is an autoimmune disease complex that involves lacrimal and salivary glands, with the typical manifestations of keratoconjunctivitis sicca and xerostomia. It is also often associated with other autoimmune or connective tissue diseases, such as rheumatoid arthritis, systemic lupus erythematosus, progressive systemic sclerosis, polymyositis/dermatomyositis, or polyarteritis nodosa. When associated with another connective tissue disease, it is referred to as *secondary Sjögren's syndrome;* in the absence of another connective tissue disease, it is called *primary Sjögren's syndrome.* Detailed discussions of the syndrome have been published (19).

Benign lymphoepithelial lesion and Sjögren's syndrome predominantly affect women in a ratio of about 3 to 1. Most lesions manifest in the fourth to seventh decades of life. Benign lymphoepithelial lesions involve the parotid glands in about 85 percent of cases and the submandibular glands in 15 percent. When the submandibular glands are affected in patients with Sjögren's syndrome, the parotid glands are also usually involved. Clinically, patients generally present with recurrent, firm swelling of the affected glands, which may or may not be associated with discomfort or pain (fig. 9-1).

Histologically, benign lymphoepithelial lesions are characterized by lymphocytic infiltration of the gland, parenchymal atrophy, and foci of epithelial proliferation referred to as epimyoepithelial islands. Immunohistochemical and electron microscopic studies have confirmed that the epimyoepithelial islands are composed of both ductal and myoepithelial differentiated cells (20,45). In the early stages of the disease, there is often multiple foci of periductal lymphoid proliferation (fig. 9-2). The disease progresses to near total or total replacement of acinar tissue of the gland lobules with lymphoreticular infiltration. The lobular architecture of the gland is usually retained and the interlobular fibrous septa are preserved (fig. 9-3). The glandular lobules are usually not equally affected. Germinal center formation within the lymphoid infiltrate varies from rare to extensive in any particular case. The polyclonal lymphoid infiltrate is primarily of mature lymphocytes with a predominance of T cells (2,12,28). In later stages of the disease, plasma cells and immunocytes are frequently conspicuous (7). The epimyoepithelial islands are formed by hyperplasia of residual foci of ductal structures. In early stages lumens persist, but in later stages the islands are irregularly shaped nests of polygonal and spindled cells in which there are often deposits of intercellular eosinophilic hyaline material, which is excessive basement membrane (fig. 9-4) (56). The epimyoepithelial islands are typically permeated by lymphocytes: these are often larger than the surrounding lymphocytes and have clear cytoplasm, features of so-called monocytoid B cells of mucosal-associated lymphoid tissue (MALT) (fig. 9-5). Immunohistochemistry confirms the B-cell lineage of these lymphocytes (2).

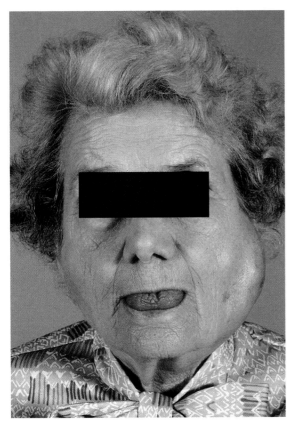
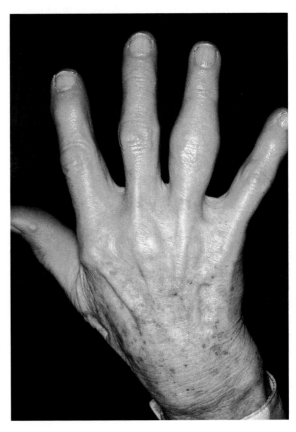

Figure 9-1
SJÖGREN'S SYNDROME

Left: Along with the symptoms of keratoconjunctivitis sicca and xerostomia this woman has marked enlargement of the left parotid gland and slight enlargement of the right parotid gland, which are features of primary Sjögren's syndrome. (Courtesy of Col. Robert Achterberg, USAF, DC.)

Right: If there is also evidence of another connective tissue disease, such as the enlarged finger joints in this patient with rheumatoid arthritis, the disease is referred to as secondary Sjögren's syndrome.

The minor salivary glands rarely manifest lymphoepithelial lesions, but they do undergo alterations in patients with Sjögren's syndrome that are indicative of the changes seen in the parotid glands. The labial minor salivary gland biopsy has become an integral part of the assessment for Sjögren's syndrome (fig. 9-6): although the labial salivary gland biopsy by itself is insufficient to establish a diagnosis of Sjögren's syndrome, an evaluation of the degree of alterations in conjunction with other clinical and laboratory parameters can be diagnostic (19).

Patients with benign lymphoepithelial lesions and Sjögren's syndrome have a markedly increased risk for developing non-Hodgkin's lymphoma (26,58,65). It has recently become evident that some lesions previously identified as benign

lymphoepithelial lesions were actually early stage MALT lymphomas (12,26). Although it was once thought that epimyoepithelial islands were indicative of benignancy, it is now recognized that they are present in low-grade MALT lymphomas of salivary glands (26). Indeed, with the recent elaboration of the concept of MALT and the recognition of MALT lymphomas, the AFIP files show an increase in the incidence of lymphomas of salivary glands and a decrease in the incidence of benign lymphoepithelial lesions. It is now realized that these low-grade lymphomas may remain localized to the salivary glands for long periods before showing evidence of extraglandular dissemination (26). Features that are indicative of the development of lymphoma include prominent aggregations of monomorphic,

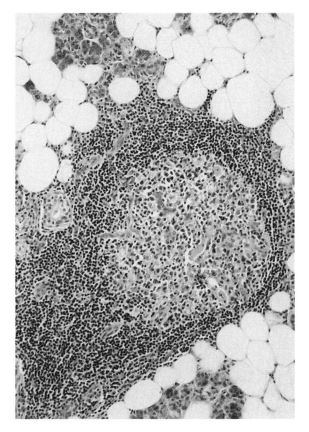

Figure 9-2
LYMPHOID PROLIFERATION IN PAROTID GLAND
In the early stages of development of benign lymphoepithelial lesion, scattered foci of lymphoid proliferation involve glandular parenchyma.

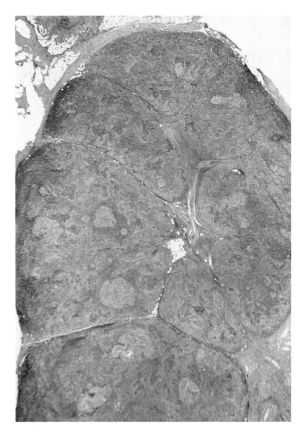

Figure 9-3
BENIGN LYMPHOEPITHELIAL LESION
The parenchyma of several lobules of the parotid gland are almost entirely replaced by lymphoid tissue, but the lobular architecture is preserved. Many epimyoepithelial islands are present within the lymphoid infiltrate, which contains several germinal centers.

medium-sized lymphoid cells that have abundant pale cytoplasm and bland, uniform nuclei (so-called monocytoid B cells); involvement of paraglandular fat or connective tissue or evidence of perineural infiltrates; and immunohistochemical demonstration of a B-cell phenotype and light chain restriction. The development of molecular techniques for the assessment of gene rearrangements and clonal proliferation of lymphocytes in formalin-fixed and paraffin-embedded tissue should aid in diagnosing these early low-grade lymphomas that either mimic or develop within the environment of benign lymphoepithelial lesions. However, distinguishing early low-grade MALT lymphoma from benign lymphoepithelial lesion can sometimes be difficult even for pathologists with expertise in lymphomas and salivary gland disease. Further investigations are needed for more definitive parameters. For a more detailed discussion see the section, Lymphomas of Salivary Glands.

NECROTIZING SIALOMETAPLASIA

Necrotizing sialometaplasia is a reactive inflammatory condition of the salivary glands that was first described as a distinct entity by Abrams et al. in 1973 (1). The principal characteristics are lobular coagulative necrosis of salivary gland acini, squamous metaplasia of salivary gland ducts, pseudoepitheliomatous hyperplasia of overlying or adjacent mucosal epithelium, and inflammation. The clinical and histopathologic features can resemble malignant neoplasia and have led to misdiagnosis and inappropriate treatment in some cases (10).

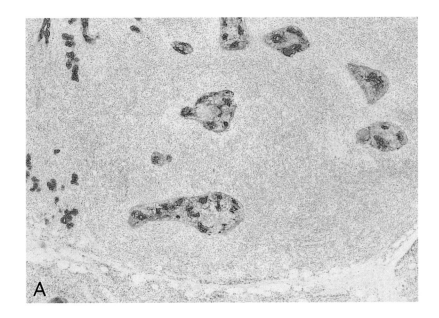

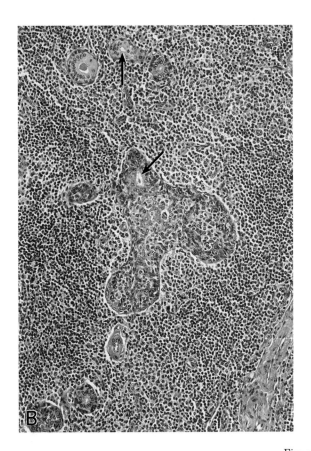

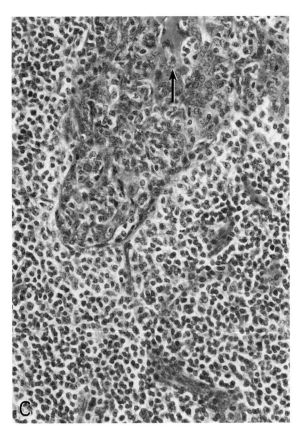

Figure 9-4
BENIGN LYMPHOEPITHELIAL LESION

A: Immunohistochemistry for cytokeratin highlights the epimyoepithelial islands within the lymphoid proliferation.

B: Several epimyoepithelial islands contain duct lumens (arrows).

C: The epimyoepithelial island at left is composed of polygonal and spindle cells and contains some eosinophilic hyaline material (arrow). Lymphocytes permeate the epithelial proliferation.

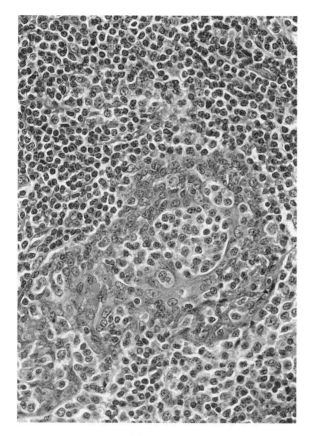

Figure 9-5
BENIGN LYMPHOEPITHELIAL LESION
The lymphocytes that infiltrate the epimyoepithelial island are larger than the surrounding lymphocytes and have pale to clear cytoplasm. These features are consistent with B-cell lymphocytes of MALT origin.

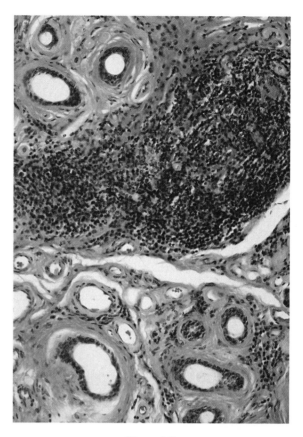

Figure 9-6
LABIAL SALIVARY GLAND BIOPSY
IN SJÖGREN'S SYNDROME
Acinar atrophy, periductal sclerosis, and lymphoid aggregates are typical alterations present in labial salivary gland biopsies in patients with Sjögren's syndrome.

In the largest study, 69 cases were reported from the AFIP and Wilford Hall USAF Medical Center and another 115 cases were reviewed from the literature (10). Patients ranged in age from 1.5 to 83 years, with an average of 46 years. Even when the male bias of military cases was eliminated from reported data, there was a nearly 2 to 1 predominance in men. Just over three fourths of all lesions involved the salivary glands of the palate, mostly the hard palate or junction of hard and soft palate. The majority of these palatal lesions were unilateral, but occasional bilateral or midline palatal lesions were noted. Other uncommon sites of occurrence in the oral cavity were the lower lip, retromolar mucosa, tongue, and buccal mucosa. Rare nonoral lesions were found in the nasal cavity, maxillary sinus, and larynx. The major salivary glands, primarily the parotid gland, were affected in 8.5 percent of cases.

Clinically, necrotizing sialometaplasia usually presents as a deep crater-like ulcer that develops rapidly over a few days and is slow to heal (fig. 9-7). Duration of the lesion before the patient seeks diagnosis and treatment has been as long as 180 days, but the average is about 21 days. Depending upon the size of the lesion, complete healing varies from 3 to 12 weeks (41). This failure to resolve in a timely fashion heightens concern about neoplasia. Some lesions present as nonulcerated swellings (fig. 9-8), some of which subsequently breakdown and ulcerate. The lesions range in size from less than 1 cm to 5 cm. A majority of patients complain of pain or numbness associated with their lesions.

Ischemic necrosis or infarction is believed to be the pathogenesis of necrotizing sialometaplasia by most investigators; however, a specific event or factor that would compromise the blood supply

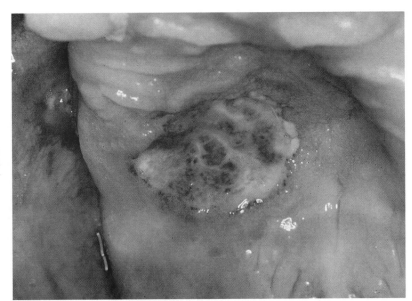

Figure 9-7
NECROTIZING
SIALOMETAPLASIA
A 2- to 3-cm unilateral ulcer of the
hard palate that is slow to heal is a
common clinical presentation for necrotizing sialometaplasia.

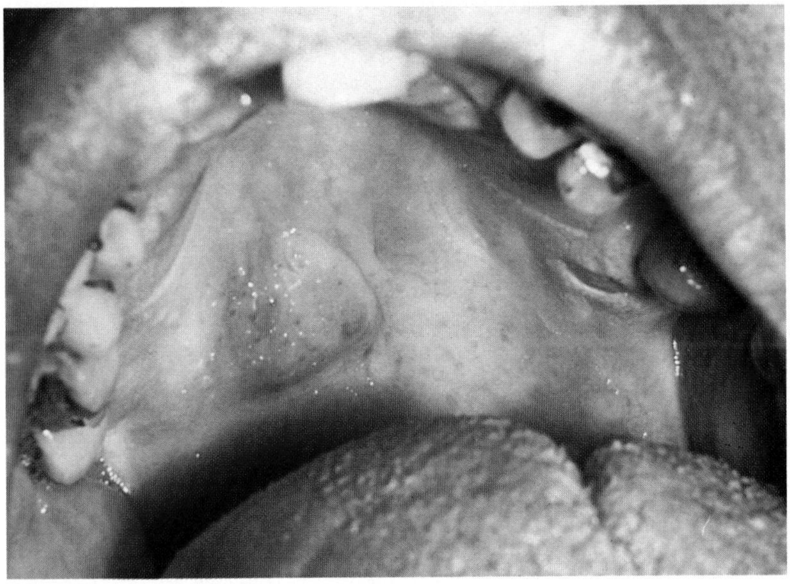

Figure 9-8
NECROTIZING
SIALOMETAPLASIA
Swelling, as shown in this photograph of a palatal lesion, is a frequent
initial clinical presentation. Many of the
swellings subsequently ulcerate and appear similar to figure 9-7. (Courtesy of
Dr. Ralph Correll, Los Angeles, CA.)

to the salivary glands is unknown in most cases.
Some cases have been associated with such predis-
posing factors as traumatic injury, dental injection,
denture use, adjacent cysts and tumors, surgery
for benign and malignant tumors, and upper respiratory infection or allergy. In cases with preceding
surgery, Brannon et al. (10) reported that the
interval from surgery to the development of necrotizing sialometaplasia ranged from 6 to 53 days,
with an average of 18 days.

Histologically, coagulative necrosis and ductal metaplasia are the principal features. The

lobular architecture of the salivary gland is preserved, but the mucous acini are necrotic (fig.
9-9). Pale outlines of the acini often persist, but
the nuclei are hypochromatic or absent. The
mucinous contents of the necrotic cells form
pools demarcated by necrotic fibrous septa (fig.
9-10). Inflammatory cells within the necrotic
lobules are frequently minimal but are usually
prominent in the surrounding tissues (fig. 9-11).
Neutrophils and lymphocytes predominate.
Mucin sometimes extends into adjacent tissues
and evokes an inflammatory reaction dominated

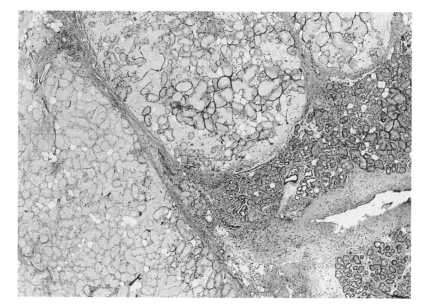

Figure 9-9
NECROTIZING
SIALOMETAPLASIA
The lobular pattern of the salivary
gland is preserved. The acini in the salivary gland lobules at the top and left of
the photomicrograph are necrotic, and
there is some spillage of mucin into the
interacinar tissue. The salivary gland at
the right and bottom is still viable.

Figure 9-10
NECROTIZING
SIALOMETAPLASIA
The necrotic mucous acini are outlined by thin septa of necrotic fibrous
tissue. A mild inflammatory infiltrate is
composed predominantly of neutrophils.

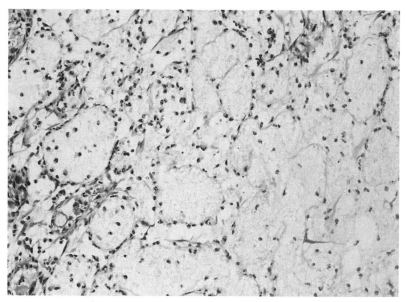

by histiocytes and granulation tissue. Squamous
metaplasia of salivary gland ducts and residual
acini is a constant finding and often quite extensive. Again, the metaplastic ducts tend to retain a
lobular pattern. The nests of squamous epithelium
occasionally have an irregular outline, but usually
the periphery is smooth. Some ducts have persistent lumens and are composed partially of squamous cells and partially of cuboidal or columnar
cells (fig. 9-12). Some mucous cells persist. The
squamous epithelium is usually cytologically
bland with little pleomorphism and hyperchromatism and few mitotic figures; however, reactive atypia that occurs in proliferating epithelium is focally evident in some lesions (fig. 9-12).

The mucosal epithelium that overlies the lesion or is adjacent to the ulcer is often hyperplastic and thickened with elongated rete pegs.
When this pseudoepitheliomatous hyperplasia
is juxtaposed to areas of prominent metaplasia
of superficial ducts, it may look malignant to the
unwary pathologist (fig. 9-13).

Brannon et al. (10) noted that the histologic
features have some relation to the duration of the
lesion. Coagulation necrosis of acini is a dominant feature in early lesions while extensive

417

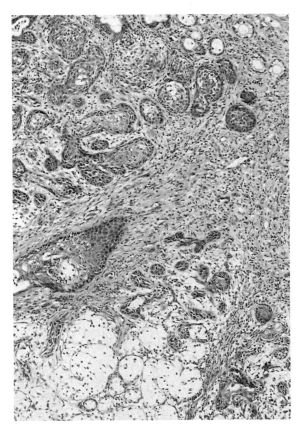

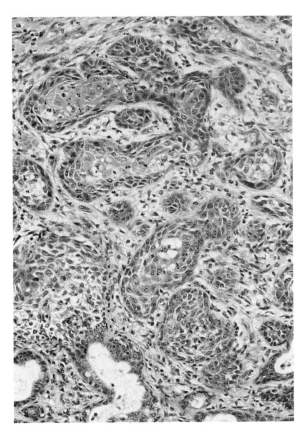

Figure 9-11
NECROTIZING SIALOMETAPLASIA
Squamous metaplasia of salivary ducts (top) is present adjacent to necrotic mucous gland lobules (bottom). There is a moderately intense inflammatory cell infiltrate in the fibrous connective tissue.

Figure 9-12
NECROTIZING SIALOMETAPLASIA
Most of the metaplastic ducts in this field are entirely squamous epithelium, but several ducts along the bottom of the field have retained a lumen and are partially composed of duct-type cuboidal epithelium. Some cytologic atypia is evident in the squamous epithelium.

Figure 9-13
NECROTIZING
SIALOMETAPLASIA
Pseudoepitheliomatous hyperplasia of mucosal surface epithelium (right) in association with squamous metaplasia of salivary gland ducts in the subjacent lamina propria resembles squamous cell carcinoma.

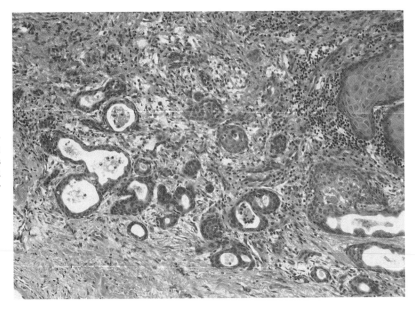

squamous metaplasia and fibrosis dominate older lesions. Necrotizing sialometaplasia of serous glands, such as the parotid gland, tends to have less coagulative necrosis and more acinar atrophy and fibrosis.

Necrotizing sialometaplasia with pseudoepitheliomatous hyperplasia and florid squamous metaplasia of ducts needs to be differentiated from mucosal squamous cell carcinoma and mucoepidermoid carcinoma. Four features help distinguish necrotizing sialometaplasia from these malignant neoplasms: 1) maintenance of the lobular architecture of the salivary gland; 2) infarctive necrosis of salivary gland lobules; 3) bland cytologic features of most of the metaplastic ducts and mucosal surface epithelium; and 4) a more intense and mixed inflammatory reaction than usually accompanies squamous cell or mucoepidermoid carcinoma. In addition, necrotizing sialometaplasia lacks the cystic epithelium that is a component of most mucoepidermoid carcinomas.

No specific therapy is necessary other than to reassure the patient of the benign nature of the lesion. Although resolution is often slow, necrotizing sialometaplasia is self-healing.

CHRONIC SCLEROSING SIALADENITIS

Chronic sclerosing sialadenitis is a chronic inflammatory disease of salivary gland that often produces a firm swelling of the gland that clinically cannot be easily distinguished from neoplasia. The submandibular gland is affected more often than any other salivary gland; it is the most common disease of the submandibular gland (17,30). The first description of a tumorous swelling of the submandibular gland due to sclerosing sialadenitis is attributed to Küttner (48), and this entity is sometimes referred to as *Küttner's tumor* (40,65,79).

Most patients experience recurrent pain and swelling that is often associated with food ingestion, but others only have asymptomatic hard swelling of the submandibular gland. Most patients seek consultation and treatment within 1 year of the appearance of their signs and symptoms, but durations up to 55 years have been reported (40). There is a slight predilection for occurrence in men. The mean age of affected patients is about 44 years, but there is a fairly uniform incidence of occurrence in the third through seventh decades of life. Although some studies have reported a preference for left over right side involvement, other investigations dispute this (40).

Sialolithiasis is the most common etiologic or pathogenic factor associated with chronic sclerosing sialadenitis of the submandibular gland, and sialoliths have been found in 50 to 83 percent of cases (38–40,46,74). In fact, Epivatianos et al. (25) found microcalculi with ultrastructural examination in all 14 cases of chronic submandibular sialadenitis they studied. Sialoliths develop by accretion of mineralized secretions within a salivary gland duct. This mineralization may develop about a nidus of exfoliated cellular debris, a mucus plug, a bacterial colony, or a foreign body, and is primarily composed of calcium salts in the form of hydroxyapatite (47). Using histochemical and biochemical methods, Harrison et al. (35) found that most salivary calcium is associated with secretory granules, and they speculated that this is the likely source of the calcium involved in salivary calcification. Most sialoliths can be detected with radiography (fig. 9-14), but up to 20 percent are radiolucent (39); sialography with contrast media can usually identify these. In addition to sialoliths, disorders of secretion and immune reactions may also be pathogenic (65).

The histopathologic features vary from mild, focal chronic inflammation, usually periductal, with periductal fibrosis and ductal ectasia to extensive fibrosis with marked acinar atrophy and ductal dilatation. The lobular architecture of the gland is usually preserved, although in older lesions marked fibrosis often distorts and disrupts the lobular pattern (fig. 9-15). The degree of fibrosis and inflammation varies from lobule to lobule within the same gland (fig. 9-16). The inflammatory infiltrate is predominantly lymphocytic and plasmacytic, and in some cases lymphoid follicle formation with reactive germinal centers is prominent (fig. 9-17). Focal granulomas, which are probably a reaction to extravasation of mucus, have been observed in some cases (73,74). Dilated excretory ducts sometimes demonstrate squamous metaplasia and an increased number of goblet-like mucous and ciliated cells (54,72).

Sialoliths more frequently develop in the extraglandular excretory ducts than within the gland. The duct lining epithelium adjacent to sialoliths

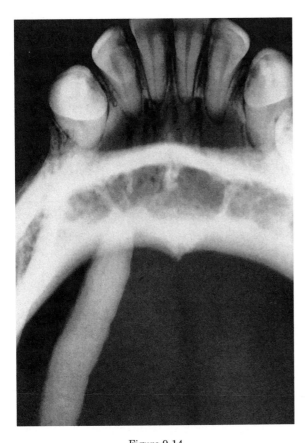

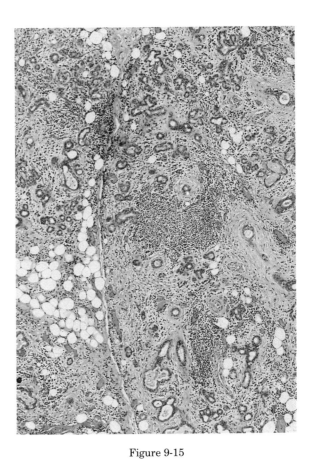

Figure 9-14
SIALOLITHIASIS
This mandibular occlusal radiograph demonstrates a large, elongated sialolith that has developed along an extensive portion of the excretory duct from the submandibular gland.

Figure 9-15
CHRONIC SCLEROSING SIALADENITIS
The normal lobular architecture of this submandibular gland is preserved although there is extensive fibrosis and inflammation.

Figure 9-16
CHRONIC
SCLEROSING SIALADENITIS
The lobular pattern of the submandibular gland is accentuated by increased fibrosis, and multifocal lymphoid infiltrates involve the salivary gland lobules in varying degrees.

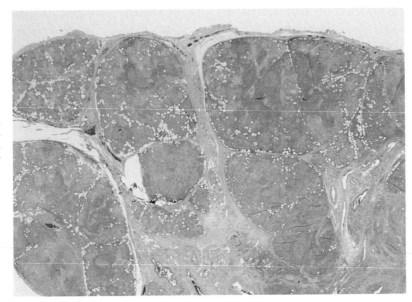

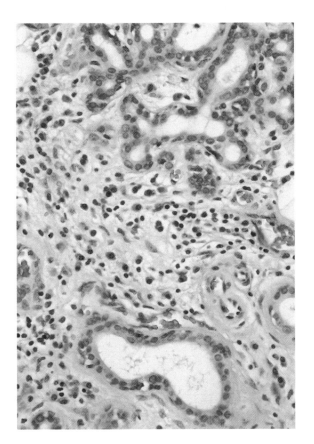 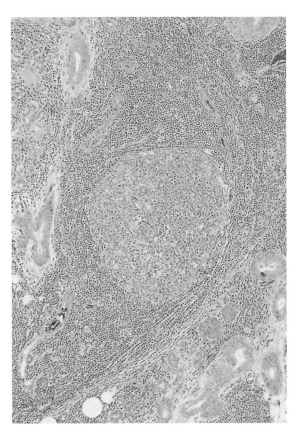

Figure 9-17
CHRONIC SCLEROSING SIALADENITIS
Left: In advanced stage disease there is nearly complete loss of acinar cells. The intercalated and intralobular ducts are dilated, and there is marked interstitial fibrosis with a lymphocytic and plasmacytic inflammatory cell infiltrate.
Right: In this submandibular gland the lymphoid infiltrate is very dense, and a germinal center is evident in the center of the field.

commonly shows squamous metaplasia, thickening, and ulceration that is associated with marked periductal inflammation (fig. 9-18).

In most cases of sialolithiasis, the submandibular gland swelling and pain resolve after removal of the salivary duct stone, especially when the sialolith is located in the distal portion of the duct. However, in about 20 percent of cases, the symptoms persist and the gland must be excised (40). In cases of immune secretory dysfunction or unknown etiology the gland is usually excised.

SALIVARY CYSTS

Mucoceles

Mucoceles are defined as the pooling of salivary mucus within a cystic cavity. They are the most common non-neoplastic lesion of salivary glands. Over the last decade they have comprised 9 to 10 percent of the salivary gland lesions reviewed at the AFIP; in the Salivary Gland Register at the University of Hamburg, Germany, they constitute about 4.5 percent of all lesions of salivary glands (65). They are reported to be the most common intraoral lesion in patients under 20 years of age (21). Two types of mucoceles are recognized: *the extravasation type* and *the retention type*. The extravasation type results from the escape of secreted salivary fluid from the salivary gland duct system into the surrounding connective tissues. Terms that have been used for this type of mucocele are *mucus escape reaction* and *mucus retention phenomenon*. Traumatic severance of a salivary gland duct, such as may result from accidental biting of the lip, is probably the most common etiology, although many patients are unable to recall a specific traumatic event (47). Praetorius and Hammarstrom

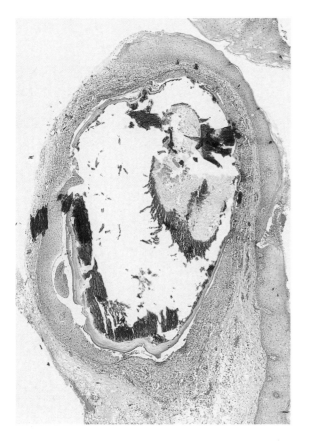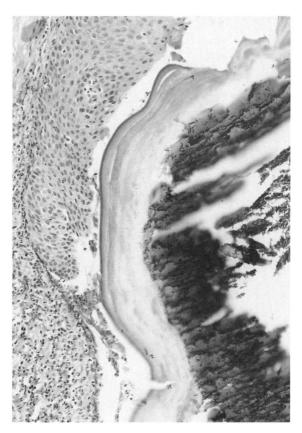

Figure 9-18
SIALOLITHIASIS

Left: A sialolith, which has partially shattered during tissue preparation, is located just beneath the oral mucosa in the submandibular excretory duct.

Right: Higher magnification of the sialolith and duct shows squamous metaplasia, ulceration of the duct-lining epithelium, and periductal inflammation.

(59) have proposed that some intraglandular mucoceles are caused by traumatic destruction of a large amount of glandular acini and continuing secretion from the remaining acini. In mucous retention cysts the mucus pools are confined within epithelial-lined cysts that are most likely markedly dilated excretory ducts. The pathogenesis may be related either to partial obstruction of a duct which results in increased intraluminal pressure and dilation or congenital or acquired weakness in the structure of a duct (47,69).

In AFIP data, mucus escape reactions outnumber mucous retention cysts by a ratio of about 10 to 1; in the University of Hamburg's Salivary Gland Register 85 percent of mucoceles were the mucous extravasation type (65). About 70 percent of extravasation mucoceles occur in the lower lip. Most of the remainder occur in other intraoral sites, such as tongue, floor of mouth, palate, and buccal mucosa. The parotid and submandibular glands are rarely involved. Mucous retention cysts are more evenly distributed among the various intraoral sites and major salivary glands. The peak incidence for mucus escape reactions is in the third decade of life and 70 percent occur in patients under 30 years of age. Slightly more men than women are affected. The mucous retention cyst occurs in all age groups, but the peak incidence is in the seventh and eighth decades.

Clinically, mucoceles are typically small, dome-shaped swellings of the mucosa (fig. 9-19). Their size ranges from about 0.2 to 1.0 cm. The exceptions are mucoceles that develop in the floor of the mouth, which may become several centimeters large and even dissect through tissue planes and

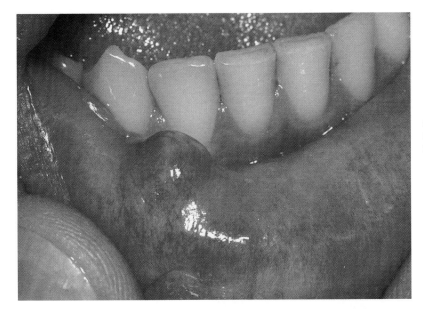

Figure 9-19
MUCOCELE
This extravasation type mucocele is a smooth-surfaced, dome-shaped nodule of the mucosa of the lower lip, the most common site for these lesions.

Figure 9-20
RANULA
This 2.5-cm ranula in the anterior floor of the mouth is not especially large, but it is larger than mucoceles that occur in most other sites. Ranulas are either extravasation type or retention cyst type mucoceles.

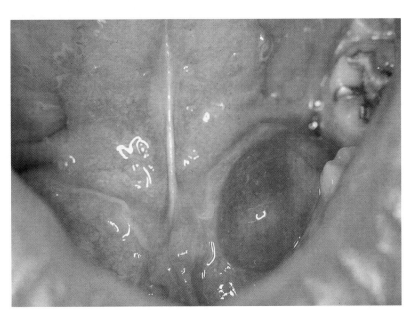

muscles of the floor of the mouth into the submandibular and upper cervical tissues. These large mucoceles are often referred to as *ranulas* (fig. 9-20), and those that extend outside the oral cavity into the cervical tissues are called *plunging ranulas*. The sublingual gland commonly supplies mucus to ranulas.

Some patients report fluctuation in size of mucoceles that is related to meals or to rupture of the overlying oral mucosa, which may be spontaneous or secondary to trauma, such as repeated lip biting (fig. 9-21). They are generally soft and fluctuant, but older lesions become firmer as organization ensues. When very superficial in the mucosa they often have a slightly translucent appearance (fig. 9-22). With deeper lesions the color of the mucosa is normal. They are usually painless and develop rapidly within hours to days.

Microscopically, the extravasation type of mucocele is a rounded pool of mucus within fibrous connective tissue (fig. 9-23). In very early lesions, the wall of the mucus pool is formed by compressed collagen, but quickly an inflammatory reaction develops around the mucus pool.

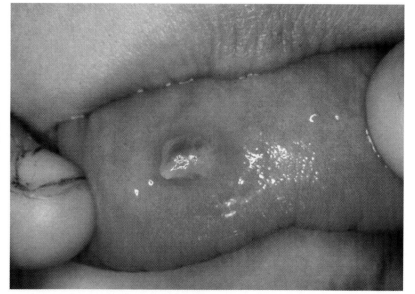

Figure 9-21
RUPTURED MUCOCELE
This mucocele of the lower lip has ruptured and collapsed due to trauma from lip biting.

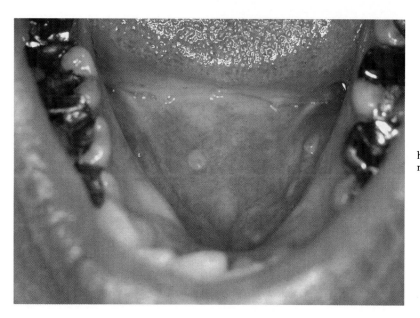

Figure 9-22
SUPERFICIAL MUCOCELE
This mucocele in the floor of the mouth has a translucent appearance because the mucosa overlying it is very thin.

This inflammatory reaction is dominated by macrophages that contain phagocytized mucus (fig. 9-24). Older lesions frequently undergo organization by granulation tissue. In older lesions that are primarily granulation tissue, it is difficult to distinguish a mucocele from an organized thrombus or small hematoma. Mucicarmine stain identifies residual mucus and can sometimes be helpful in diagnosis. In the retention cyst type of mucocele, an epithelial-lined fibrous tissue wall surrounds the mucus pool (fig. 9-25).

As long as the epithelial lining remains intact, there is little or no inflammatory reaction. The epithelium of the cyst varies from simple cuboidal to columnar to stratified squamous.

Mucoceles are usually treated by local excision. It is desirable to remove the glandular tissue that supplies mucus to the mucocele. Failure to identify and remove the associated gland or severance of another salivary duct during the excision of a mucocele probably accounts for some of the frequent recurrences of these lesions.

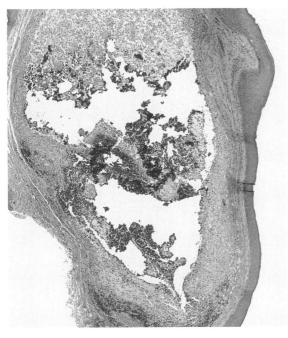

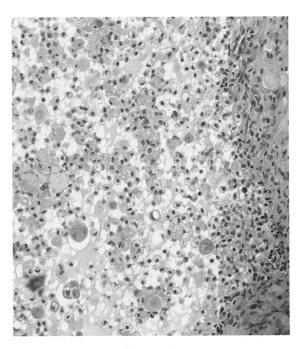

Figure 9-23
MUCUS ESCAPE REACTION

Within the lamina propria is a pool of mucus and hemorrhage (some was lost during processing of the tissue) that is surrounded by inflamed fibrous tissue. Inflammatory cells have migrated into the mucus pool.

Figure 9-24
MUCUS ESCAPE REACTION

Granulation tissue borders the mucus cavity (left) and numerous phagocytic macrophages have migrated into the mucus.

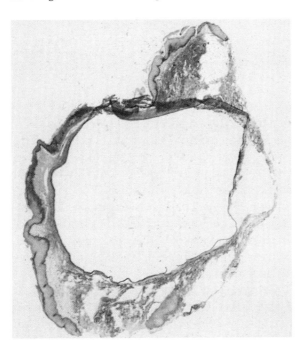

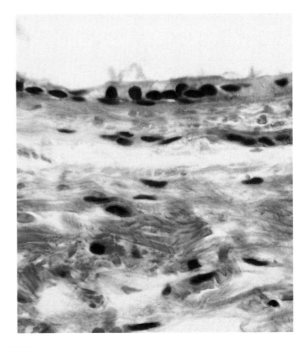

Figure 9-25
MUCUS RETENTION CYST

Left: The mucus in this retention cyst from the floor of the mouth was lost during tissue processing.

Right. High magnification of the wall of the cyst shows that it is lined by a thin layer of cuboidal epithelium and that there are no inflammatory cells.

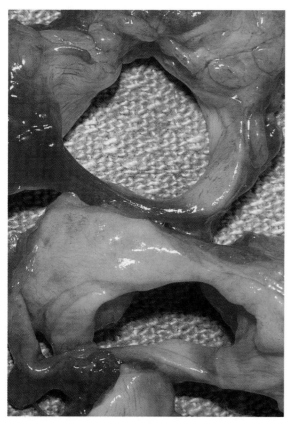

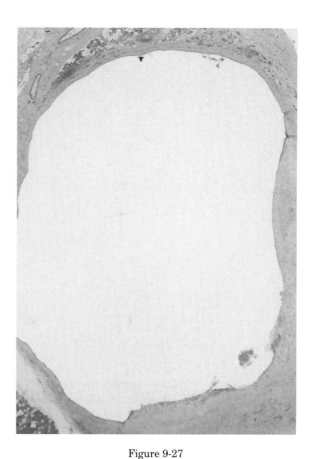

Figure 9-26
SALIVARY DUCT CYST
Gross specimen of a partial parotid gland resection shows a smooth-surfaced, unilocular cyst.

Figure 9-27
SALIVARY DUCT CYST
A rounded, smooth-surfaced cystic cavity is sharply separated from the adjacent parotid gland parenchyma by dense fibrous connective tissue.

Salivary Duct Cysts

Salivary duct cysts are acquired cysts that are believed to develop from marked cystic dilation of a salivary gland duct. The majority occur in the parotid gland, and ductal obstruction is thought to be a principal etiologic factor. Therefore, some investigators consider these to be a form of retention cyst (41,60). They are distinguished from mucus retention cysts because they typically do not contain mucus pools or plugs, occur primarily in the parotid gland, and on average are larger than mucus retention cysts of the minor salivary glands. Specific causes of obstruction are often not recognized although some cysts have been associated with benign and malignant neoplasms, postinflammatory sequela, calculi, and mucus plugs.

In the experience of the AFIP, 85 percent of salivary duct cysts occur in the parotid gland, 10 percent in the submandibular gland, and the remainder in various other salivary gland sites. These cysts constitute 2 to 3 percent of all parotid gland lesions. Others report a similar incidence (16,57) although Richardson et al. (60) reported only 5 salivary duct cysts among 708 parotidectomy specimens. There is no sex predilection. Children to older adults are affected, but most patients are over 30 years old. The cysts are unilateral, painless, compressible swellings that are as large as 10 cm, but the majority are 1 to 3 cm (41).

Grossly and microscopically, salivary duct cysts are well circumscribed and usually unilocular (figs. 9-26, 9-27). The fluid content varies in amount and consistency, from thin and watery to viscous and brownish. The cyst wall is a dense fibrous connective tissue that is usually 1 to 3 mm thick. It often contains a mild to moderate chronic inflammatory cell infiltrate but not the

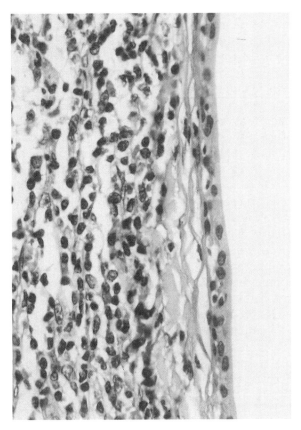

Figure 9-28
SALIVARY DUCT CYST
Thin, flattened, cuboidal or squamous epithelium covers the luminal surface of this parotid cyst, which has a lymphocytic and plasmacytic inflammatory cell infiltrate in the wall.

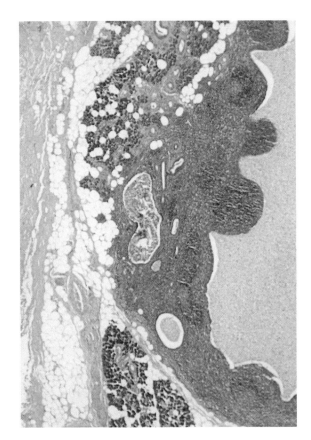

Figure 9-29
LYMPHOEPITHELIAL CYST
This parotid gland cyst has an undulating luminal surface, thin epithelial lining, and a wall of dense lymphoid tissue with several follicular centers. It is moderately well demarcated from the adjacent parotid parenchyma.

dense lymphoid tissue of lymphoepithelial cysts or Warthin's tumor. The luminal surface of the cyst wall is lined by epithelium that is stratified squamous, flattened squamous, cuboidal, or columnar (fig. 9-28). Occasionally, goblet-type mucous cells or oncocytic cells are present. The parotid parenchyma immediately peripheral to the cyst wall is usually compressed and atrophic, and in some cases mild sialadenitis and duct ectasia with inspissated secretions are evident. Surgical excision is curative.

Lymphoepithelial Cyst

Lymphoepithelial cysts are similar to salivary duct cysts in their clinical presentation and they share some histologic features. Nearly all occur in the parotid gland as compressible to firm, unilateral and unicystic masses, with the excep-

tion of human immunodeficiency virus (HIV)-associated lymphoepithelial cysts, which are discussed separately. A few lymphoepithelial cysts occur in the floor of the mouth and lateral tongue, but these cysts are probably related to ectopic tonsillar tissue and tonsillar crypt epithelium rather than salivary gland tissue. Histologically, parotid lymphoepithelial cysts typically have a more uneven or irregular luminal surface than salivary duct cysts (fig. 9-29). In some cysts this is observed grossly as a granular surface texture. The characteristic feature is dense lymphoid tissue in the cyst wall. Germinal centers are usually conspicuous in the lymphoid tissue, which is generally well demarcated from the adjacent parotid gland parenchyma. The epithelial lining of the cysts is of squamous, cuboidal, columnar, or pseudostratified ciliated type,

427

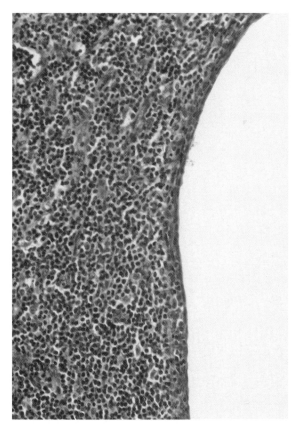

Figure 9-30
LYMPHOEPITHELIAL CYST

Thin, lumen-lining, stratified squamous epithelium and dense lymphocytes form the wall of a lymphoepithelial cyst of the parotid. The demarcation of epithelium and lymphoid tissue is somewhat obscure because many lymphocytes penetrate the epithelium.

but stratified squamous epithelium is the most common (fig. 9-30). Columnar epithelium also sometimes contains a few goblet-like mucous cells. Sebaceous cells have rarely been observed in the wall of lymphoepithelial cysts (32,57).

Salivary duct cysts are twice as common as lymphoepithelial cysts in the Salivary Gland Register of the University of Hamburg, Germany (65); however, at the AFIP they occur with about equal frequency. Richardson et al. (60), on the other hand, found that lymphoepithelial cysts occur more frequently than salivary duct cysts of the parotid gland. Similar to the AFIP's experience, they also found that lymphoepithelial cysts comprised 2 to 3 percent of all parotid surgical specimens. Peiterse and Seymour (57) and Katz (42) found an incidence closer to 1 percent in resected parotid glands.

After eliminating the male bias of military cases, the male to female ratio in cases submitted to the AFIP in the last decade was 3 to 1, which is similar to that found by Fujibayashi and Itoh (29). Lymphoepithelial cysts are rare in children. The peak incidence is in the fourth decade of life, and the average age of patients is about 45 years. Most of these cysts are asymptomatic, but occasionally patients report tenderness, pain, or even facial nerve dysfunction (41).

There have been two principal proposals on the pathogenesis of lymphoepithelial cysts. One theory is that they develop from remnants of the embryonic branchial apparatus, and the term *branchial cleft cyst* has been used (3). The more popular proposal is that they develop from cystic proliferation of salivary gland epithelium entrapped in intraparotid and paraparotid lymph nodes (15,29,41).

Lymphoepithelial cysts are distinguished from Warthin's tumor by their unilocular nature, minimal to mild papillary configuration, and absence of oncocytic columnar cells, although this is not of significant therapeutic importance. More serious is the distinction between lymphoepithelial cyst and cystic metastatic squamous cell carcinoma. The latter is commonly associated with a primary nasopharyngeal squamous cell carcinoma. The absence of significant cytologic atypia in the cyst-lining epithelial cells differentiates lymphoepithelial cyst from cystic carcinoma.

Lymphoepithelial cysts are not known to recur and are treated by surgical excision.

Polycystic (Dysgenetic) Disease of the Parotid Gland

Polycystic (dysgenetic) disease of the parotid gland is a rare developmental malformation of the duct system, similar to polycystic disease of the kidney. However, at this time an association between polycystic disease of the parotid and dysgenetic cysts of either the kidney, liver, lung, or pancreas is unknown. It appears that the developmental defect occurs in the intercalated ducts, and these ducts become markedly distended. The striated and interlobular ducts do not appear to be involved. Seifert et al. (66) provided the first description of this disease in 1981. There have been eight documented cases reported in the literature (9,23,66,68), and an additional two cases have been examined at the

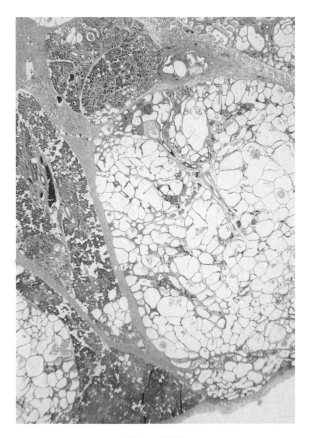

Figure 9-31
POLYCYSTIC (DYSGENETIC) DISEASE
OF PAROTID GLAND
Honeycomb-like, cystic lobules of parotid tissue are separated by collagenous septa. The degree of cystic change varies from lobule to lobule.

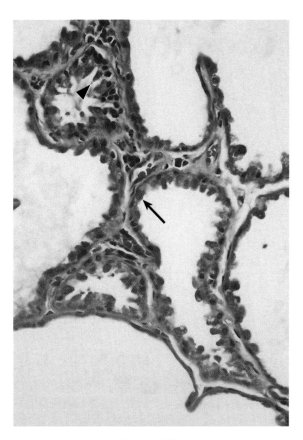

Figure 9-32
POLYCYSTIC (DYSGENETIC) DISEASE
OF PAROTID GLAND
In most areas the cysts are lined by cuboidal or flattened epithelium (arrow), but in focal areas the epithelial cells have rounded, bulging luminal surfaces and eosinophilic, apocrine-like cytoplasm (arrowhead).

AFIP. A case reported by Mandel and Kaynar (52) was based solely on radiographic findings without histopathologic verification. Smyth et al. (68) reported the familial occurrence of the disease in a mother and daughter. All but one of the known lesions occurred in females. Most lesions first manifested in childhood, but in three cases the lesions did not become apparent until adulthood. Recurrent swelling of the parotid glands is the typical clinical history. Other salivary glands have not been involved, and the patients have not experienced abnormal salivation.

Grossly and microscopically, the involved parotid gland maintains its lobular architecture, which is often emphasized by thickened fibrous septa. The lobules are distended by a honeycomb of variably sized epithelial-lined cysts (fig. 9-31).

The lining of the cysts is flattened cuboidal or low columnar epithelium. In some areas the columnar epithelium has abundant eosinophilic cytoplasm and rounded luminal borders, similar in appearance to apocrine type cells (fig. 9-32). Many of the epithelial cells have cytoplasmic vacuolation. The cysts are often interconnected. Occasional striated ducts open directly into cysts, and some acinar units also appear to communicate with cysts (fig. 9-33). These findings strongly suggest that the cystic structures involve the intercalated ducts. The largest cysts are generally not more than a few millimeters in greatest dimension. The cysts are irregular in shape, and many have spur-like or incomplete septa that extend into the lumens (fig. 9-33). Most of the lumens contain a flocculent, proteinaceous,

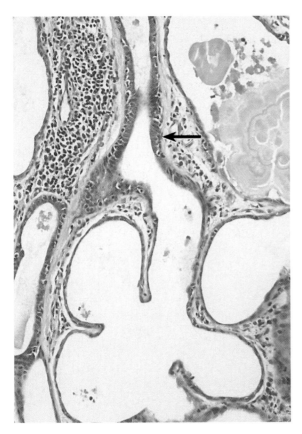

Figure 9-33
POLYCYSTIC (DYSGENETIC)
DISEASE OF PAROTID GLAND
A striated duct (arrow) opens into markedly dilated intercalated ducts. The cysts interconnect to one another, and spur-like, incomplete septa project into the lumens.

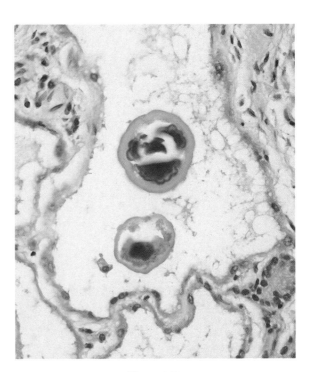

Figure 9-34
POLYCYSTIC (DYSGENETIC)
DISEASE OF PAROTID GLAND
Two small laminated microliths sit in a cystic lumen, which also contains eosinophilic, proteinaceous material that is present in many cysts.

eosinophilic material. Some macrophages are evident in this material. Inflammatory cells of varying density are present in the fibrous walls and septa of the cysts, but the overall intensity of this reaction is mild and not in proportion to the cystic changes in the gland, indicating that the cystic alterations are not secondary to sialadenitis. Some cysts also contain circular, laminated, eosinophilic or calcified bodies similar to small sialoliths (fig. 9-34).

Although the cystic process is diffuse in the gland, the extent of involvement varies from lobule to lobule. Some lobules appear to be entirely involved by cystic structures, but even in these areas small foci of residual acinar tissue are found between cysts (fig. 9-35); in other lobules, areas of apparently uninvolved acinar tissue are evident; still other lobules have only a few cysts.

The differential diagnosis principally includes salivary gland adenocarcinomas that have a prominent cystic component, such as cystadenocarcinoma, mucoepidermoid carcinoma, and acinic cell adenocarcinoma. The widespread involvement of the parotid gland, persistence of the lobular architecture, absence of a significant stromal or inflammatory reaction, and microliths distinguish polycystic disease from neoplasm.

Surgical resection is limited to diagnostic procedures or cosmetic recontouring.

HIV-ASSOCIATED SALIVARY GLAND DISEASE (MULTIPLE LYMPHOEPITHELIAL CYSTS OF THE PAROTID GLAND)

Persistent generalized lymphadenopathy is one of the early manifestations of HIV infection and subsequent development of the acquired immunodeficiency syndrome (AIDS). A less well-recognized but related manifestation of HIV infection is lymphoid hyperplasia of the salivary

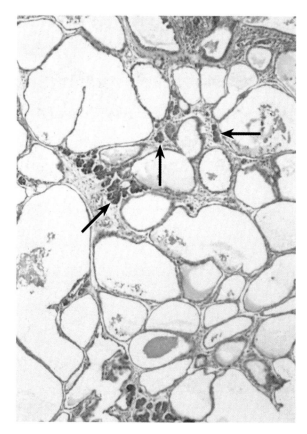

Figure 9-35
POLYCYSTIC (DYSGENETIC) DISEASE
OF PAROTID GLAND
Scattered foci of acinar tissue (arrows) are evident in
some of the intercystic areas.

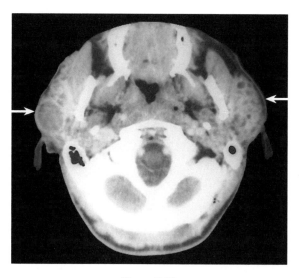

Figure 9-36
HIV-ASSOCIATED PAROTID GLAND DISEASE
Bilateral, multicystic disease is evident in the parotid
gland (arrows) in this CT image of an HIV-infected man.
(Courtesy of Dr. Angelo DelBalso, Buffalo, NY.)

glands, especially the parotid glands. The associated proliferation of ductal epithelium that gives rise to cysts and epithelial islands is reminiscent of that seen with Sjögren's syndrome. Since the recognition of HIV infection and AIDS in the early 1980s, over 200 cases of HIV-associated parotid adenopathy have appeared in the literature (6,18,34,36,53,67,70,71). The exact incidence of parotid gland enlargement in HIV-infected patients is not known, but Schiodt et al. (62) found it to be about 5 percent in their series of adult patients. HIV-infected children seem to have parotid enlargement much more frequently than adults, 47 percent in the series of Katz et al. (43), but most of these enlargements are probably acute infections rather than lymphoepithelial cysts (50). Terry et al. (71) found that 38 of 60 consecutive patients with lymphoepithelial lesions were HIV infected.

Parotid disease is the first clinical manifestation of HIV infection in some patients. Parotid involvement is seven times more frequent in men than women. The majority of patients are intravenous drug users, but many are homosexual men (61). It is likely that all HIV risk groups are affected. Parotid gland swelling typically manifests early in the course of HIV disease, before the development of AIDS. It is usually bilateral but can be unilateral and it is usually accompanied by cervical lymphadenopathy. Computed tomographic scans are frequently able to demonstrate multiple parotid cysts (fig. 9-36). The parotid enlargement is generally painless and slow.

Histopathologically, the features are similar to those in lymph nodes of persistent generalized lymphadenopathy. There is florid follicular hyperplasia of lymphoid tissue that disrupts and replaces the normal parotid parenchyma. The lymphoid follicles are typically larger and more irregularly shaped than unreactive follicles in normal lymph nodes (fig. 9-37). The germinal centers often contain numerous macrophages that bear tingible bodies, and mitotic figures are plentiful. The interfollicular lymphoid tissue contains many histiocytes and large monomorphic round cells with pale cytoplasm that are often clustered. Neutrophils and plasma cells

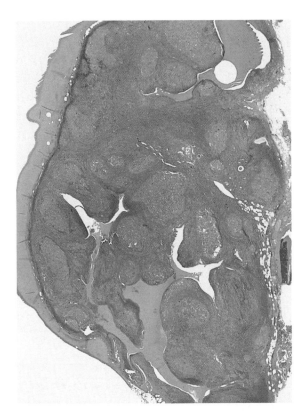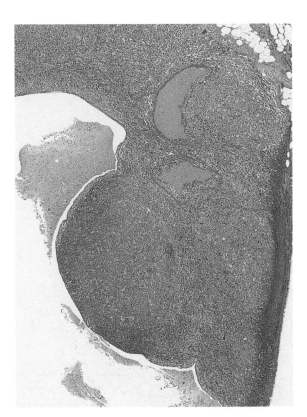

Figure 9-37

HIV-ASSOCIATED PAROTID GLAND DISEASE

Left: Prominent intraparotid lymphoid tissue with multiple, irregular-shaped cysts has displaced much of the parotid gland parenchyma.

Right: Higher magnification shows large, hyperplastic germinal centers in the lymphoid tissue adjacent to two small and one large cyst.

are also often conspicuous. Some of the germinal centers have an attenuated mantle of small lymphocytes that invaginates into the follicle, termed follicle lysis (fig. 9-38). Squamous epithelial-lined cysts and epimyoepithelial islands that are reminiscent of those seen in Sjögren's syndrome occur within the lymphoid proliferation (fig. 9-39). While these features together are indicative of HIV infection, they are not pathognomonic since similar features have been observed in HIV-negative individuals. However, some patients that initially were HIV negative subsequently became seropositive (36).

While lymphoepithelial cysts are not a typical feature of Sjögren's syndrome, the lymphoepithelial lesions of the parotid gland and some clinical symptoms of HIV-associated salivary gland disease are similar to Sjögren's syndrome. HIV patients lack the serum autoantibodies (antinuclear antibodies, anti-SSA, anti-SSB, rheu-

matoid factor) frequent in Sjögren's syndrome, and the parotid lymphoid proliferation is predominantly CD8 rather than CD4 positive, as in Sjögren's syndrome. A reversed T4/T8 ratio of peripheral blood lymphocytes is usually present in patients with HIV-associated salivary gland disease (62). HIV-infected lymphoid cells but not epithelial cells have been demonstrated in parotid tissue from patients with HIV-associated parotid adenopathy (78).

Therapeutic recommendations for HIV-related multicystic lymphoepithelial lesions of the parotid have been parotidectomy, conservative excision, curettage, radiation, and periodic reexamination (27,34,36,67). Therapy seems to be mostly for cosmetic reasons. Parotid enlargement does not appear to have any significance for the course of HIV infection or progression to AIDS other than that associated with persistent generalized lymphadenopathy.

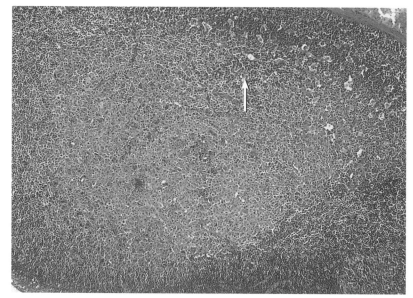

Figure 9-38
HIV-ASSOCIATED PAROTID
GLAND DISEASE
A lymphoid follicle has an irregular outline, poorly defined mantle zone, and focal follicle lysis (arrow).

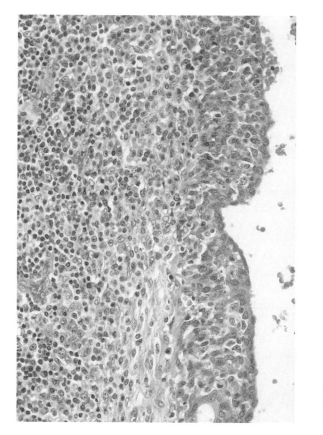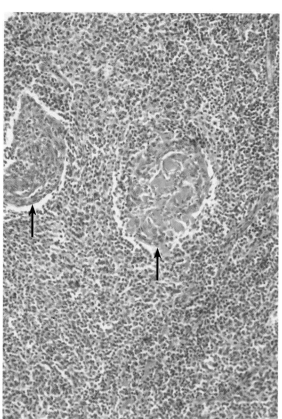

Figure 9-39
HIV-ASSOCIATED PAROTID GLAND DISEASE
Left: The squamous epithelial lining of a parotid cyst is penetrated by many lymphocytes. The subepithelial lymphoid tissue contains many large mononuclear cells and plasma cells as well as small lymphocytes.
Right: Two epimyoepithelial islands (arrows) within the lymphoid tissue are penetrated by many lymphocytes.

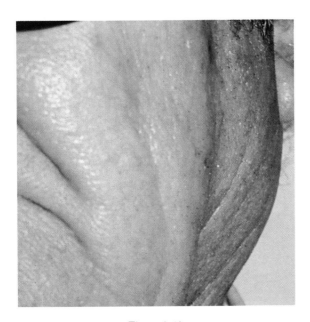

Figure 9-40
SIALADENOSIS
Enlargement of the left parotid gland is evident in a man with chronic alcoholism and cirrhosis of the liver.

SIALADENOSIS

Sialadenosis is the non-neoplastic and noninflammatory enlargement of salivary glands due to metabolic factors or secretory dysfunction. The parotid glands are typically affected and produce painless bilateral swellings. This salivary gland enlargement is nearly always related to a systemic condition and has been most often associated with diabetes mellitus, thyroid insufficiency, malnutrition, alcoholism and liver cirrhosis, sex hormone changes (puberty and menopause), drug reactions (commonly antihypertensive medications), and neurogenic disorders (fig. 9-40) (8,44,49,51,55,64, 65,76). The basic underlying problem is thought to be a disorder of salivary gland innervation due to peripheral autonomic neuropathy (65).

According to data from the Salivary Gland Register at the University of Hamburg, which has the largest known collection of cases of sialadenosis (388 cases), the peak incidence is in the fifth and sixth decades of life, with a slight female predominance (65). Clinically, parotid gland swelling develops as slow, intermittent, nonpainful enlargement that is frequently accompanied by decreasing saliva secretion.

In the early stages of the disease, acinar hypertrophy characterizes the histopathologic fea-

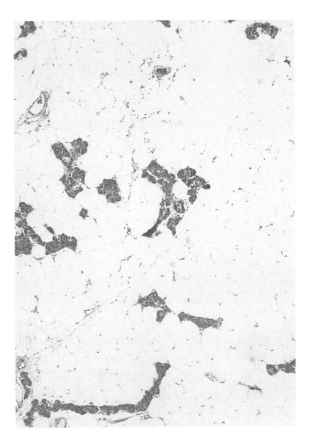

Figure 9-41
SIALADENOSIS
In long-term sialadenosis there is eventually atrophy of the parotid parenchymal tissue and increase in intraglandular fat.

tures. Although few patients have their parotid glands excised during this phase of the disease, Seifert (65) was able to describe three types of acinar cell swelling: granular with densely packed periodic acid–Schiff (PAS)-positive granules in the cytoplasm; honeycomb with vacuolated cytoplasm; and mixed. The character of the acinar swelling does not seem to be related to the associated systemic condition. Paradoxically, as the disease persists, there is eventual atrophy of the parenchymal tissue, but the glands remain clinically enlarged because there is a compensatory increase in the amount of intraglandular adipose tissue (fig. 9-41) (8). Inflammatory cell infiltrates are absent.

Treatment of sialadenosis is directed toward the underlying systemic disorder. Glandular swelling associated with drugs or sex hormone changes may resolve with withdrawal of the drug or resolution of the hormonal imbalance

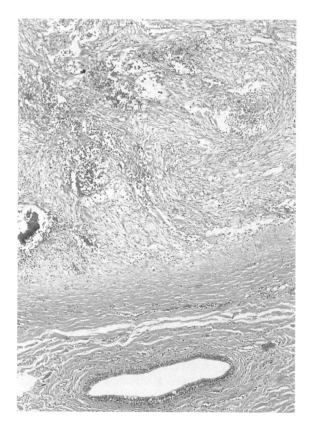 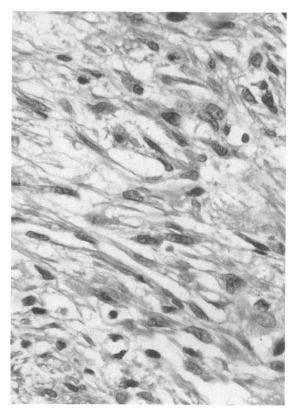

Figure 9-42
NODULAR FASCIITIS
Left: This intraparotid circumscribed lesion is composed of a spindle cell proliferation in a richly mucinous stroma.
Right: The immature fibroblasts have ovoid or fusiform nuclei with occasional nucleoli and are more haphazardly arranged than in myoepitheliomas. Limited amounts of collagen fibrils are present.

(51). Sialadenosis associated with diabetes mellitus or other endocrine disorders, cirrhosis, or neurogenic abnormalities is resistant to treatment. Orally administered pilocarpine hydrochloride has been used to successfully treat sialadenosis in bulimic patients (55). Cosmetic surgery is sometimes employed in severe cases.

NODULAR FASCIITIS

Nodular fasciitis presents in the parotid gland or parotid region as a tender, rapidly growing mass, which clinically is often thought to be a parenchymal salivary neoplasm. Because of its rapid growth, composition of immature spindle fibroblasts, and mitotic activity, it may be mistaken for a sarcoma (24,75). When located within the salivary glands, its spindle cell component, combined with a richly myxoid stroma, suggest

a tumor derived from myoepithelial cells (fig. 9-42). Additionally, because the lesion is not encapsulated, a spindle cell carcinoma may also be considered. Nodular fasciitis does not contain chondroid zones or small duct-like structures characteristic of mixed tumors. Immunohistochemical studies demonstrate that the spindle cells in nodular fasciitis, unlike those seen in myoepithelioma, are not immunoreactive with cytokeratin, although the lesional cells in both react with antibodies to smooth muscle actin.

INFLAMMATORY PSEUDOTUMOR

Inflammatory pseudotumors are reactive fibroinflammatory lesions that produce dense, hard, nodular swellings that can simulate neoplasia in their clinical presentation. They have been described under various terms in a wide

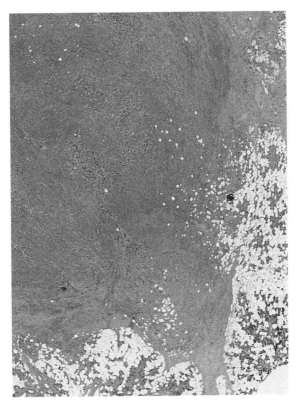

Figure 9-43
INFLAMMATORY PSEUDOTUMOR
This low-magnification micrograph shows an inflammatory pseudotumor in the parotid gland that is densely cellular, nodular, and unencapsulated.

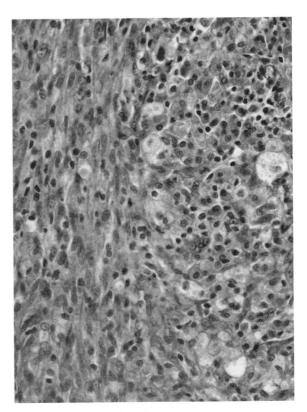

Figure 9-44
INFLAMMATORY PSEUDOTUMOR
Plump, spindled and rounded cells have abundant eosinophilic cytoplasm and round to oval, lightly basophilic nuclei without cytologic atypia or mitotic figures. Some larger xanthoma type cells have pale, foamy cytoplasm. Plasma cells and lymphocytes are scattered throughout the tissue.

variety of tissues, including lung, liver, spleen, skin, lymph nodes, and soft tissues. Williams et al. (77) described six cases from the AFIP files that involved the parotid glands. The lesions presented clinically as firm, nodular swellings in the parotid glands and were apparent to the patients for several months. Men and women were equally affected. The patients were all adults over 45 years of age, with a mean of 70 years, which is older than has been described for this entity in other sites. Antibiotic therapy prior to surgical excision was ineffective. Grossly, the lesions were circumscribed but unencapsulated, yellowish tan nodules within the body of the parotid gland (fig. 9-43). Histologically, they were composed of plump, spindled and rounded cells in poorly formed fascicles and storiform arrays and had the general characteristics of fibrohistiocytic, fibroblastic, and myofibroblastic cells (fig. 9-44). There was abundant eosinophilic cytoplasm that was frequently granular. Abundant PAS-positive cytoplasmic granules were seen in many cells (fig. 9-45). Some cells were larger, with foamy cytoplasm, and consistent with xanthoma cells. Occasional multinucleated giant cells were found. Diffusely distributed but low-density inflammatory cells were predominantly plasma cells and lymphocytes with a few neutrophils. Strong immunohistochemical reactions for both CD68 (KP1) and smooth muscle actin were consistent with histiocytic and myofibroblastic differentiation (fig. 9-46).

Specific etiologies for inflammatory pseudotumors are usually unknown. Although focal salivary duct rupture was evident in two of the parotid lesions, these were believed to be a result rather than a cause of the pseudotumors (77). Surgery was curative, and there was no complication or recurrence up to 8 years after excision.

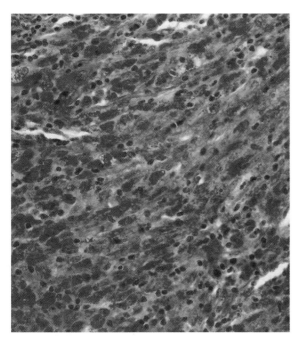

Figure 9-45
INFLAMMATORY PSEUDOTUMOR
Many of the cells are packed with diatase-resistant PAS-positive cytoplasmic granules. (PAS stain)

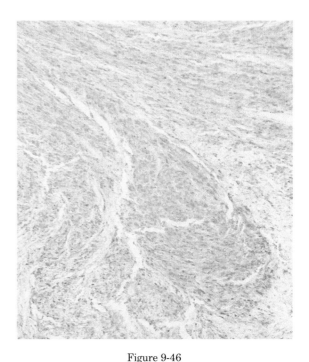

Figure 9-46
INFLAMMATORY PSEUDOTUMOR
The immunohistochemical reaction for CD68 is strong, and similar results were obtained for smooth muscle actin. Immunoreactions for cytokeratin, desmin, and S-100 protein were negative.

ADENOMATOID HYPERPLASIA OF MUCOUS SALIVARY GLANDS

Adenomatoid hyperplasia of minor salivary glands is a rare clinicopathologic entity characterized by a clinically evident nodular mass that histologically is composed of normal-appearing minor salivary gland lobules. Fifty-eight cases have been documented in the literature since the first report by Giansanti et al. (4,5,11,13,14,22, 31). The two largest series have been 10 cases from the AFIP files (4) and 40 cases from the University of the Pacific (14).

Clinically, these lesions present as 0.5- to 3.0-cm nodular mucosal swellings. Most lesions are 1.0 to 1.5 cm, normal colored, and asymptomatic (fig. 9-47). In fact, many patients are unaware of the lesion until noted by their dentists, so determination of the duration of the lesions has been difficult. At least two patients claimed durations of 20 and 40 years, but most patients report durations of weeks to several years (14). Eighty-five percent of the lesions occur on the palate, mostly the hard palate. Other sites are the mandibular retromolar area, buccal mucosa, lips, and tongue. Male patients outnumber female patients in a ratio of about 1.5

to 1. Lesions have been reported in patients of all ages, but the majority are 30 to 60 years old.

Most frequently considered in the clinical differential diagnosis is benign salivary gland neoplasm, but histologically, normal-appearing mucous salivary glands in fibrous tissue are found (fig. 9-48). The salivary gland tissue has the ductal and lobular structure of normal minor salivary glands. In some cases the glandular tissue has been described as hypertrophic, but this has been a subjective appraisal without quantitative morphometric analysis (14). Inflammation is minimal or absent.

Once adenomatoid hyperplasia of minor salivary gland has been identified in a biopsy or excisional specimen, no further treatment is needed since these lesions do not recur. None of the conditions that are associated with sialadenosis of the parotid glands is associated with minor salivary gland hyperplasia. Since these are only isolated focal lesions it is doubtful that there is any connection to a systemic condition. No specific local or systemic etiologic factors have been identified in most cases but local chronic irritation or trauma may have been a factor in some (14).

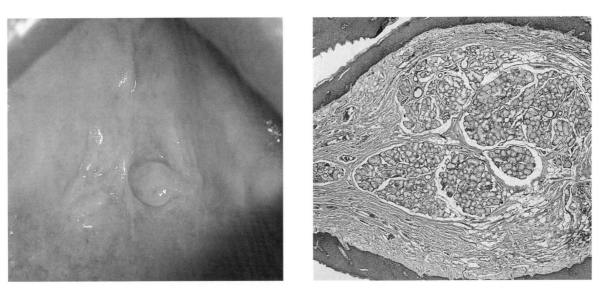

Figure 9-47
ADENOMATOID HYPERPLASIA OF MUCOUS SALIVARY GLANDS

A 0.5 cm, smooth surfaced, normal colored nodule of the posterior hard palate (left) was found to be composed of normal-appearing mucous salivary gland when examined microscopically (right).

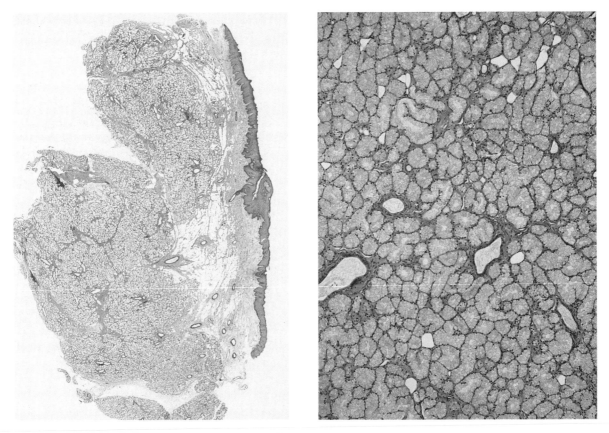

Figure 9-48
ADENOMATOID HYPERPLASIA OF MUCOUS SALIVARY GLANDS

An increase in the amount of otherwise normal minor salivary gland tissue apparently produced this swelling of the soft palate (left). Higher magnification (right) shows a normal ductal and acinar structural relationship.

REFERENCES

1. Abrams AM, Melrose RJ, Howell FV. Necrotizing sialometaplasia. A disease simulating malignancy. Cancer 1973;32:130–5.

2. Andrade RE, Hagen KA, Manivel JC. Distribution and immunophenotype of the inflammatory cell population in the benign lymphoepithelial lesion (Mikulicz's disease). Hum Pathol 1988;19:932–41.

3. Antoniadis K, Karakasis D, Tzarou V, Skordalaki A. Benign cysts of the parotid gland. Int J Oral Maxillofac Surg 1990;19:139–40.

4. Arafat A, Brannon RB, Ellis GL. Adenomatoid hyperplasia of mucous salivary glands. Oral Surg Oral Med Oral Pathol 1981;52:51–5.

5. Aufdemorte TB, Ramzy I, Holt GR, Thomas JR, Duncan DL. Focal adenomatoid hyperplasia of salivary glands. A differential diagnostic problem in fine needle aspiration biopsy. Acta Cytol 1985;29:23–8.

6. Barr LC, Cox PJ, Maskell GF, Thomas JM. Benign parotid cysts associated with human immunodeficiency virus infection. Br J Surg 1993;80:39.

7. Batsakis JG. Lymphoepithelial lesion and Sjögren's syndrome. Ann Otol Rhinol Laryngol 1987;96:354–5.

8. Batsakis JG. Pathology consultation. Sialadenosis. Ann Otol Rhinol Laryngol 1988;97:94–5.

9. Batsakis JG, Bruner JM, Luna MA. Polycystic (dysgenetic) disease of the parotid glands. Arch Otolaryngol Head Neck Surg 1988;114:1146–8.

10. Brannon RB, Fowler CB, Hartman KS. Necrotizing sialometaplasia. A clinicopathologic study of sixty-nine cases and review of the literature. Oral Surg Oral Med Oral Pathol 1991;72:317–25.

11. Brannon RB, Houston GD, Meader CL. Adenomatoid hyperplasia of mucous salivary glands: a case involving the retromolar area. Oral Surg Oral Med Oral Pathol 1985;60:188–90.

12. Bridges AJ, England DM. Benign lymphoepithelial lesion: relationship to Sjögren's syndrome and evolving malignant lymphoma. Semin Arthritis Rheum 1989;19:201–8.

13. Brown FH, Houston GD, Lubow RM, Sagan MA. Adenomatoid hyperplasia of mucous salivary glands. Report of two cases. J Periodontol 1987;58:125–7.

14. Buchner A, Merrell PW, Carpenter WM, Leider AS. Adenomatoid hyperplasia of minor salivary glands. Oral Surg Oral Med Oral Pathol 1991;71:583–7.

15. Cleary KR, Batsakis JG. Lymphoepithelial cysts of the parotid region: a new face on an old lesion. Ann Otol Rhinol Laryngol 1990;99:162–4.

16. Cohen MN, Rao U, Shedd DP. Benign cysts of the parotid gland. J Surg Oncol 1984;27:85–8.

17. Crabtree GM, Yarington CT. Submandibular gland excision. Laryngoscope 1988;98:1044–5.

18. d'Agay MF, de Roquancourt A, Peuchmaur M, Janier M, Brocheriou C. Cystic benign lymphoepithelial lesion of the salivary glands in HIV-positive patients. Report of two cases with immunohistochemical study. Virchows Arch [A] 1990;417:353–6.

19. Daniels TE. Benign lymphoepithelial lesion and Sjgren's syndrome. In: Ellis GL, Auclair PL, Gnepp DR, eds. Surgical pathology of the salivary glands. Philadelphia: WB Saunders, 1991:83–106.

20. Dardick I, van Nostrand AW, Rippstein P, Skimming L, Hoppe D, Dairkee SH. Characterization of epimyoepithelial islands in benign lymphoepithelial lesions of major salivary gland: an immunohistochemical and ultrastructural study. Head Neck Surg 1988;10:168–78.

21. Das S, Das AK. A review of pediatric oral biopsies from a surgical pathology service in a dental school. Pediatr Dent 1993;15:208–11.

22. Devildos LR, Langlois CC. Minor salivary gland lesion presenting clinically as tumor. Oral Surg Oral Med Oral Pathol 1976;41:657–9.

23. Dobson CM, Ellis HA. Polycystic disease of the parotid glands: case report of a rare entity and review of the literature. Histopathology 1987;11:953–61.

24. Enzinger FM, Weiss SW. Soft tissue tumors. 2nd ed. St. Louis: CV Mosby. 1988:102–12.

25. Epivatianos A, Harrison JD, Dimitriou T. Ultrastructural and histochemical observations on microcalculi in chronic submandibular sialadenitis. J Oral Pathol 1987;16:514–7.

26. Falzon M, Isaacson PG. The natural history of benign lymphoepithelial lesion of the salivary gland in which there is a monoclonal population of B cells. A report of two cases. Am J Surg Pathol 1991;15:59–65.

27. Ferraro FJ Jr, Rush BF Jr, Ruark D, Oleske J. Enucleation of parotid lymphoepithelial cyst in patients who are human immunodeficiency virus positive. Surg Gynecol Obstet 1993;177:524–6.

28. Freimark B, Fantozzi R, Bone R, Bordin G, Fox R. Detection of clonally expanded salivary gland lymphocytes in Sjögren's syndrome. Arthritis Rheum 1989;32:859–69.

29. Fujibayashi T, Itoh H. Lymphoepithelial (so-called branchial) cyst within the parotid gland. Report of a case and review of the literature. Int J Oral Surg 1981;10:283–92.

30. Gallina E, Gallo O, Boccuzzi S, Paradiso P. Analysis of 185 submandibular gland excisions. Acta Otorhinolaryngol Belg 1990;44:7–10.

31. Giansanti JS, Baker GO, Waldron CA. Intraoral, mucinous, minor salivary gland lesions presenting clinically as tumors. Oral Surg Oral Med Oral Pathol 1971;32:918–22.

32. Gnepp DR, Sporck FT. Benign lymphoepithelial parotid cyst with sebaceous differentiation—cystic sebaceous lymphadenoma. Am J Clin Pathol 1980;74:683–7.

33. Godwin JT. Benign lymphoepithelial lesion of the parotid gland (adenolymphoma, chronic inflammation, lymphoepithelioma, lymphocytic tumor, Mikulicz disease): report of eleven cases. Cancer 1952;5:1089–103.

34. Goldstein J, Rubin J, Silver C, et al. Radiation therapy as a treatment for benign lymphoepithelial parotid cysts in patients infected with human immunodeficiency virus-1. Int J Radiat Oncol Biol Phys 1992;23:1045–50.

35. Harrison JD, Triantafyllou A, Baldwin D, Schafer H. Histochemical and biochemical determination of calcium in salivary glands with particular reference to chronic submandibular sialadenitis. Virchows Arch [A] 1993;423:29–32.

36. Huang RD, Pearlman S, Friedman WH, Loree T. Benign cystic vs. solid lesions of the parotid gland in HIV patients. Head Neck 1991;13:522–7.

37. Hyjek E, Smith WJ, Isaacson PG. Primary B-cell lymphoma of salivary glands and its relationship to myoepithelial sialadenitis. Hum Pathol 1988;19:766–76.

38. Isacsson G, Ahlner B, Lundquist PG. Chronic sialadenitis of the submandibular gland. A retrospective study of 108 case. Arch Otorhinolaryngol 1981;232:91–100.

39. Isacsson G, Isberg A, Haverling M, Lundquist PG. Salivary calculi and chronic sialoadenitis of the submandibular gland: a radiographic and histologic study. Oral Surg Oral Med Oral Pathol 1984;58:622–7.

40. Isacsson G, Lundquist PG. Salivary calculi as an aetiological factor in chronic sialadenitis of the submandibular gland. Clin Otolaryngol 1982;7:231–6.

41. Jensen JL. Idiopathic diseases. In: Ellis GL, Auclair PL, Gnepp DR, eds. Surgical pathology of the salivary glands. Philadelphia: WB Saunders, 1991:60–82.

42. Katz AD. Unusual lesions of the parotid gland. J Surg Oncol 1975;7:219–35.

43. Katz MH, Mastrucci MT, Leggott PJ, Westenhouse J, Greenspan JS, Scott GB. Prognostic significance of oral lesions in children with perinatally acquired human immunodeficiency virus infection. Am J Dis Child 1993;147:45–8.

44. Kinzl J, Biebl W, Herold M. Significance of vomiting for hyperamylasemia and sialadenosis in patients with eating disorders. Int J Eat Disord 1993;13:117–24.

45. Kjorell U, Ostberg Y, Virtanen I, Thornell LE. Immunohistochemical analyses of autoimmune sialadenitis in man. J Oral Pathol 1988;17:374–80.

46. Kondratowicz GM, Smallman LA, Morgan DW. Clinicopathological study of myoepithelial sialadenitis and chronic sialadenitis (sialolithiasis). J Clin Pathol 1988;41:403–9.

47. Koudelka BK. Obstructive disorders. In: Ellis GL, Auclair PL, Gnepp DR, eds. Surgical pathology of the salivary glands. Philadelphia: WB Saunders, 1991:26–38.

48. Küttner H. Über entzndliche Tumoren der Submaxillarspeicheldrüse. Beitr Klin Chir 1896;15:815–34.

49. Lamey PJ, Darwazeh AM, Frier BM. Oral disorders associated with diabetes mellitus. Diabet Med 1992;9:410–6.

50. Leggott PJ. Oral manifestations of HIV infection in children. Oral Surg Oral Med Oral Pathol 1992;73:187–92.

51. Loria RC, Wedner HJ. Facial swelling secondary to inhaled bronchodilator abuse: catecholamine-induced sialadenosis. Ann Allergy 1989;62:289–93.

52. Mandel L, Kaynar A. Polycystic parotid disease: a case report. J Oral Maxillofac Surg 1991;49:1228–31.

53. Mandel L, Reich R. HIV parotid gland lymphoepithelial cysts. Review and case reports. Oral Surg Oral Med Oral Pathol 1992;74:273–8.

54. Matthews TW, Dardick I. Morphological alterations of salivary gland parenchyma in chronic sialadenitis. J Otolaryngol 1988;17:385–94.

55. Mehler PS, Wallace JA. Sialadenosis in bulimia. A new treatment. Arch Otolaryngol Head Neck Surg 1993;119:787–8.

56. Palmer RM, Eveson JW, Gusterson BA. Epimyoepithelial' islands in lymphoepithelial lesions. An immunocytochemical study. Virchows Arch [A] 1986;408:603–9.

57. Pieterse AS, Seymour AE. Parotid cysts. An analysis of 16 cases and suggested classification. Pathology 1981;13:225–34.

58. Pisa EK, Pisa P, Kang HI, Fox RI. High frequency of t(14;18) translocation in salivary gland lymphomas from Sjögren's syndrome patients. J Exp Med 1991;174:1245–50.

59. Praetorius F, Hammarstrom L. A new concept of the pathogenesis of oral mucous cysts based on a study of 200 cases. J Dent Assoc S Afr 1992;47:226–31.

60. Richardson GS, Clairmont AA, Erickson ER. Cystic lesions of the parotid gland. Plast Reconstr Surg 1978;61:364–70.

61. Schiodt M. HIV-associated salivary gland disease: a review. Oral Surg Oral Med Oral Pathol 1992;73:164–7.

62. Schiodt M, Greenspan D, Daniels TE, et al. Parotid gland enlargement and xerostomia associated with labial sialadenitis in HIV-infected patients. J Autoimmun 1989;2:415–25.

63. Schmid U, Lennert K, Gloor F. Immunosialadenitis (Sjögren's syndrome) and lymphoproliferation. Clin Exp Rheumatol 1989;7:175–80.

64. Scott J, Burns J, Flower EA. Histological analysis of parotid and submandibular glands in chronic alcohol abuse: a necropsy study. J Clin Pathol 1988;41:837–40.

65. Seifert G. Tumour-like lesions of the salivary glands. The new WHO classification. Pathol Res Pract 1992;188:836–46.

66. Seifert G, Thomsen S, Donath K. Bilateral dysgenetic polycystic parotid glands. Morphological analysis and differential diagnosis of a rare disease of the salivary glands. Virchows Arch [A] 1981;390:273–88.

67. Shaha AR, DiMaio T, Webber C, Thelmo W, Jaffe BM. Benign lymphoepithelial lesions of the parotid. Am J Surg 1993;166:403–6.

68. Smyth AG, Ward-Booth RP, High AS. Polycystic disease of the parotid glands: two familial cases. Br J Oral Maxillofac Surg 1993;31:38–40.

69. Tal H, Altini M, Lemmer J. Multiple mucous retention cysts of the oral mucosa. Oral Surg Oral Med Oral Pathol 1984;58:692–5.

70. Tao LC, Gullane PJ. HIV infection-associated lymphoepithelial lesions of the parotid gland: aspiration biopsy cytology, histology, and pathogenesis. Diagn Cytopathol 1991;7:158–62.

71. Terry JH, Loree TR, Thomas MD, Marti JR. Major salivary gland lymphoepithelial lesions and the acquired immunodeficiency syndrome. Am J Surg 1991;162:324–9.

72. Testa Riva F, Riva A, Puxeddu P. Ciliated cells in the main excretory duct of the submandibular gland in obstructive sialadenitis: a SEM and TEM study. Ultrastruct Pathol 1987;11:1–10.

73. Therkildsen MH, Nielsen BA, Krogdahl A. A case of granulomatous sialadenitis of the submandibular gland. APMIS 1989;97:75–8.

74. van der Walt JD, Leake J. Granulomatous sialadenitis of the major salivary glands. A clinicopathological study of 57 cases. Histopathology 1987;11:131–44.

75. Werning JT. Nodular fasciitis of the orofacial region. Oral Surg Oral Med Oral Pathol 1979;48:441–6.

76. Werning JT. Infectious and systemic diseases. In: Ellis GL, Auclair PL, Gnepp DR, eds. Surgical pathology of the salivary glands. Philadelphia: WB Saunders, 1991:39–59.

77. Williams SB, Foss RD, Ellis GL. Inflammatory pseudotumors of the major salivary glands. Clinicopathologic and immunohistochemical analysis of six cases. Am J Surg Pathol 1992;16:896–902.

78. Yeh CK, Fox PC, Goto Y, Austin HA, Brahim JS, Fox CH. Human immunodeficiency virus (HIV) and HIV infected cells in saliva and salivary glands of a patient with systemic lupus erythematosus. J Rheumatol 1992;19:1810–2.

79. Yoshihara T, Kanda T, Yaku Y, Kaneko T. Chronic sialadenitis of the submandibular gland (so-called Kuttner tumor). Auris Nasus Larynx 1983;10:117–23.

FINE-NEEDLE ASPIRATION BIOPSY OF SALIVARY GLANDS

Fine-needle aspiration biopsy (FNAB) has gained popularity as a technique for the evaluation of salivary gland lesions, particularly those of the parotid and submandibular glands. Several amply illustrated, comprehensive reviews are available (15,23,41,50,53,61). The advantages of FNAB over frozen section are that it provides a preoperative rather than intraoperative diagnosis, eliminates the need for general anesthesia, offers the possibility of using special stains if necessary, and reduces costs (11,13,24). There is general agreement that FNAB is free of the complications associated with the use of larger bore needles, such as tumor seeding and significant hemorrhage (6,38,54,59, 64). Nevertheless, there remain some questions about its accuracy in recognizing malignant salivary gland tumors and its value in the clinical management of patients. Some investigators advocate its routine systematic use for the evaluation of all salivary gland lesions whereas others contend that, except in certain situations, it is a cost-added procedure. Those that support its routine use agree that there is a slightly increased cost for the majority of patients for whom FNAB merely confirms the correct clinical diagnosis (16). A review of its accuracy and clinical utility is followed by brief descriptions of the FNAB characteristics of some of the most common neoplasms.

ACCURACY OF FNAB IN ASSESSING SALIVARY GLAND LESIONS

Accuracy rates of FNAB reported in published studies are often difficult to compare to one another. Some studies have included cases that were not histologically verified, some do not inform the reader whether or not unsatisfactory smears were included, some do not attempt to specifically diagnose malignant tumors, and the definitions for false-positive and false-negative results are often not precisely defined (6,15,64). Although much of the literature on the subject espouses high accuracy for FNAB of all salivary masses, critical review shows that this is not always the case.

The success rate of correctly predicting whether a mass is benign or malignant ranges between 81 and 98 percent in most recent reports whereas a specific diagnosis can be established in about 60 to 75 percent of cases (6,13,35,40,48,54,60,63-65,67). Benign tumors are much more often correctly classified than malignant ones (54,55). Some studies have shown a false-negative (histologically malignant cases in which the cytologic diagnosis was benign or insufficient) rate of 5 to 10 percent and a false-positive (histologically benign lesions designated as suspicious of malignancy) rate of 0 to 6 percent (13,24,48,73). However, the diagnostic accuracy is unquestionably related to the experience of the cytopathologist and the type and quality of the case material (20).

For instance, in a study by Pitts et al. (59) in a community hospital setting, the sensitivity (the number of positive FNAB results in patients that were confirmed to have the lesion) was 88.4 percent for benign neoplasms and 58.3 percent for malignant neoplasms. The overall false-negative rate was 26.4 percent, but the authors noted that this had decreased with experience from a rate early in the study of 50 percent (59). For non-neoplastic salivary disease the sensitivity was 35.3 percent. The misdiagnoses of the malignant salivary neoplasms included their interpretation as normal salivary tissue, non-neoplastic salivary disease, and benign salivary neoplasms. The conclusion of the authors of this study was that FNAB of suspected malignant lesions should not be depended on for diagnosis or surgical planning. They suggested that intraoperative frozen sections also be performed.

The false-negative rate of other studies has been as high as 47 percent (43). In the study by O'Dwyer et al. (54) only 46 of 63 (73 percent) aspirates from malignant tumors were recognized as such. In this same study 16 of 265 aspirates of benign tumors were erroneously diagnosed as malignant. Zurrida et al. (77) reported that of 36 malignant tumors in their series, malignancy was recognized in only 22 (61.1 percent). Low sensitivity has been reported in other studies (31,49,66). Guyot et al. (30) concluded that the false-negative and false-positive rates severely diminish the value of salivary gland FNAB and preclude its use for major clinical decisions.

As discussed elsewhere (see Malignant Lymphoma), the major gland parenchyma is often the site first involved by lymphomas of mucosa-associated lymphoid tissue. Advocates of FNAB claim it is especially valuable in recognizing disease such as malignant lymphoma that is not primarily treated by surgery. However, in one study all seven low-grade lymphomas were underdiagnosed with FNAB (77). Shaha et al. (65) recommend that even if an aspiration suggests lymphoma, confirmation should be obtained by open biopsy.

Peters and colleagues (58) studied the interobserver variability in the interpretation of FNAB of masses of the head and neck and found salivary gland lesions the most difficult to agree upon. Of 82 parotid and submandibular masses, two observers disagreed in 10 percent of the cases. Dejmek and Lindholm (19) also found that of aspirations of cystic head and neck lesions, diagnostic problems were greatest with those in the salivary glands.

The problem of inaccurate FNAB interpretation of salivary gland lesions is not surprising. Salivary glands harbor a number of developmental, inflammatory, and neoplastic diseases. Primary salivary gland neoplasms have an exceptionally diverse range of morphologic growth patterns, and their diagnosis depends largely on the recognition of these patterns in addition to the presence or absence of invasion. Squamous, mucous, ductal, clear, and oncocytoid cells as well as lymphocytes and hyaline material are found in a variety of benign and malignant salivary gland tumors, so they are nonspecific in an aspirate. Distinction among the various tumors, as the collective experience indicates, in many instances is beyond the scope of FNAB. Most salivary carcinomas have relatively uniform cytologic features that, by themselves, do not facilitate accurate diagnosis. Unlike exfoliative cytology, FNAB diagnosis is based in part on the pattern of the aspirated cells, but it discloses no information about the nature of the tumor interface with surrounding tissues (53).

Some investigators consider FNAB to be a diagnostic tool that aids in evaluation of salivary gland masses and not a histologic procedure on which detailed operative decisions can be based because it is not highly accurate (54). When used for diagnosis, incorrect FNAB interpretation has led to unnecessary wider excision and facial nerve damage (55). In some instances, even distinguishing between obstructive sialadenitis and malignancy has been difficult (65). As noted by Layfield and Glasgow (46), careful attention to the clinical findings, smear cellularity, background, and cytologic features may help reduce misinterpretation. Young (74) has detailed the lesions most likely to cause diagnostic problems.

CLINICAL UTILITY

For many patients with masses in the major salivary glands, distinction between neoplastic and non-neoplastic salivary disease is possible on the basis of clinical history; radiologic, computerized tomographic (CT), and magnetic resonance (MR) images; and physical examination. However, most parotid tumors are asymptomatic, and pain may be experienced in both neoplastic and non-neoplastic conditions. In the submandibular gland episodic pain and swelling are often considered the hallmark of inflammatory disease. Nonetheless, in some patients it is difficult to clinically differentiate neoplastic from non-neoplastic lesions, and in these cases some have proposed a role for FNAB.

There are two basic opinions regarding the utility of FNAB in the diagnosis and treatment planning of major salivary gland tumors. Spiro (69) suggests that FNAB is unnecessary most of the time for the evaluation of swelling near the ear. He notes that FNAB can be helpful when there is suspicion of an inflammatory or neoplastic process in parotid lymph nodes or when the size and location of the mass indicate that a particularly tedious facial nerve dissection is likely. Additionally, when a parotid mass is suspected but no external swelling is evident, CT scan followed by FNAB may be helpful.

Like Spiro, other investigators question the routine use of FNAB in the systematic evaluation of salivary masses but believe it has a role in certain situations (7,30,73). Batsakis et al. (7) suggest that its value is unquestioned when: 1) the probability of a neoplasm is low, such as in a pediatric population; 2) the likelihood of an inflammatory or immune sialadenitis is high; 3) the salivary lesions are suspected of being a manifestation of systemic disease, such as lymphoma; 4) surgical exploration would severely challenge a patient's health; or 5) metastasis or direct invasion of the gland is more likely than primary salivary disease. These investigators observe that the extent of parotid gland surgery is primarily determined by the size of the tumor and the presence or absence of local extension rather than the histologic type. Decisions about facial nerve preservation or sacrifice are often made during surgery and prior FNAB diagnosis, even if a specific diagnosis is confidently established, is not helpful. Batsakis et al. believe that if a parotid neoplasm is likely, FNAB becomes a procedure that increases rather than contains costs. Johns and Kaplan (36) note that the lack of a preoperative tissue diagnosis does not alter the surgical approach.

In contrast to these investigators, others believe FNAB frequently provides valuable clinical information, largely because in many cases differentiation between a neoplastic or non-neoplastic disorder is difficult even for the experienced clinician. In a study of the incidence of neoplastic versus inflammatory disease in major salivary gland masses diagnosed by surgery, 27 percent of parotid masses and 85 percent of submandibular masses were non-neoplastic (27). Surgery is often not indicated for non-neoplastic disease, malignant lymphoma, and some metastatic cancers (55). In a study by Qizilbash et al. (60) surgery was not performed in 45 of 122 patients (36.8 percent) because the cytologic diagnosis suggested a benign lesion that was later confirmed by the clinical course. Frable and Frable (24) reported that 298 of 350 patients who clinically had salivary gland masses but no evidence of tumor or inflammation cytologically, were spared surgical procedures at a great savings in cost and surgical complications. Heller et al. (31) reported that surgery was avoided in 27 percent of 101 patients while 7 patients, who might have simply been observed based on clinical findings alone, received necessary surgery. Layfield (16) believes FNAB should be employed in the investigation of all salivary gland lesions and observes that it is precisely when the aspirate provides a diagnosis not anticipated by the clinical findings that it can play a critical role in patient management. Kocjan et al. (40), while recognizing the shortfalls of FNAB, have observed that it helped one third of their patients avoid surgery. They found that in the majority of cases FNAB helped

determine if a lesion was neoplastic and had a role in planning therapy.

There has been some debate regarding the histopathologic effects of FNAB on tissue that is later excised (7,16). At the AFIP, tissue sections from major gland lesions that had FNAB frequently have shown hemorrhage, focal epithelial proliferation, or tumor infarction (fig. 10-1). These changes have been observed in tissue removed as long as 30 days after the aspiration. Usually these changes are focal and do not hinder diagnosis, but occasionally a large part of the tumor is affected and the diagnostic histopathologic features are obscured. Other investigators have noted alterations in tissues following FNAB of salivary glands and other tissues (7,37,71,72). While not usually a serious consequence of FNAB, pathologists should be aware of these adverse affects.

In summary, diagnosis with FNAB can only be made when the cytologic findings fit the clinical picture and when long-term clinical follow-up is feasible for patients who are not treated operatively (24). Koss et al. (41) suggest that the relative rarity of salivary gland tumors makes it difficult to obtain FNAB experience, and accurate interpretation may be difficult even for the most experienced. If there is doubt about specific classification of an FNAB, it is best to give a differential diagnosis and recommend excision (51). The value of FNAB seems to be in indicating whether definitive surgery is needed or not rather than establishing a specific diagnosis. The surgical procedure, possibly with the aid of CT or MRI, then provides information regarding anatomic relationships of the tumor to the facial nerve and other structures. If no evidence of a tumor or cyst is found with FNAB, communication between the pathologist and surgeon is critical in the decision to either follow the patient or perform exploratory surgery. If cautiously and carefully implemented, FNAB may yield important benefits to the patient (41).

Normal Gland

The aspirates from normal salivary gland contain small aggregates of cohesive but distinctive serous or mucous acini that frequently have adherent adipose tissue and associated ductal epithelium (fig. 10-2). Layfield et al. (47) have discussed potential problems in distinguishing

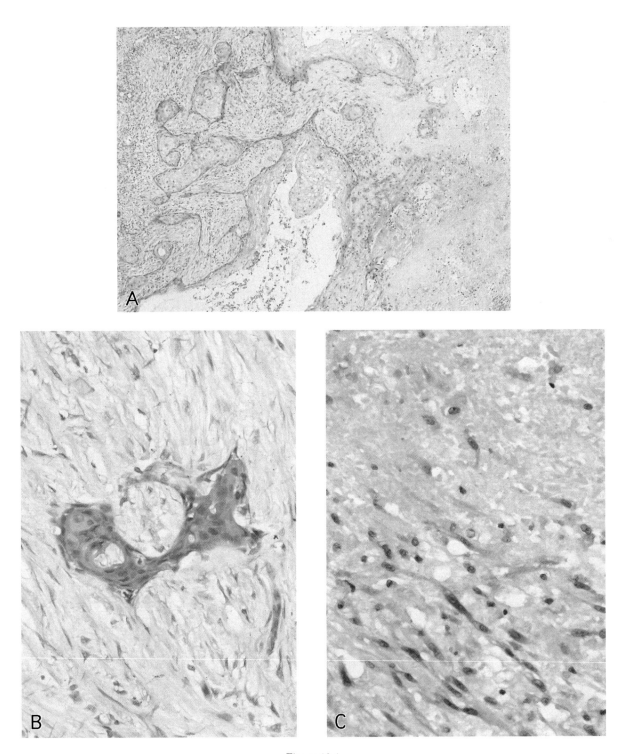

Figure 10-1
POSSIBLE EFFECTS OF FNAB

A: Surgical excision of a parotid mass following fine-needle aspiration biopsy shows a pale-staining, necrotic, largely unrecognizable lesion that focally is consistent with mixed tumor. In this field prominent squamous metaplasia obscures the typical epithelial characteristics.

B: A different example of an excised, infarcted tumor contains small, proliferative epithelial islands that demonstrate morphologic atypia.

C: In this infarcted mixed tumor, scattered, spindled epithelial cells are embedded within zones of prominent hyalinization.

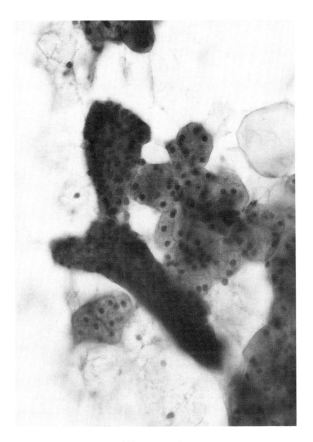

Figure 10-2
FNAB OF NORMAL PAROTID GLAND
Acini are associated with branching ductal elements and adipose tissue (X100). (Papanicolaou stain)

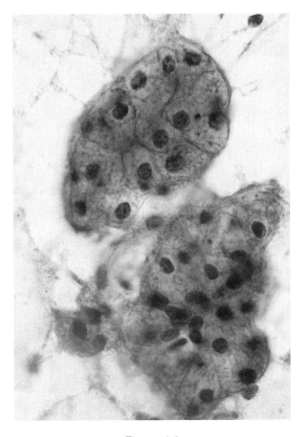

Figure 10-3
NORMAL PAROTID GLAND
High magnification shows an abundant, granular cytoplasm and uniformly round nuclei that have a basal orientation (X250). (Papanicolaou stain)

lipomatous lesions from the fat in normal gland. Acini have abundant granular or vacuolated cytoplasm and small, round nuclei that are typically located in a peripheral position (fig. 10-3).

Mixed Tumor

Mixed tumor is the most common salivary gland tumor and represents a large proportion of FNAB samples. Similar to the histomorphology of tissue specimens, FNAB of mixed tumor demonstrates wide morphologic diversity (fig. 10-4). The aspirates are characterized by the presence of coherent clusters or branching trabeculae of ovoid, plasmacytoid or spindle cells that focally are associated with fibrillar myxoid or myxochondroid stroma (fig. 10-5). The epithelial cells have round, ovoid or fusiform nuclei and fine chromatin. The stroma stains pale green

with Papanicolaou and intensely magenta to purple with Romanowsky-type (Giemsa) stains. The striking metachromatic staining with the Giemsa stain is often helpful in the recognition of this tumor (fig. 10-6). Squamous cells or areas of keratinization are sometimes evident. Spindle cells typically are more widely separated than other epithelial cells and are usually embedded within the adjacent stroma (fig. 10-7). Because cellular mixed tumors have a limited stromal element and occasional nuclear atypia they are less easily recognized (21). The atypia normally occurs in cell clusters (fig. 10-8) but is seen in single cells as well (13). It has resulted in misdiagnoses as mucoepidermoid carcinoma, carcinoma ex mixed tumor, and other carcinomas (13,48,54,73). Layfield et al. (48) recommended that highly cellular lesions that lack the expected stroma of mixed tumor and do not show

445

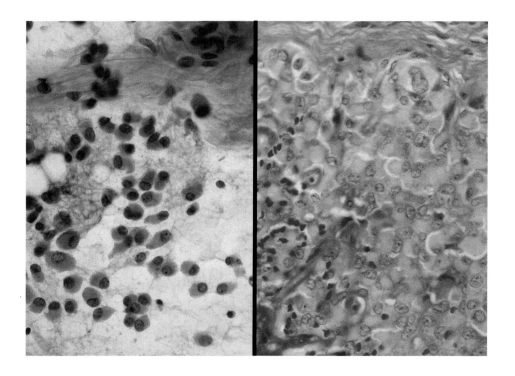

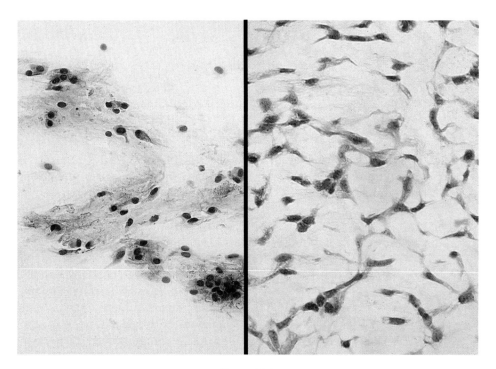

Figure 10-4
MIXED TUMOR

Two examples of mixed tumor show that the variation in the tissue specimen is reflected in the FNAB appearance.

Top: The FNAB (left) shows a cellular sample that contains numerous, large plasmacytoid cells representative of the solid sheets of similar cells present in the tissue (right).

Bottom: FNAB shows less cellular fragments with spindle and stellate cells (left) that were taken from a tumor that is largely comprised of a similar cell population (right) (X100). (Papanicolaou stain)

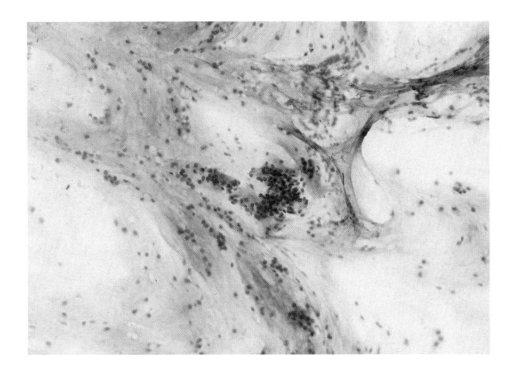

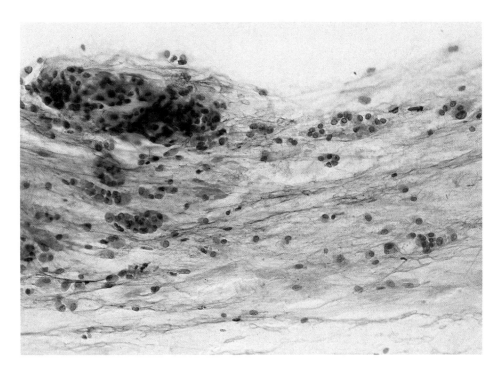

Figure 10-5
MIXED TUMOR

Top: Several clusters of epithelial cells are closely associated with an abundant myxoid stroma.

Bottom: Higher magnification of a different case demonstrates the fibrillar nature of the stroma that contains clusters as well as individual epithelial cells (X100). (Papanicolaou stain)

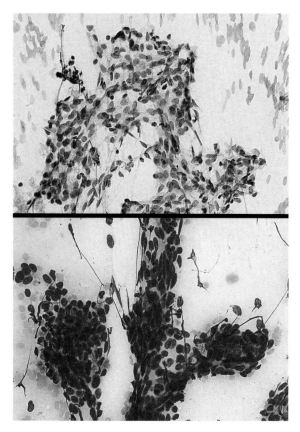

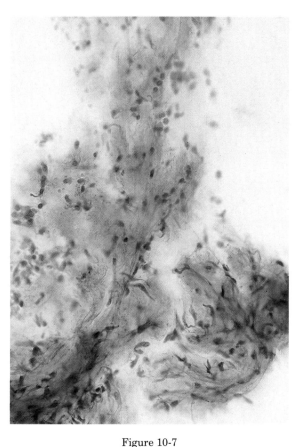

Figure 10-6
MIXED TUMOR

These illustrations contrast staining of the same mixed tumor with Papanicolaou (top) and Giemsa (bottom) stains. The nuclear features, especially the chromatin pattern, are easier to assess with the Papanicolaou stain because the Giemsa stain often obscures much of the nuclear detail.

Figure 10-7
MIXED TUMOR

Spindle cells are widely separated by abundant myxoid stroma. (Papanicolaou stain)

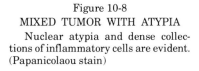

Figure 10-8
MIXED TUMOR WITH ATYPIA

Nuclear atypia and dense collections of inflammatory cells are evident. (Papanicolaou stain)

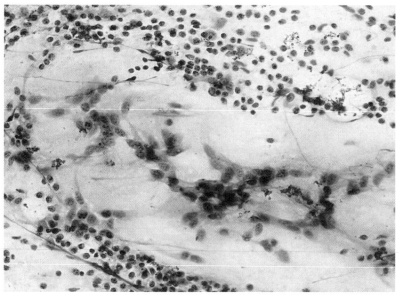

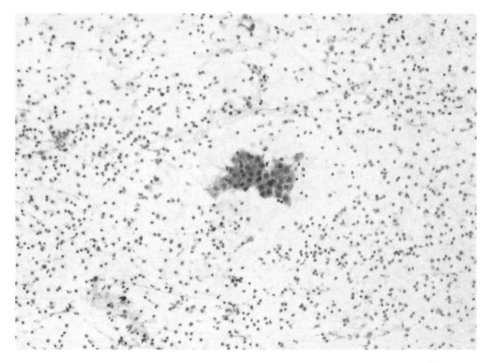

Figure 10-9
WARTHIN'S TUMOR
A single fragment of neoplastic epithelium is surrounded by numerous inflammatory cells (X25). (Papanicolaou stain)

nuclear atypia be classified as salivary gland neoplasm, not otherwise specified. This encourages the surgeons to perform limited dissections with frozen-section analysis. The presence of small tubular structures with central hyalinized spherical cores in some mixed tumors has lead to misinterpretation as adenoid cystic carcinoma (15,23,55,63).

Warthin's Tumor

Aspirates of Warthin's tumor show small fragments of oncocytic epithelium that have a honeycomb arrangement and are partially surrounded by lymphocytes (fig. 10-9). The clustered epithelial cells (fig. 10-10), as well as scattered individual cells (fig. 10-11), have distinct cell borders. The epithelial clusters do not contain lymphocytes. The epithelial cells have moderate to abundant finely granular cytoplasm and uniform round nuclei that are often centrally placed and have small nucleoli (22). Mast cells are often present (9). Squamous metaplasia occasionally develops within Warthin's tumor and aspirates in such instances show single,

atypical squamous cells with no cellular associations. This finding has led to misinterpretation as carcinoma (15,24,44).

Basal Cell Adenoma

Familiarity with the FNAB features of basal cell adenoma is important because the tumor often mimics adenoid cystic carcinoma (8,32,45,55, 63,68). Irregular solid sheets and branching trabeculae are formed by numerous small cells that have uniformly dense, round to ovoid nuclei and limited cytoplasm (fig. 10-12). Tubular structures are present in some. Amorphous eosinophilic intercellular material is often seen. In some cases this material is present as spherical globules that are surrounded by adherent basaloid cells (fig. 10-13). Layfield (45) has noted that in both basal cell adenoma and adenoid cystic carcinoma these globules stain red to red-blue with the May-Grünwald-Giemsa stain but the spheres are less numerous and have a bluer appearance in basal cell adenoma. This is a difficult distinction. He also noted that there is minimally greater nuclear atypia in adenoid cystic carcinoma. Canalicular

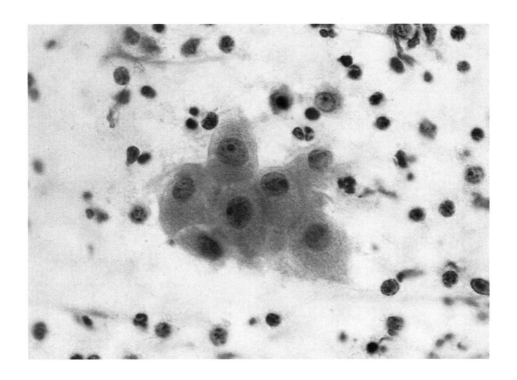

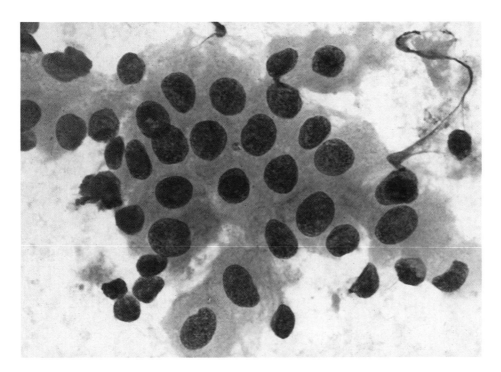

Figure 10-10
WARTHIN'S TUMOR

The epithelial clusters in these two different examples are composed of cells with abundant cytoplasm, distinct borders, and relatively large, centrally placed nuclei. Small nucleoli are present in both cases but are more readily apparent with the Papanicolaou (top) than with the Giemsa (bottom) stain.

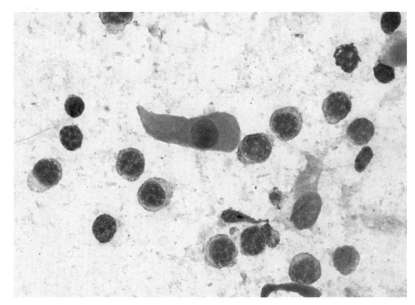

Figure 10-11
WARTHIN'S TUMOR
A single columnar neoplastic cell is
evident among numerous lymphocytes.
(Giemsa stain)

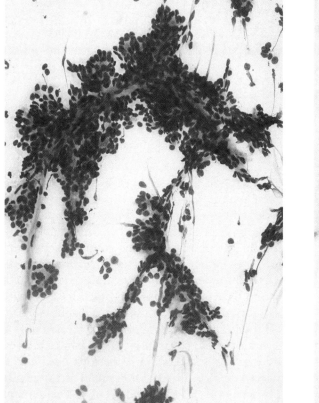
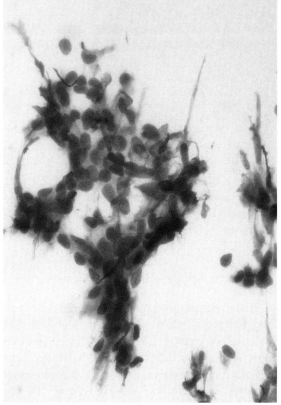

Figure 10-12
BASAL CELL ADENOMA
Left: Trabecular collections of small, cohesive basaloid cells that lack a stromal element are characteristic of basal cell adenoma (X50).
Right: Higher magnification shows cells with uniformly round nuclei and sparse, indistinct cytoplasm (X100). (Giemsa stain)

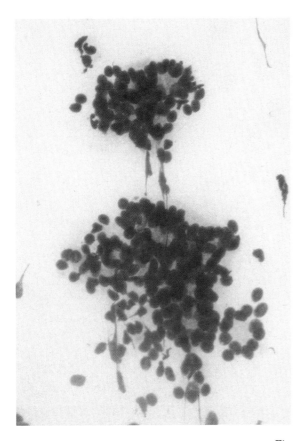 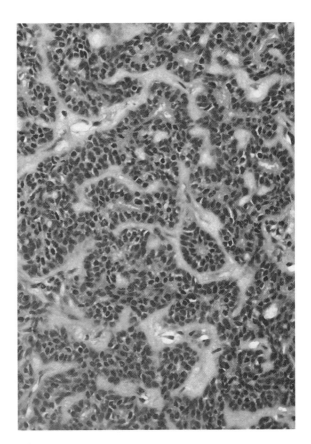

Figure 10-13
BASAL CELL ADENOMA
Left: Small cores of amorphous, amphophilic material surround basaloid cells. In the lower right area a single row of cells surrounds a core of material (X100). (Giemsa stain)
Right: The histologic appearance of the excised specimen correlates well with FNAB.

adenoma also consists of small basaloid cells but, unlike basal cell adenoma, has epithelial fragments that are partially lined by a layer of tall columnar cells (fig. 10-14); papillae are occasional (33).

Mucoepidermoid Carcinoma

Mucoepidermoid carcinoma presents the most frequent problems in interpretation of aspirates of the salivary glands (14,34,35,42,48,76). It is the most common of all malignant salivary gland tumors and second in frequency of occurrence only to mixed tumor. It is often cystic and frequently yields only acellular mucoid material (15, 55). The low-grade variant lacks nuclear atypia and is far more common than the high-grade type in which the cytomorphologic features alone are suspicious for malignancy. The characteristic

FNAB features of low-grade mucoepidermoid carcinoma include the presence of aggregates of cells with dense, green-blue waxy cytoplasm on Papanicolaou stain (fig. 10-15) and light pink-purple cytoplasm with the Romanowski stain (15). Cells thought to represent the intermediate cells characteristic of this tumor have bland, round to ovoid nuclei surrounded by moderate cytoplasm. Mucus-containing cells have intracellular, red granular material on Romanowsky-stained slides, often have cytoplasm distended by mucin (fig. 10-16) or numerous perinuclear vacuoles (fig. 10-17), and have eccentrically placed nuclei (23,42). Cohen et al. (14) noted that finely vacuolated cells are not specific for mucoepidermoid carcinoma because they are found in a small percentage of other lesions. In histologic sections, mucous cells account for a very small proportion of most mucoepidermoid

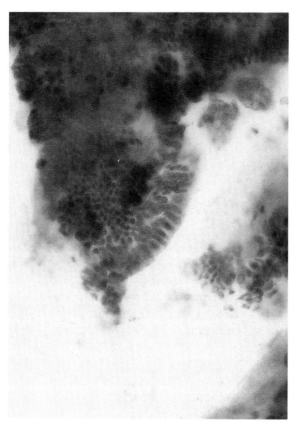

Figure 10-14
CANALICULAR ADENOMA
The epithelial fragments in this tumor consisted principally of basaloid cells but focally were lined by columnar cells, as shown here. (Papanicolaou stain)

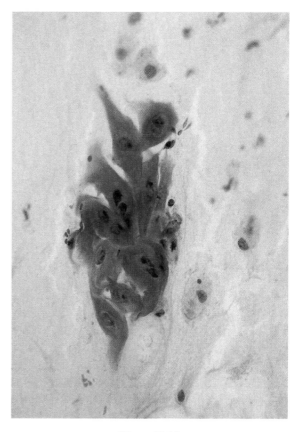

Figure 10-15
MUCOEPIDERMOID CARCINOMA
This cluster of tumor cells is formed by cohesive, fusiform cells that have small, round to ovoid nuclei (X100). (Papanicolaou stain)

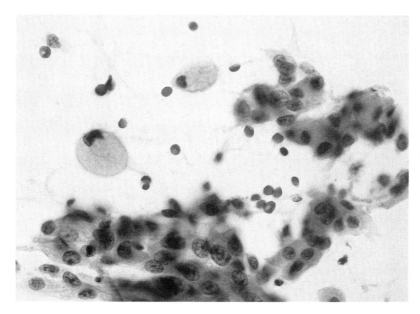

Figure 10-16
MUCOEPIDERMOID CARCINOMA
Two large, pale-staining mucous cells are adjacent to a cluster of intermediate cells. (Papanicolaou stain)

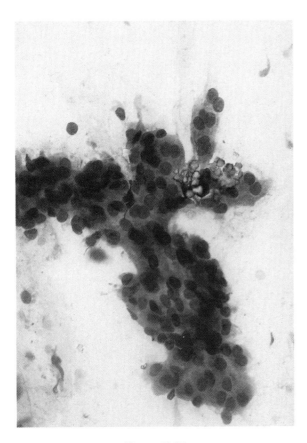

Figure 10-17
MUCOEPIDERMOID CARCINOMA
This aspirate has clusters of intermediate cells that contain several mucous cells with large, cytoplasmic vacuoles. (Giemsa stain)

carcinomas so, understandably, in some aspirates they are sparse or altogether absent. Prominently cystic lesions, however, have greater numbers of mucous cells than more solid tumors. Extracellular mucin is also often abundant (fig. 10-18) and mimics the mesenchymal element in mixed tumors. In contrast to its appearance in mixed tumor, mucin is not as fibrillar and does not usually stain as intensely (46,51). Its nature is best appreciated with air-dried Romanowsky stains. Squamous cells are often present (14) and distinction from mixed tumor, Warthin's tumor with squamous metaplasia, and primary and metastatic squamous cell carcinomas is necessary (55,75). Cohen and colleagues (14) have suggested that overlapping of nuclei within the epithelial groups (fig. 10-19) is also characteristic of mucoepidermoid carcinoma and helps distinguish it from Warthin's tumor.

Acinic Cell Adenocarcinoma

Aspirates of acinic cell adenocarcinomas that have well-differentiated acinar structures show either clusters or individual uniform cells with abundant cytoplasm and scattered cellular formations that resemble normal acini. The cells have finely granular cytoplasm which is not as sharply defined as in normal cells and small dark nuclei. Unlike normal acini that have basally oriented nuclei, those in the neoplastic cells often are centrally located and lack nuclear polarity (fig. 10-20) (57). Additionally, unlike normal gland, close association with ductal and fat cells is not evident. The cytoplasm may contain periodic acid–Schiff (PAS)-positive granules that are resistant to diastase digestion (fig. 10-21) (15, 57). The presence of numerous lymphocytes in some has lead to consideration of Warthin's tumor, sialadenitis, and malignant lymphoma (55,57,73). The granular neoplastic cells often resemble oncocytes, a feature that can lead to misinterpretation as oncocytoma (55).

Adenoid Cystic Carcinoma

As previously noted, adenoid cystic carcinoma, mixed tumor, and basal cell adenoma occasionally share features that complicate FNAB interpretation (1,28,51,55,63,75). The characteristic cytologic features of adenoid cystic carcinoma are aggregates of small, relatively uniform, round to ovoid cells that surround scattered spheres of mucopolysaccharide material (15,23,52). The purplish pink hyaline cores seen with the Giemsa stain (fig. 10-22) are more easily visualized than the clear, pale green or light orange material evident with the Papanicolaou stain. In some cases isolated cores of the mucoid material are surrounded by rows of adherent cells (fig. 10-23), whereas in others multiple closely associated cores simulate the cribriform duct–like structures from which they are derived (fig. 10-24). Because these structures are also seen in some mixed tumors, basal cell adenoma, acinic cell adenocarcinoma, and epithelial-myoepithelial carcinoma (3,12,19,39), some investigators have urged caution in making a definitive diagnosis unless evidence of peripheral nerve involvement is found (50). Although polymorphous low-grade adenocarcinomas are nearly always limited to the minor glands, similar structures have also

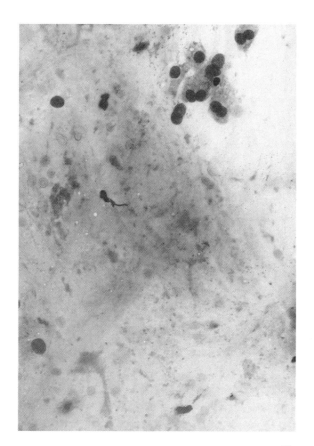
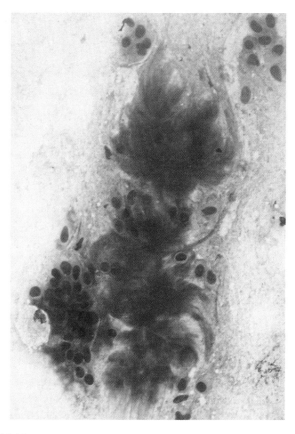

Figure 10-18
MUCOEPIDERMOID CARCINOMA
Left: Pools of mucoid material in mucoepidermoid carcinoma contain scattered individual and groups of tumor cells.
Right: The mucoid material in mucoepidermoid carcinoma does not usually demonstrate the focal, densely metachromatic staining typically present in mixed tumors (X100). (Giemsa stain)

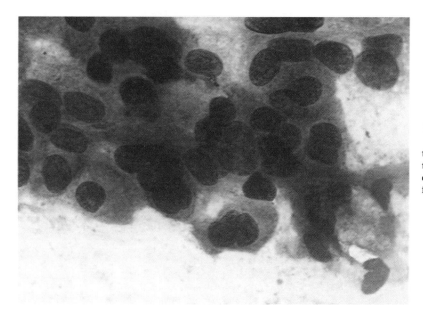

Figure 10-19
MUCOEPIDERMOID CARCINOMA
Overlapping of nuclei is evident in the cluster of tumor cells. Compared to the cell clusters in Warthin's tumor, the cells are noticeably more crowded (see figure 10-10). (Giemsa stain)

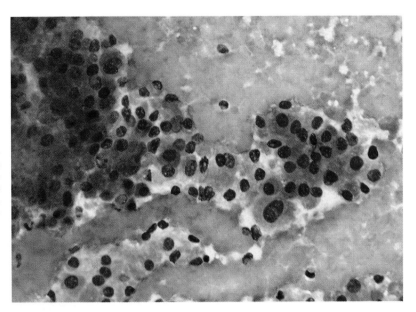

Figure 10-20
ACINIC CELL
ADENOCARCINOMA
Aggregates of large cells with granular cytoplasm are evident. The cells have a vague "acinar" arrangement but compared to normal gland the nuclei are more variable and not basally located, and the cell borders are not sharply demarcated (X100). (Giemsa stain)

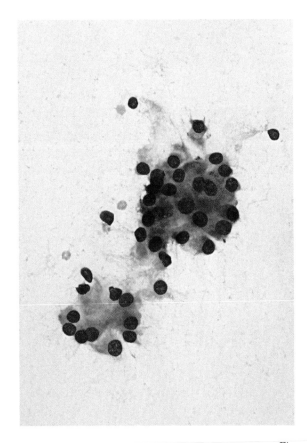

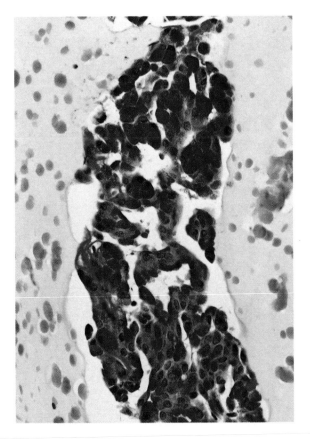

Figure 10-21
ACINIC CELL ADENOCARCINOMA
Left: This aspirate contains clusters of large cells with abundant granular cytoplasm. (Giemsa stain)
Right: Periodic acid–Schiff stain with diastase shows many of the cells are strongly positive and enzyme resistant.

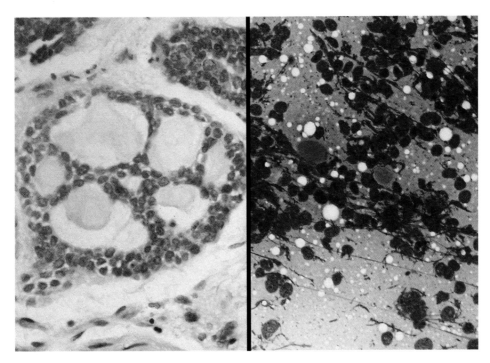

Figure 10-22
ADENOID CYSTIC CARCINOMA
Aspiration from an adenoid cystic carcinoma that demonstrated cribriform growth in the tissue sections (left) shows aggregates of cells that have indistinct cell borders and round nuclei. The nuclei have coarse chromatin but no nucleoli. Two purplish hyaline spheres are evident. (Right: Giemsa stain)

been described in association with them (25). Small fragments of myxoid stroma suggest mixed tumor (13). The cells of adenoid cystic carcinoma have limited cytoplasm, indistinct cytoplasmic borders, and nuclei with evenly distributed chromatin. In the solid type there is cellular overlapping, and the nuclei are larger and more variable, with visible nucleoli (15,23). The use of immunohistochemical stains for glial fibrillary acidic protein (GFAP) to distinguish mixed tumor from adenoid cystic carcinoma is, in our opinion, not sufficiently reliable. Some cellular mixed tumors are GFAP negative (46,56) and, conversely, some adenoid cystic carcinomas are focally positive.

Other Malignant Tumors

Other salivary gland tumors diagnosed by FNAB include epithelial-myoepithelial carcinoma (3,12,39), oncocytic carcinoma (2,5,62), salivary duct carcinoma (18,26), polymorphous low-grade adenocarcinoma (25), primary squamous cell carcinoma (13), small cell carcinoma (10), and carcinosarcoma (29). In some cases the aspirates have nuclear characteristics of an epithelial tumor that indicate frank malignancy but lack cellular features that allow a specific diagnosis (fig. 10-25). These cases often represent high-grade adenocarcinoma, not otherwise specified, or undifferentiated carcinoma (13,60,75).

Comparison with Frozen Section Interpretation

Frozen section often complements FNAB and is used routinely by those who perform outpatient parotidectomy (13,70). However, as with FNAB, the difficulty of interpreting frozen sections warrants considerable caution when used to determine therapy. In a review of 21 series with a total of 1,898 cases, excluding deferred diagnoses, and in two recent studies, the accuracy rate was about 96 percent (4,13,17). More importantly, however, when salivary gland lesions are divided into benign and malignant groups it becomes apparent that the accuracy rate for the two groups is significantly different. The average false-positive

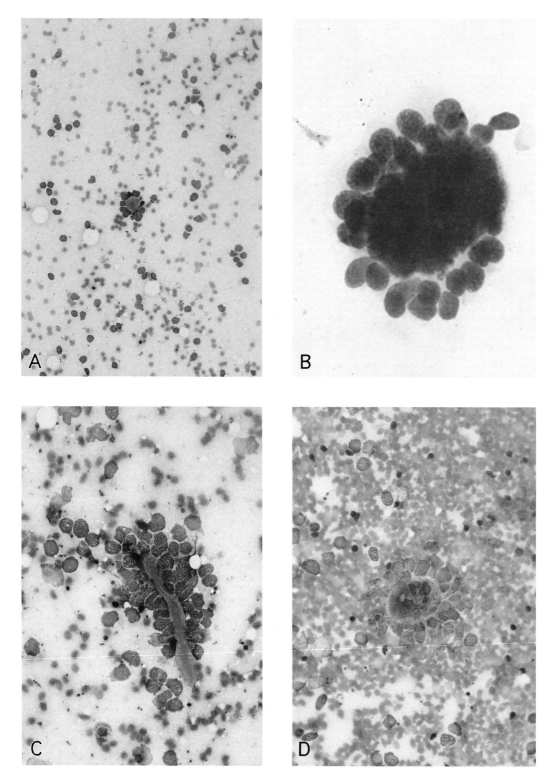

Figure 10-23
ADENOID CYSTIC CARCINOMA

Isolated hyaline cores are numerous and often surrounded by several layers of tumor cells resembling rosettes. Compared to the nuclei of the basaloid cells of basal cell adenoma (see fig. 10-13), the nuclei in adenoid cystic carcinoma are typically slightly larger and show mild atypia. (Giemsa stain)

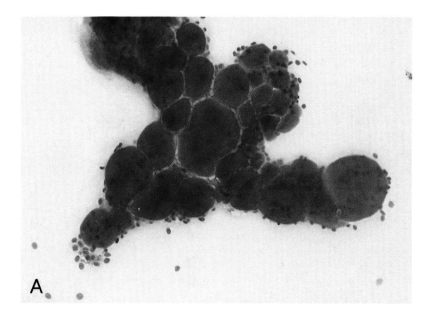

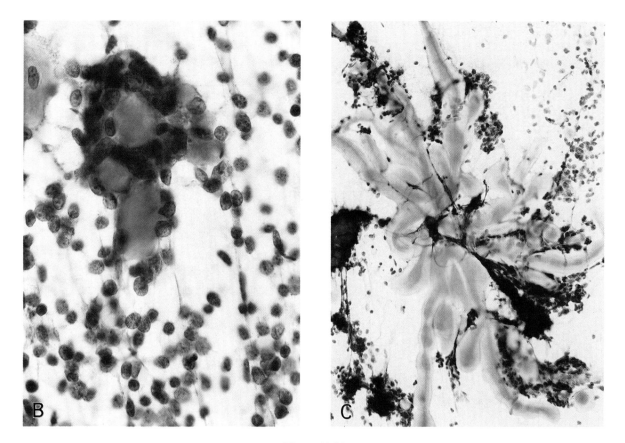

Figure 10-24
ADENOID CYSTIC CARCINOMA
A: With Giemsa stain numerous adherent purplish cores of hyaline material are arranged in a cribriform pattern.
B,C: Contrast the appearance of the cores with the two Papanicolaou-stained aspirates.

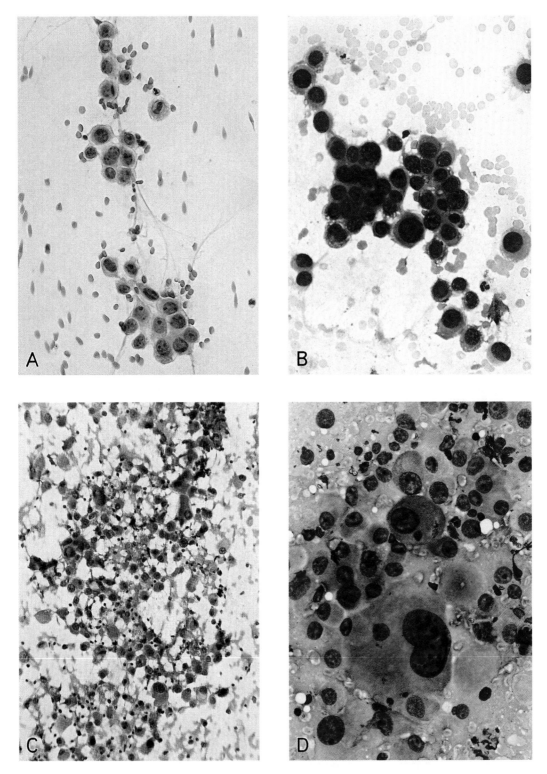

Figure 10-25
ADENOCARCINOMA, NOT OTHERWISE SPECIFIED: HIGH GRADE

A,B: This parotid aspirate reveals loosely cohesive, clustered and dissociated cells with atypical, variable nuclei. Cells with multiple nucleoli are evident with the Papanicolaou stain (A), but little nuclear detail is evident with the Giemsa stain (B).
C,D: These two smears were from a FNAB of a high-grade adenocarcinoma, not otherwise specified, of the submandibular gland.

rate for the benign groups was 1.2 percent, most often resulting from misinterpretation of cellular mixed tumors that contained atypical cells. Cysts and lesions with a prominent lymphoid element also were often confused with mucoepidermoid carcinoma and malignant lymphoma, respectively. The malignant group had a false-negative rate of 14.3 percent and, similar to fine-needle aspiration biopsy, misinterpretation frequently involved mucoepidermoid carcinoma, acinic cell adenocarcinoma, adenoid cystic carcinoma, and malignant mixed tumor (4).

As with FNAB, false negatives are sometimes related to poor sampling of lesional tissue. Un-like FNAB, however, the surgeon and the pathologist have the opportunity to directly visualize the lesion and its relationship to surrounding tissues. After careful examination of the entire specimen, solid, cystic, and necrotic foci are separately sampled. Sections should include lesional and adjacent tissues so that the interface between the two can be evaluated. Because there are focal variations in cellular composition and architectural configuration in any single salivary gland tumor, it is often necessary to sample multiple areas. Sometimes adequately sampled lesions are nondiagnostic and deferral to permanent sections is prudent.

REFERENCES

1. Abad MM, G-Macias C, Alonso MJ, et al. Statistical evaluation of the predictive power of fine needle aspiration (FNA) of salivary glands. Results and cytohistological correlation. Pathol Res Pract 1992;188:340–3.
2. Abdul-Karim FW, Weaver MG. Needle aspiration cytology of an oncocytic carcinoma of the parotid gland. Diagn Cytopathol 1991;7:420–2.
3. Arora VK, Misra K, Bhatia A. Cytomorphologic features of the rare epithelial-myoepithelial carcinoma of the salivary gland. Acta Cytol 1990;34:239–42.
4. Auclair PL, Ellis GL, Gnepp DR, Wenig BM, Janney CG. Salivary gland neoplasms: general considerations. In: Ellis GL, Auclair PL, Gnepp DR, eds. Surgical pathology of the salivary glands. Philadelphia: WB Saunders, 1991:135–64.
5. Austin MB, Frierson HF Jr, Feldman PS. Oncocytoid adenocarcinoma of the parotid gland. Cytologic, histologic and ultrastructural findings. Acta Cytol 1987;31:351–6.
6. Barnard NA, Paterson AW, Irvine GH, Mackenzie ED, White H. Fine needle aspiration cytology in maxillofacial surgery—experience in a district general hospital. Br J Oral Maxillofac Surg 1993;31:223–6.
7. Batsakis JG, Sneige N, el-Naggar AK. Fine-needle aspiration of salivary glands: its utility and tissue effects. Ann Otol Rhinol Laryngol 1992;101:185–8.
8. Bedrossian CW, Martinez F, Silverberg AB. Fine needle aspiration. In: Gnepp DR, ed. Pathology of the head and neck. New York: Churchill Livingstone, 1988:25–99.
9. Bottles K, Lowhagen T, Miller TR. Mast cells in the aspiration cytology differential diagnosis of adenolymphoma. Acta Cytol 1985;29:513–5.
10. Cameron WR, Johansson L, Tennvall J. Small cell carcinoma of the parotid. Fine needle aspiration and immunochemical findings in a case. Acta Cytol 1990;34:837–41.
11. Cardillo MR. Ag-NOR technique in fine needle aspiration cytology of salivary gland masses. Acta Cytol 1992;36:147–51.
12. Carrillo R, Poblet E, Rocamora A, Rodriguez-Peralto JL. Epithelial-myoepithelial carcinoma of the salivary gland. Fine needle aspiration cytologic findings. Acta Cytol 1990;34:243–7.
13. Chan MK, McGuire LJ, King W, Li AK, Lee JC. Cytodiagnosis of 112 salivary gland lesions. Correlation with histologic and frozen section diagnosis. Acta Cytol 1992;36:353–63.
14. Cohen MB, Fisher PE, Holly EA, Ljung BM, Löwhagen T, Bottles K. Fine needle aspiration biopsy diagnosis of mucoepidermoid carcinoma. Statistical analysis. Acta Cytol 1990;34:43–9.
15. Cohen MB, Reznicek MJ, Miller TR. Fine-needle aspiration biopsy of the salivary glands. Pathol Annu 1992;27(Pt. 2):213–45.
16. Cramer H, Layfield L, Lampe H. Fine-needle aspiration of salivary glands: its utility and tissue effects [Letter]. Ann Otol Rhinol Laryngol 1993;102:483–5.
17. Cross DL, Gansler TS, Morris RC. Fine needle aspiration and frozen section of salivary gland lesions. South Med J 1990;83:283–6.
18. Dee S, Masood S, Issacs JH Jr, Hardy NM. Cytomorphologic features of salivary duct carcinoma on fine needle aspiration biopsy. A case report. Acta Cytol 1993;37:539–42.
19. Dejmek A, Lindholm K. Fine needle aspiration biopsy of cystic lesions of the head and neck, excluding the thyroid. Acta Cytol 1990;34:443–8.
20. Eneroth CM, Franzén S, Zajicek J. Aspiration biopsy of salivary gland tumors. A critical review of 910 biopsies. Acta Cytol 1967;11:470–2.
21. Eneroth CM, Zajicek J. Aspiration biopsy cytology of salivary gland tumors. III. Morphologic studies on smears and histologic sections from 368 mixed tumors. Acta Cytol 1966;10:440–54.

22. Eneroth CM, Zajicek J. Aspiration biopsy of salivary gland tumors. II. Morphologic studies on smears and histologic sections from oncocytic tumors (45 cases of papillary cystadenoma lymphomatosum and 4 cases of oncocytoma). Acta Cytol 1965;9:355–61.

23. Feldman PS, Covell JL, Kardos TF. Fine needle aspiration cytology. Lymph node, thyroid, and salivary gland. Chicago: ASCP Press, 1989:165–238.

24. Frable MA, Frable WJ. Fine-needle aspiration biopsy of salivary glands. Laryngoscope 1991;101:245–9.

25. Frierson HF Jr, Covell JL, Mills SE. Fine-needle aspiration cytology of terminal duct carcinoma of minor salivary gland. Diagn Cytopathol 1987;3:159–62.

26. Gal R, Strauss M, Zohar Y, Kessler E. Salivary duct carcinoma of the parotid gland. Cytologic and histopathologic study. Acta Cytol 1985;29:454–6.

27. Gallia LJ, Johnson JT. The incidence of neoplastic versus inflammatory disease in major salivary gland masses diagnosed by surgery. Laryngoscope 1981;91:512–6.

28. Geisinger KR, Reynolds GD, Vance RP, McGuirt WF. Adenoid cystic carcinoma arising in a pleomorphic adenoma of the parotid gland. An aspiration cytology and ultrastructural study. Acta Cytol 1985;29:522–6.

29. Granger JK, Houn HY. Malignant mixed tumor (carcinosarcoma) of parotid gland diagnosed by fine-needle aspiration biopsy. Diagn Cytopathol 1991;7:427–32.

30. Guyot JP, Auberson S, Obradovic D, Lehmann W. Fine-needle aspiration in the diagnosis of head and neck growths: the pitfalls of false-positive diagnosis. ORL J Otorhinolaryngol Relat Spec 1993;55:41–4.

31. Heller KS, Dubner S, Chess Q, Attie JN. Value of fine needle aspiration biopsy of salivary gland masses in clinical decision-making. Am J Surg 1992;164:667–70.

32. Hood IC, Qizilbash AH, Salama SS, Alexopoulou I. Basal-cell adenoma of parotid. Difficulty of differentiation from adenoid cystic carcinoma on aspiration biopsy. Acta Cytol 1983;27:515–20.

33. Hruban RH, Erozan YS, Zinreich SJ, Kashima HK. Fine-needle aspiration cytology of monomorphic adenomas. Am J Clin Pathol 1988;90:46–51.

34. Jacobs JC. Low grade mucoepidermoid carcinoma ex pleomorphic adenoma. A diagnostic problem in fine needle aspiration biopsy. Acta Cytol 1994;38:93–7.

35. Jayaram N, Ashim D, Rajwanshi A, Radhika S, Banerjee CK. The value of fine-needle aspiration biopsy in the cytodiagnosis of salivary gland lesions. Diagn Cytopathol 1989;5:349–54.

36. Johns ME, Kaplan MJ. Malignant neoplasms. In: Cummings CW, Fredrickson JM, Harker LA, Krause CJ, Schuller DE, eds. Otolaryngology—head and neck surgery. St Louis: CV Mosby, 1986:1035–69.

37. Kern SB. Necrosis of a Warthin's tumor following fine needle aspiration. Acta Cytol 1988;32:207–8.

38. Kline TS, Merriam JM, Shapshay SM. Aspiration biopsy cytology of the salivary gland. Am J Clin Pathol 1981;76:263–9.

39. Kocjan G, Milroy C, Fisher EW, Eveson JW. Cytological features of epithelial-myoepithelial carcinoma of salivary gland: potential pitfalls in diagnosis. Cytopathology 1993;4:173–80.

40. Kocjan G, Nayagam M, Harris M. Fine needle aspiration cytology of salivary gland lesions: advantages and pitfalls. Cytopathology 1990;1:269–75.

41. Koss LG, Woyke S, Olszewski W. Aspiration biopsy. Cytologic interpretation and histologic bases. New York: Igaku-Shoin, 1984.

42. Kumar N, Kapila K, Verma K. Fine needle aspiration cytology of mucoepidermoid carcinoma. A diagnostic problem. Acta Cytol 1991;35:357–9.

43. Lau T, Balle VH, Bretlau P. Fine needle aspiration biopsy in salivary gland tumours. Clin Otolaryngol 1986;11:75–7.

44. Laucirica R, Farnum JB, Leopold SK, Kalin GB, Youngberg GA. False-positive diagnosis in fine-needle aspiration of an atypical Warthin's tumor: histochemical differential stains for cytodiagnosis. Diagn Cytopathol 1989;5:412–5.

45. Layfield LJ. Fine needle aspiration cytology of a trabecular adenoma of the parotid gland. Acta Cytol 1985;29:999–1002.

46. Layfield LJ, Glasgow BJ. Diagnosis of salivary gland tumors by fine-needle aspiration cytology: a review of clinical utility and pitfalls. Diagn Cytopathol 1991;7:267–72.

47. Layfield LJ, Glasgow BJ, Goldstein N, Lufkin R. Lipomatous lesions of the parotid gland. Potential pitfalls in fine needle aspiration biopsy diagnosis. Acta Cytol 1991;35:553–6.

48. Layfield LJ, Tan P, Glasgow BJ. Fine-needle aspiration of salivary gland lesions. Comparison with frozen sections and histologic findings. Arch Pathol Lab Med 1987;111:346–53.

49. Lindberg LG, Akerman M. Aspiration cytology of salivary gland tumors: diagnostic experience from six years of routine laboratory work. Laryngoscope 1976;86:584–94.

50. Löwhagen T, Tani EM, Skoog L. Salivary glands and rare head and neck lesions. In: Bibbo M, ed. Comprehensive cytopathology. Philadelphia: WB Saunders, 1991:621–48.

51. MacLeod CB, Frable WJ. Fine-needle aspiration biopsy of the salivary gland: Problem cases. Diagn Cytopathol 1993;9:216–25.

52. Nguyen G, Kline TS. Essentials of aspiration biopsy cytology. New York: Igaku-Shoin, 1991:43–53.

53. Nguyen G, Kline TS. Essentials of aspiration biopsy cytology. New York: Igaku-Shoin, 1991.

54. O'Dwyer P, Farrar WB, James AG, Finkelmeier W, McCabe DP. Needle aspiration biopsy of major salivary gland tumors. Its value. Cancer 1986;57:554–7.

55. Orell SR, Nettle WJ. Fine needle aspiration biopsy of salivary gland tumours. Problems and pitfalls. Pathology 1988;20:332–7.

56. Ostrzega N, Cheng L, Layfield L. Glial fibrillary acid protein immunoreactivity in fine-needle aspiration of salivary gland lesions: a useful adjunct for the differential diagnosis of salivary gland neoplasms. Diagn Cytopathol 1989;5:145–9.

57. Palma O, Torri AM, de Cristofaro JA, Fiaccavento S. Fine needle aspiration cytology in two cases of well-differentiated acinic-cell carcinoma of the parotid gland. Discussion of diagnostic criteria. Acta Cytol 1985;29:516–21.

58. Peters BR, Schnadig VJ, Quinn FB Jr, et al. Interobserver variability in the interpretation of fine-needle aspiration biopsy of head and neck masses. Arch Otolaryngol Head Neck Surg 1989;115:1438–42.

59. Pitts DB, Hilsinger RL, Jr, Karandy E, Ross JC, Caro JE. Fine-needle aspiration in the diagnosis of salivary gland disorders in the community hospital setting. Arch Otolaryngol Head Neck Surg 1992;118:479–82.

60. Qizilbash AH, Sianos J, Young JE, Archibald SD. Fine needle aspiration biopsy cytology of major salivary glands. Acta Cytol 1985;29:503–12.

61. Qizilbash AH, Young JE. Guides to clinical aspiration biopsy. Head and neck. New York: Igaku-Shoin, 1988.

62. Rajan PB, Wadehra V, Hemming JD, Hawkesford JE. Fine needle aspiration cytology of malignant oncocytoma of the parotid gland—a case report. Cytopathology 1994;5:110–3.

63. Rodriguez HP, Silver CE, Moisa II, Chacho MS. Fine-needle aspiration of parotid tumors. Am J Surg 1989;158:342–4.

64. Roland NJ, Caslin AW, Smith PA, Turnbull LS, Panarese A, Jones AS. Fine needle aspiration cytology of salivary gland lesions reported immediately in a head and neck clinic. J Laryngol Otol 1993;107:1025–8.

65. Shaha AR, Webber C, DiMaio T, Jaffe BM. Needle aspiration biopsy in salivary gland lesions. Am J Surg 1990;160:373–6.

66. Silver CE, Koss LG, Brauer RJ, et al. Needle aspiration cytology of tumors at various body sites. Curr Probl Surg 1985;22:1–67.

67. Sismanis A, Merriam JM, Kline TS, Davis RK, Shapshay SM, Strong MS. Diagnosis of salivary gland tumors by fine needle aspiration biopsy. Head Neck Surg 1981;3:482–9.

68. Sparrow SA, Frost FA. Salivary monomorphic adenomas of dermal analogue type: report of two cases. Diagn Cytopathol 1993;9:300–3.

69. Spiro RH. Diagnosis and pitfalls in the treatment of parotid tumors. Semin Surg Oncol 1991;7:20–4.

70. Steckler RM. Outpatient parotidectomy. Am J Surg 1991;162:303–5.

71. Tabbara SO, Frierson HF, Fechner RE. Diagnostic problems in tissues previously sampled by fine-needle aspiration. Am J Clin Pathol 1991;96:76–80.

72. Tsang WY, Chan JK. Spectrum of morphologic changes in lymph nodes attributable to fine needle aspiration. Hum Pathol 1992;23:562–5.

73. Weinberger MS, Rosenberg WW, Meurer WT, Robbins KT. Fine-needle aspiration of parotid gland lesions. Head Neck 1992;14:483–7.

74. Young JA. Diagnostic problems in fine needle aspiration cytopathology of the salivary glands. J Clin Pathol 1994;47:193–8.

75. Young JA, Smallman LA, Thompson H, Proops DW, Johnson AP. Fine needle aspiration cytology of salivary gland lesions. Cytopathology 1990;1:25–33.

76. Zajicek J, Eneroth CM, Jakobsson P. Aspiration biopsy of salivary gland tumors. VI. Morphologic studies on smears and histologic sections from mucoepidermoid carcinoma. Acta Cytol 1976;20:35–41.

77. Zurrida S, Alasio L, Tradati N, Bartoli C, Chiesa F, Pilotti S. Fine-needle aspiration of parotid masses. Cancer 1993;72:2306–11.

---

*Numbers in boldface indicate table and figure pages.

✧✧✧